Informatik aktuell

Herausgeber: W. Brauer
im Auftrag der Gesellschaft für Informatik (GI)

Thomas Tolxdorff Jürgen Braun
Thomas M. Deserno Heinz Handels
Alexander Horsch Hans-Peter Meinzer (Hrsg.)

Bildverarbeitung für die Medizin 2008

Algorithmen – Systeme – Anwendungen

Proceedings des Workshops
vom 6. bis 8. April 2008 in Berlin

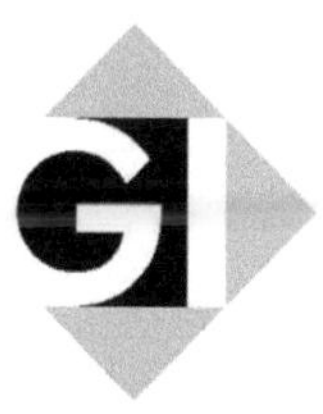

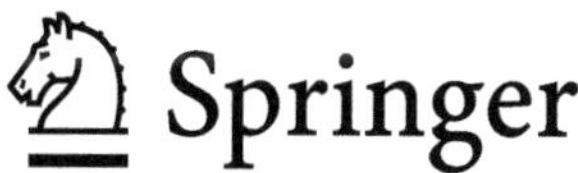

Herausgeber

Thomas Tolxdorff
Jürgen Braun
Charité – Universitätsmedizin Berlin
Campus Benjamin Franklin
Institut für Medizinische Informatik
Hindenburgdamm 30, 12200 Berlin

Thomas M. Deserno
Rheinisch-Westfälische Technische Hochschule Aachen
Institut für Medizinische Informatik
Pauwelsstraße 10, 52074 Aachen

Alexander Horsch
Technische Universität München, Klinikum rechts der Isar
Institut für Medizinische Statistik und Epidemiologie
Ismaninger Straße 22, 81675 München

Heinz Handels
Universitätsklinikum Hamburg-Eppendorf
Institut für Medizinische Informatik
Martinistraße 52, 20246 Hamburg

Hans-Peter Meinzer
Deutsches Krebsforschungszentrum
Abteilung für Medizinische und Biologische Informatik / H0100
Im Neuenheimer Feld 280, 69120 Heidelberg

Bibliographische Information der Deutschen Bibliothek
Die Deutsche Bibliothek verzeichnet diese Publikation in der Deutschen Nationalbibliografie; detaillierte bibliografische Daten sind im Internet über http://dnb.ddb.de abrufbar.

CR Subject Classification (1998): A.0, H.3, I.4, I.5, J.3, H.3.1, I.2.10, I.3.3, I.3.5, I.3.7, I.3.8, I.6.3

ISSN 1431-472-X
ISBN-13 978-3-540-78639-9 Springer Berlin Heidelberg New York

Springer Berlin Heidelberg New York
Springer ist ein Unternehmen von Springer Science+Business Media

springer.de

Satz: Reproduktionsfertige Vorlage vom Autor/Herausgeber
Gedruckt auf säurefreiem Papier SPIN: 11240937 33/3142-543210

Bildverarbeitung für die Medizin 2008

Veranstalter

IMI	Institut für Medizinische Informatik Charité - Universitätsmedizin Berlin und Freie Universität
BVMI	Berufsverband Medizinischer Informatiker e.V.
DAGM	Deutsche Arbeitsgemeinschaft für Mustererkennung
DGBMT	Fachgruppe Medizinische Informatik der Deutschen Gesellschaft für Biomedizinische Technik im VDE
GI	Fachgruppe Imaging und Visualisierungstechniken der Gesellschaft für Informatik
GMDS	Arbeitsgruppe Medizinische Bild- und Signalverarbeitung der Gesellschaft für Medizinische Informatik, Biometrie und Epidemiologie
IEEE	Joint Chapter Engineering in Medicine and Biology, German Section

Tagungsvorsitz

Priv.-Doz. Dr. Jürgen Braun
Prof. Dr. Thomas Tolxdorff

Institut für Medizinische Informatik
Charité - Universitätsmedizin Berlin
Hindenburgdamm 30, 12200 Berlin

Lokale Organisation

Jürgen Braun
Egbert Gedat
Holger Kunz
Birgit Porsch
Thorsten Schaaf
Sabine Sassmann
Dagmar Stiller
Sabine Hanß
Dagmar Krefting
Michael Vossberg
u.v.m.

Institut für Medizinische Informatik
Charité - Universitätsmedizin Berlin
Hindenburgdamm 30, 12200 Berlin

Verteilte BVM-Organisation

Prof. Dr. Thomas M. Deserno, Jens Hoffmann
Rheinisch-Westfälische Technische Hochschule Aachen (Tagungsband)

Prof. Dr. Heinz Handels, Dipl.-Ing. Martin Riemer
Universitätsklinkum Hamburg-Eppendorf (Begutachtung)

Prof. Dr. Hans-Peter Meinzer, Dipl.-Ing. Matthias Baumhauer
Deutsches Krebsforschungszentrum Heidelberg (Anmeldung)

Prof. Dr. Thomas Tolxdorff, Dagmar Stiller
Charité – Universitätsmedizin Berlin (Internetpräsenz)

Programmkomitee

Prof. Dr. Til Aach, RWTH Aachen
Prof. Dr. Dr. Johannes Bernarding, Universität Magdeburg
Priv.-Doz. Dr. Jürgen Braun, Charité – Universitätsmedizin Berlin
Prof. Dr. Thorsten M. Buzug, Universität zu Lübeck
Prof. Dr. Thomas M. Deserno, RWTH Aachen
Prof. Dr. Hartmut Dickhaus, Universität Heidelberg
Dr. Jan Ehrhardt, Universitätsklinkum Hamburg-Eppendorf
Prof. Dr. Dr. Karl-Hans Englmeier, GSF Forschungszentrum Neuherberg
Prof. Dr. Bernd Fischer, Universität zu Lübeck
Prof. Dr. Heinz Handels, Universitätsklinkum Hamburg-Eppendorf
Priv.-Doz. Dr. Peter Hastreiter, Universität Erlangen-Nürnberg
Prof. Dr. Joachim Hornegger, Universität Erlangen-Nürnberg
Prof. II Dr. Alexander Horsch, TU München & Universität Tromsø, Norwegen
Prof. Dr. Frithjof Kruggel, University of California, Irvine, USA
Prof. Dr. Dr. Hans-Gerd Lipinski, Fachhochschule Dortmund
Prof. Dr. Hans-Peter Meinzer, Deutsches Krebsforschungszentrum Heidelberg
Prof. Dr. Heinrich Müller, Universität Dortmund
Prof. Dr. Nassir Navab, Technische Universität München
Dr. Stephan Nekolla, Technische Universität München
Prof. em. Dr. Heinrich Niemann, Universität Erlangen-Nürnberg
Prof. Dr. Dietrich Paulus, Universität Koblenz-Landau
Prof. Dr. Heinz-Otto Peitgen, Universität Bremen
Prof. Dr. Dr. Siegfried J. Pöppl, Universität zu Lübeck
Prof. Dr. Bernhard Preim, Universität Magdeburg
Dr. habil. Karl Rohr, Universität Heidelberg & DKFZ Heidelberg
Prof. Dr. Georgios Sakas, Fraunhofer Institut Darmstadt
Prof. Dr. Dietmar Saupe, Universität Konstanz
Prof. Dr. Rainer Schubert, UMIT Innsbruck
Prof. Dr. Thomas Tolxdorff, Charité – Universitätsmedizin Berlin
Prof. Dr. Axel Wismüller, University of Rochester, New York, USA
Dr. Thomas Wittenberg, Fraunhofer Institut Erlangen
Dr. Ivo Wolf, Deutsches Krebsforschungszentrum Heidelberg

Preisträger des BVM-Workshops 2007 in München

Die je mit einem Preisgeld von bis zu 250 € dotierten BVM-Preise zeichnen besonders hervorragende Arbeiten aus.

BVM-Preis 2007 für die beste wissenschaftliche Arbeit

1. Preis: *Christian Schumann, Steffen Oeltze, Ragnar Bade, Bernhard Preim*
Visualisierung von Gefäßsystemen mit MPU Implicits

2. Preis: *Florian Jäger, László Nyúl, Bernd Frericks, Frank Wacker, Joachim Hornegger* Whole Body MRI Intensity Standardization

3. Preis: *Heike Hufnagel, Xavier Pennec, Jan Ehrhardt, Heinz Handels, Nicholas Ayache* Point-Based Statistical Shape Models with Probabilistic Correspondences and Affine EM-ICP

BVM-Preis 2007 für den besten Vortrag

1. Preis: *Tobias Heimann, Sascha Münzing, Ivo Wolf, Hans-Peter Meinzer*
Freiheit für Formmodelle! Eine robuste Erweiterung der Deformationsgleichung

2. Preis: *Thomas Rehn, Thorsten Zerfaß, Thomas Wittenberg*
Berandungsgenaue Segmentierung von Plasma und Nucleus bei Leukozyten

3. Preis: *Nils Papenberg, Hanno Schumacher, Stefan Heldmann, Stefan Wirtz, Silke Bommersheim, Konstantin Ens, Jan Modersitzki, Bernd Fischer*
A Fast and Flexible Image Registration Toolbox: Design and Implementation of the General Approach

3. Preis: *Anja Borsdorf, Rainer Raupach, Joachim Hornegger*
Separate CT-Reconstruction for Orientation and Position Adaptive Wavelet Denoising

BVM-Preis 2007 für die beste Posterpräsentation

1. Preis: *Lena Maier-Hein, Frank Pianka, Sascha Müller, Alexander Seitel, Urte Rietdorf, Ivo Wolf, Bruno Schmied, Hans-Peter Meinzer*
Atembewegungssimulator für die in-vitro Evaluation von Weichgewebe-Navigationssystemen in der Leber

2. Preis: *Rüdiger Bock, Stefan Hoppe, Holger Scherl, Joachim Hornegger*
Beam Hardening Correction with an Iterative Scheme Using an Exact Backward Projector and a Polychromatic Forward Projector

3. Preis: *Stefan Wörz, Karl Rohr*
Hybrid Spline-based Elastic Image Registration using Analytic Solutions of the Navier Equation

Vorwort

Nach vielen Jahren rasanter Entwicklung hat sich die digitale Bildverarbeitung in der Medizin als zentraler Bestandteil diagnostischer und therapeutischer Verfahren fest etabliert. Von der Industrie kontinuierlich fortentwickelte Gerätetechnik sorgt für eine stetig steigende Bilddatenkomplexität. Diese Informationsvielfalt, gepaart mit ständig wachsender Verarbeitungsgeschwindigkeit von Rechnersystemen, verlangt neue Methoden, um die möglich gewordenen Vorteile zum Wohl von Patienten erschließen zu können. Die computergestützte Bildverarbeitung wird mit dem Ziel eingesetzt, Strukturen automatisch zu erkennen und insbesondere pathologische Abweichungen aufzuspüren und zu quantifizieren, um so beispielsweise zur Qualitätssicherung in der Diagnostik beizutragen. Doch die Anforderungen sind hoch, um die visuellen Fähigkeiten eines Experten bei der Begutachtung von medizinischem Bildmaterial nachzubilden. Dennoch gelingt die wichtige Unterscheidung von Strukturen durch zielgerichtete Algorithmen in Kombination mit der Leistungsfähigkeit moderner Computer. So wird es möglich, die Algorithmen und Technologien der medizinischen Bildverarbeitung zur Unterstützung der Medizin und zum Nutzen des Patienten einzusetzen. Der Workshop *Bildverarbeitung für die Medizin* (BVM) bietet hier ein Podium zur Präsentation und Diskussion neuer Algorithmen, Systeme und Anwendungen.

Ein Workshop *Digitale Bildverarbeitung in der Medizin* fand zum ersten Mal 1993 am Universitätsklinikum Freiburg statt. Er war Ausdruck des Bedarfs, die im Bereich der medizinischen Bildverarbeitung tätigen Kollegen aus den medizinischen und ingenieurwissenschaftlichen Fakultäten der Universitäten und Großforschungseinrichtungen, aber auch der Industrie im deutschsprachigen Raum zusammen zu bringen. Die Idee, nicht nur Raum für Präsentationen zu schaffen, sondern auch eine intensive Fachdiskussion anzuregen, trägt erheblich zum Erfolg dieser Veranstaltungsreihe bei. Um der wachsenden überregionalen Bedeutung nachzukommen, wurden ab 1998 wechselnde Veranstaltungsorte gewählt. Die Workshops *Bildverarbeitung für die Medizin* 1998 in Aachen, 1999 und 2005 in Heidelberg, 2000 und 2007 in München, 2001 in Lübeck, 2002 in Leipzig, 2003 in Erlangen, 2004 in Berlin und 2006 in Hamburg setzten das durch steigende Teilnehmerzahlen dokumentierte wachsende Interesse an dieser Veranstaltung fort. Ziel des Workshops ist auch in diesem Jahr wieder die Darstellung aktueller Forschungsergebnisse und die Vertiefung der Gespräche zwischen Wissenschaftlern, Industrie und Anwendern. Der Workshop wendet sich ausdrücklich auch an Nachwuchswissenschaftler, die über ihre Diplom/Master-, Promotions- und Habilitationsprojekte berichten wollen.

Die Vorbereitungen des Workshops werden von einem dezentral agierenden und überregional etablierten Organisationsteam vorgenommen, das von den Fachkollegen aus Aachen, Berlin, Hamburg, Heidelberg und München getragen wird. Damit ist gewährleistet, dass Erfahrungen und Traditionen vergangener BVM-Workshops mit eingebracht werden.

Am Tag vor dem wissenschaftlichen Programm werden zwei Tutorials abgehalten. Sie richten sich an Mediziner, Ingenieure, Informatiker und Naturwissenschaftler. Das erste Tutorial trägt den Titel „Visualisierung und virtuelle Realität in der Medizin“ und wird von den Kollegen Bernhard Preim aus Magdeburg und Dirk Bartz aus Leipzig gehalten. In diesem Tutorial werden Grundlagen und ausgewählte Spezialgebiete der Visualisierung medizinischer Bilddaten behandelt. Es werden die grundlegenden 3D-Visualisierungsmethoden vorgestellt: die Visualisierung auf Basis von Oberflächen durch Varianten des Marching Cubes-Verfahrens und die direkte Volumenvisualisierung, bei der auf Basis einer Transferfunktion ein 3D-Datensatz ohne Umwandlung in eine Zwischenrepräsentation dargestellt wird. Als Spezialgebiete werden die Gefäßvisualisierung, die virtuelle Endoskopie und die intraoperative Visualisierung behandelt. Die Behandlung der Spezialgebiete ist verknüpft mit einer Diskussion von Anwendungsgebieten in der Diagnostik, Therapieplanung beziehungsweise der medizinischen Ausbildung.

Das zweite Tutorial behandelt Aspekte der Bereitstellung einer neuen diagnostischen Technik, die auf der Extraktion mechanischer Gewebeeigenschaften aus Bilddaten beruht. Es wird von Jürgen Braun und Ingolf Sack von der Charité Berlin gehalten. Behandelt werden methodische Grundlagen zur Generierung neuer, bislang nicht verfügbarer Bildinformationen, darauf aufbauend die bildgestützte und modellbasierte Extraktion mechanischer Gewebeeigenschaften, sowie der klinische Einsatz des ”bildgestützten Tastbefundes”. Dazu werden praktische Anwendungen aus den Bereichen Leberzirrhose, Multipler Sklerose und Herzfunktionsmessungen demonstriert, und es wird die Möglichkeit geboten, an einer halbstündigen Untersuchung eines Probanden teilzunehmen.

Alle für den Workshop zur Präsentation ausgewählten 92 Beiträge für den Workshop sind in diesem Tagungsband abgedruckt. Die Internetseiten des Workshops bieten ausführliche Informationen über das Programm und organisatorische Details rund um den Workshop. Sie sind abrufbar unter der Adresse:

http://www.bvm-workshop.org

Wie schon in den letzten Jahren, wurde der Tagungsband auch diesmal als LaTeX-Projekt erstellt und in dieser Form an den Verlag übergeben. Von den 92 Beiträgen wurden erfreulicherweise 90 von den Autoren bereits im LaTeX-Format eingereicht. Die zwei im Winword-Format abgefassten Arbeiten wurden konvertiert und nachbearbeitet. Die Vergabe von Schlagworten nahmen die Autoren selbst vor. Die Literaturverzeichnisse sämtlicher Beiträge wurden wieder mit BibTeX generiert. Der gesamte Erstellungsprozess erfolgte ausschließlich über das Internet.

Die Herausgeber dieser Proceedings möchten allen herzlich danken, die zum Gelingen des BVM-Workshops 2008 beigetragen haben: den Mitarbeitern des Instituts für Medizinische Informatik der Berliner Charité für ihre tatkräftige Unterstützung bei der Organisation und Durchführung des Workshops. Insbesondere Sabine Saßmann und Birgit Porsch gebührt große Anerkennung für die

Unterstützung während der gesamten organisatorischen Vorbereitung. Dagmar Stiller danken wir für die Erstellung und fortwährende Aktualisierung der Internetpräsentation und Michael Engelhorn für die Organisation der Industrieausstellung. Herrn Matthias Baumhauer vom DKFZ Heidelberg danken wir für die Pflege des BVM-Emailverteilers und der webgestützten Worshopanmeldung. Für die web-basierte Durchführung des Reviewingprozesses gebührt Herrn Dipl-Ing. Martin Riemer vom Institut für Medizinische Informatik der Universität Hamburg unser Dank. Jens Hoffmann vom Institut für Medizinische Informatik der RWTH Aachen danken wir für die tatkräftige Unterstützung bei der Erstellung des Proceedingsbandes. Dem Springer-Verlag, der nun schon die elften Proceedings zu den BVM-Workshops herausbringt, wollen wir für die gute Kooperation ebenfalls unseren Dank aussprechen. Für die finanzielle Unterstützung bedanken wir uns herzlich bei unserem Hauptsponsor Siemens.

Wir wünschen allen Teilnehmerinnen und Teilnehmern des Workshops BVM 2008 lehrreiche Tutorials, viele interessante Vorträge, Gespräche an den Postern und der Industrieausstellung sowie interessante neue Kontakte zu Kolleginnen und Kollegen aus dem Bereich der Medizinischen Bildverarbeitung.

Januar 2008

Thomas Tolxdorff
Jürgen Braun
Thomas Deserno, geb. Lehmann
Heinz Handels
Alexander Horsch
Hans-Peter Meinzer

Inhaltsverzeichnis

Die fortlaufende Nummer am linken Seitenrand entspricht den Beitragsnummern, wie sie im endgültigen Programm des Workshops zu finden sind. Dabei steht V für Vortrag, P für Poster und S für Softwaredemonstration.

Segmentierung 1

Methodik 1

Segmentierung I (Poster)

Methodik I (Poster)

Registrierung

Methodik 2

Registrierung I (Poster)

3D Navigation (Poster)

Registrierung II (Poster)

Methodik II (Poster)

Segmentierung 2

Anwendungen 1

Segmentierung 3

Methodik 3

Visualisierung

Anwendungen 2

Visualisierung (Poster)

Methodik III (Poster)

Anwendungen (Poster)

Software-Demonstrationen

Segmentierung 4

Anwendungen 3

4D Endocardial Segmentation Using Spatio-temporal Appearance Models and Level Sets

Karl Fritscher[1], Rainer Schubert[1]

[1]Institute for Biomedical Image Analysis,
University for Health Sciences, Medical Informatics and Technology, Hall in Tirol
karl.fritscher@umit.at

Abstract. In this paper a framework for the segmentation of cardiac MR image sequences using spatio-temporal appearance models is presented. The method splits the 4D space into 2 separate subspaces, one for changes in appearance and one subspace for changes in motion. Using the 4D appearance models in combination with a level set framework combines the robustness of model based segmentation with the flexibility of level sets. The method is tested on the first two time frames of 10 cardiac MR sequences leading to promising results. Further tests using a larger training set for the segmentation of the whole cardiac cycle shall be performed in the near future.

1 Introduction

During the last years advances in the development of magnetic resonance imaging (MRI) have enabled the acquisition of cardiac 4D image sequences. These sequences can be very valuable for the treatment and early diagnosis of cardiovascular diseases. On the other hand the amount of data to be interpreted by clinicians drastically increases. Therefore methods and algorithms for the automatic and objective segmentation of 4D image sequences become increasingly important. Especially for the heart a number of approaches for volumetric modeling have been developed [1]. Most of these approaches use statistical shape models (e.g. Active Shape Models) of the heart ventricles. Some approaches have been proposed for the creation of 3D appearance models of the heart especially for segmentation [2, 3, 4, 5]. In [6, 7] and [8] 4D shape models of the right and left ventricle for the segmentation of the chambers of the heart have been introduced. In this work we propose a method for the segmentation of the ventricles and atria of the heart by using a spatio-temporal (4D) appearance model in combination with a level sets framework. The main contributions of this work are the combination of a 3D appearance model with a motion-model of the cardiac movement of the whole heart and the integration of these models in a maximum a posteriori level set framework.

2 Methods

For the creation of 3D appearance models, correspondences are achieved by finding an optimal transformation T_i: x $\rightarrow x'$, which maps a point x of the reference subject Sr onto the corresponding point x' of another subject S_i. The transformation T_{spatial} consists of a global rigid transformation T_{global} and a local nonrigid transformation T_{local}:

$$T_{\text{spatial}}(x) = T_{\text{global}}(x) + T_{\text{local}}(x) \tag{1}$$

For global rigid alignment, a signed distance map of an atlas subject S_r, on which the signed distance map representations of all other subjects S_i are mapped, is used as reference image. For the work presented herein the reference subject S_r was chosen arbitrarily. In order to compensate local differences in shape, diffeomorphic demons registration introduced by Vercauteren [9] was used. A statistical appearance model using the joint shape-intensity pair can then be computed using principal component analysis (PCA) [4]. For the creation of the motion model each point of a new image sequence $I(x, y, z, t)$ is mapped to its corresponding point in a reference sequence $I'(x', y', z', t')$ using the global part of the transformation T_{spatial} acquired from the 3D registration. Unlike Perperidis proposed in [6] proposed, this transformation is calculated individually for each time frame. Analogously each point of image $I_t(x, y, z)$ of time frame t of a sequence is mapped to its corresponding point in the reference image $I_{t+1}(x, y, z)$ of time frame t+1 of the same sequence resulting in n temporal transformations T_{temp}. Using the local part of the transformation T_{spatial} the temporal deformations are mapped onto the shape of the reference subject. This set of transformed motion fields can then be used for the creation of a statistical motion model using PCA. By performing the division of the space of cardiac shapes in two subspaces, an individual motion pattern can be applied to any joint shape-intensity instance caused by inter subject variability. Figure 1 is illustrating this pipeline. Using an adaption of the MAP level set framework described in [4] this spatio-temporal appearance model can be used for cardiac 4D segmentation.

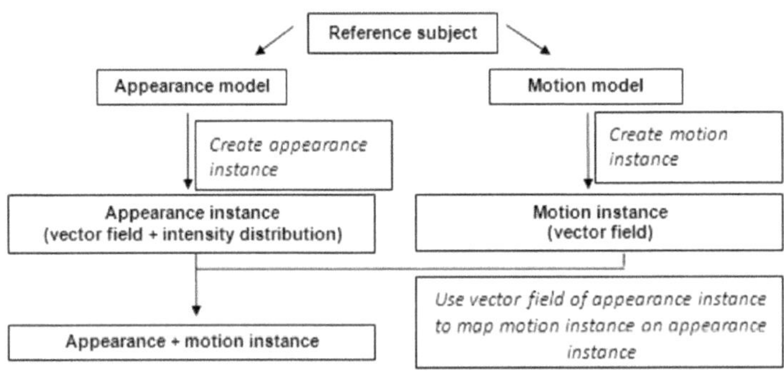

Fig. 1. Pipeline to create appearance-motion instance

Fig. 2. Significant modes of variation of the endocardial appearance (coronal cut)

	σ=-2	σ=-1	Mean	σ=1	σ=2
PC1					
PC2					

3 Results

In a first test scenario the approach described in Section 2 has been applied using the first 2 time frames of 10 cardiac MR sequences with an initial resolution of 1.56mm^3. The images for the time frames are acquired 0 ms and 100ms after the R peak of the ECG. The appearance for the first time frame and the motion of the endocardium between these two time frames was modeled. Figure 2 shows the first 2 modes of variation of the endocardial appearance within 2 standard deviations (represented by one coronal slice of the 3D volume). The time frames have not been corrected in the temporal domain regarding different pulse rates. However, all the patients roughly had the same pulse rates and the differences in the first time frames can be assumed to be rather low.

Figure 3 shows the first 2 modes of variation of the endocardial motion (respectively the shapes of the blood pool enclosed by the endocardium in time frame 2) within 2 standard deviations. The different grey levels illustrate the

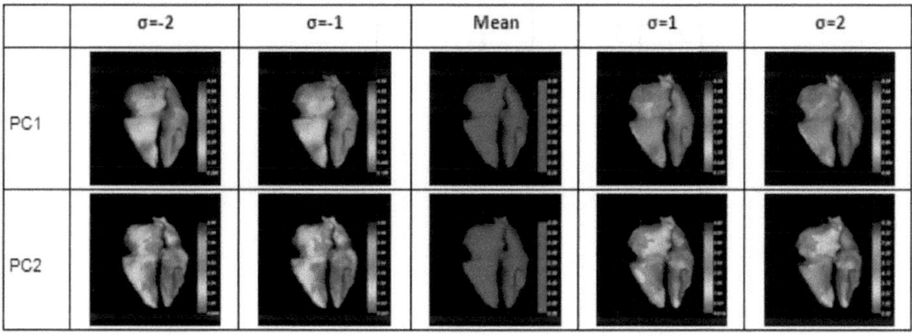

Fig. 3. Significant modes of variation for the endocardial motion

Table 1. Results of automatic segmentation compared to manual labels

Dataset	1	2	3	4	5	6	7	8	9	10
SI	0.93	0.93	0.92	0.95	0.93	0.94	0.93	0.94	0.90	0.95
HD(mm)	8.7	9.9	12.5	8.0	9.9	9.6	9.4	9.9	12.6	12.6
MD(mm)	0.96	0.93	0.93	0.7	1.0	0.84	1.00	0.90	1.28	0.89

distance to the corresponding point on the average shape of the endocardium in time frame 2. The opaque surface is representing the mean shape of the endocardium in time frame 2.

For the evaluation of the segmentation process leave all in tests for all 10 sequences using the 7 first modes of both models (covering more than 90 percent of the appearance and motion variations) have been performed. The results of the automatic segmentation were compared with manual expert segmentation of the endocardium by calculating the undirected Hausdorff distance (HD), mean distance (MD) and a similarity index (SI) between the corresponding labels. Table 1 is summing up the results of these calculations.

Note that the largest segmentation faults are situated in the area of the left atrial ear, a small processus in the left atrium. However, the average segmentation fault between the two surfaces is only between 0.75 and 1.29 mm, which is less than one pixel (pixel spacing 1.56 mm). Figure 4 is showing the result of an automatic segmentation for the first 2 time frames compared to the manual segmentation. The circle is illustrating the area of the left atrial ear.

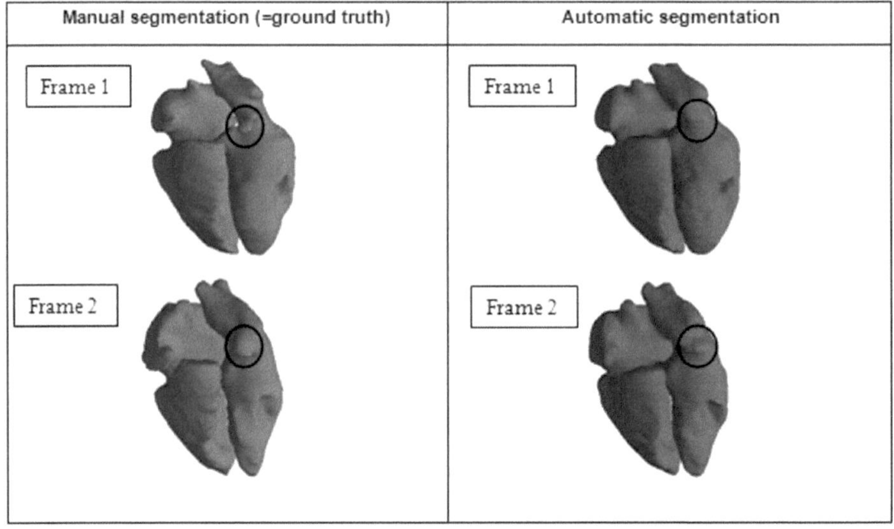

Fig. 4. Comparison of manually corrected semi-automatic (left) and automatic (right) segmentation of the endocardium

4 Discussion

In this paper we presented a novel method for the segmentation of 4D MR sequences of the heart using spatio-temporal appearance models and level sets. Compared to the usage of 4D shape models as presented in [6, 7] and [8] the usage of appearance model offers the possibility to use information about the spatial intensity distribution of an organ in order to find a proper model instance for an unseen dataset. Using segmented labels for the training set, the modeling process as well as the segmentation itself can be performed unsupervised. In first test using the first two time frames of 10 MR sequences the spatio-temporal model turned out to be adequate to model the characteristic variations concerning the appearance and motion within the training set. Moreover, the model lead to satisfying results when used for 4D segmentation. Note, however, that the size of the training set, especially for modeling the cardiac motion is extremely small and the results for the segmentation are expected to be even better when using a larger training set. This is especially true, when segmenting new unseen images. Therefore one necessary step for further improvements and more sophisticated testing scenarios would be a larger training set. Moreover, especially for modeling the endocardial motion, non-linear alternatives to PCA like LLE or kernel PCA should be tested. Moreover, all these methods will be tested for the whole cardiac cycle and with compensation of variation of individual pulse rates.

References

1. Frangi AF, Niessen WJ, Viergever MA. Three-dimensional modeling for functional analysis of cardiac images: A review. IEEE Trans Med Imaging. 2001;20(1):2–25.
2. Mitchell SC, Bosch JG, Lelieveldt BP, et al. 3-D active appearance models: Segmentation of cardiac MR and ultrasound images. IEEE Trans Med Imaging. 2002;21(9):1167–78.
3. Mitchell SC, Lelieveldt BP, van der Geest RJ, et al. Multistage hybrid active appearance model matching: segmentation of left and right ventricles in cardiac MR images. IEEE Trans Med Imaging. 2001;20(5):415–23.
4. Fritscher KD, Grünerbl A, Schubert R. 3D image segmentation using combined shape-intensity prior models. Int J Comp Assist Radiol Surg. 2007;1(6):341–50.
5. Stegmann MB, Ersboll BK, Larsen R. FAME: A flexible appearance modeling environment. IEEE Trans Med Imaging. 2003;22(10):1319–31.
6. Perperidis D, Mohiaddin RH, Rueckert D. Spatio-temporal free-form registration of cardiac MR image sequences. Med Image Anal. 2005;9(5):441–56.
7. von Berg J, Lorenz C. A geometric model of the beating heart. Methods Inf Med. 2007;46(3):282–6.
8. Montagnat J, Delingette H. 4D deformable models with temporal constraints: Application to 4D cardiac image segmentation. Med Image Anal. 2005;9(1):87–100.
9. Vercauteren T, Pennec X, Perchant A, et al. Non-parametric diffeomorphic image registration with the demons algorithm. Proc MICCAI. 2007;10(2):319–26.

3D Segmentation of the Left Ventricle Combining Long- and Shortaxis Views

Jatin Relan[1], Dennis Säring[1], Michael Groth[2], Kai Müllerleile[3], Heinz Handels[1]

[1]Department of Medical Informatics
[2]Department of Diagnostic and Interventional Radiology
[3]Department of Cardiology/Angiology
University Medical Center Hamburg-Eppendorf, 20246 Hamburg, Germany
jatinralhan@hotmail.com

Abstract. Segmentation of the left ventricle (LV) is required to quantify LV remodeling after myocardial infarction. Therefore spatiotemporal Cine MR sequences including longaxis and shortaxis images are acquired. In this paper a new segmentation method for fast and robust segmentation of the left ventricle is presented. The new approach considers the position of the mitral valve and the apex as well as the longaxis contours to generate a 3D LV surface model. The segmentation result can be checked and adjusted in the shortaxis images. Finally quantitative parameters were extracted. For evaluation the LV was segmented in eight datasets of the same subject by two medical experts using a contour drawing tool and the new segmentation tool. The results of both methods were compared concerning interaction time and intra- and interobserver variance. The presented segmentation method proved to be fast. The intra- and interobserver variance is decreased for all extracted parameters.

1 Introduction

Cardiovascular disease is reported as the number one cause of death globally. Approximately 280,000 Germans suffer from a myocardial infarction each year. The infarcted area of the myocardium loses its ability to contract and the remaining healthy muscle needs to compensate for that weakened area. This yields to left ventricle (LV) remodeling which is characterized by e.g. decreased LV ejection fraction. The quantification of LV remodeling based on volume and mass paramters is an indicator for diagnosis and treatment planing. Säring [1] (2006) presented a software system HeAT (Heart Analysis Tool) for the quantitative analysis of 4D MR image sequences. The analysis was based on a manual LV segmentation where the user has to define endocardial and epicardial structures in all shortaxis images. This segmentation process is time-consuming and observer-dependent.

In this paper a new semi-automatic segmentation method for the detection of myocardial structure combining longaxis (LA) and shortaxis (SA) images is presented. Recently several approaches for the LV segmentation were published. These approaches can be divided in intensity, shape and model based methods

[2, 3]. Generally these methods operate on shortaxis images (Fig. 1(c)) only. Due to the slice thickness of 10mm and the orientation of SA images in clinical Cine MR datasets the definition of the ending (mitral valve) slice is ambiguous. So the number of slices for calculating the volume or mass parameters are user-dependent. Therefore longaxis views (Fig. 1(a+b)) have to be included to identify the position of the mitral valve plane in 3D space. Goshtaby et al. [4] show the fusing of LA and SA images into an isotropic volume image using voxel interpolation without posterior LV segmentation. In van Geuns et al. [5] SA contours are generated based on LA contours using spline interpolation. Here the global parameters are computed using the Simpson rule on the number of SA contours without including information concerning mitral valve position.

2 Materials and Methods

The goal of this work is to develop a fast segmentation method with reduced interobserver variability. Therefore LA information about position and orientation of the mitral valve plane (MVP) and the apex as well as the myocardial contours (endocardium, epicardium) are used to generate a 3D surface model of the left ventricle. Due to the fact that only 4 LA contours have to be outlined the time for the segmentation process will be decreased. In SA images the shape of the model can be visually inspected and if needed manually adjusted.

2.1 Material

Unfortunately no gold standard for LV segmentation exists and software phantoms are commonly used to evaluate new methods [6]. In this paper four datasets ($D_{1,2,3,4}$) from the same subject but in different subject position are acquired. The slice thickness s is changed in comparison to the clinical standard ($D_{1,2} : s =$ 6mm, no gap; $D_3 : s =$ 8mm, gap = 2mm; $D_4 : s =$ 10mm, gap = 2mm; standard: $s =$ 8mm, gap = 2mm). Now two of these datasets D_k with ($k = 1, 2$) were divided into subdatasets with different number of slices and different startslices and different s.

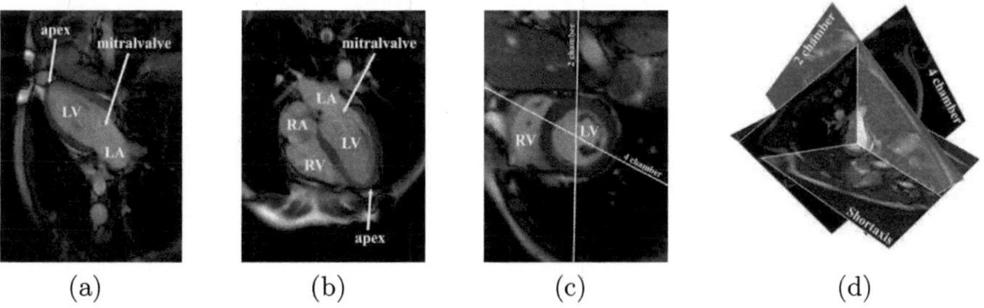

(a) (b) (c) (d)

Fig. 1. 4D Cine MR sequence in vertical longaxis (a) and horizontal longaxis (b) and a midventricular shortaxis (c) 2D views and transferred in 3D coordinate system (d). (LV: left ventricle; LA: left atrium; RV: right ventricle; RA: right atrium)

- D_k^1 is build by appending all odd numbered slices of D_k
- D_k^2 is build by appending all even numbered slices of D_k

Optimally the calculated volume and mass parameters for all datasets are equal. $D_{1,2,3,4}$ are acquired in vertical longaxis (2 chamber view) and horizontal longaxis (4 chamber view) and shortaxis (SA) views.

2.2 Methods

In this paper LA and SA images are transferred from 2D in a 3D coordinate system based on the DICOM header information solving a linear equation [4] (Fig. 1(c)). Mitral valve and apex as well as endocardial and epicardial contours are outlined in vertical and horizontal LA 2D view (Fig. 2(a)). The mitral valve plane (MVP) is build in 3D using position information of both LA views. Then intersection planes (ISP_i with $i = 1, ..., n$) with a distance of 1mm are generated automatically parallel to the MVP covering the whole left ventricle from apex to mitral valve (Fig. 2(b)). For each plane ISP_i the four endocardial $endo_i^j$ and four epicardial epi_i^j ($j = 1, ..., 4$) intersection points are calculated (Fig. 2(c)). Defining these intersection points as seedpoints enable the generation of smooth in-plane contours C_i^{endo} and C_i^{epi} using Bezier interpolation. 3D surface models for endocardium and epicardium are constructed based on LA contours and all in-plane contours C_i^{endo} and C_i^{epi} for $i = 1, ..., n$. Additionally contours in the original shortaxis views are extracted by cutting the surface models in 3D space with the image plane. These contours can be reviewed and adjusted. Mass and volume parameters are calculated using the adjusted 3D surface models.

2.3 Evaluation

For the evaluation process endocardial and epicardial contours of the datasets $D_{1,2,3,4}$ in end-diastolic and end-systolic phase in all shortaxis MR images are

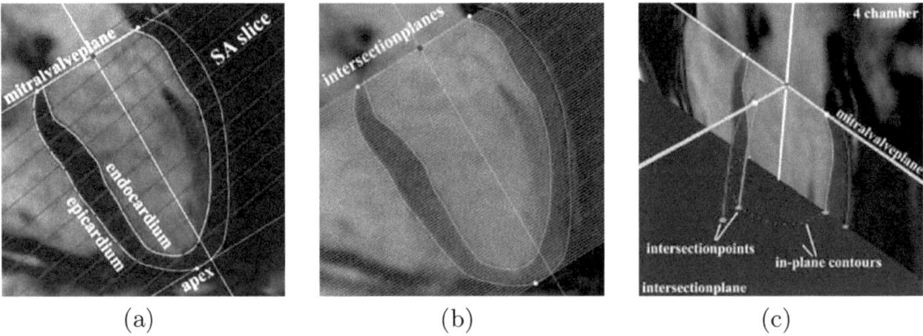

Fig. 2. Position of the mitral valve plane and SA images (a) and the intersection planes covering the whole LV (b). Intersection points and in-plane contour generation (c)

outlined by two medical experts using a contour drawing tool [1]. Each observer traced the contours of each dataset two times with the manual segmentation. Therfore approx. 500 contours have to be defined. Based on these contours five global parameters (e.g. end-diastolic Volume (EDV), LV-ejection fraction (LVEF)) were extracted for each dataset using Simpson rule. Then the presented segmentation method is used to compute the same global parameters including LA information. For each dataset only 4 LA contours need to be defined. If needed the shape of the generated model is manually adjusted. To evaluate intra- and interobserver difference the mean and standard deviation of the differences of the extracted parameters were compared.

At last the variance of the extracted parameters for MR datasets of the same subject but with different slice thickness ($s = 6, 8, 10, 12$mm) are evaluated (Fig. 3(a)). Here the parameters for each observer are compared separately to avoid interobserver variability.

3 Results

Four 4D Cine MR image sequences were obtained at the Department of Diagnostic and Interventional Radiology from one subject in different positions using a Siemens 1.5T MR scanner. Longaxis and shortaxis images were aquired by using electrocardiographically triggered breath-hold imaging techniques according to the American Heart Assiciation (AHA) scientific statement. For each slice 20 phases provided the complete coverage of the cardiac cycle resulting in a total of 380 cardiac images per sequence. The intra- and interobserver difference comparison between global LV function for manually and semi-automatically segmented images are shown in Tab. 1. The mean difference and standard deviation of all parameters is decreased. In case of intraobserver comparison e.g. the mean EDV difference is reduced from 13.7% to 2.3%. Concerning slice thickness the mean difference of EDV (14.1% to 5.8%) and ESV (18.8% to 4.9%) are decreased but SV (10.7% to 20.7%) and LVEF (4.3% to 11.6%) are increased.

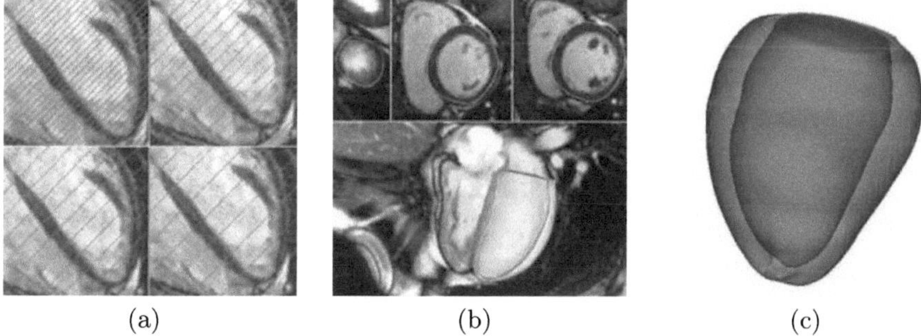

(a) (b) (c)

Fig. 3. LA view of dataset D_2, D_2^1, D_3 and D_4. Position of the SA images with different slicethickness s are overlayed (a) and 2D/3D segmentation results (b-c)

Table 1. Inter- and intraobserver difference comparison between global LV function for manually and semi-automatically segmented images. (EDV: end-diastolic volume; ESV: end-systolic volume; SV: stroke volume; LVEF: left ventricular ejection fraction; Mass: mass of the myocardium)

	intra observer				inter observer			
	manual		semi-automatic		manual		semi-automatic	
	value	[%]	value	[%]	value	[%]	value	[%]
EDV	6.4 ± 0.5	4.5 ± 0.8	1.7 ± 0.1	1.3 ± 0.0	17.8 ± 11.7	13.7 ± 9.5	2.9 ± 2.1	2.3 ± 1.7
ESV	5.9 ± 7.5	8.8 ± 11.2	0.3 ± 0.2	0.5 ± 0.3	7.9 ± 8.0	11.3 ± 11.6	3.1 ± 2.0	4.9 ± 3.1
SV	5.5 ± 1.6	7.3 ± 1.1	2.9 ± 0.6	4.0 ± 0.3	13.0 ± 13.4	22.7 ± 25.9	5.6 ± 6.1	9.1 ± 2.6
LVEF	4.2 ± 2.7	7.6 ± 4.5	1.5 ± 2.6	0.8 ± 1.2	9.4 ± 2.7	20.9 ± 8.2	3.1 ± 4.1	6.3 ± 8.4
Mass	7.8 ± 5.3	7.5 ± 4.7	6.2 ± 6.1	4.8 ± 4.7	15.5 ± 13.7	6.3 ± 5.0	1.1 ± 0.8	0.6 ± 0.5

4 Discussion

A semi-automatic LV segmentation method has been developed that combines LA information and intersection planes as well as SA images.

In the presented work global parameters including position and orientation of the mitral valve and the apex are extracted. The generation of intersection planes and in-plane contours covering the whole left ventricle enable the construction of a surface model (Fig. 3(b+c)). The intra- and interobserver difference can be decreased for all extracted parameters. Using the presented approach the time for the segmentation process is decreased from 60 minutes to 10 minutes including manual adjustment. So the semi-automatic segmentation using LA information proved to be fast and robust for the quantification of LV mass and volume properties.

In future the variability concerning slice thickness has to be evaluated. Also new MR protocols enable the acquisition of a third LA image called 3 chamber view. This image can be used to increase the number of in-plane seedpoints which can improve the quality of the initial surface model.

References

1. Säring D, et al. Computer-assisted analysis of 4D cardiac MR image sequences after myocardial infarction. Methods Inf Med. 2006;45(4):377–83.
2. Rueckert D, et al. Shape-based segmentation and tracking in 4D cardiac MR images. In: CVRMed; 1997. p. 43–52.
3. Spreeuwers LJ, et al. Myocardial boundary extraction using coupled active contours. In: Computers in Cardiology, 2003; 2003. p. 745–8.
4. Goshtasby AA, et al. Fusion of short-axis and long-axis cardiac MR images. Comput Med Imaging Graph. 1996;20(2):77–87.
5. van Geuns RJM, et al. Automatic quantitative left ventricular analysis of cine MR images by using three-dimensional information for contour detection. Radiology. 2006;240(1):215–21.
6. Segars WP, et al. A realistic spline-based dynamic heart phantom. IEEE Trans Nuc Sci. 1999;46(3):503–6.

Computer-Aided Diagnosis in Breast MRI: Do Adjunct Features Derived from T_2-weighted Images Improve Classification of Breast Masses?

Willem van Aalst[1], Thorsten Twellmann[1], Hans Buurman[2], Frans A. Gerritsen[1,2], Bart M. ter Haar Romeny[1]

[1]Dept. of Biomedical Engineering, Eindhoven University of Technology, NL
[2]Philips Medical Systems, Healthcare Informatics - Advanced Development, Best, NL
t.twellmann@tue.nl

Abstract. In the field of dynamic contrast-enhanced magnetic resonance imaging (DCE-MRI) of breast cancer, current research efforts in computer-aided diagnosis (CADx) are mainly focused on the temporal series of T_1-weighted images acquired during uptake of a contrast agent, processing morphological and kinetic information. Although static T_2-weighted images are usually part of DCE-MRI protocols, they are seldom used in CADx systems. The aim of this work was to evaluate to what extent T_2-weighted images provide complementary information to a CADx system, improving its performance for the task of discriminating benign breast masses from life-threatening carcinomas. In a preliminary study considering 64 masses, inclusion of lesion features derived from T_2-weighted images increased the classification performance from A_z=0.94 to A_z=0.99.

1 Introduction

In recent years, dynamic contrast-enhanced magnetic resonance imaging (DCE-MRI) has evolved to a powerful tool for detection, diagnosis and management of breast cancer [1]. A temporal series of 3D T_1-weighted MR images is acquired during the uptake of a contrast agent based on gadolinium chelates. This enables radiologists to localize suspicious tissue areas and to further assess their likelihood of malignancy by means of their morphologic and kinetic characteristics. Static T_2-weighted images provide complementary information for discriminating benign fibroadenoma from malignant cancers, as both expose similar enhancement patterns in the DCE T_1-weighted images. Furthermore, several secondary signs such as edemas, which frequently accompany pathological tissue growth, are accentuated in T_2-weighted images [2].

The role of T_2-weighted images for the general discrimination of benign and malignant findings was investigated in several studies, e.g. [3, 4]. In the majority of studies, suspicious masses were initially located by means of the DCE T_1-weighted images. Subsequently, the brightness of the corresponding region in the T_2-weighted image was visually rated as hypo-, iso- or hyperintense to a reference region, e.g. the tissue surrounding the mass or air. In summary, the different studies reached different conclusions allowing no clear statement about the added value of T_2-weighted images for the discrimination of benign and malignant breast masses.

Computer-aided diagnosis (CADx) systems supporting radiologists in detecting and assessing suspicious tissue regions in DCE-MRI data are expected to improve the reliability of clinical decisions and, therewith, to potentially decrease the number of unnecessary biopsies. (Semi-)automatic discrimination of benign and malignant masses in breast MRI was investigated by several authors [5, 6, 7]. The proposed approaches have in common that they solely concentrate on processing of kinetic and morphologic features as depicted in the DCE T_1-weighted images, which are, without doubt, the most important source of information in breast MRI. However, the inclusion of the frequently acquired T_2-weighted images might be beneficial in the context of CADx.

This work investigates for the first time whether adjunct features derived from static T_2-weighted images improve the performance of computer-aided classification of benign and malignant breast masses based on supervised pattern recognition techniques.

2 Methods

In bilateral DCE-MRI studies[1] of 50 patients, $N = 64$ breast masses (28 benign and 36 malignant) were segmented in the T_1-weighted images with a semi-automatic segmentation algorithm [8]. Additionally, binary masks separating breasts from thoraces were computed by applying a sequence of smoothing, thresholding and morphological operators. To adjust for the different voxel size in the T_1- and T_2-weighted images, the latter were resampled by tri-linear interpolation. Sufficient spatial alignment between the dynamic T_1-weighted series and between T_1- and T_2-weighted images was verified by visual inspection.

2.1 T_1- and T_2-weighted Lesion Features

A total of 22 morphological and kinetic T_1-weighted features described in [5, 6, 7] were evaluated for all binary lesion segmentations. Due to the limited space we have to refer the reader to the corresponding articles for more information about these features. In addition to the T_1-weighted features, the following T_2-weighted lesion features were computed: Let Γ_{L_i} be the set of grey values in the T_2-weighted image corresponding to the voxels as marked by a binary segmentation of lesion i, Γ_{B_i} the set of grey values in the left or right breast (depending on the location of the lesion i) excluding the lesion and $\Gamma_{S_i^t}$ the set of grey values in a t

[1] Dynamic T_1-weighted images: TR=4.4-6.9ms, TE=2.1-3.4ms, FA=10°, Δt=60-90s, 6-7 dynamics, fat-suppressed, transversal orientation. Static T_2-weighted image: TR=6.7-16.9s, TE=120ms, FA=90°, transversal orientation.

mm thick shell enclosing the segmentation of lesion i. The *normalized intensity mean* and *variance* features are defined as

$$f_{\mu}^{T_2}(\Gamma_{L_i}, \Gamma_{R_i}) = \frac{\mu_{\Gamma_{L_i}}}{\mu_{\Gamma_{R_i}}} \quad \text{and} \quad f_{\sigma^2}^{T_2}(L_i, R_i) = \frac{\sigma^2_{\Gamma_{L_i}}}{[\mu_{\Gamma_{R_i}}]^2},$$

with μ and σ^2 being the intensity mean and variance of the lesion set Γ_{L_i} or one of the reference regions $\Gamma_{R_i} \in \{\Gamma_{B_i}, \Gamma_{S_i^t}\}$. By normalizing with respect to the mean intensity of a reference region, we take into account the qualitative nature of MR images and resemble the clinical practice of rating lesions as hypo-, iso- or hyperintense with respect to some reference region.

The *normalized α-percentile* is defined as

$$f_{perc_\alpha}^{T_2}(\Gamma_{L_i}, \Gamma_{B_i}, \alpha) = \frac{H^{\alpha}_{\Gamma_{L_i}}}{\mu_{\Gamma_{B_i}}},$$

with $H^{\alpha}_{\Gamma_{L_i}}$ being the intensity threshold in the cumulative relative frequency histogram H of lesion Γ_L for which the cumulative relative frequency exceeds α percent. A second normalized α-percentile is computed for the enclosing shell, reflecting potential bright regions (caused e.g. edema) in the tissue surrounding the lesion:

$$f_{perc_\alpha}^{T_2}(\Gamma_{S_i^t}, \Gamma_{B_i}, \alpha) = \frac{H^{\alpha}_{\Gamma_{L_i}}}{\mu_{\Gamma_{B_i}}}.$$

Both α-percentiles were normalized with respect to the mean breast intensity.

The aforementioned features were evaluated for the sets Γ_{L_i} containing voxels as marked by the binary segmentation of lesion i and for the subsets $\Gamma^*_{L_i} \subset \Gamma_{L_i}$ of lesion voxels as marked after applying a morphological erosion operator to the binary lesion mask. The free parameters t and α were varied in reasonable ranges ($t \in \{2, 4, \ldots, 20\}$ in mm, $\alpha \in \{0, 2, \ldots, 20, 80, 82, \ldots, 100\}$ in %), considering each setting as a new feature.

The sharpness of the lesion margin in the T_2-weighted image is quantified by evaluating the *mean* and *variance of the margin gradient* as described for DCE T_1-weighted images in [5] in the static T_2-weighted images. These features reflect the mean and variance of gradient magnitudes computed with Gaussian derivatives of reasonable scale for all voxels in a three voxels thick shell centered on the lesion segmentation's surface.

2.2 Feature Selection and Classification

Due to the limited number of lesions, feature selection is a mandatory step to avoid overfitting of the data. For the final classification of lesions we selected two sets of features, each containing five features in total. A linear classification function was estimated by Fisher linear discriminant analysis (FDA) [9].

To determine the baseline performance of a CADx system based on T_1-weighted information only, a set of three T_1-weighted features was selected by exhaustive search and subsequently extended to a size of five features by forward-backward feature selection. At each iteration, the performance of the FDA after including a new candidate feature was evaluated in a leave-one-lesion-out scheme. For all permutations of the N lesions, the FDA was trained with data of $N-1$ lesions and subsequently applied to the omitted unseen lesion. The final performance was quantified by estimating the area-under-the-ROC-curve (A_z) computed for the FDA output [10].

The same feature selection process was repeated a second time, this time selecting candidate features from the pooled set of T_1- and T_2-weighted features.

3 Results

Figure 1 shows the ROC curves for the FDA evaluating the selected set of five DCE T_1-weighted features (dashed line) and the mixed set of DCE T_1- and static T_2-weighted features (solid lines). The non-parametric estimates of the area-under-the-ROC curve are $A_z = 0.94$ and $A_z = 0.99$, respectively. Though inclusion of the T_2-weighted features leads to a considerable improvement of $\Delta A_z = 0.05$, a statistical test for the significance of the difference between the A_z values of the two correlated ROC curves [11] failed with $p = 0.064$ (CI=95%).

4 Discussion

After feature selection from the pooled set, the final set consists of two DCE T_1-weighted and three T_2-weighted features. The DCE T_1-weighted features are *circularity* and *variance of the radial gradient histogram* as described in [5], reflecting the lesion shape and the sharpness of its margin, respectively. The

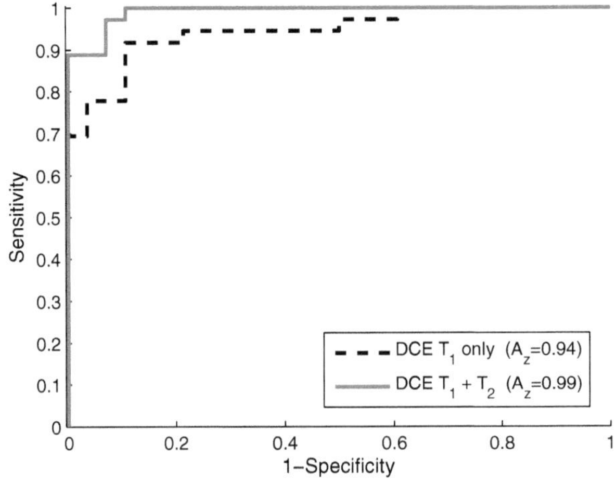

Fig. 1. Results

three T_2-weighted features are the normalized α-percentile for the eroded lesion segmentation ($\alpha = 20\%$) and the normalized α-percentile for the lesion shell with ($\alpha = 92\%, t = 2$mm) and ($\alpha = 98\%, t = 20$mm). The latter features resemble clinical practice of rating the intensities within the lesion and within the enclosing shell of non-lesion tissue.

For the considered set of lesions, inclusion of T_2-weighted features improved the performance of the classification of breast masses by $\Delta A_z = 0.05$ to $A_z = 0.99$, yet a statistical test for significance failed. In consideration of the low power of the test, we nevertheless belief that inclusion of information derived from the T_2-weighted images, which are usually part of today's breast MRI protocols, provides valuable complementary information to CADx systems and we will reinvestigate this issue in a future larger study.

Acknowledgement. This work was conducted in cooperation with the University of Chicago; the authors are grateful to Dr. Gillian Newstead (UoC) and Ursula Kose (PMS) for their support.

References

1. Kuhl CK. The current status of breast MR imaging (Part I). Radiology. 2007;244(2):356–78.
2. Fischer DR, Wurdinger S, Boettcher J, et al. Further signs in the evaluation of magnetic resonance mammography: A retrospective study. Invest Radiol. 2005;40(7):430–5.
3. Kuhl CK, Klaschik S, Mielcarek P, et al. Do T2-weighted pulse sequences help with the differential diagnosis of enhancing lesions in dynamic breast MRI? J Magn Reson Imaging. 1999;9(2):187–96.
4. Kelcz F. Quantitative assesment of T2 imaging information in differential diagnosis of enhancing breast lesons. Eur Radiol. 2006;16 (Suppl 5):E51–E53.
5. Gilhuijs KGA, Giger ML, Bick U. Computerized analysis of breast lesions in three dimensions using dynamic magnetic-resonance imaging. Med Phys. 1998;25:1647–54.
6. Chen W, Giger ML, Lan L, et al. Computerized interpretation of breast MRI: Investigation of enhancement-variance dynamics. Med Phys. 2004;31(5):1076–82.
7. Arbash-Meinel L, Stolpen AH, Berbaum KS, et al. Breast MRI lesion classification: Improved performance of human readers with a backpropagation neural network computer-aided diagnosis (CAD) system. J Magn Reson Imaging. 2007;25:89–95.
8. Bülow T, Meinel LA, Wiemker R, et al. Segmentation of suspicious lesions in dynamic contrast-enhanced breast MR images. In: Proc. of SPIE Medical Imaging 2006; 2006.
9. Duda RO, Hart PE. Pattern Classification and Scene Analysis. Wiley; 1973.
10. Swets JA, Pickett RM. Evaluation of Dignostic Systems. Academic Press; 1982.
11. DeLong ER, DeLong DM, Clarke-Pearson DL. Comparing the areas under two or more correlated receiver operating characteristics curves: A nonparametric approach. Biometrics. 1988;44:837–45.

Halbautomatische Segmentierung von Pulmonalgefäßen in CT Daten als Referenz zur Validierung automatischer Verfahren

Jens N. Kaftan[1,2], Annemarie Bakai[2], Florian Maier[3], Til Aach[1]

[1]Lehrstuhl für Bildverarbeitung, RWTH Aachen
[2]Siemens Medical Solutions, Computed Tomography Division, Forchheim
[3]Institut für Technische Informatik, Universität Karlsruhe (TH)
jens.kaftan@lfb.rwth-aachen.de

Kurzfassung. Das Segmentieren von Pulmonalgefäßen in Computertomographie (CT) Daten wurde schon vielfach behandelt und wird z.B. bei der computerunterstützten Detektion von Lungenembolien angewendet. Vielen Segmentierverfahren fehlt jedoch eine quantitative Validierung aufgrund mangelnder Referenzsegmentierungen. Wir stellen ein System zur halbautomatischen Segmentierung von Blutgefäßen in definierten Bereichen der Lunge basierend auf dem Random-Walker-Algorithmus vor. Durch Initialisierung der Methode mittels automatisch generierter Saatpunkte wird die Effizienz des Verfahrens erhöht und die erforderliche Benutzerinteraktion reduziert. Die resultierenden Segmentierungen können zur Validierung von automatischen Verfahren verwendet werden. Exemplarisch evaluieren wir ein vollautomatisches Segmentierverfahren basierend auf dem Fuzzy-Connectedness-Algorithmus.

1 Einleitung

Pulmonalgefäßsegmentierung in kontrastverstärkten CT Daten (z.B. [1, 2, 3]) ist Grundlage für Anwendungen wie z.B. die Detektion von Lungenembolien. Üblicherweise werden solche Segmentierverfahren lediglich qualitativ validiert, da das Erzeugen von manuellen Referenzen aufgrund der Komplexität des Gefäßbaumes schwierig ist. Darüber hinaus kann man die Genauigkeit eines Verfahrens abschätzen, indem man die Anzahl von manuell markierten Mittellinien-Punkten, die von der Segmentierung beinhaltet werden, prozentual bestimmt [1], was aber keinerlei Rückschlüsse auf fehlerhaft positive Regionen zulässt. Wu et al. [2] vergleichen ihre Segmentierergebnisse aus künstlich verrauschten, klinischen Daten mit dem Ergebnis aus den Originaldaten. Damit lässt sich zwar die Robustheit des Verfahrens zeigen, nicht aber die Genauigkeit selbst bewerten.

Wir stellen ein schnelles, halbautomatisches Verfahren zur Erzeugung von Referenzsegmentierungen in definierten Bereichen der Lunge, basierend auf dem Random-Walker-Algorithmus [4, 5], vor. Durch Initialisierung des Verfahrens mit effizient generierten Saatpunkten wird die Interaktionszeit soweit reduziert, dass das Verfahren anwendbar für diese ansonsten langwierige Aufgabe wird. Das Ergebnis kann interaktiv so lange verfeinert werden, bis es zufriedenstellend präzise ist, wobei jedes beliebige Segmentierergebnis durch Definition ausreichend vieler Saatpunkte erzeugt werden kann. Das Resultat kann dann zur Validierung und Optimierung automatischer Verfahren herangezogen werden.

2 Material und Methoden

Halbautomatische Segmentierverfahren erlauben eine schnellere und reproduzierbarere Segmentierung als manuelle Verfahren. Dabei verbleibt die Aufgabe der Detektion (z.B. von Saatpunkten) beim Benutzer, wobei die Delineation vom Computer übernommen wird.

Der Random-Walker-Algorithmus [4, 5] ist ein graphbasierter Ansatz zur interaktiven Segmentierung, bei dem die Voxel Knoten entsprechen und banachbarte Voxel durch gewichtete Kanten verbunden sind

$$w_{ij} = \exp\left(-\beta \cdot d_{ij} \cdot |I(\mathbf{x}_i) - I(\mathbf{x}_j)|\right) \tag{1}$$

wobei $I(\mathbf{x}_i)$ der Intensitätswert des Voxels i in HU-Werten, d_{ij} dem Abstand zwischen i, j in mm entsprechen und β ein frei wählbarer Parameter ist, der angibt wie stark die Bildkanten berücksichtigt werden sollen (hier: $\beta = 150$). Unter der Vorraussetzung, dass ein Benutzer einen Teil der Voxel bereits als Vorder- und Hintergrund Saatpunkte definiert hat, berechnet er anschaulich gesehen die Wahrscheinlichkeit für jeden verbleibenden Knoten, dass ein sich auf dem Graphen zufällig fortbewegender Spaziergänger zuerst einen Saatpunkt des Vorder- oder Hintergrunds erreicht, wobei Kanten mit höherer Gewichtung wahrscheinlicher passiert werden.

Es kann gezeigt werden, dass die gesuchten Wahrscheinlichkeiten sich durch Lösen des diskretisierten Dirichletproblems berechnen lassen. Numerisch kann dies effizient durch das Konjugierte-Gradienten-Verfahren gelöst werden. Um dieses Verfahren anwendbar bezüglich Interaktionsaufwand und Rechenzeit für die Erzeugung von Referenzsegmentierungen der Pulmonalgefäße zu machen, haben wir es um automatische Initialisierungsschritte erweitert.

2.1 Initialisierung

Um das zu segmentierende Volumen überschaubar zu halten und den Rechenaufwand zu begrenzen, wird zunächst eine 3D Region of Interest (ROI) ausgewählt und automatisch Saatpunkte generiert. Zusätzlich werden Initialisierungswahrscheinlichkeiten abhängig vom Intensitätswert jedes Voxels berechnet um die Konvergenzgeschwindigkeit des numerischen Verfahrens zu erhöhen. Um eine sinnvolle Wahrscheinlichkeitsfunktion aufzustellen haben wir verschiedene, mit diesem Verfahren segmentierte ROIs unterschiedlicher Patienten bezüglich ihrer Intensitätsverteilung untersucht (Abb. 1a). Unter der Annahme, dass die Intensitätswerte $I(\mathbf{x})$ einer Verteilung G entspricht, die sich aus zwei Gauss-Verteilungen G_{VG} und G_{HG} für Blutgefäße (Vordergrund) und Nicht-Blutgefäße (Hintergrund) zusammensetzt, können die Parameter μ, σ der bedingten Wahrscheinlichkeitsdichtefunktion geschätzt werden. Daraus lässt sich eine Wahrscheinlichkeitsverteilung definieren, in der die Hintergrundwahrscheinlichkeit $P(HG|\mathbf{x}) = 1$ für $I(\mathbf{x}) \leq \mu_{HG}$ und die Vordergrundwahrscheinlichkeit $P(VG|\mathbf{x}) = 1$ für $I(\mathbf{x}) \geq \mu_{VG}$ ist (Abb. 1b). Alle Voxel, die eines dieser Kriterien erfüllen werden als Vorder- bzw. Hintergrundsaatpunkte definiert. Dazwischen fällt die Wahrscheinlichkeit entsprechend einer Gaussfunktion mit den bestimmten Parametern μ, σ ab, wobei Vorder- und Hintergrundwahrscheinlichkeit komplementär sein müssen. Zusätzlich erlauben wir einen Bereich, für den keine der beiden Klassen bevorzugt wird: $P(VG|\mathbf{x}) = P(HG|\mathbf{x}) = 0.5$.

2.2 Anwendung

Die mit dem vorgestellten Verfahren erzeugten Segmentierungen können vom Benutzer so lange verfeinert werden, bis das Resultat qualitativ als Referenz genügt und damit zur Validierung automatischer Verfahren herangezogen werden kann. Exemplarisch zeigen wir eine quantitative Validierung für ein automatisches Verfahren [3]. Zur automatischen Segmentierung werden zunächst Blutgefäßregionen mit sehr hoher Spezifität schwellwertbasiert detektiert und jeder resultierende, zusammenhängende Teilbaum wird zu einem oder mehreren Saatpunkten reduziert. Anschließend wird ein Fuzzy-Connectedness-Regionenwachstum [6] gestartet, dass jedem Voxel ein wahrscheinlichkeits-ähnliches Maß zuweist, welches angibt wie stark ein Voxel mit einem der Saatpunkte verbunden ist und damit zum Blutgefäßbaum gehört. Die Zusammengehörigkeit benachbarter Voxel i, j berechnet sich mittels einer intensitätsbasierten Wahrscheinlichkeitsfunktion:

$$g\left(I(\mathbf{x}_i), I(\mathbf{x}_j)\right) = \exp\left(-\frac{1}{2\sigma^2}\left(\frac{I(\mathbf{x}_i) - I(\mathbf{x}_j)}{2} - \mu\right)^2\right) \tag{2}$$

wobei μ hier dem mittleren HU-Wert der Saatpunkte entspricht und σ frei wählbar ist (hier: $\sigma = 250$). Das Wachstum wird abgebrochen, wenn die Wahrscheinlichkeit unter eine bestimmte Schwelle sinkt. Abschließend erhält man eine bi-

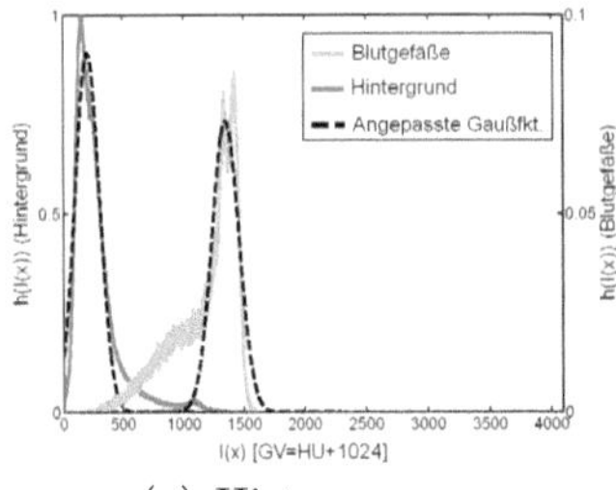

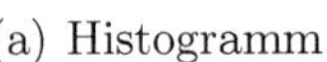

(a) Histogramm

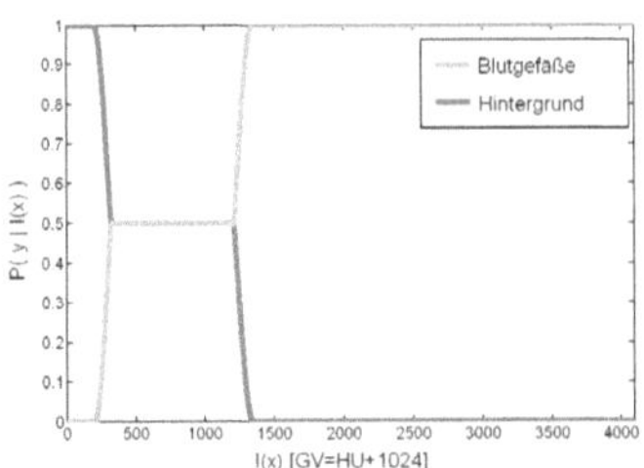

(b) Wahrscheinlichkeitsverteilung

Abb. 1. (a) Histogramm über verschiedene ROIs getrennt nach Blutgefäße (hellgrau) und Hintergrund (dunkelgrau) und die entsprechenden angepassten Gaußfunktionen mit $\mu_{HG} = -826$ HU, $\sigma_{HG} = 102$ HU und $\mu_{VG} = 322$ HU, $\sigma_{VG} = 111$ HU. Man beachte die unterschiedliche Achsenskalierung für beide Klassen. (b) Wahrscheinlichkeitsverteilung zur Initialisierung des Random-Walker-Algorithmus

Abb. 2. (a) Lungenausschnitt mit ROI (gelb). (b) Initiale Segmentierung ohne manuelle Nachverarbeitung. Vorder- und Hintergrundsaatpunkte sind opak blau bzw. grün dargestellt, während die resultierende Segmentierung halbtransparent gezeigt wird. (c) Segmentierung nach Hinzufügen weiterer Saatpunkte. (d) 3D Darstellung

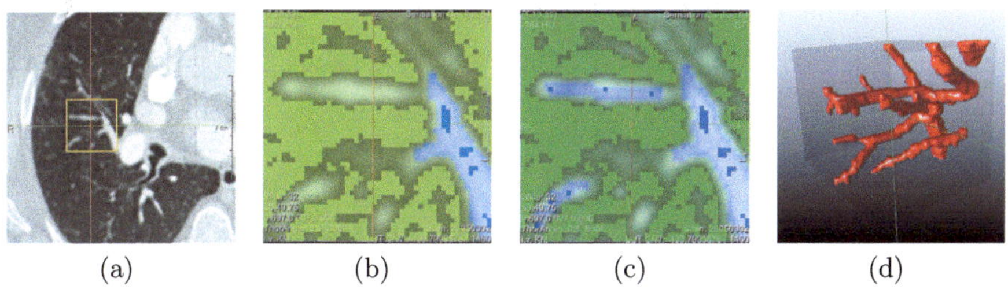

(a) (b) (c) (d)

näre Segmentierung durch Anwendung eines Schwellwerts auf die Wahrscheinlichkeitskarte, welcher die Sensitivität/Spezifität des Verfahrens beeinflusst.

3 Ergebnisse

Das vorgestellte Verfahren erlaubt eine schnelle und präzise halbautomatische Segmentierung der Blutgefäße innerhalb der ROI. Das Segmentierergebnis ist exemplarisch in Abbildung 2 dargestellt, basierend lediglich auf der automatischen Initialisierung und einer Random-Walker-Anwendung (b) und nach weiterer Benutzerinteraktion (c-d). Während die automatische Detektion von Saatpunkten den Interaktionsaufwand erheblich reduziert, bewirkt die Vor-Initialisierung mit der Wahrscheinlichkeitsfunktion aus Abb. 1b lediglich eine Zeitersparnis von maximal 4-5% für die erste Random-Walker Berechnung.

Mit dem neuen Verfahren können Segmentierergebnisse im Detail (fehlerhaft positiv/negativ segmentierte Voxel) untersucht werden (Abb. 3). Das automatische Verfahren erreicht eine Sensitivität von 80% bei einer Spezifität von 95%.

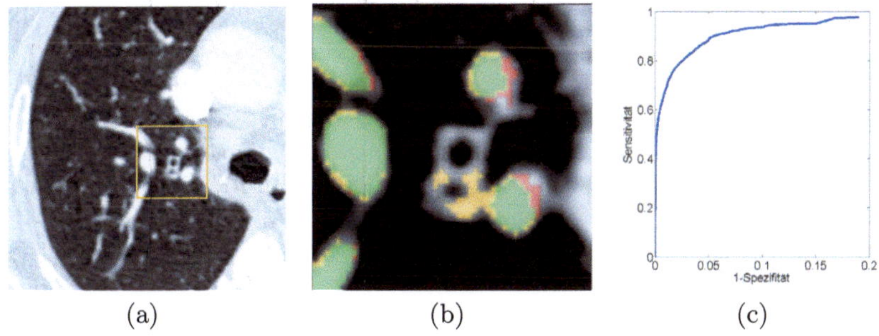

(a) (b) (c)

Abb. 3. (a) ROI. (b) Vergleich automatischer mit Referenzsegmentierung. Korrekt positive Regionen sind grün, fehlerhaft positive gelb und fehlerhaft negative rot dargestellt. (c) ROC Kurve über 5 Patienten mit je 3 ROIs der Größe 50^3 Voxel

4 Diskussion

Wir haben ein halbautomatisches Verfahren zur Erzeugung von Referenzsegmentierungen des Blutgefäßbaumes in definierten Bereichen der Lunge vorgestellt. Wir nutzen dabei den Random-Walker-Algorithmus, den wir um automatische Initialisierungsschritte erweitert haben, wodurch das Verfahren anwendbar für diese ansonsten langwierige Aufgabe wird.

Streng genommen müsste die Qualität der so erzeugten Referenzsegmentierungen ebenfalls untersucht werden, was aus Mangel an einem exakten Goldstandard für klinische Daten wiederum nicht möglich ist. Das vorgestellte Verfahren weist jedoch einige Merkmale auf, die darauf hindeuten, dass die so erzeugten Segmentierungen zur Validierung genutzt werden können:

- Mit dem Random-Walker-Algorithmus lässt sich jede beliebige Segmentierung durch Definition ausreichend vieler Saatpunkte erzeugen [5].
- Es wird nur eine kleine Zahl von Saatpunkten benötigt um eine Segmentierung zu erzeugen, die einer Manuellen nahezu identisch ist [4].
- Änderungen an der Anordnung der Saatpunkte resultieren nur in einer kleinen Änderung des Segmentierergebnisses [4], wodurch das Verfahren reproduzierbarere Ergebnisse liefert als manuelle Methoden.

Aufgrund der Automatisierung beider Teilschritte – Saatpunktgewinnung und Strukturdelineation – kann ein präzises Segmentierergebnis mit akzeptablem Zeitaufwand erzielt werden, welches als Referenz zur Optimierung und Validierung automatischer Verfahren genutzt werden kann. Durch Wahl mehrerer Referenzregionen pro Lunge, randomisiert oder systematisch in verschiedenen Bereichen, kann die Relevanz der Vergleichskriterien weiter erhöht werden.

Literaturverzeichnis

1. Zhou C, Chan HP, Hadjiiski LM, et al. Automatic pulmonary vessel segmentation in 3D computed tomographic pulmonary angiographic (CTPA) images. Proc SPIE. 2006;6144:1524–30.
2. Wu C, Agam G, Roy AS, et al. Regulated morphology approach to fuzzy shape analysis with application to blood vessel extraction in thoracic CT scans. Proc SPIE. 2004;5370:1262–70.
3. Kaftan JN, Kiraly AP, Bakai A, et al. Fuzzy pulmonary vessel segmentation in contrast enhanced CT data. Proc SPIE. 2008;6914. To appear.
4. Grady L, Schiwietz T, Aharon S, et al. Random walks for interactive organ segmentation in two and three dimensions: Implementation and validation. Lec Note Comp Sci. 2005;3750(2):773–80.
5. Grady L. Random walks for image segmentation. IEEE Trans Pattern Anal Mach Intell. 2006;28(11):1768–83.
6. Udupa JK, Samarasekera S. Fuzzy connectedness and object definition: Theory, algorithms, and applications in image segmentation. Graph Models Image Process. 1996;58(3):246–61.

Non-equispaced Fourier Transform Vs. Polynomial-Based Metal Artifact Reduction in Computed Tomography

Bärbel Kratz, Tobias Knopp, Jan Müller, May Oehler, Thorsten M. Buzug

Institute of Medical Engineering, University of Lübeck, 23538 Lübeck, Germany
kratz@imt.uni-luebeck.de

Abstract. We propose a method, which treats metal artifact reduction in CT by sinogram restoration as a problem of scattered data interpolation. Corrupted sinogram entries are discarded and replaced with artificially generated values. The presented interpolation algorithm is based on the 2D non-equispaced fast Fourier transform (NFFT). Results are compared to two common polynomial interpolation schemes.

1 Introduction

The non-equispaced fast Fourier transform (NFFT) [1] is a generalization of the fast Fourier transformation (FFT) for data located on non-equispaced grids. It has several applications in medical imaging, such as for instance it is used in magnetic resonance imaging for reconstruction of data located on spiral or radial trajectories. Further, NFFT can be used for direct reconstruction methods [2], exploiting the well known Fourier-slice theorem. Beside these applications, the NFFT can be generally used for multidimensional interpolation of scattered data as described in [3]. In the present work we propose to apply NFFT-based scattered data interpolation to metal artifact reduction in CT, where inconsistent data needs to be replaced by interpolated one.

If one or more metal objects, e.g. dental fillings or hip prosthesis are present in the field of view of a CT scanner, the reconstructed images are often severely degraded by bright star-shaped artifacts (Fig. 1). The main cause of these metal artifacts is the so called beam hardening effect, where photons of high and low energies are attenuated differently. Due to the highly non-linear nature of this process, this results in inconsistent projection data. These artifacts impare the diagnostic value of the reconstructed images and, therefore, give rise to the introduction of correction methods into the reconstruction schemes.

A common method for metal artifact reduction consists of two parts: First, the inconsistent data is removed from the sinogram. Afterwards, the resulting gap is to be filled with surrogate values. The first step can be accomplished by segmentation of the regions containing metal in a preliminary reconstruction. After forward projection of the resulting binary label image, the resulting mask can then be used to remove metal traces from the initial sinogram. In literature, several approaches to complete the sinogram are known. One popular method is proposed in [4] and [5], in which the gap is filled with interpolated values from adjacent detector elements. The interpolation is done independendly for each view.

In the present paper it is shown, how the computation of the discarded values can be interpreted as a problem of scattered data interpolation. Additionally it is shown, how this very problem can be solved using an NFFT based approach.

2 Materials and Methods

The FFT provides a method for interpolation of multidimensional data. By zero padding the vector of Fourier coefficients, the number of elements of an pixel grid can be increased. However, the FFT is limited to equispaced voxel positions and cannot be applied directly for interpolation of the gap in a sinogram. Therefore, we propose to use a generalization of the FFT, the so called NFFT that can handle non-equispaced voxel positions in the image domain. In the following we describe the application of NFFT interpolation to the gap filling problem in CT.

Let $p(\boldsymbol{r})$, $\boldsymbol{r} = (\theta, r)^T$ denote the measured projection that depends on the angle θ and on the position r. The projections are sampled on N equispaced positions $\boldsymbol{r}_\rho$ that are located on a grid of size $N_1 \times N_2$. For simplicity let the positions $\boldsymbol{r}_\rho$ be scaled to fit into the torus $[-\frac{1}{2}, \frac{1}{2})^2$. After detection of metal traces, located on N_{gap} positions $\bar{\boldsymbol{r}}_n$, only a subset of $M = N - N_{\text{gap}}$ projections are available located on non-equispaced positions $\tilde{\boldsymbol{r}}_j$.

In order to interpolate the missing values necessary for the reconstruction, a Fourier decomposition of the projections p is performed, i.e. the complex coefficients $\hat{f}_\kappa$ are computed, such that

$$p(\tilde{\boldsymbol{r}}_j) = \sum_{\kappa=0}^{N-1} \hat{f}_\kappa e^{2\pi i \boldsymbol{k}_\kappa^T \tilde{\boldsymbol{r}}_j}, \quad \text{for} \quad j = 0, \ldots, M-1 \tag{1}$$

where $\boldsymbol{k}_\kappa \in [-\frac{N_1}{2}, \frac{N_1}{2}) \times [-\frac{N_2}{2}, \frac{N_2}{2})$ denote equispaced frequencies. Then, the missing values can be interpolated by evaluating (1) at the missing positions $\bar{\boldsymbol{r}}_n$

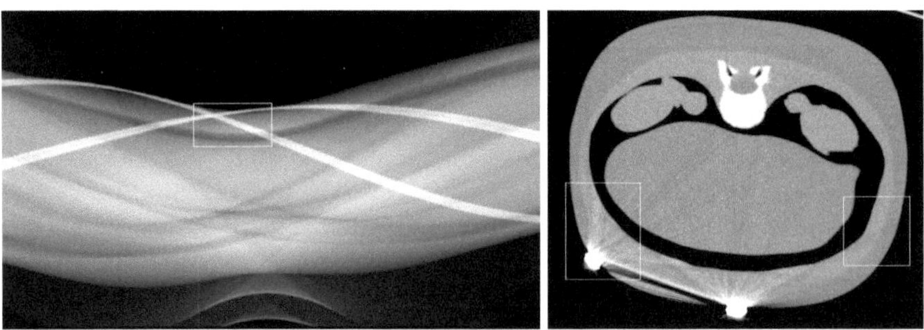

Fig. 1. Measured data (left) and reconstructed image (right) after filtered backprojection. Close-up regions for the results in Fig. 2 are marked

for $n = 0, \ldots, N_{\text{gap}}$. Turning (1) into matrix vector notation yields

$$\boldsymbol{p} = \boldsymbol{A}\hat{\boldsymbol{f}} \tag{2}$$

with vectors $\boldsymbol{p} := (p_j)_{j=0}^{M-1}$, $\hat{\boldsymbol{f}} := (\hat{f}_\kappa)_{\kappa=0}^{N-1}$ and the non-equispaced Fourier matrix $\boldsymbol{A} := (\mathrm{e}^{2\pi\mathrm{i}\boldsymbol{k}_\kappa^T \tilde{\boldsymbol{r}}_j})_{j=0,\ldots,M-1;\kappa=0,\ldots,N-1}$. Since $M < N$, the system (2) is under-determined and, as proposed in [3], it can be solved by the minimization problem

$$\|\hat{\boldsymbol{f}}\|_{\hat{\boldsymbol{w}}}^2 = \sum_{\kappa=0}^{N-1} \frac{|\hat{f}_\kappa|^2}{\hat{w}_\kappa} \xrightarrow{\hat{\boldsymbol{f}}} \min \quad \text{subject to} \quad \boldsymbol{p} = \boldsymbol{A}\hat{\boldsymbol{f}} \tag{3}$$

where the damping factors $\hat{\boldsymbol{w}} = (\hat{w}_\kappa)_{\kappa=0}^{N-1}$ can be used to incorporate knowledge on the decay of the Fourier coefficients. In that way, we can choose a "smooth" solution of the under-determined system (2). As proposed in [3] the minimization problem (3) can be solved efficiently by a variant of the conjugated gradient (CG) method in combination with the NFFT. The CG algorithm proceeds iteratively performing multiple matrix-vector multiplications. Every matrix-vector multiplication can be performed by the NFFT, which is an approximative algorithm for the evaluation of (1) that needs only $\mathcal{O}(N \log N + \varepsilon M)$ operations, where ε denotes the desired accuracy. In summary, the vector of Fourier coefficients $\hat{\boldsymbol{f}}$ can be calculated with $\mathcal{O}(\lambda(N \log N + \varepsilon M))$ operations, where λ denotes the number of CG iterations. To compute the missing values from the Fourier coefficients $\hat{\boldsymbol{f}}$, an ordinary FFT can be used.

To demonstrate the interpolation approach, the projection data of a slice through an anthromorphic torso phantom with two externally attached steel markers was used. The uncorrected dataset is shown in Fig. 1. In order to provide ground truth data for error assessment, the phantom was additionally scanned without markers. The image, which masks the metal traces, was generated by applying a simple threshold segmentation to a preliminary reconstructed image and a subsequent forward projection of this binary image.

Two different interpolation methods were applied for comparison with the proposed NFFT method: A linear and a cubic spline interpolation along single projections. For the implementation of the NFFT interpolation method, we use the software package described in [6]. The damping factors $\hat{\boldsymbol{w}}$ were chosen as the absolute value of the Fourier coefficients of the spline interpolated image. In this way, an appropriate weighting in Fourier space is enforced.

3 Results

The restorated sinograms and their corresponding reconstructed images are shown in Fig. 2. Visual inspection of the singoram data after interpolation suggests that the NFFT approach outperforms the two other methods. However, for regions in the reconstructed images in the vicinity of the metal markers, the spline based method seems to perform best. Streak artifacts situated further away from the markers are significantly reduced when using the NFFT approach.

Fig. 2. Detailed view of the results. From top to bottom: Uncorrected dataset, a scan of the torso phantom without markers, linear sinogram interpolation, spline sinogram interpolation, and NFFT sinogram interpolation

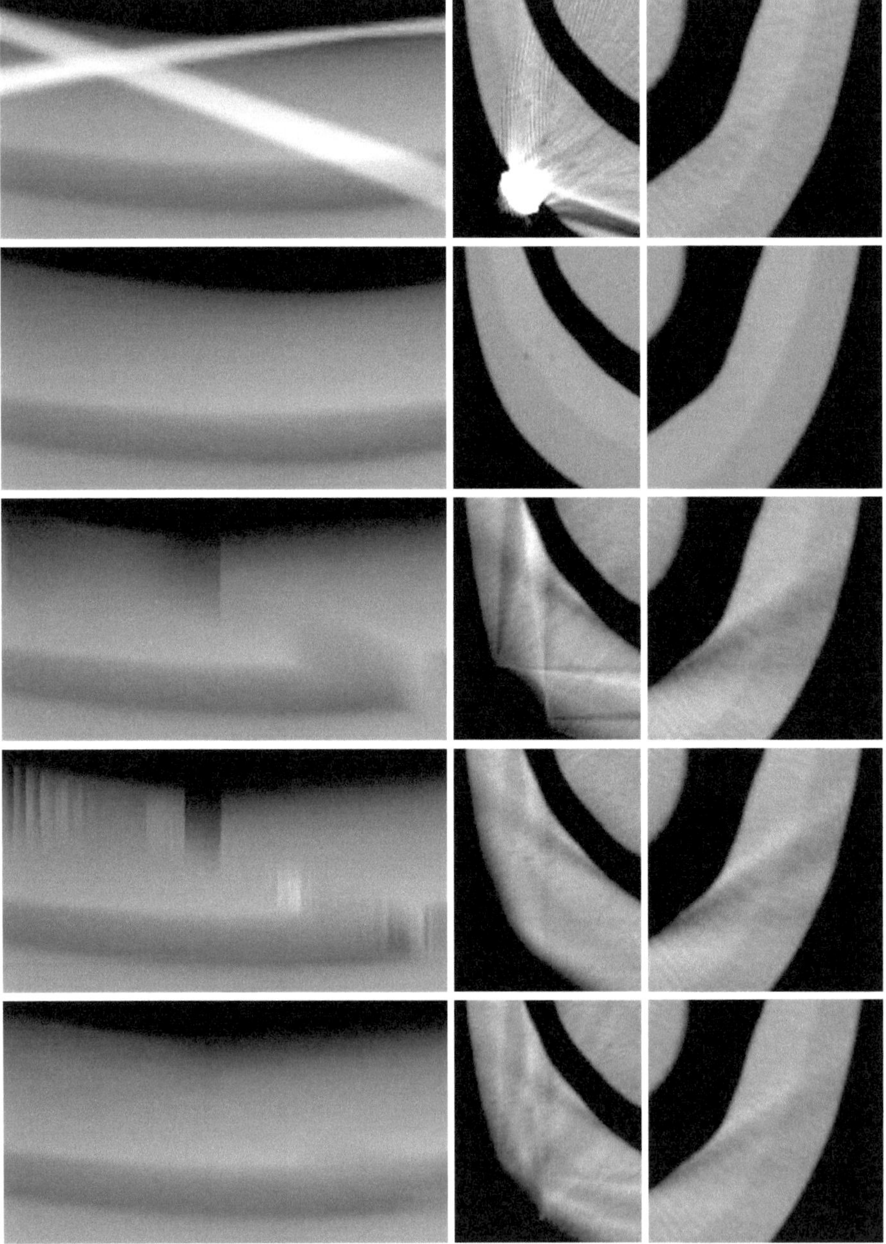

Table 1. Relative error of different interpolation methods

Relative Error	Linear	Spline	NFFT
Gap in Radon Space	0.0681	0.0566	0.0316
Image Space	0.0978	0.0699	0.0668

Linear interpolation performs worst in all cases. For error analysis the relative error $\|\boldsymbol{f} - \tilde{\boldsymbol{f}}\|_2 / \|\boldsymbol{f}\|_2$ is computed, where $\boldsymbol{f}$ denotes the ground truth data and $\tilde{\boldsymbol{f}}$ the data obtained by interpolation. For the sinogram data only the gap of missing values was taken into account for computation of the error. Results are listed in Tab. 1. As already seen in the close-up views, the NFFT provides the lowest error in Radon space, while the improvement for the reconstructed images is only marginal compared to the spline method.

4 Discussion

In the present work a new algorithm for metal artifact reduction based on two-dimensional interpolation by means of non-equispaced Fourier transform was proposed. Missing sinogram values were filled with interpolated values, significantly reducing metal artifacts in the reconstructed images. For comparison, two polynomial algorithms were used. In the sinogram we achieved an improvement of the image quality using the NFFT interpolation. However, in the reconstructed images we obtained only a marginal improvement compared to spline based interpolation. This behavior may be due to the smoothness of the NFFT interpolation, since the filtered backprojection includes a high pass filtering. Taking this into account, an appropriate choice of the damping factors $\hat{\boldsymbol{w}}$ may yield better reconstruction results.

References

1. Potts D, Steidl G, Tasche M. Fast Fourier transforms for non-equispaced data: A tutorial. In: Modern Sampling Theory: Mathematics and Applications. Birkhäuser, Boston; 2001. p. 247–70.
2. Potts D, Steidl G. New Fourier reconstruction algorithms for computerized tomography. Proc SPIE. 2000;4119:13–23.
3. Kunis S, Potts D. Stability results for scattered data interpolation by trigonometric polynomials. SIAM J Sci Comput. 2007;29:1403–19.
4. Glover G H, Pelc N J. An algorithm for the reduction of metal clip artifacts in CT reconstructions. Med Phys. 1981;8(6):799–807.
5. Kalender W A, Hebel R, Ebersberger J. Reduction of CT artifacts caused by metallic implants. Radiology. 1987;164(2):576–7.
6. Keiner J, Kunis S, Potts D. NFFT3.0, Softwarepackage, C subroutine library; 2006. http://www.tu-chemnitz.de/~potts/nfft.

Variationeller Ansatz für eine integrierte Segmentierung und nicht-lineare Registrierung

Alexander Schmidt-Richberg[1,2], Jan Ehrhardt[1], Heinz Handels[1]

[1]Institut für Medizinische Informatik, Universitätsklinikum Hamburg-Eppendorf
[2]Institut für Künstliche Intelligenz, Technische Universität Dresden
s3704637@inf.tu-dresden.de

Kurzfassung. Vierdimensionale tomographische Bilddaten ermöglichen neuartige Therapie- und Diagnoseverfahren in der medizinischen Praxis. Voraussetzung dafür sind oft die räumlich-zeitliche Segmentierung anatomischer Strukturen in den 4D- Daten und die Bestimmung ihrer dynamischen Eigenschaften durch Schätzung der 3D-Bewegungsfelder mittels nicht-linearer Registrierungsverfahren. In dieser Arbeit wird ein Ansatz vorgestellt, mit dem sich Level-Set-Segmentierung und diffusive, nicht-lineare Registrierung unter Berücksichtigung ihrer wechelseitigen Abhängigkeiten integriert lösen lassen. Die Aufgabe wird als Energieminimierung formuliert und ein variationelles Lösungsverfahren angegeben. Anschließend wird der Ansatz an Phantom- und CT-Patientendaten am Beispiel der Leber validiert.

1 Einleitung

Mit der Entwicklung tomographischer räumlich-zeitlicher Bilddaten, wie 4D-CT oder dynamischer MRT, wurden Voraussetzungen für die Erstellung vierdimensionaler Organmodelle und die Analyse derer Bewegungen geschaffen. In der Strahlentherapie zur Behandlung thorakaler Tumore werden solche Modelle beispielsweise genutzt, um durch Prädiktion der Atembewegung eine zeitlich modellierte Bestrahlung zu ermöglichen [1]. Dabei treten hauptsächlich zwei Problemstellungen auf: Zum einen ist die Abgrenzung (Segmentierung) der relevanten Organe in den 4D-Daten erforderlich, zum anderen die Analyse der Organbewegung mittels nicht-linearer Registrierung der einzelnen Bilder der Sequenz.

In vielen bestehenden Ansätzen werden diese Aufgaben separat betrachtet und gelöst, z.B. [2]. Weitere Arbeiten zielen hingegen auf die Ausnutzung der wechselseitigen Abhängigkeiten beider Verfahren ab, also die Verwendung der Segmentierungsinformationen zur Verbesserung der Bewegungsanalyse und gleichzeitig die Erleichterung der Segmentierung durch Einbeziehung der Registrierungsergebnisse. Viele dieser Ansätze sind jedoch nicht für die Segmentierung und Bewegungsanalyse von 4D-Bilddaten geeignet, da sie affine Bewegungsmodelle voraussetzen [3, 4], nur Deformationen der Objektoberflächen erlauben [5] oder spezifische Atlasinformationen erfordern [6], die oft nicht vorliegen.

In dieser Arbeit wird ein neuer Ansatz zur simultanen Segmentierung und Registrierung räumlich-zeitlicher Bildfolgen präsentiert.

2 Material und Methoden

Ziel des vorgeschlagenen Verfahrens ist zum einen die Level-Set-Segmentierung der relevanten anatomischen Strukturen (Leber, Lunge, Tumor, etc.) in den Bildern einer räumlich-zeitlichen Sequenz, zum anderen die Bewegungsschätzung durch nicht-rigide Registrierung der Bilder der Folge mit einem Referenzbild.

Ausgegangen wird von einer bekannten Segmentierung des Objektes im Referenzbild. Die Segmentierungen der weiteren Bilder der Sequenz (Ziel- oder Target-Bilder) können damit auf zwei unterschiedlichen Wegen berechnet werden: Zum einen ist eine direkte Segmentierung des Zielbildes denkbar, zum Beispiel mithilfe des Level-Set-Verfahrens. Zum anderen ist es möglich, das Referenz- mit dem Target-Bild zu registrieren und mit dem berechneten Bewegungsfeld die bekannte Referenzsegmentierung auf das Target-Bild zu übertragen.

Die daraus deutlich werdende Abhängigkeit der beiden Verfahren voneinander soll für eine wechselseitige Verbesserung der Ergebnisse von Registrierung und Segmentierung genutzt werden. Zu diesem Zweck werden beide Verfahren verknüpft, indem zusätzlich eine Konformität der Ergebnisse gefordert wird, d.h. eine Übereinstimmung der direkten Segmentierung mit der entsprechend des Bewegungsfeldes transformierten Initialsegmentierung.

Nachfolgend werden zunächst die verwendeten Methoden für die Level-Set-Segmentierung und die nicht-rigide Registrierung erläutert. Im Anschluss wird auf die Verknüpfung der Verfahren eingegangen und eine numerische Lösung skizziert.

2.1 Variationelle Level-Set-Segmentierung

Für die Segmentierung wurde ein Level-Set-Ansatz gewählt [7, 8], d.h. die Oberfläche des Objektes wird implizit mithilfe einer Level-Set-Funktion $\phi(x) : \mathbb{R}^3 \rightarrow \mathbb{R}$ mathematisch beschrieben. Die Funktion ϕ, die das Objekt bestmöglich beschreibt, wird dabei durch Minimierung des Energiefunktionals

$$\mathcal{J}_{Seg}[\phi] := \mathcal{I}[\phi] \; + \; \mathcal{E}[T;\phi] = \min!$$

ermittelt. Dieses Funktional besteht aus der Internen Energie

$$\mathcal{I}[\phi] := \int_{\Omega} \delta_\alpha(\phi(x)) \; \|\nabla\phi(x)\| \; dx$$

die eine Glättung der Segmentgrenze bewirkt, und der Externen Energie

$$\mathcal{E}[T;\phi] := \int_{\Omega} H_\alpha(\phi(x)) \cdot \log p_{\text{out}}(T(x)) + (1 - H_\alpha(\phi(x))) \cdot \log p_{\text{in}}(T(x)) \; dx$$

welche die Segmentgrenze in Richtung der Objektoberfäche im Bild lenkt. Dabei bezeichnet $\delta_\alpha(x)$ eine stetige Approximation der Dirac-Distribution und $H_\alpha(x)$ die approximierte Heaviside-Funktion [8]. Die Wahrscheinlichkeitsdichten der Grauwerte p_{in} bzw. p_{out} werden anhand der bekannten Segmentierung des Referenzbildes geschätzt.

2.2 Variationelle nicht-rigide Registrierung

Ziel der Registrierung ist die Bestimmung eines Vektorfeldes $u(x)$, das die Bewegung der Bildpunkte von Bild R nach T wiedergibt, so dass $R(x - u(x))$ in möglichst großem Ausmaß $T(x)$ ähnelt. Das hierfür zu minimierende Energiefunktional [9] lautet

$$\mathcal{J}_{Reg}[u] := \mathcal{D}[R, T; u] \; + \; \mathcal{S}[u] = \min!$$

Dabei bewertet das Distanzmaß

$$\mathcal{D}[R, T; u] := \frac{1}{2} \int_{\Omega} (R(x - u(x)) - T(x))^2 \; dx$$

die Ähnlichkeit von Target-Bild und transformiertem Referenzbild, während die diffusive Regularisierung

$$\mathcal{S}[u] := \frac{1}{2} \sum_{l=1}^{d} \int_{\Omega} \|\nabla u_l\|^2 \; dx$$

für eine Glättung des Vektorfeldes sorgt und so Unstetigkeiten vermeidet.

2.3 Integrierung von Segmentierung und Registrierung

Die Segmentierung des Target-Bildes und die Registrierung von Referenz- und Target-Bild werden verknüpft, indem zusätzlich eine möglichst große Übereinstimmung der transformierten Referenzsegmentierung $\hat{\phi}(x - u(x))$ mit der direkten Segmentierung $\phi(x)$ gefordert wird. Zu diesem Zweck wird ein Shape-Prior-Term eingeführt, durch den der SSD-Abstand der Level-Set-Funktionen berücksichtigt wird:

$$\mathcal{P}[\hat{\phi}; \phi, u] := \frac{1}{2} \int_{\Omega} \delta_{\alpha}(\phi(x)) \; (\hat{\phi}(x - u(x)) - \phi(x))^2 \; dx$$

Damit kann ein gemeinsames Energiefunktional für die integrierte Segmentierung und Registrierung definiert werden:

$$\mathcal{J}[u, \phi] := \mathcal{D}[R, T; u] \; + \; \mathcal{S}[u] \; + \; \mathcal{I}[\phi] \; + \; \mathcal{E}[R; \phi] \; + \; \mathcal{P}[\hat{\phi}; u, \phi] \; = \min! \qquad (1)$$

Die numerische Umsetzung der Energieminimierung erfolgt über einen variationellen Ansatz. Durch ein Zeitschrittverfahren erhält man schließlich ein Iterationsschema, mit dem Segmentierung und Registrierung abwechselnd und in Wechselwirkung schrittweise berechnet werden können. Eine effiziente Implementierung wurde durch Verwendung von Sparse-Field-Level-Sets [10] und Additive Operator Splitting (AOS) [9] realisiert.

2.4 Methodik der Evaluation

Der vorgeschlagene Ansatz wurde durch Gegenüberstellung der Ergebnisse von drei Algorithmen evaluiert. Das Ergebnis der herkömmlichen Level-Set-Segmentierung nach Abschnitt 2.1 (Alg. I) und die mit dem integrierten Verfahren (Alg.

III) ermittelte Segmentierung wurden mit der manuellen Segmentierung eines Spezialisten (Goldstandard) verglichen. Dabei wurde der Überlappungs-Koeffizient $\frac{A \cap B}{A \cup B}$ der Segmentierungen als Gütemaß herangezogen. Die Güte der Ergebnisse der herkömmlichen (Abschnitt 2.2, Alg. II) und der integrierten Registrierung (Alg. III) wurde durch den Vergleich der mit dem berechneten Bewegungsfeld transformierten Referenzsegmentierung mit dem Goldstandard bewertet.

3 Ergebnisse

Mit den beschriebenen Algorithmen wurden Segmentierung und Registrierung an den synthetischen Daten eines Software-Phantoms des menschlichen Thorax und an vier 4D-CT-Patientendatensätzen am Beispiel der Leber berechnet und die Ergebnisse einander gegenübergestellt.

In allen Fällen belegt eine Untersuchung des Überlappungs-Koeffizienten eine Verbesserung der Ergebnisse durch den integrierten Ansatz (Abb. 1). Weitere untersuchte Metriken wie die mittlere Oberflächendistanz (Verbesserung der Seg. im Mittel um 1,8% bzw. der Reg. um 16,3%), der maximale Abstand (Seg. um durchschnittlich 7% bzw. Reg. um 22,8%) und das MSD-Maß der Registrierung (im Mittel um 1,9%) bestätigen diese Resultate.

4 Diskussion

Die Ergebnisse belegen eine Verbesserung der Resultate sowohl der Segmentierung, als auch der Registrierung. Besonders signifikant sind die Verbesserungen bei der Registrierung, da diese durch den geringen Grauwertunterschied zwischen Leber und umliegendem Gewebe erschwert ist und deutlich von der Kenntnis der Segmentierung profitiert (Abb. 2). Bei der Segmentierung kann hauptsächlich ein Auslaufen in benachbarte Strukturen und durch die Glättung bedingte Fehlklassifizierungen schlanker Strukturen vermieden werden.

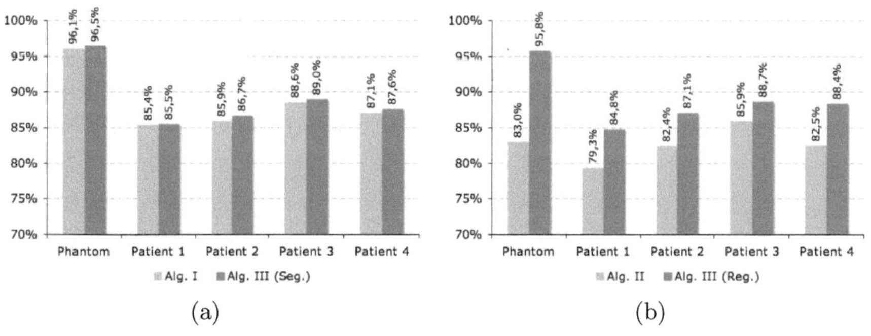

Abb. 1. Evaluation der Segmentierung: (a): Überlappungs-Koeffizient der Segmentierungen nach Alg. I und Alg. III mit dem Goldstandard und des Goldstandards mit der mit Alg. II bzw. Alg. III transformierten Referenzsegmentierung

Abb. 2. Checkerboard-Darstellung des Target-Bildes mit dem transformierten Referenzbild nach Alg. II (links) und Alg. III (rechts)

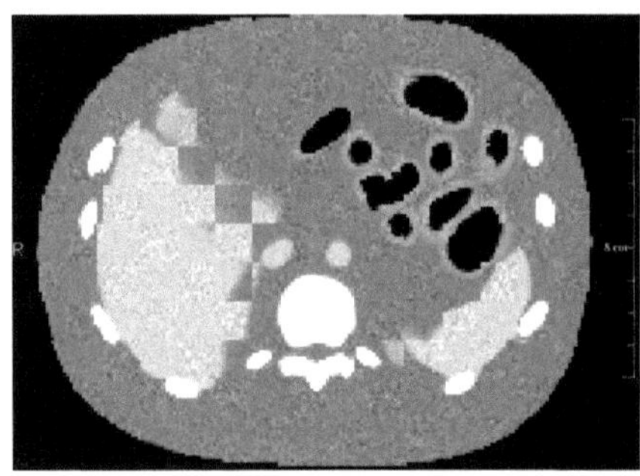
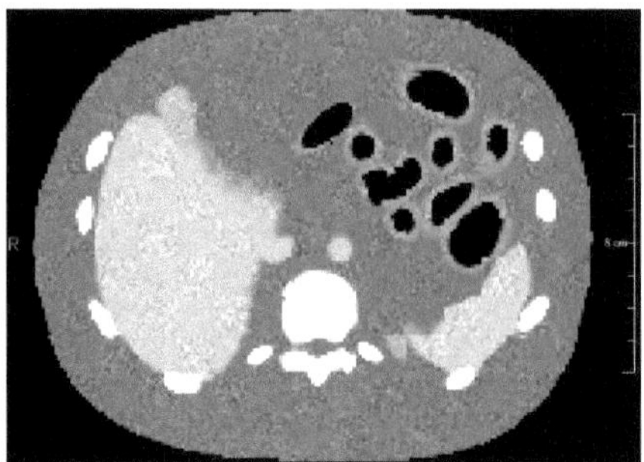

Als aufwändig stellt sich die geeignete Wahl der fünf Modellparameter dar, wobei auch bei der separaten Segmentierung und Registrierung drei der Parameter benötigt werden. In dieser Arbeit wurden die Werte empirisch bestimmt.

Der vorgeschlagene Ansatz erwies sich in allen untersuchten Fällen als geeignet für die integrierte Segmentierung und Registrierung thorakaler CT-Daten.

Danksagung. Ich danke Herrn PD Dr. Boris Flach für viele fruchtbare Diskussionen.

Literaturverzeichnis

1. Sarrut D, Boldea V, Ayadi M, et al. Nonrigid registration method to assess reproducibility of breath-holding with ABC in lung cancer. Int J Radiat Oncol Biol Phys. 2005;61(2):594–607.
2. Ehrhardt J, Werner R, Säring D, et al. An optical flow based method for improved reconstruction of 4D CT data sets acquired during free breathing. Med Phys. 2007;34(2):711–21.
3. Paragios N, Rousson M, Ramesh V. Knowledge-based registration and segmentation of the left ventricle: A level set approach. Proc IEEE Comput Graph Appl. 2002; p. 37–42.
4. Yezzi A, Zollei L, Kapur T. A variational framework for integrating segmentation and registration through active contours. Med Image Anal. 2003;7(2):171–85.
5. An JH, Chen Y, Huang F, et al. A variational PDE based level set method for a simultaneous segmentation and non-rigid registration. Proc MICCAI. 2005; p. 286–93.
6. Ashburner J, Friston KJ. Unified segmentation. NeuroImage. 2005;26(3):839–51.
7. Sethian JA, Osher S. Level Set Methods and Fast Marching Methods. Cambridge University Press; 2002.
8. Chan TF, Vese LA. Active contours without edges. IEEE Trans Image Process. 2001;10(2):266–77.
9. Modersitzki J. Numeric Meth Image Regist. Oxford University Press; 2004.
10. Whitaker RT. A level-set approach to 3D reconstruction from range data. Int J Comp Vis. 1998;29(3):203–31.

Hatch Textures for Virtual Endoscopy

C. Schaller[1], D. Wellein[2], S. Born[2], D. Bartz[2]

[1] WSI/GRIS, University of Tübingen
[2] Visual Computing for Medicine, ICCAS, University of Leipzig
daniela.wellein@iccas.de

Abstract. We present an illustrative rendering extension for virtual endoscopy to enhance depth perception. For this purpose different hatch textures are applied and their ability to enhance 3D shape estimation is discussed. The stroke directions of the textures are aligned to the principal curvature directions of the surface. Starting with two patterns suggested by Kim et al. [1], we developed texture patterns for the use in our virtual endoscopy system. Altogether five different hatch textures are integrated within the framework and OpenGL-generated mipmaps are applied to account for aliasing effects on the textured surfaces.

1 Introduction

Virtual endoscopy can provide a fast non-invasive exploration method suited for screening, diagnosis, access planning and post-operative evaluation, depending on the clinical application area. While only minimal patient preparation is needed, it even can allow virtual access to obstructed or otherwise physically unreachable regions. Clinical application areas are amongst others virtual bronchoscopy, colonoscopy, and ventriculoscopy. A general overview can be found in [2]. Our framework for virtual endoscopy supports multiple applications such as cardio-vascular [3] or neuroendoscopic [4] exploration. It allows interactive and

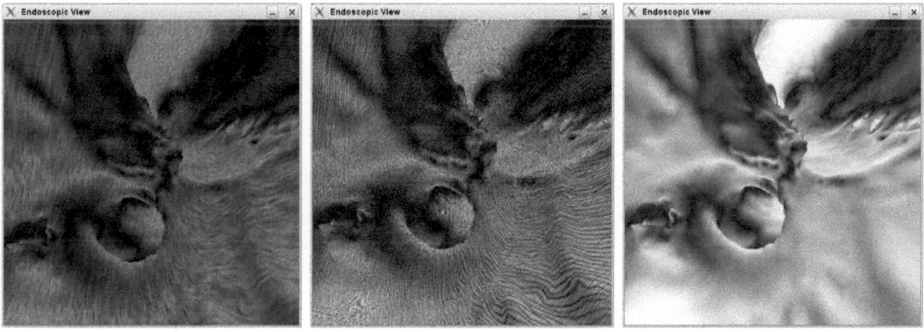

Fig. 1. Screenshot of our virtual endoscopy framework. Scene with texture a (left), with texture b (middle) and, with no texture (right). For the textures see Fig. 2

intuitive handling on a common PC by combining polygonal surface rendering with a guided-navigation paradigm.

In virtual endoscopy, crucial depth information is significantly reduced by projecting a 3D scene onto a 2D screen. One of the main ideas of illustrative rendering is to provide additional visual cues for the interpretation of a scene. The most important source of depth cues in virtual endoscopy is the relative movement of objects due to shifts in perspective (motion parallax). Appropriate texturing, like with hatch textures, can provide additional depth cues and therefore enhances the perception of 3D shapes.

Ritter et. al [5] describe a hatching algorithm along with shadow-like depth indicators, that is used to increase depth perception for vascular structures. This visualization technique is validated by a large scale user study. Zander et al. [6] direct hatching strokes along the surface curvature. Their approach may be suitable for medical scenarios in general but proves to be problematic for real-time applications. Kim et al. demonstrate in [1] that hatch textures following one or two principal curvature directions of an 3D object facilitate the perception of 3D object geometry.

The remainder of this paper is structured as follows. In Section 2 we will introduce the textures utilized within our framework and their applicability to virtual endoscopy. Section 3 presents our results and in Section 4 we will discuss these results and give a brief outlook.

2 Material and Methods

All applied textures are depicted in Figure 2. In [1] the authors compared the subjects' ability to correctly estimate surface orientation of bumps on a landscape in four different conditions (no texture and three different textures). The textures a and c (Fig. 2) lead to the most accurate estimation of 3D objects and therefore will be used for texturing in our virtual environment system. Texture mapping is done with standard openGL functions. In openGL the textures are aligned orthogonal to the surface normals. This automatically leads to an alignment of the hatches along the curvature of the object surfaces.

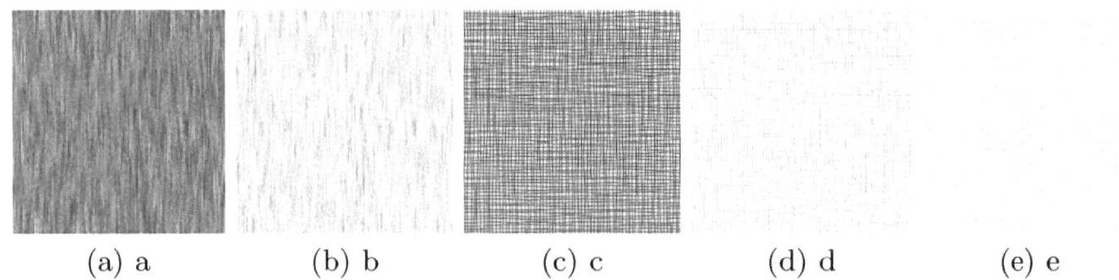

(a) a (b) b (c) c (d) d (e) e

Fig. 2. Textures. a) lic-like, one principal curvature direction b) contrast-reduced version of a c) grid, two principal curvature directions d) contrast-reduced version of c e) diamond pattern, principal curvature directions

Due to the high contrast of both textures (a, c) the endoscopic scene is significantly darkened (Fig. 2). When these textures are mapped on distant structures the resulting aliasing-effects are quite strong. This produces an especially interfering flickering effect when navigating within the endoscopic view. Therefore, we adapted the original textures by lowering contrast and luminance, obtaining textures b and d. While aliasing is reduced when applying the low-contrast textures b and d, nevertheless it is still perceivable. To account for this, we applied OpenGL-generated mipmaps. A mipmap is a downscaled versions of the original texture with reduced level of detail. The size of the object on the screen determines which downscaled version of the texture map is used.

We additionally created a fifth texture, the rectilinear diamond texture (Fig. 2 e). Like texture c and d it is bi-directional, which is – according to Kim et al. [1] – slightly superior to uni-directional hatch textures (a, b). The regularity of the strokes and its low contrast draws less visual attention and is therefore more suitable for virtual endoscopy than the textures a and c and their derivatives b and d.

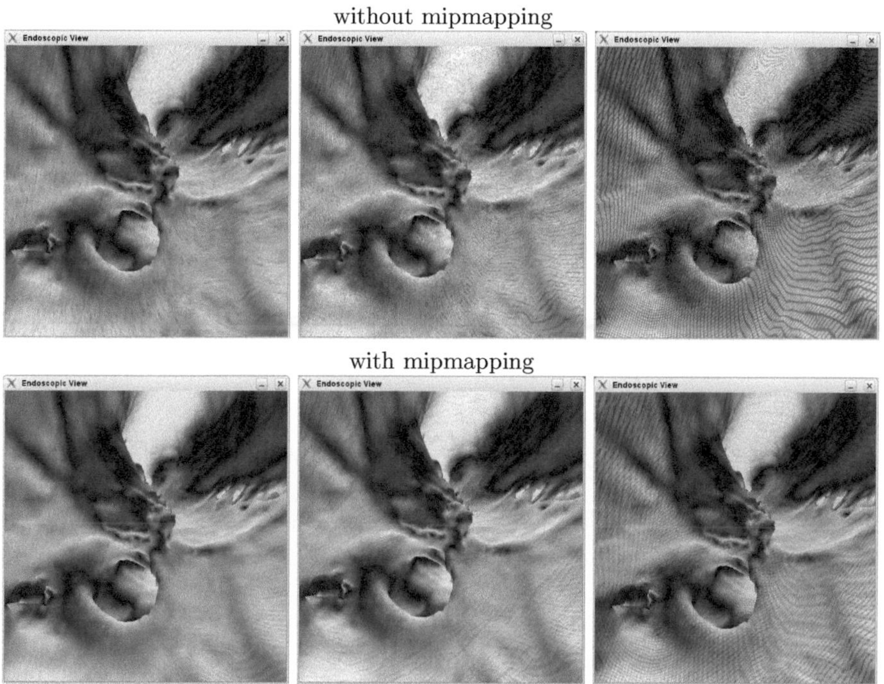

Fig. 3. The application of different textures (Fig. 2 b, d and e), with and without mipmapping. Texture b (left), texture d (middle) and, texture e (right)

3 Results

Figure 1 displays the application of the original textures to our virtual endoscopy framework together with a non-textured scene. High-contrast textures result in a relatively dark endoscopic view (Fig. 1 left, middle) and aliasing leads to a flicker-effect on distant objects while navigating through the scene. Using the contrast-reduced textures the scenes are lightened up (Fig. 3). Simultaneously the aliasing effects, while still perceptible, are considerably reduced. The contrast-reduced textures permit to blend texture and surface, rather than completely replacing it. This allows for additional accuracy due to the underlying lighting. The OpenGL-intrinsic mipmapping turns out to be a mixed blessing. While aliasing effects are significantly reduced, the down-scaled mipmaps produce additional artifacts due to discontinuities between different resolutions at texture patch boundaries (see Fig. 4).

4 Discussion

We extended our framework for virtual endoscopy by hatching. The applied textures were chosen because they facilitate 3D shape perception. Luminance and stroke thickness have a huge influence on the quality of the visualization. Hence, textures b and d result in lighter representations than textures a and c, whereas texture e offers a smoother and more regular appearance. In summary, hatch textured surfaces bear an advantage over non-textured surfaces in 3D shape estimation, but have to be carefully selected and at present manually adapted for any given data set.

The attainment of an optimal texture depends largely on the artifacts that need to be accounted for. Aliasing effects, like described above, can be mostly eliminated by using mipmaps, but this technique in turn causes artifacts of its own. First, in some scenarios the boundaries between different texture maps

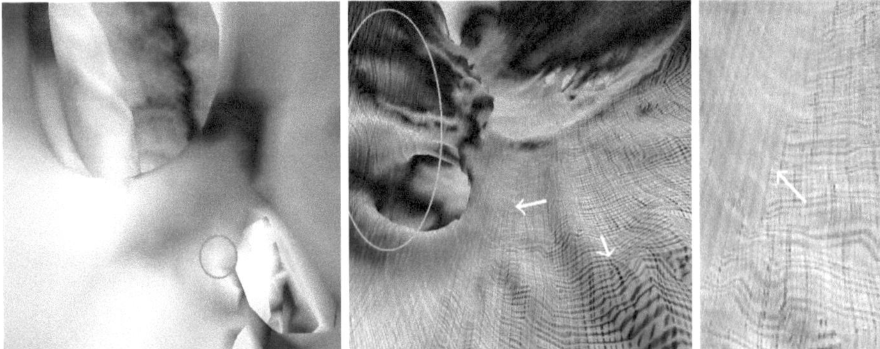

Fig. 4. Visualization artifacts. Diamond artifact (circle, left), blurred textures at an acute angle (ellipse, middle) visible texture boundaries (arrow, middle and right)

are visible (Fig. 4 right, circle). Second, when using OpenGL-generated texture maps, boundaries between texture patches of differing level of detail become visible and, within the texture patch itself the strokes become discontinuous for the smaller texture maps. Smooth transitions between texture patches require manual adaptation. Weighting of the texture maps by contrast can account for smoother boundaries between different mipmap resolutions. A general problem is that OpenGL does not allow for anisotropic filtering. This leads to a blurring of textured surfaces when observed from an acute angle (Fig. 4 middle, green ellipse). A general advantage of texturing is, that diamond artifacts (Fig. 4 left, red circle) caused by insufficient triangle subdivision during 3D model generation is masked.

The next steps will include the weighting the textures according to vertex lighting and the integration of tonal art maps (TAM) like proposed by Praun et al. [7]. We also plan a psychophysical user-study to more accurately specify the benefits of hatch textures for virtual endoscopy.

References

1. Kim S, Hagh-Shenas H, Interrante V. Showing shape with texture: Two directions seem better than One. Proc HVEI. 2003;5007:332–339.
2. Bartz D. Virtual endoscopy in research and clinical practice. Comput Grap Forum. 2005;24(1):111–26.
3. Bartz D, Gürvit O, Lanzendörfer M, et al. Virtual endoscopy for cardio vascular exploration. Proc CARS. 2001; p. 960–4.
4. Bartz D, Straßer W, Gürvit O, et al. Interactive and multi-modal visualization for neuroendoscopic interventions. Proc Eurographics Symp Data Vis. 2001; p. 157–64.
5. Ritter F, Hansen C, Dicken V, et al. Real-time illustration of vascular structures. Proc IEEE Vis. 2006; p. 877–84.
6. Zander J, Isenberg T, Schlechtweg S, et al. High quality hatching. Comp Graph Forum. 2004;23(3):421–30.
7. Praun E, Hoppe H, Webb M, et al. Real-time hatching. Proc ACM SIGGRAPH. 2001; p. 579–84.

A Comparison of Five Methods for Signal Intensity Standardization in MRI

Jan-Philip Bergeest, Florian Jäger

Lehrstuhl für Mustererkennung, Friedrich-Alexander-Universität Erlangen-Nürnberg
jan.p.bergeest@informatik.stud.uni-erlangen.de

Abstract. A major problem in magnetic resonance imaging (MRI) is the lack of a pulse sequence dependent standardized intensity scale like the Hounsfield units in computed tomography. This affects the post processing of the acquired images as, in general, segmentation and registration methods depend on the observed image intensities. Different approaches dealing with this problem were proposed recently. In this article we will describe and compare five state-of-the-art standardization methods regarding speed, applicability and accuracy. As a quality measure the mean distance and the Kullback-Leibler divergence are considered. For the experiments 28 MRI head volume images, acquired during clinical routine, were used.

1 Introduction

MRI has the drawback of having intensity variations due to magnetic field inhomogeneities and scanner-related intensity artifacts. Thus, it is not possible to create a pulse sequence dependent, general intensity scale. Algorithms dealing with the problem of the correction of signal intensity inhomogeneities usually focus on intra-volume signal intensity distortions and do not correct the inherently non-standardness. Hence, intensities obtained from the same or different patients have no meaning related to a specific anatomical tissue even if they are acquired on the same MRI scanner. This implies a significant affect on the accuracy and precision of following image processing, analysis, segmentation and registration methods relying on intensity similarity. Furthermore, standard presets cannot be used to display MR images or to visualize certain tissue classes and/or pathologies. These settings have to be adjusted for every single case.

First we will give a brief overview of the intensity standardization method described in Florian Jäger et al. [1] that basically performs a registration of joint histograms. Further, we will discuss 1-d histogram based approaches presented in Nyúl et al. [2] that matches landmarks on histograms, in [3] a method is introduced that is based on histogram estimation using Gaussian mixtures, as well as an algorithm adapted from dynamic histogram warping [4]. In addition we will have a brief look at the algorithm proposed by Weisenfeld and Warfield [5], in which a multiplicative correction field is estimated. Finally the experimental setup is described and the evaluation results are presented and discussed.

2 Methods

2.1 MRI Intensity Standardization by Non-rigid Registration of Joint Histograms

The idea proposed in [1] is that a normalization can be achieved by finding a deformation of the joint histograms of two sets of images with respect to a certain distance measure. Each of these histograms is at least two dimensional and contains the intensity information of two or more MRI sequences (e.g. T1 or T2 weighted images). If the probability density functions are considered as images, the normalization can be treated as a registration problem. The resulting non-linear correction function is used to adjust the image intensities of the MRI image series. In [6] this approach is extended to be applicable to a whole body MRI scan. Therefore, the volume is split up into K sub volumes which are corrected separately. In order to include the influence of small local structures the other $K - 1$ sub volumes are used as regularizer.

2.2 Landmark-Based MRI Scale Standardization

The basic idea of the method presented in [2] is to find a mapping that deforms the template intensity histogram of an input image so that it matches a reference histogram based on landmarks. In the first step the landmarks of the mean histogram are detected which has to be done only once for each given protocol and body region (training). Second, the real image-dependent normalization is applied to a given volume image, of the same body region and protocol as used in the training step, by matching its detected landmarks to the standard positions (transformation). Hence each segment, between two landmarks, is mapped linearly and independently. The resulting transformation is nonlinear.

2.3 MRI Intensity Correction Using Mixture Mapping

A normalization that is only applicable to images of the head region is described in [3]. This is done by matching intensities of head specific anatomical tissue classes. Therefore five main classes are used: background, cerebrospinal fluid (CSF), gray matter (GM), white matter (WM) and a mixture of fat and muscle. In the first step the histograms from a source and a target data set, i.e. two 3D images, are approximated by a Gaussian mixture. Each tissue class k is modeled by a Gaussian probability density function which has a mean μ_k that is approximated using the Expectation-Maximization (EM) algorithm. In the second step a polynomial correction function f^p of order p is used to interpolate the correction of the intensities smoothly: $f^p(x) = \sum_{i=0}^{p} \Theta_i x^i$. By minimizing the cost function $\sum_{k=1}^{n}(f^p(\mu_k) - \upsilon_k)^2$ the coefficients Θ_i are obtained, where μ_k and υ_k are the means of the reference and template image respectively.

2.4 Dynamic Programming Applied to Intensity MRI Correction

Dynamic programming can be used to find an optimal alignment between two sequences of data of different length with respect to a monotonic and separable cost function. Furthermore, this function is constrained to hold the principle of optimality. In [4], one histogram is mapped to another by a one-to-one, one-to-many and many-to-one mapping. Let f_i^t denote the frequency of occurrence in the i-th bin of the template histogram, respectively f_j^r of the j-th bin in the reference histogram. A plausible cost function $c(i,j)$ for two intensities is the difference $\left|f_i^t - f_j^r\right|$. In order to find an appropriate mapping a cost matrix C is defined where $C(i,j)$ corresponds to a optimal sub path and $C(i_{max}, j_{max})$ contains the minimal distance of the histograms. The cheapest path and the corresponding mapping can be computed efficiently using dynamic programming.

2.5 Intensity Normalization by Minimizing the Kullback-Leibler Divergence

A multiplicative correction field is estimated in [5] to match a template histogram to a reference model density. The observed image O is composed of a multiplicative pixelwise intensity corruption field F, additional acquisition noise n and the correct image I in the following way: $O = FI + n$. After neglecting n for having only little influence on the problem of intensity normalization and solving the equation for I the uncorrupted image is obtained as $I \approx F^{-1}O$. The parameter field F^{-1} has to be chosen in a way that the Kullback-Leibler divergence between source and target sets is minimized. The Simultaneous Perturbation Stochastic Approximation (SPSA) is used to generate the gradient estimate.

3 Results

The images used for evaluation were T1- and T2/FLAIR images. The T2-weighted FLAIR datasets were acquired on a Siemens Avanto 1.5 T scanner with $408 \times 512 \times 19$, pixel size of 0.43 mm^2 and 7.2 mm slice thickness and TE = 143 and TR = 9000. The T1-weighted images had a resolution of $208 \times 256 \times 19$ with 0.86 mm^2 and 7.2 mm slice thickness and TE = 14 and TR = 510. In total 28 volumes from eleven different patients were used. Since the methods need to be applicable for medical diagnosis in a real clinical environment, all images used were chosen to be real patient data including evolving lesions.

For the evaluation, T1-weighted volumes and the appropriate FLAIR data sets were evaluated separately. A single reference image was chosen for each patient. Then the follow-up studies were standardized to the intensities of the corresponding reference images. As a measure for the quality of the standardization the absolute mean (Equation 1) and the average Kullback-Leibler (KL) divergence (Equation 2) were computed. In order to minimize the influence of changing anatomy on the evaluation, lesions were segmented and removed beforehand. However, the normalization was applied to the original images since

Table 1. The measurement before standardization is given in parenthesis and the methods are numbered in the same order as described above. μ_{kl} is the average KL divergence and μ_{m} is the overall mean distance

Method	T1		FLAIR	
	μ_{m} (32.62)	μ_{kl} (0.46)	μ_{m} (53.22)	μ_{kl} (0.61)
2.1	6.82	0.12	7.47	0.16
2.2	10.41	0.14	10.30	0.27
2.3	14,69	0.16	12,33	0.56
2.4	7.65	0.07	5.99	0.30
2.5	8.25	0.07	16.79	0.15

the pathological distortions should be considered in the evaluation of the robustness of the algorithm. As quality measure the average absolute distance between all reference and template volumes, is given by:

$$\mu_{\mathrm{m}} = \frac{1}{N} \sum_{i} |x_i - y_i| \tag{1}$$

with N being the number of compared images, x_i being the mean intensity of the reference and as y_i the corresponding template mean is used. As a measure of the difference between two probability densities, the overall average KL divergence between the reference and template images is computed as follows:

$$\mu_{\mathrm{kl}} = \frac{1}{N} \sum_{i} \sum_{j} p_{ij} \log(p_{ij}/q_{ij}) \tag{2}$$

where p_{ij} is the probability of occurrence of intensity j in the template image i and q_{ij} is the probability of occurrence of intensity j in the reference image i.

In Figure 3 an example for the standardization is given. All images were binarized and displayed at the same threshold value. It can be seen that the intensities vary globally and become more similar regarding similar tissue classes. In Table 1 a quantitative overview of the computed distance measures is given. As mentioned above these values were computed after removal of the lesions but without any additional inhomogeneity correction. Thus, the difference between

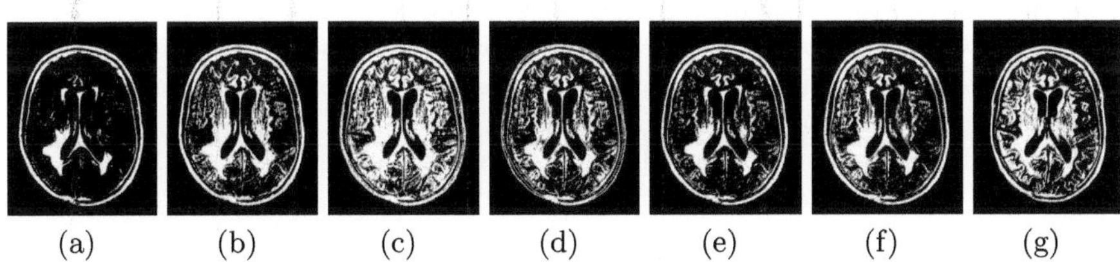

(a) (b) (c) (d) (e) (f) (g)

Fig. 1. Binary FLAIR image slices of two data sets from the same patient where (a) is standardized on (g) the reference image. (b) corresponds to the corrected image gained by the algorithm presented in 2.1, respectively (c) to 2.2, (d) to 2.3, (e) to 2.4 and (f) to 2.5

Table 2. General overview: + is good, o is average and – is below average

Method	Speed	Applicability	Accuracy
2.1	o (≈ 1 minute)	+	+
2.2	+ (≈ 2 seconds)	o	+
2.3	o (≈ 5 minutes)	–	0
2.4	+ (≈ 2 seconds)	o	+
2.5	– (≈ 30 minutes)	o	+

the volumes will never become zero. A short overview of the methods for comparison can be found in Table 2, where applicability means that the algorithm can be easily adapted to different regions of the body. Accuracy refers to robustness and improvement of the image quality. The runtime measurements were performed on a Intel Core2 CPU T5500 with 1.66GHz and 2 gigabyte RAM.

4 Discussion

In this article we have compared five MRI signal intensity standardization methods in terms of speed, applicability and accuracy. More sophisticated methods that make use of all image sequences or do a pixelwise correction estimation are of course slower but lead to better results (approaches 2.1 and 2.5), whereas approach 2.3 leads to worse results. Algorithm 2.2 and 2.4 are fast and in general provide good results but 2.2 is vulnerable to distortions in the histograms due to the fact that it is piecewise linear and relies on a learned histogram shape. All methods can be potentially applied to every body area excepting 2.3 which uses head specific tissue classes.

References

1. Jäger F, Deuerling-Zheng Y, Frericks B, et al. A new method for MRI intensity standardization with application to lesion detection in the brain. In: Kobbelt L, et al, editors. Vision Modeling and Visualization. Köln: Aka GmBH; 2006. p. 269–76.
2. Nyúl LG, Udupa JK, Zhang X. New variants of a method of MRI scale standardization. IEEE Trans Med Imaging. 2000;19(2):143–50.
3. Hellier P. Consistent intensity correction of MR images. Proc ICIP. 2003;1:1109–12.
4. Cox IJ, Roy S, Hingorani SL. Dynamic histogram warping of image pairs for constant image brightness. Proc ICIP. 1995; p. 2366–9.
5. Weisenfeld N, Warfield S. Normalization of joint image-intensity statistics in MRI using the Kullback-Leibler divergence. Proc IEEE Int Symp Biomed Imaging. 2004;1:101–4.
6. Jäger F, Nyul L, Frericks B, et al. Whole body MRI intensity standardization. Proc BVM. 2007; p. 459–63.

Wissensakquisition mit Methoden der Mustererkennung zur wissensbasierten Segmentierung von Risikoorganen in CT-Bilddaten

Armin Stoll[1], Thomas Wetter[2], Rolf Bendl[1,3]

[1]Abteilung für Medizinische Physik in der Strahlentherapie, DKFZ Heidelberg
[2]Institut für Medizinische Biometrie und Informatik, Universität Heidelberg
[3]Fakultät für Informatik, Hochschule Heilbronn
a.stoll@dkfz-heidelberg.de

Kurzfassung. In diesem Beitrag werden vier Mustererkennungsmethoden vorgestellt und bewertet die für die Bestimmung der kranial-kaudalen Korrespondenz von transversalen CT-Schnittbildern evaluiert wurden. Die Klassifikationsleistungen sind an insgesamt 13 Datensätzen bestimmt worden. Fünf intensitätsbasierte Merkmale und ein anatomisches Vermessungsmaß spannen einen 6-dimensionalen Merkmalsraum auf und ermöglichen eine robuste Klassifikation. Es werden Klassifikationsleistungen mit Sensitivität > 0.9 erzielt. Die resultierende Detektion und Abgrenzung von Körperregionen in beliebigen CT-Bilddaten ermöglicht es Segmentierungsaufgaben auf bestimmte Bereiche zu begrenzen. Semi-automatische Segmentierungsalgorithmen können anschließend automatisch initialisiert und ohne Benutzerinteraktion ausgeführt werden.

1 Einleitung

Das wichtigste bildgebende Verfahren für die computergestützte Strahlentherapieplanung ist die Computertomographie (CT). Mit dieser Modalität können nicht-invasiv sehr hochauflösende und kontrastreiche Schnittbilder von der Anatomie des Menschen rekonstruiert werden. Die Schnittbilder bilden eine wichtige Grundlage, auf der eine Strahlentherapie geplant, simuliert und evaluiert werden kann. Alle therapierelevanten Strukturen (Risikoorgane, Gewebe und Zielvolumen) müssen jedoch zuvor in den Bilddaten segmentiert werden. Dieses geschieht häufig manuell, indem der Bestrahlungsplaner die Konturen in den Transversalschichten mit einfachen grafischen Hilfsmitteln einzeichnet. Um diesen Vorgang zu beschleunigen, werden semi-automatische Segmentierungsverfahren entwickelt. Hierzu gehören z.B. Bereichswachstumsverfahren, Aktive Konturen oder Formmodelle.

Mit dem Ziel die Segmentierungsaufgabe weiter zu automatisieren, werden in zahlreichen Publikationen wissensbasierte Systeme (WBS) vorgestellt. Sie zeigen, dass semi-automatische Segmentierungsalgorithmen automatisch parametrisiert werden können, so dass sie ohne Benutzerinteraktion anwendbar werden

[1]. Zhou et al. [2], Braun et al. [3] und Hu et al. [4] präsentieren Ansätze für das automatische Erkennen und Segmentieren von Strukturen der Lunge. In den Arbeiten von Brown et al. [5] und Lin et al. [6] werden WBS zur Segmentierung von Nieren vorgestellt. Alle Arbeiten zeigen, dass es möglich ist Risikoorgane automatisch zu segmentieren, indem etablierte Segmentierungsverfahren automatisch parametrisiert und ausgeführt werden. Ein wichtiges Kriterium hierfür ist die Bestimmung der kranial-kaudalen Korrespondenz, um beispielsweise ein Bereichswachstumsverfahren auf eine bestimmte Körperregion zu begrenzen.

In diesem Beitrag werden Mustererkennungsmethoden vorgestellt und bewertet, um die kranial-kaudale Korrespondenz für transversale CT-Schnittbilder zu bestimmen. Ziel ist es, Körperregionen in beliebigen CT-Bilddaten präzise abzugrenzen und somit das Segmentierungsproblem auf eine Teilregion (engl. clipping area) innerhalb des gesamten Datensatzes zu begrenzen. Das individuell akquirierte Wissen kann dann in die Parametrisierung von Segmentierungsalgorithmen einfließen.

2 Material und Methoden

Für die Präzisionsstrahlentherapie existieren verschiedene Immobilisationstechniken und stereotaktische Rahmensysteme, welche die Fixierung der Patienten und die Definition eines Koordinatensystems ermöglichen. Diese technischen Hilfsmittel sind als zusätzliche Objekte in den Schnittbildern enthalten. Sie wechseln in Abhängigkeit von der Indikation und erschweren die Bildverarbeitung. Um das im Folgenden vorgestellt Verfahren unabhängig von diesen Nebenbedingung anwenden zu können, wird in einem Vorverarbeitungsschritt eine anatomische Maske generiert. Sie begrenzt den Blick auf die Anatomie des Patienten. Das allgemeine Vorgehen wird von Hu et al. [4] beschrieben, wobei für die Binarisierung jedes Schnittbildes der dynamische Schwellwert nach der Methode von Otsu et al. [7] bestimmt wird. Aus den anatomischen Bilddaten werden im Anschluss fünf Gewebemerkmale und ein Vermessungsmaß abgeleitet. Abbildung 1 gibt einen qualitativen Eindruck der Merkmale. Der 6-dimensionale Merkmalsraum $\boldsymbol{m}$ wird anschließend mit den im Folgenden beschriebenen Mustererkennungsmethoden nach den Körperregionen $\Omega = \{$Kopf, Hals, Schulter, Thorax, Abdomen, Becken$\}$ klassifiziert.

2.1 Quadratische Diskriminanzanalyse

Die Quadratische Diskriminanzanalyse (QDA) ist dadurch gekennzeichnet, dass sie unter der Verwendung von Gauß-Normalverteilungsannahmen $N(\mu, \sigma)$ eine Schätzung der klassenbedingten Verteilungsdichte $p(\boldsymbol{m}|\Omega_i)$ vornimmt. Das Problem der Bestimmung der klassenbedingten Wahrscheinlichkeitsdichten wird auf die Schätzung der Verteilungsparameter reduziert. Für die QDA wird angenommen, dass die Kovarianz-Matrizen Σ_i für die Klassen i verschieden und somit unterschiedlich standardnormalverteilt sein können.

2.2 k-nächste Nachbarn Klassifikator

Der k-nächste Nachbarn Klassifikator (kNN) weist einem Merkmalsvektor $\boldsymbol{m}$ diejenige Klasse Ω_i zu, zu der die Mehrzahl der k-nächsten Nachbarn gehören. Als Abstandmaß wird die Euklidische Distanz $d(\boldsymbol{m}, \boldsymbol{x}) = \sqrt{\sum_{i=1}^{n} (\boldsymbol{m}_i - \boldsymbol{x}_i)^2}$ berechnet.

2.3 Perzeptron

Das Perzeptron ist ein einfaches künstlich neuronales Netz. Es stellt ein zweilagiges feed-forward Netzwerk dar bei dem jedes Neuron der Eingabeschicht mit allen Neuronen der Ausgabeschicht verbunden ist. Die Anzahl der Eingabe-Neuronen n entspricht der Anzahl der Merkmale. Die Anzahl der Ausgabe-Neuronen k korrespondiert mit der Anzahl an Klassenausprägungen $|\Omega|$. Jede Verbindung zwischen Eingabe- und Ausgabeschicht ist mit einem Gewicht $w_{ij} \in \mathbb{R}$ mit $i \in \{1, \ldots, n\}$ und $j \in \{1, \ldots, k\}$ belegt. In der Lernphase werden die Gewichte w_{ij} angepasst, so dass der Merkmalsraum linear getrennt wird.

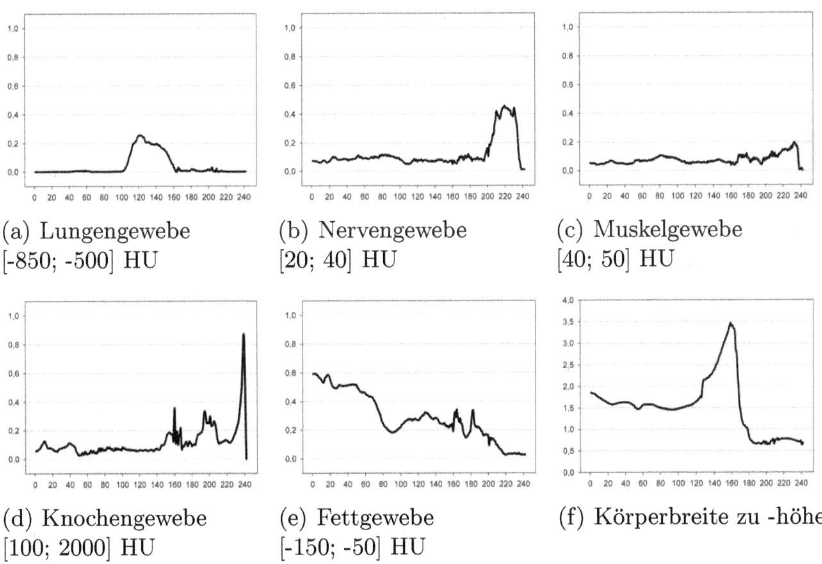

(a) Lungengewebe [-850; -500] HU

(b) Nervengewebe [20; 40] HU

(c) Muskelgewebe [40; 50] HU

(d) Knochengewebe [100; 2000] HU

(e) Fettgewebe [-150; -50] HU

(f) Körperbreite zu -höhe

Abb. 1. Die Abbildungen (a) bis (e) zeigen die Ausprägungen der Gewebeklassen. Zu jeder Abbildung ist der entsprechende Intensitätsbereich in Hounsfield-Units gegeben. Der Flächeninhalt, den ein Gewebe in einer Transversalschicht einnimmt, ist auf den gesamten Flächeninhalt, den der Körper in derselben Transversalschicht einnimmt, normiert. Abbildung (f) zeigt das Verhältnis Körperbreite zur -höhe. Auf der x-Achse sind die Transversalschichten entlang der Körperachse dargestellt. Der Datensatz beginnt im Bereich des Beckens (in Höhe der Femurköpfe, slice=0) und endet mit der Schädelkalotte (slice=244)

2.4 Support Vector Machine Klassifikator

Ein weiterer Klassifikator ist die Support Vector Machine (SVM). Anhand einer vorklassifizierten Stichprobe $S = \{\boldsymbol{x}_i, y_i\}$, bestehend aus $i = 1, \ldots, l$ Beobachtungen $\boldsymbol{x}_i$ und den Klassenzugehörigkeiten $y_i \in \{+1, -1\}$, wird eine Hyperebene $(\boldsymbol{w} \cdot \boldsymbol{x} + b) = 0$ bestimmt, welche die Klassen y_i optimal trennt. Nicht-linear separierbare Merkmalsräume können mit verschiedenen Kernelfunktionen (z.B. die Radiale Basis Funktion) getrennt werden. Die SVM unterscheidet sich von anderen Klassifikatoren dadurch, dass von allen möglichen Hyperebenen diejenige mit minimaler quadratischer Norm bestimmt wird, so dass die einzelnen Klassen optimal getrennt werden [8].

3 Ergebnisse

Für die Bewertung der Klassifikationsleistung wurde zwischen männlichen und weiblichen Patienten unterschieden. Es standen sieben CT-Datensätze von Männern zur Verfügung, woraus sich aus den einzelnen Transversalschichten insgesamt 909 Muster ergaben. Fünf CT-Datensätze von Frauen führten zu 650 Muster. Die Schätzung der Klassifikationsleistung wurde mit der Hold-out-Methode vorgenommen. Hierfür wurden die Stichproben S_M und S_W im Verhältnis $5:1$ zufällig und vollständig in eine Lern- und eine Teststichprobe zerlegt. Die resultierenden Klassifikationsleistungen sind in Abbildung 3 dargestellt.

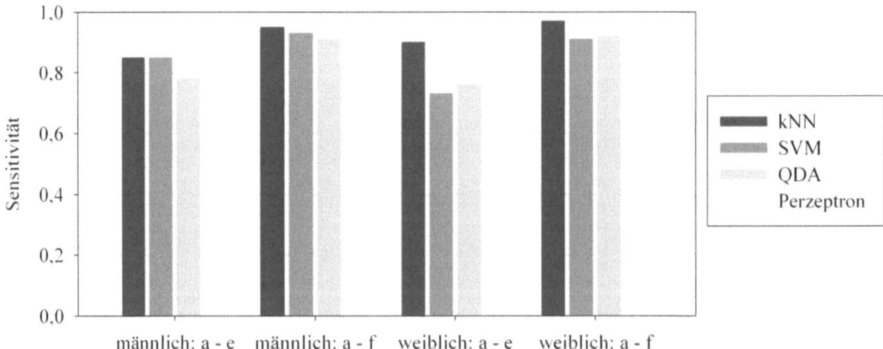

Abb. 2. Das Balkendiagramm veranschaulicht die Sensitivitäten, mit denen Transversalschichten einer Körperregion zugeordnet werden. Gegenübergestellt sind die Differenzierung nach dem Geschlecht (männlich, weiblich) und die Auswirkung verschiedener Merkmale (Abb. 1). Das Vermessungsmaß (Abb. 1(f)) verbessert die Klassifikationsleistung deutlich

4 Diskussion

In diesem Beitrag wurde gezeigt, dass individuell gegebenes, anatomisches Wissen aus beliebigen CT-Bilddaten mit Methoden der Mustererkennung akquiriert werden kann. Dieses Wissen kann verwendet werden, um semi-automatische Segmentierungsalgorithmen automatisch zu parametrisieren und in ihrem Aktionsbereich entlang der Longitudinalachse einzugrenzen. Dabei wird berücksichtigt, dass es sich um nicht statisch formulierbares Wissen handelt. Das heißt, dass es für jeden Patient individuell akquiriert werden muss. In der Bewertung der verschiedenen Klassifikationsleistungen zeigt der k-nächste Nachbarn Klassifikator die besten Ergebnisse. Aus Gründen der Performance und unwesentlich schlechteren Klassifikationsleistungen ist die SVM oder QDA dem kNN-Klassifikator vorzuziehen. Das Perzeptron zeigt bei dieser Klassifikationsaufgabe kein zufriedenstellendes Ergebnis. Dieses lässt darauf schließen, dass die Diskriminierungsaufgabe nicht-linear separierbar ist.

Die verwendeten Merkmale sind ausreichend, um mehr als 90% der Transversalschichten richtig zu klassifizieren. Einzelne Fehlklassifikationen konnten mit einem kantenerhaltenden Medianfilter korrigiert werden. Eine zusätzliche Konsistenzprüfung, in der eine bestimmte Abfolge von Körperregionen eingehalten werden muss, erhöht ebenfalls die Sicherheit. Im Falle stark verrauschter oder anormalen anatomischen Bedingungen (z.B. durch Vorerkrankung oder Implantate) kann die Weiterverarbeitung an dieser Stelle frühzeitig gestoppt werden.

Literaturverzeichnis

1. Faiß K, Oertel S, Schlegel W, et al. Wissensbasierte Segmentierung von Risikoorganen in der Strahlentherapieplanung. Proc BVM. 2005; p. 193–7.
2. Zhou X, Hayashi T, Hara T, et al. Automatic segmentation and recognition of anatomical lung structures from high-resolution chest CT images. Comput Med Imaging Graph. 2006;30(5):299–13.
3. Brown MS, Goldin JG, McNitt-Gray MF, et al. Knowledge-based segmentation of thoracic computed tomography images for assessment of split lung function. Med Phys. 2000;27(3):592–8.
4. Hu S, Hoffman EA, Reinhardt JM. Automatic lung segmentation for accurate quantitation of volumetric X-ray CT images. IEEE Trans Med Imaging. 2001;20(6):490–8.
5. Brown MS, Feng WC, Hall TR, et al. Knowledge-based segmentation of pediatric kidneys in CT for measurement of parenchymal volume. J Comput Assist Tomogr. 2001;25(4):639–48.
6. Lin DT, Lei CC, Hung SW. Computer-aided kidney segmentation on abdominal CT images. IEEE Trans Inf Technol Biomed. 2006;10(1):59–5.
7. Otsu N. A threshold selection method from gray-level histograms. IEEE Trans System Man Cybern. 1979;9(1):62–6.
8. Chang CC, Lin CJ. LIBSVM: A library for support vector machines; 2001. Software available at http://www.csie.ntu.edu.tw/cjlin/libsvm.

Level Set Segmentation of Lumbar Vertebrae Using Appearance Models

Karl Fritscher[1], Stefan Leber[1], Werner Schmölz[2], Rainer Schubert[1]

[1]Institute for Biomedical Image Analysis,
University for Health Sciences, Medical Informatics and Technology, Hall in Tirol
[2]University Clinic of Diagnostical Radiology, Medical University of Innsbruck
karl.fritscher@umit.at

Abstract. For the planning of surgical interventions of the spine exact knowledge about 3D shape and the local bone quality of vertebrae are of great importance in order to estimate the anchorage strength of screws or implants. As a prerequisite for quantitative analysis a method for objective and therefore automated segmentation of vertebrae is needed. In this paper a framework for the automatic segmentation of vertebrae using 3D appearance models in a level set framework is presented. In this framework model information as well as gradient information and probabilities of pixel intensities at object edges in the unseen image are used. The method is tested on 29 lumbar vertebrae leading to accurate results, which can be useful for surgical planning and further analysis of the local bone quality.

1 Introduction

For surgical interventions at the spine after vertebral instability exact preoperative surgical planning is crucial. It is highly important for the surgeon to gain insight into the exact 3D shape and the local quality of vertebrae in order to estimate the anchorage strength of screws or implants that are planned to be inserted into the vertebra. For this purpose the calculations of features which are able to asses the local bone quality in predefined regions of interest (ROIs) is necessary. Ideally these ROIs should be placed automatically in order to guarantee reproducible and objective results concerning the placement, size and – possibly – shape of the ROIs. For this purpose an – ideally – automatic segmentation of the vertebra is needed. In the last decade geometric deformable models based on level sets [1] became a widely used methods in medical segmentation pipelines. In [2] Leventon combined geometric deformable models with prior shape information in the level set evolution process. By introducing geodesic active regions [3] Paragios et al. also used texture information for the level set segmentation process. In [4] an approach based on level set segmentation, which is especially focusing on the segmentation of syndesmophytes in the vertebral body is introduced. In [5] a method based on the usage of shape models was proposed for the segmentation of a vertebra. In this paper we propose an approach which uses a level set framework in combination with appearance models for the segmentation of lumbar vertebrae. By combining level sets and appearance models the robustness of model based segmentation shall be combined with the flexibility of level set segmentation. Based on the work presented in [6] a cost function using a non-parameteric kernel based method to assess the intensity distribution at object edges will be proposed. It is the purpose of this paper to investigate if the proposed methods are feasible to provide a segmentation which can be used for further tasks concerning the planning of surgical interventions at the lumbar spine.

2 Methods

For the creation of the model pre-segmented images of the organ of interest are needed in order build 3D appearance models as described in [6]. Moreover, the level-set segmentation framework presented in [6] was used as a basis to combine model and image gradient based segmentation. In this work, the same speed function as in [6] was used. However, the grey scale statistics term for the MAP estimation presented in [6] was replaced by a term based on a nonparametric kernel-based method as presented in [7]. This term uses a Gaussian kernel which enables the calculation of the probability of a pixel's intensity i of belonging to a given region. This probability can be calculated as follows

$$p(i\,|\phi_M) = \frac{1}{V(R)} \iint_R \frac{1}{\sqrt{2\pi}\sigma} e^{\frac{-(i-I(y))^2}{2\sigma^2}} \tag{1}$$

where V(R) is the volume of the region R and σ specifies the width of the Gaussian kernel. I(y) represents the intensity of a pixel at index y. ϕ_M stands for the current zero level set. In contrast to [7] where this kernel-based method is used to calculate the probability of a pixels intensity to be consistent with the whole interior of a deformable contour, in our implementation the probabilities for a given pixel intensity are calculated within 2 regions P_{in} and P_{out}. These regions are represented by a narrow band [8] at the inside and outside of the propagating level set front. If the probability of a pixel with intensity i lying on the evolving front is higher for the narrow band inside the evolving region than the probability of belonging to the outside region, the front expands outwards. If the probabilities are vice versa the front moves inwards. The speed of the evolution is proportional to the calculated difference of the two probabilities P_{in} and P_{out}. The curve stops if the probability for a pixel with intensity i for belonging to P_{in} is equally high as the probability for belonging to P_{out}. In practice the pixels in the regions are converted to 8 bit (256 grey values). Moreover, this intensity statistics term (IST) is calculated independently in different sub-regions of the evolving front since it has to be assumed that the pixel intensities at the edge of the object of interest are not homogeneous throughout the whole surface. Furthermore the width of the narrow band in which the probabilities are calculated can be parameterized as well as the amount of the influence of the intensity statistics term on the propagation of the level set front using a weighting factor.

Table 1. Segmentation results for datasets included in model

	Known vertebrae using IST			Known vertebrae without IST		
Dataset	SI	HD (mm)	MD (mm)	SI	HD (mm)	MD (mm)
Average:	0.932	6.722	0.512	0.922	6.746	0.586
Sigma:	0.013	2.970	0.130	0.017	2.553	0.113

3 Results

The proposed algorithm was tested using 29 CT datasets of specimen of the spine and its surrounding muscles having an image resolution of 0.7 mm^3. 19 of these datasets have been used to create statistical appearance model of the third lumbar vertebra (L3) as described in [6]. Figure 1 shows the first two modes of variation for the shape of L3 within 2 standard deviations. The first 10 modes which are representing 92 percent of the appearance variations of L3 were used for the segmentation.

The 19 datasets used to build the model and the 10 unseen datasets have been segmented twice: One time using the new intensity statistics term and one time without this term. As gold standard a manual segmentation of the vertebra performed by a medical expert was used. The initialization for the automatic segmentation was performed by manually defining a rectangular region around the vertebra of interest. Tables 1 and 2 are showing the mean value and standard deviation of three common metric values – similarity index (SI), contour mean distance (MD) and Hausdorff distance (HD) – for the comparison of automatically segmented vertebra and the gold standard. It can be observed that the usage of the intensity statistics term improved the results of the segmentation.

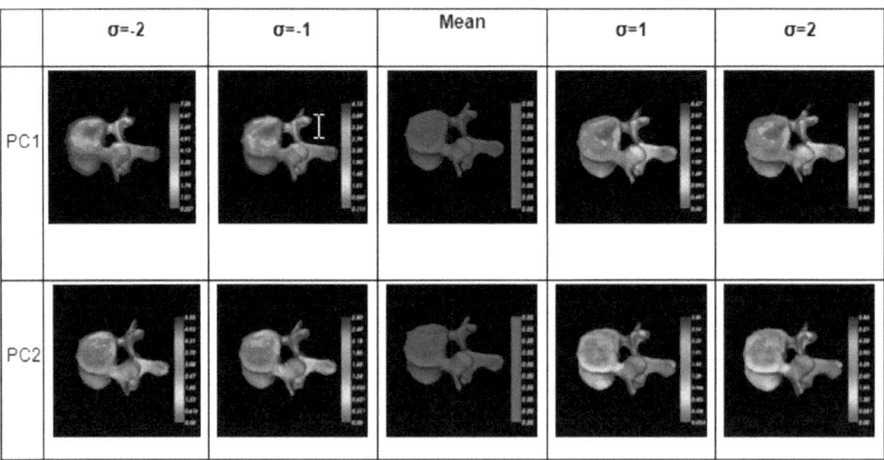

Fig. 1. First 2 modes of variation for the shape of L3 within 2 standard deviations from the mean (axial cut)

Table 2. Segmentation results for unseen datasets

	Unseen vertebrae using IST			Unseen vertebrae without IST		
Dataset	SI	HD (mm)	MD (mm)	SI	HD (mm)	MD (mm)
Average:	0.918	9.249	0.625	0.903	9.405	0.8
Sigma:	0.025	2.638	0.149	0.032	2.603	0.282

Figure 2 is showing two segmentation results. The left image is showing a vertebra that has been included in the model, the right image shows the segmentation result for a new vertebra.

4 Discussion

In this paper a way to combine the framework presented in [6] with a non parametric kernel based intensity statistics term was introduced. The segmentation for both the included as well as for the unseen datasets showed satisfying results with an average mean distance of 0.59 mm between automatic and manual segmentation performed by an expert. This is below the pixel spacing of 0.7 mm and the true 3D shape of the vertebra can be reconstructed with high accuracy suitable for surgical planning. It could be shown that the results of the segmentation could be improved by using the intensity statistics term. The segmentation faults were mainly situated in the transverse process. Since this is typically not a region, where the local bone quality must be known for surgical interventions, the segmentation is also highly suitable for the placement of adaptive ROIs using a method like e.g. presented in [9]. Since the appearance model is also reproducing the intensity distribution of the vertebra in high detail, the possibility of

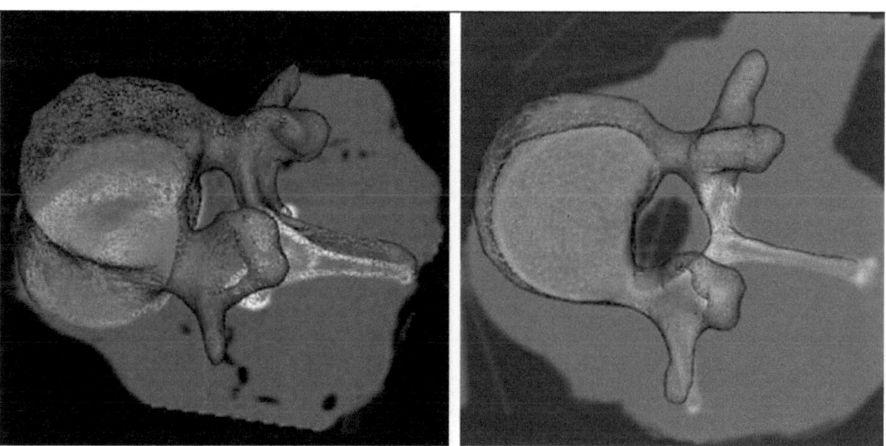

Fig. 2. Result of automatic segmentation for vertebra included in the model (left) and for unseen vertebra

using the final estimate of the appearance parameters at the end of the segmentation process directly for further analysis of the local bone quality should be considered.

References

1. Osher S, Sethian J, James A. Fronts propagating with curvature-dependent speed: Algorithms based on Hamilton-Jacobi formulations. J Comput Phys. 1988;79:12–49.
2. Leventon ME, Grimson WEL, Faugeras O. Statistical shape influence in geodesic active contours. IEEE Comp Vis Pattern Recognit. 2000;01:1316.
3. Paragios N, Deriche R. Geodesic active regions: A new framework to deal with frame partition problems in computer vision. J Vis Commun Image Represent. 2002;13:249–68.
4. Tan S, Jinhua Y, Ward M, et al. Level set based vertebra segemntation for the evaluation of ankylosing spondylitis. Proc SPIE. 2006;6144:07/01–10.
5. Fritscher KD, Schubert R. 3D image segmentation by using statistical deformation models and level sets. J Comp Assist Radiol Surg. 2006;1:123–35.
6. Fritscher KD, Gruenerbl A, Schubert R. 3D image segmentation using combined shape-intensity prior models. J Comp Assist Radiol Surg. 2007;1:341–50.
7. Huang X, Metaxas D, Chen T. Metamorphs: Deformable shape and texture models. IEEE Comp Vis Pattern Recognit. 2004;1:496–503.
8. Chopp DL. Computing minimal surfaces via level set curvature flow. J Comput Phys. 1993;106(1):77–91.
9. Fritscher KD, Schuler B, Grünerbl A, et al. Assessment of femoral bone quality using co-occurrence matrices and adaptive regions of interest. Proc SPIE. 2007;6514:1K1–9.

Segmentierung von Aortenaneurysmen in CTA-Bildern mit dem statistischen Verfahren der Active Appearance Models

Katharina Greiner[1,3], Jan Egger[2,3], Stefan Großkopf[3], Jens N. Kaftan[3,4], Ralf Dörner[1], Bernd Freisleben[2]

[1]Fachhochschule Wiesbaden, FB Design Informatik Medien
[2]Philipps-Universität Marburg, FB Mathematik und Informatik
[3]Siemens Computed Tomography, Forchheim
[4]RWTH Aachen, Lehrstuhl für Bildverarbeitung
stefan.grosskopf@siemens.com

Kurzfassung. In diesem Beitrag werden Active Appearance Models (AAMs) zur Segmentierung der äußeren Kontur von Aortenaneurysmen eingesetzt. Diese Aufgabe ist wegen des geringen Kontrastes zum umliegenden Gewebe und des Aufbaus der teils thrombotisierten oder kalzifizierten Gefäßwände im Bereich eines Aneurysmas so komplex, dass sie aufgrund der Vielgestalt der Kontur in CT-Angiographie-Bildern die Verwendung eines statistischen Modells für Form und eingeschlossene Textur rechtfertigt. Für die Evaluation des Verfahrens wurden verschiedene statistische Modelle aus Schichten von neun CTA-Datensätzen trainiert und die Segmentierung anhand von Leave-One-Out-Tests überprüft.

1 Einleitung

Ein Aortenaneurysma (AA) ist eine Erkrankung der Aorta, bei der eine dauerhafte lokale Dilatation des Gefäßes besteht. Die Ruptur eines Aneurysmas führt zu schweren inneren Blutungen und endet auch bei sofortiger Behandlung oft tödlich [1]. Eine präventive Therapiemöglichkeit ist das Einsetzen von Gefäßprothesen, die im Aneurysmenbereich den Blutfluss übernehmen [2] und die Größenzunahme des Aneurysmensacks stoppen bzw. sein Schrumpfen bewirken. Zur Therapieplanung und in der postoperativen Nachuntersuchungsphase werden CTA-Bilder des Gefäßes gescannt, um Änderungen festzustellen. Dazu wird das Aneurysma in einer zeitaufwändigen manuellen Prozedur Schicht für Schicht vermessen. Ein automatisches Verfahren kann dies nicht nur beschleunigen, sondern führt auch zu reproduzierbaren Ergebnissen.

In der Literatur finden sich verschiedene Verfahren zur automatischen Segmentierung von AAs. Lu et al. stellen einen Ansatz vor, der auf Aktiven Konturen aufbaut [3]. Subasic et al. beschreiben einen auf der Level-Set-Methode basierenden Algorithmus [4]. Das Verfahren von Olabarriaga et al. basiert auf einem deformierbaren 3D-Ansatz, wobei externe Kräfte aus einem statistischen Modell abgeleitet werden [5]. Ein bildmerkmalsgetriebenes Graph-Cut-Verfahren, das runde Strukturen bevorzugt, wurde von Bodur et al. entwickelt [6]. De Bruijne et al. führen die Segmentierung mit einem Active Shape Model durch [7].

2 Methoden

Für das Training des AAM [8] wurden Lumen und äußere Kontur der Aneurysmen manuell in den CTA-Schichtbildern konturiert. Zur Generierung der Annotation arbeitet das Trainingsmodul auf zum Gefäß orthogonalen MPRs (Multi Planar Reformatting). Durch eine strahlbasierte Suche werden – ausgehend von der Gefäßmittellinie – in gleichen Winkelabständen Pseudo-Landmarken für die Thrombus- bzw. Lumenkontur generiert (Abb. 1). Jede Annotation im Trainingsset wird durch einen Shape-Vektor repräsentiert, der die Koordinaten der Landmarken enthält. Diese Shape-Vektoren werden für das AAM-Training mit Hilfe der Procrustes-Analyse aneinander ausgerichtet um Variation durch euklidische Transformationen zu eliminieren, was im so genannten Point Distribution Model (PDM) resultiert. Aus dem PDM wird die durchschnittliche Form (Mean Shape) berechnet. Die Texturen werden durch Triangulation der Shapes und anschließendes stückweise affines Image Warping uniform aus den Bildern extrahiert. Durch Hauptkomponentenanalyse kann die Variation der Form und Textur auf wenige Parameter reduziert werden, die zur Abdeckung eines vorgegebenen Anteils der Varianz im Trainingsset geeignet sind. Das AAM ist nach erfolgtem Training in der Lage, durch Modifikation dieser Parameter MPRs zu segmentieren, indem der Texturfehler des parametrisierten AAMs von einer initialen Vorgabe ausgehend iterativ minimiert wird. Als Fehlermaß wird die Differenz zwischen der vom Modell generierten Textur und der aus dem Bild gesampelten Textur herangezogen.

Wir stellen verschiedene Trainingsmethoden vor, die unterschiedliche Konfigurationen der Annotation (Abb. 2) und unterschiedliches Vorgehen bei der Berechnung des Texturmodells beinhalten (normalisierte bzw. nicht normalisierte Grauwerte). Das Einbeziehen eines Randbereiches durch entsprechende Annotation dient dazu, dem Modell spezifischere Texturinformationen zum Erschei-

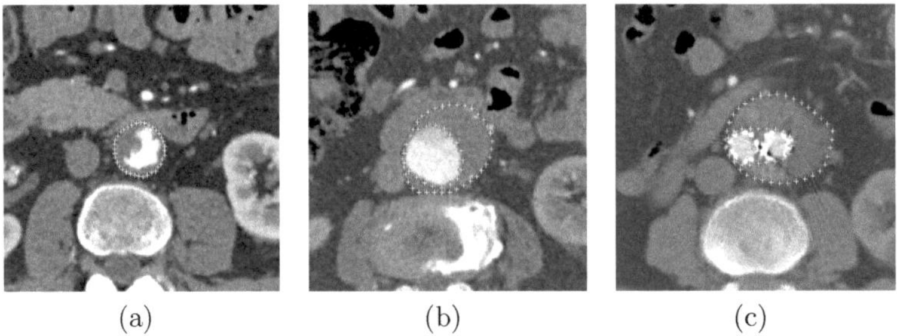

(a) (b) (c)

Abb. 1. Präoperative CT-Aufnahmen von Aortenaneurysmen mit Annotation der Thrombuskontur (a) bzw. des Thrombus und Lumen (b). Postoperative CT-Aufnahme mit Y-Stent und Annotation des Thrombus und des geteilten Lumen (c)

Abb. 2. Unterschiedliche Konfigurationen der Annotation für das Training der AAMs

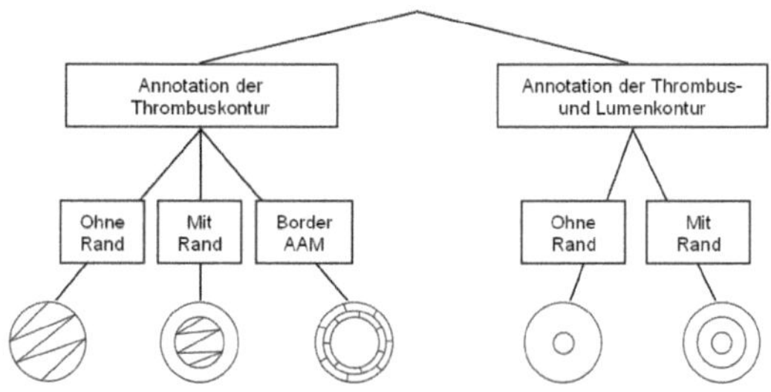

nungsbild der äußeren Aneurysmenkontur zur Verfügung zu stellen. Bezüglich des Texturmodells wurde der Einfluss der in der AAM-Formulierung enthaltenen Texturnormalisierung untersucht, die bei Anwendung auf CT-Daten dem Modell Informationen über die tatsächlichen Intensitätswerte entzieht. Zum Vergleich dieser unterschiedlichen Vorgehensweisen wurde der Point-to-Curve-Fehler für die Schichten der einzelnen Datensätze (Leave-One-Out-Methode) bestimmt.

Um einen CT-Datensatz zu segmentieren, wird das erste MPR-Bild manuell segmentiert (bei den automatisierten Tests wurde die vorhandene Referenzsegmentierung verwendet) und daraus die initiale Modellparameterkonfiguration gewonnen. Unter Ausnutzung der Ähnlichkeit von benachbarten Bildern wird die resultierende Parameterkonfiguration jeweils zur Initialisierung im benachbarten Bild verwendet.

Zum Training der AAMs wurden aus jedem der neun prä- und postoperativen CT-Datensätze, die unterschiedliche klinische Grade aufweisen, im Durchschnitt 26 MPR-Bilder verwendet. Die Modelle für die Leave-One-Out-Tests wurden jeweils aus Bildern aus acht Datensätzen berechnet und weisen ca. 80 signifikante Eigenwerte auf, die mindestens 98% der Varianz repräsentieren.

Die Methoden aus diesem Beitrag wurden innerhalb der MeVisLab-Plattform teilweise unter Verwendung einer Open-Source-Bibliothek[1] [9] realisiert.

3 Ergebnisse

Abbildung 3 zeigt Segmentierungsergebnisse unserer Modelle für prä- und postoperative CT-Aufnahmen. In einzelnen Fällen konnte der komplette Datensatz zufriedenstellend segmentiert werden, in einigen Fällen war jedoch die beim Training gewonnene Information zur Parameteroptimierung nicht ausreichend, um die Segmentierung zu optimieren (hohe Fehlerwerte in Abb. 5). Außerdem konnte gezeigt werden, dass ohne Texturnormalisierung im Schnitt bessere Segmentierungsergebnisse erreicht werden (Abb. 5(a)). Bei einem Vergleich der verwendeten Trainingsmethoden erzielte das Border-AAM, bei dem nur die Textur in einem schmalen Bereich um die äußere Kontur berücksichtigt wird, die stabilsten Ergebnisse. In Abbildung 5(b) sind die Point-to-Curve-Fehler für die verschiedenen Modelle dargestellt.

[1] AAM-API, Mikkel B. Stegmann, Technical University of Denmark

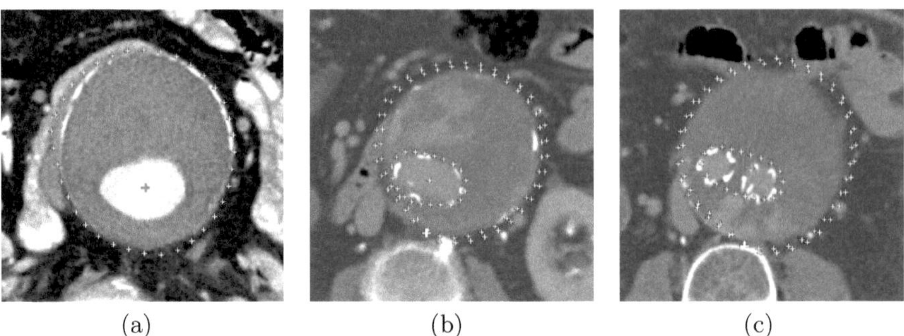

(a) (b) (c)

Abb. 3. Segmentierungsergebnis der Thrombuskontur in einer präoperativen CT-Aufnahme eines AA (a). Segmentierungsergebnis der Thrombuskontur und des Lumen bei einer postoperativen CT-Aufnahme mit implantiertem Stent (b) bzw. Y-Stent (c)

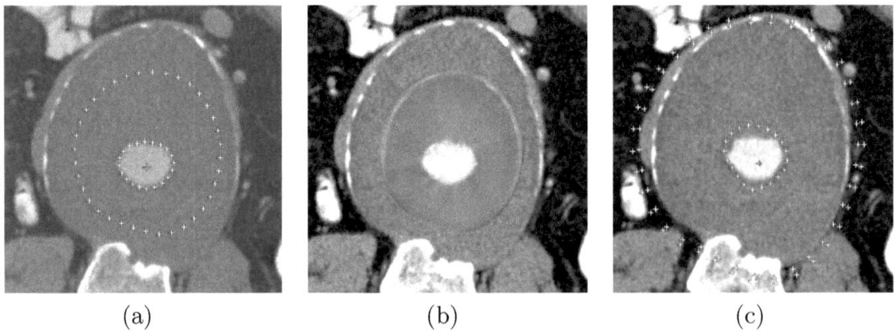

(a) (b) (c)

Abb. 4. Beispiel, bei dem die äußere Kontur fehlerhaft innerhalb des Thrombus liegt (a). (b) zeigt die zu (a) gehörige generierte Textur und (c) das entsprechende Ergebnis bei Ergänzung des Modells und der Segmentierung um einen Randbereich von 10 Pixeln

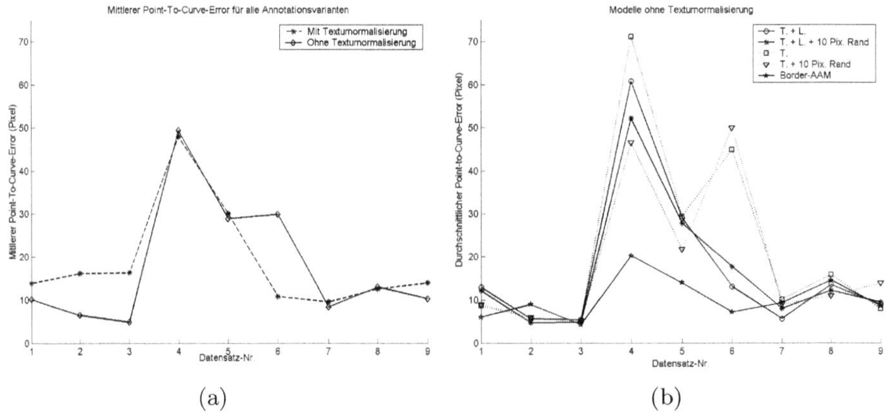

(a) (b)

Abb. 5. Mittlerer Point-to-Curve-Fehler für Modelle mit bzw. ohne Texturnormalisierung (a). Point-to-Curve-Fehler bei unterschiedlichen Trainingsmethoden für Modelle ohne Texturnormalisierung (b). (T.: Annotation der Thrombuskontur, L.: Annotation der Lumenkontur)

4 Diskussion

In diesem Beitrag wurde ein statistisches Verfahren zur automatischen Segmentierung von Aortenaneurysmen vorgestellt. Ziel war es, die aufwändige manuelle Segmentierung zu beschleunigen und reproduzierbare Ergebnisse zu erzeugen.

Zielsetzung war in erster Linie eine Segmentierung der äußeren Kontur des Aneurysmas. Die Problematik der Thrombussegmentierung liegt insbesondere im geringen Kontrast zwischen Thrombusgewebe und den umliegenden Gewebestrukturen (Abb. 1), so dass ein Ansatz beispielsweise auf Basis von Level-Sets ohne trainiertes a priori-Wissen bei solchen CTA-Aufnahmen dazu tendiert, in das umliegende Gewebe auszulaufen. Hieraus rechtfertigt sich der Einsatz der mit hohem Trainingsaufwand verbundenen statistischen Methode der AAMs.

Im Zuge unserer Versuchsreihen hat sich herausgestellt, dass das Modell aufgrund des verwendeten Fehlermaßes (Texturdifferenz) bei einigen CT-Schichten dazu tendiert, die generierte Textur vorrangig auf das Lumen anzupassen, so dass die äußere Kontur innerhalb des Thrombus liegt (Abb. 4). Dies ist auf den hohen Kontrast zwischen Thrombus und Lumen zurückzuführen. Diesem Problem kann dadurch entgegengewirkt werden, dass ein schmaler Rand vom umgebenden Gewebe in das Modell einbezogen wird. Dieser zusätzliche Rand enthält Texturinformationen, die ein Kantenmodell realisieren.

Unsere Tests haben gezeigt, dass die Segmentierung von Aortenaneurysmen mit AAMs möglich ist, eine Evaluation der Methode auf einem größeren Trainingsset steht jedoch noch aus. Als nächster Schritt ist eine Erweiterung auf 3D-Modelle geplant, so dass zusätzlich zur aktuell zu segmentierenden Schicht auch Informationen aus den benachbarten Schichten berücksichtigt werden.

Literaturverzeichnis

1. Treska V, Novak M. Rupture of abdominal aortic aneurysm: Factors of mortality. Bratisl Lek Listy. 2006;107(1-2):22–5.
2. Blankensteijn JD, de Jong SECA, Prinssen M, et al. Two-Year Outcomes after conventional or endovascular repair of abdominal aortic aneurysms. N Engl J Med. 2005;352:2398–405.
3. Lu J, Egger J, Wimmer A, et al. Segmentierung und Visualisierung von Lumen und Thrombus bei thorakalen Aortenaneurysmen. Proc CURAC. 2007; p. 251–4.
4. Subasic M, Loncaric S, Sorantin E. 3-D Image analysis of abdominal aortic aneurysm. Proc SPIE. 2002;4684:1681–9.
5. Olabarriaga SD, Rouet JM, Fradkin M, et al. Segmentation of thrombus in abdominal aortic aneurysms from CTA with nonparametric statistical grey level appearance modeling. IEEE Trans Med Imaging. 2005;24(4):477–85.
6. Bodur O, Grady L, Stillman A, et al. Semi-automatic aortic aneurysm analysis. Proc SPIE. 2007 3;6511:1G.
7. de Bruijne M, van Ginneken B, Viergever MA, et al. Interactive segmentation of abdominal aortic aneurysms in CTA images. Med Image Anal. 2004;8(2):127–38.
8. Cootes TF, Edwards GJ, Taylor CJ. Active appearance models. IEEE Trans Pattern Anal Mach Intell. 2001;23(6):681–5.
9. Stegmann MB, Ersbøll BK, Larsen R. FAME: A flexible appearance modelling environment. IEEE Trans Med Imaging. 2003;22(10):1319–31.

Automatic Liver Segmentation Using the Random Walker Algorithm

F. Maier[1,2], A. Wimmer[2,3], G. Soza[2], J.N. Kaftan[2,4], D. Fritz[1,2], R. Dillmann[1]

[1]Universität Karlsruhe (TH),
[2]Siemens Medical Solutions, Forchheim,
[3]Friedrich–Alexander University Erlangen–Nuremberg,
[4]RWTH Aachen University
maier@ira.uka.de

Abstract. In this paper we present a new method for fully automatic liver segmentation in computed tomography images. First, an initial set of seed points for the random walker algorithm is created. In this context, voxels belonging to air, fat tissue and ribcage are labeled as background. Furthermore, depending on the shape of the ribcage and voxel intensities, several seed points inside the liver are automatically selected as foreground. This seed mask is then used to initialize the segmentation algorithm. Our method was successfully tested on data of 22 patients.

1 Introduction

Liver segmentation is an important prerequisite for a variety of applications. Surgery planning, image guided liver surgery and computed tomography (CT) perfusion examinations benefit from an accurate segmentation.

Fully automatic and at the same time accurate liver segmentation is an unsolved problem by now, despite several diverse attempts exist. Soler et al. [1] presented an algorithm for a segmentation of the liver using a reference 3-d model. After estimation of the liver contour, the model is improved by means of topological and geometrical analysis. With this approach, however, the segmentation is constrained by the reference model, which can be adapted to the real image information only in a restricted way. Lamecker et al. [2] presented an approach for liver segmentation using a 3-d statistical shape model built from a training set of semi-automatically segmented livers. This technique also suffers from restricted flexibility in shape adaptation. Lim et al. [3] use their deformable contour model for segmentation.

A drawback common to most approaches is a lack of interactive controllability if the automatic segmentation has failed. Grady et al. [4, 5] introduced the random walker (RW) algorithm, which is a general segmentation technique based on graph theory. It allows image segmentation given fore- and background seed points. A big advantage of the algorithm is that the calculated results can be easily corrected in a semi-automatic way.

2 Materials and Methods

A new fully automatic algorithm for liver segmentation is introduced. The presented algorithm extends and adapts the general graph theoretic image segmentation [4] to the liver segmentation problem. Within our approach, several seed points inside and outside of the liver are automatically detected. These seeds are then supplied as input to the RW algorithm.

2.1 Generation of Seed Points

In the first step, seed points within different abdominal structures are automatically detected. All seed points lying within structures outside the liver are then labeled as background and seed points within the liver are labeled as foreground. Seed point detection is performed for each slice separately. A polar coordinate system is associated with each axial slice. The center of the polar coordinate system is set to the barycenter of the body. The advantage of such a polar coordinate system is that the angle coordinate can be easily correlated with the anatomy to make restrictions which part of the body can comprise the liver (e.g., left, right, anterior, posterior, see Fig. 1(a)).

Several different structures are considered for automatic seed detection. The details are provided below.

Generation of ribcage seed points To prevent oversegmentation of the liver into the adjacent muscle tissue between the ribs, the shape of the ribcage is estimated. For this purpose, anatomical knowledge is used. First assumption is that the liver is located on the right side of the body near the bottom of the ribcage. It is also assumed that some liver tissue touches or is very close to the ribcage. The rib detection algorithm works as follows.

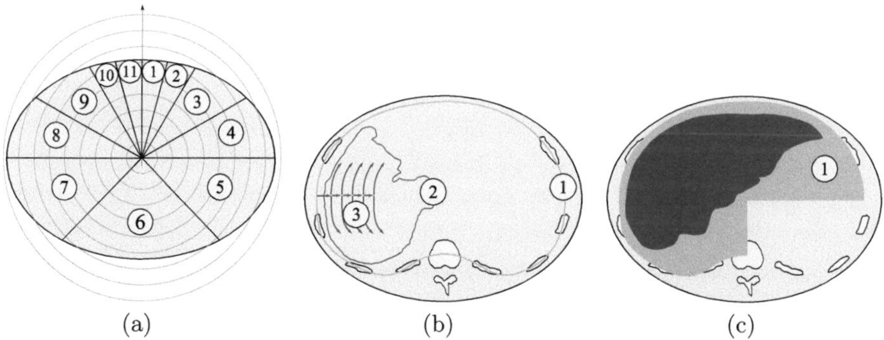

Fig. 1. Segmentation: (a) Polar coordinate system and angle depended sector sizes. Anterior: small sectors (1, 2, 10, 11), posterior: large sector (6). (b) Liver seed point creation. Spline (1), contour of liver (2), liver seed search paths (3). (c) Histogram analysis area (1). The area for histogram analysis is defined by the interior of the ribcage spline in the posterior and anterior right part of the abdomen

First, intensity differences on each radius for all angles are checked to detect the body surface and the boundary between fat and muscle tissue (Fig. 2(a)). Median filters with angle dependent kernel sizes are applied to all determined radii in order to eliminate outliers. Based on the detected boundary and an angle dependent maximum rib depth, a search area is defined (Fig. 2(b)). Voxels therein with high intensities (e.g., > 300 HU) are classified as bone (Fig. 2(c)). Positions of ribs are stored in a separate list (Fig. 2(d)). Then, all detected rib positions are clustered with hierarchical clustering depending on radius and angle of the voxel positions belonging to the ribs. The final cluster centers are stored as the outer rib positions, one for each rib (Fig. 2(e)).

Starting with the outer rib positions, the corresponding inner rib positions are estimated by analysis of the intensity profile into the direction of the body barycenter (Fig. 2(f)). The inner rib positions shifted away from the body center by some small safety distance are used as support points for a cubic spline (Fig. 1(b)). If there are not enough support points in a given sector (Fig. 1(a)), positions from neighboring slices are used. In this case, a new rib point is placed into the current slice by interpolating the corresponding lower and upper rib positions. If there are no rib points that can be used, points from the fat/muscle boundary are taken as substitute. This prevents the spline from passing through the liver. The ribcage points lying on the generated spline curve are taken as background seeds for each slice. This information prevents the RW algorithm from oversegmentation of the liver into the surrounding muscle or fat regions.

Generation of liver seed points An intensity histogram is built from voxels in the anterior and right posterior part of the abdomen that are enclosed by the cubic spline (Fig. 1(c)). Known background voxels like air, fat or bone are thereby excluded. HU value distributions of the liver and stomach are assumed to be Gaussians. Hence, mean and variance of these Gaussians are estimated by a bimodal distribution analysis. Mean and variance of the Gaussian of the liver are used to define the intensity range of liver pixels. On the right side of the body

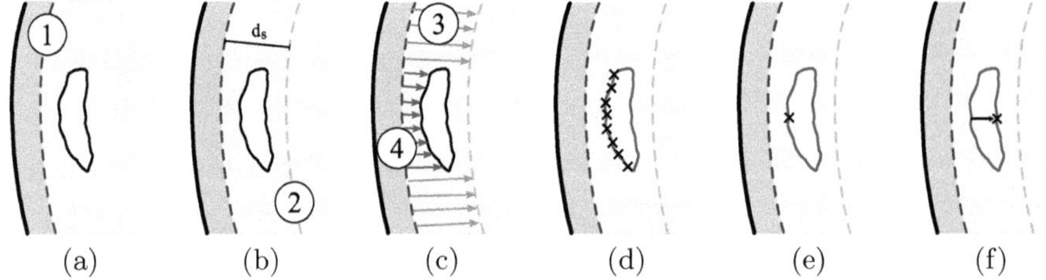

Fig. 2. Rib detection: Right part of the body including fat tissue (dark gray) and rib (white). (a) Fat/muscle boundary (line 1). (b) Maximum search depth d_s (line 2) from fat/muscle boundary. (c) Search for bone failed on bright paths (3). Search was successful on dark paths (4). (d) Marked points: detected outer bone positions. (e) Marked point: Center of bone position cluster, outer rib position. (f) Marked point: Inner rib position, corresponding to outer position of (e) detected on search path

the right turning point of the spline is used to start foreground seed generation (Fig. 1(b)). The radius is reduced in given steps and the corresponding pixels are checked if they lie within the range calculated from the histogram. If they fulfill this criterion, they are labeled as foreground seeds. The angle is then changed iteratively in the clockwise and counter-clockwise direction. The progression of each line will stop if a group of pixels is outside the intensity interval or a stop position is reached. Stop positions are defined by the last visible rib.

Generation of air, bone and fat seeds Air and any other gases are clearly delineated in CT data and are used to generate background seeds. All voxels with a lower intensity than a predefined threshold (e.g., −460 HU) are marked as air. All voxels with a higher intensity than a given threshold (e.g., 325 HU) are classified as bone. Fat tissue inside the body is also labeled as background. For this purpose, the image is first filtered with a median filter (e.g., 9×9 pixel), which reduces noise. After filtering, an interval threshold (e.g., −117 HU to −53 HU) is applied and the result is classified as fat tissue.

3 Results

In order to prove the stability of the method with respect to varying liver shapes and contrast enhancements, the algorithm has been evaluated with 22 CT liver perfusion datasets comprising native, arterial and venous enhancement phases. Since perfusion scans require a high temporal resolution, they are acquired without CT table movement. The maximum number of slices is consequently limited by detector width and reconstruction settings and was less or equal 12 in our experiments. Slice distance and slice thickness were equal in all datasets and varied between 2.4 and 6 mm. The axial resolution of all slices was 512×512 voxels of size varying between 0.64×0.64 mm^2 and 0.72×0.72 mm^2.

The automatic results have been quantitatively compared to manual segmentations performed by medical experts using the dice similarity coefficient (DSC), the average contour distance ($\overline{d}$) and the Hausdorff distance (H). Mean values and standard deviations over all 22 patients are $\mu_{DSC} = 91.9\%$, $\sigma_{DSC} = 7.2\%$, $\mu_{\overline{d}} = 4.6$ mm, $\sigma_{\overline{d}} = 3.7$ mm, $\mu_H = 34.3$ mm and $\sigma_H = 14.53$ mm. Table 1 shows more detailed numerical results for seven randomly selected patients. Additionally, visual analysis of the segmentation results has been conducted, which confirmed the overall good quality of the results. The resulting liver contours and probabilities for each voxel to be part of the liver are presented in Fig. 3.

Execution of the RW algorithm on downsampled (256×256) 3-d images required between 1.63 s (1 slice) up to 19.56 s (12 slices) on an Intel Pentium 4 CPU (3.4 GHz, 1 GB RAM). The seed point creation algorithm needed 7.7 s per slice. The software has been developed with MeVisLab 1.4 (VC++ 6).

Table 1. Results: dataset (D), vol. of dataset (V), vol. of RW segmentation (RWV), vol. of manual segmentation (MV), vol. of overlap (OLV), vol. of oversegmentation (OSV), vol. of undersegmentation (USV), all volumes in ml, $\overline{d}$, and H in mm

D	V	RWV	MV	OLV	OSV	USV	DSC	$\overline{d}$	H
1	1075,8	155,1	147,9	145,6	9,5	2,3	96,1%	2,1	14,2
2	3232,1	439,6	441,4	394,1	45,5	47,3	89,5%	5,9	36,9
3	3465,6	778,6	771,7	760,3	18,3	11,3	98,1%	1,7	56,0
4	3270,8	606,2	662,8	585,0	21,1	77,8	92,2%	5,4	49,4
5	3232,1	769,9	757,1	731,8	38,1	25,3	95,9%	1,7	13,5
6	3290,2	279,8	256,4	238,1	41,7	18,3	88,8%	4,4	28,8
7	3270,8	675,2	695,8	637,5	37,8	58,4	93,0%	5,3	47,5

4 Discussion

In this paper, a fully automatic liver segmentation algorithm, based on the general RW approach and customized automatic seed point creation, has been proposed. Using the presented approach, it is possible to generate robust liver segmentations. There are only few assumptions about the shape and size of the liver. Therefore, it is possible to reach high segmentation quality on abnormal livers, in contrast to model based approaches. Small intensity differences, caused e.g. by liver tumors, do not corrupt the segmentation results.

The segmentation algorithm reaches an average DSC value of 91.9%, which shows the high concordance between automatic and manual segmentation. The large mean value of H is caused by oversegmentation of small areas between the lobes of the liver. Oversegmentation of these small gaps causes high peaks in the surface distance between manual and automatic segmentation. The significantly lower value of $\overline{d}$ shows that most of the distances between the surfaces are smaller than the peaks. In difficult cases, the new algorithm allows intuitive interactive correction of its results. Users that are capable to use a simple paint application will be able to quickly edit the results in a semi-automatic way.

Improvements of our approach can be attained by integrating additional background seed points using existing organ segmentations (e.g., heart). Furthermore, a more efficient implementation of the seed point creation algorithms would bring improvement in execution times.

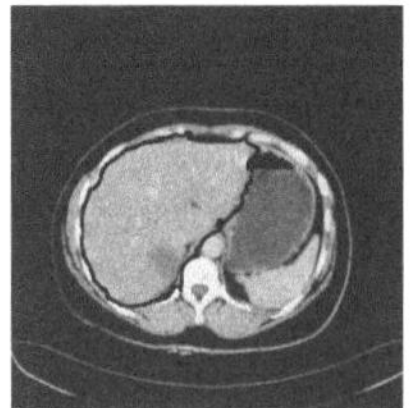
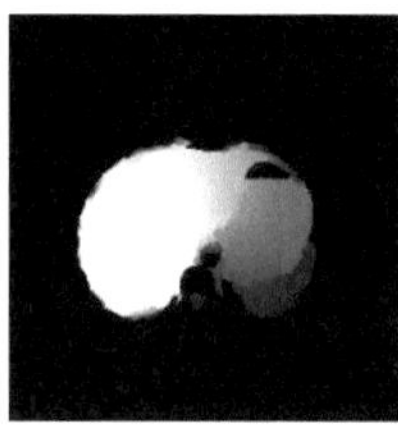
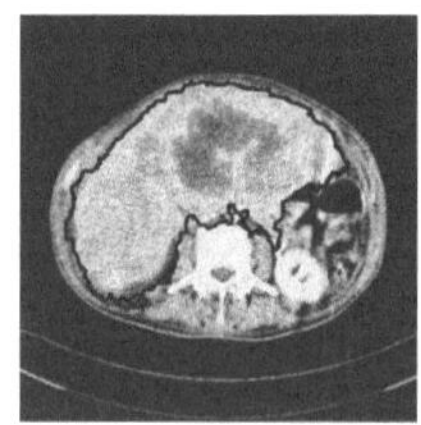
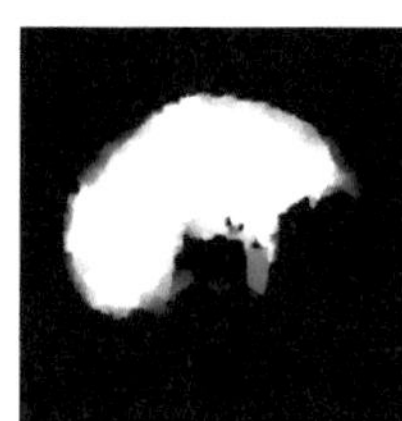

Fig. 3. CT image slices with determined liver contours (black) and corresponding probabilities (white=100%, black=0%)

References

1. Soler L, Delingette H, Malandain G, et al. Fully automatic anatomical, pathological, and functional segmentation from CT scans for hepatic surgery. Comput Aided Surg. 2001;6:131–42.
2. Lamecker H, Lange T, Seebaß M. A statistical shape model for the liver. Proc MICCAI. 2002;2489:421–27.
3. Lim SJ, Jeong YY, Ho YS. Segmentation of the liver using the deformable contour method on CT images. Proc SPIE. 2005;3767:570–81.
4. Grady L. Random walks for image segmentation. IEEE Trans Pattern Anal Mach Intell. 2006;28(11):1768–83.
5. Grady L, Schiwietz T, Aharon S, et al. Random walks for interactive organ segmentation in two and three dimensions: Implementation and validation. Proc MICCAI. 2005;3750:773–80.

Simulation of Contrast Agent Enhanced Ultrasound Imaging Based on Field II

Tobias Gehrke, Heinrich M. Overhoff

Medical Engineering Laboratory, University of Applied Sciences Gelsenkirchen
tobias.gehrke@fh-gelsenkirchen.de

Abstract. Pulse-echo ultrasound signal formation can be simulated by numerical emulation of the process chain: emit signal – electromechanical emit transformation – wave propagation and scattering – electromechanical receive transformation – receive signal. The simulation software Field II is indented for simulation of linear ultrasound systems. We present an extension to Field II that enables the inclusion of nonlinear oscillations of ultrasound contrast agent bubbles into the simulation. An example is given for contrast agent enhanced imaging of a virtual vessel phantom probed by a linear array transducer.

1 Introduction

Ultrasound contrast agents consist of gas-filled microbubbles whose radii oscillate when exposed to sonic waves emitted from an ultrasound transducer. Simulation enables evaluation of novel contrast imaging modalities with respect to different transducer geometries, electronic settings and irradiated phantoms as well as various concentrations and types of contrast agent, without costly experiments.

The software package Field II [1] has become a standard tool in the simulation of ultrasonic pulse echo imaging. This software is limited to the simulation of linear passive scattering from tissue inhomogeneities. However, the physics of bubble dynamics is nonlinear and can therefore not be modelled within the Field II framework. Approaches to overcome this limitation have been undertaken, but are either limited to linear bubble oscillation [2] or rely on empirical data that has to be acquired prior to the simulation [3]. We present an extension to Field II that enables inclusion of signals originating from nonlinear contrast agent bubble oscillations. Our approach is entirely derived from basic physical relations what makes empirical modification dispensable.

2 Materials and Methods

2.1 Basic Physical Relations

The process of contrast agent enhanced medical ultrasound imaging is determined by the physical relations in three coupled physical domains: The ultrasound transducer, the propagation medium, i. e. the human body, and the gas phase inside the contrast agent bubbles.

Electromechanical Transducer Behaviour Assuming linearity, an ultrasound transducer can be characterized by a four pole model that relates the force $F(\omega)$ onto and the velocity $\bar{V}(\omega)$ of the transducer's front face $\mathcal{S}_{\mathrm{t}}$, to voltage $E(\omega)$ and current $I(\omega)$ at its electrodes [4]. For a fix electrical impedance and a time invariant radiation impedance, it can be reduced to a two pole model. Making a distinction between transmission and reception for convenience it reads

$$\bar{V}(\omega) = H_{\mathrm{trm}}(\omega)E_{\mathrm{exc}}(\omega) \quad \Rightarrow \quad \bar{v}(t) = h_{\mathrm{trm}}(t) * e_{\mathrm{exc}}(t) \tag{1}$$

$$E_{\mathrm{rec}}(\omega) = H_{\mathrm{rec}}(\omega)F(\omega) \quad \Rightarrow \quad e_{\mathrm{rec}}(t) = h_{\mathrm{rec}}(t) * f(t), \tag{2}$$

with $*$ denoting convolution [1]. Voltage and force are coupled by the electromechanical transfer functions $H_{\mathrm{trm}}(\omega)$ and $H_{\mathrm{rec}}(\omega)$ for transmission and reception respectively in frequency domain or the corresponding impulse responses $h_{\mathrm{trm}}(t)$ and $h_{\mathrm{rec}}(t)$ in time domain.

Wave Propagation Under linear conditions, propagation of pressure waves $p(\boldsymbol{r},t)$ inside a medium with density $\rho(\boldsymbol{r})$ and compressibility $\kappa(\boldsymbol{r})$ is described by [5]

$$\nabla\left(\rho(\boldsymbol{r})^{-1}\nabla p(\boldsymbol{r},t)\right) - \kappa(\boldsymbol{r})\ddot{p}(\boldsymbol{r},t) = 0 \tag{3}$$

For a homogeneous medium with density $\bar{\rho}$, compressibility $\bar{\kappa}$, and speed of sound $\bar{c} = (\bar{\rho}\bar{\kappa})^{-\frac{1}{2}}$ wave equation (3) reduces to

$$\nabla^2 p(\boldsymbol{r},t) - \bar{c}^{-2}\ddot{p}(\boldsymbol{r},t) = 0 \tag{4}$$

Bubble Dynamics Under equilibrium conditions $p(\boldsymbol{r},t) = p_0$, the radius of a single spherical gas-bubble immersed in an incompressible homogeneous fluid is $R(t) = R_0$. The bubble dynamics is modelled by the Rayleigh-Plesset equation

$$\bar{\rho}\left(R(t)\ddot{R}(t) + \tfrac{3}{2}\dot{R}(t)^2\right) = \left(p_0 + \frac{2\sigma}{R_0} - p_{\mathrm{v}}\right)\left(\frac{R_0}{R(t)}\right)^{3\gamma} - \frac{2\sigma + 4\eta\dot{R}(t)}{R(t)} + p_{\mathrm{v}} - p(\boldsymbol{r},t) \tag{5}$$

which relates a varying pressure $p(\boldsymbol{r},t)$ to oscillation of $R(t)$ [4]. Besides its density $\bar{\rho}$, the surrounding liquid is characterized by its dynamic viscosity η and vapour pressure p_{v}. The quantity σ is the surface tension of the liquid-gas interface, and γ denotes the polytropic exponent of the gas inside the bubble.

2.2 System Model

To model the process of pulse-echo signal formation, the pressure field $p(\boldsymbol{r},t)$ is decomposed into three different fields: The incident pressure $p_{\mathrm{i}}(\boldsymbol{r},t)$ would be present in a homogeneous i. e. scatterer and bubble free medium due to radiation from the transducer, the fields $p_{\mathrm{s}}(\boldsymbol{r},t)$ and $p_{\mathrm{b}}(\boldsymbol{r},t)$ are the additional pressures from passive scattering and active bubble emission.

[1] The function arguments t on the right hand side indicate that two functions of time are convolved. This notation shall not imply that the convolution at time t is computed solely from the function values at time t.

Incident Pressure Field The incident pressure $p_\mathrm{i}(\boldsymbol{r},t)$ originating from a transducer at position $\boldsymbol{r}_\mathrm{t}$ is calculated by a Green's function solution to the homogeneous wave equation (4). If the transducer is assumed to be placed in an infinite rigid baffle $\mathcal{S}_\mathrm{b}$, the boundary conditions are

$$\frac{\partial}{\partial \boldsymbol{n}} p_\mathrm{i}(\boldsymbol{r},t)\Big|_{\boldsymbol{r}=\boldsymbol{r}_\mathrm{t}+\boldsymbol{s}} = \begin{cases} -\bar{\rho} w(\boldsymbol{s}) \frac{\partial \bar{v}(t)}{\partial t}, & (\boldsymbol{r}_\mathrm{t}+\boldsymbol{s}) \in \mathcal{S}_\mathrm{t} \\ 0, & (\boldsymbol{r}_\mathrm{t}+\boldsymbol{s}) \in (\mathcal{S} \setminus \mathcal{S}_\mathrm{t}) \end{cases} \tag{6}$$

Here $\boldsymbol{n}$ denotes the normal vector onto transducer surface $\mathcal{S}_\mathrm{t}$ and $\boldsymbol{s}$ points towards any position on the transducer surface or baffle. Position dependency of the transducer displacement is accounted for by the surface velocity distribution function $w(\boldsymbol{s})$. The Green's function solution to this problem is [6]

$$p_\mathrm{i}(\boldsymbol{r},t) = \iint_{\mathcal{S}_\mathrm{t}} \int_0^t 2w(\boldsymbol{s}) \frac{\partial \bar{v}(\tau)}{\partial \tau} \frac{\delta(t-\tau-|\boldsymbol{r}-(\boldsymbol{r}_\mathrm{t}+\boldsymbol{s})|/\bar{c})}{4\pi|\boldsymbol{r}-(\boldsymbol{r}_\mathrm{t}+\boldsymbol{s})|} \,\mathrm{d}\tau\, \mathrm{d}\boldsymbol{s} \tag{7}$$

By defining a spatial impulse response

$$h_\mathrm{spt}(\boldsymbol{r},t) = \iint_{\mathcal{S}_\mathrm{t}} w(\boldsymbol{s}) \frac{\delta(t-\tau-|\boldsymbol{r}-(\boldsymbol{r}_\mathrm{t}+\boldsymbol{s})|/\bar{c})}{4\pi|\boldsymbol{r}-(\boldsymbol{r}_\mathrm{t}+\boldsymbol{s})|} \,\mathrm{d}\boldsymbol{s} \tag{8}$$

and using the electromechanical relation (1), the incident pressure is given by

$$p_\mathrm{i}(\boldsymbol{r},t) = 2\bar{\rho} e(t) * h_\mathrm{trm}(t) * \frac{\partial}{\partial t} h_\mathrm{spt}(\boldsymbol{r},t) \tag{9}$$

Scattered Pressure Field The left hand side of the homogeneous wave equation (4) is subtracted on both sides of its inhomogeneous counterpart (3) to derive the component of the pressure field due to an inhomogeneity q [7]:

$$\begin{aligned} \nabla^2 p_{\mathrm{s}q}(\boldsymbol{r},t) - \bar{c}^{-2} \ddot{p}_{\mathrm{s}q}(\boldsymbol{r},t) &= \bar{c}^{-2} \left(\tfrac{\kappa(\boldsymbol{r})}{\bar{\kappa}} - 1\right) \ddot{p}(\boldsymbol{r},t) - \nabla \left[\left(\tfrac{\bar{\rho}}{\rho(\boldsymbol{r})} - 1\right) \nabla p(\boldsymbol{r},t)\right] \\ &\approx V_q \bar{c}^{-2} \left[\left(\tfrac{\kappa(\boldsymbol{r}_q)}{\bar{\kappa}} - 1\right) + \left(\tfrac{\bar{\rho}}{\rho(\boldsymbol{r}_q)} - 1\right) \cos \Theta_q\right] \ddot{p}(\boldsymbol{r}_q,t) \end{aligned} \tag{10}$$

Comparison with (4) shows that the scatter act as a source to the homogeneous wave equation. The approximation has been made by lumping the scatterer with volume V_q and irradiation angle Θ_q into a single point at $\boldsymbol{r}_q$ [7] and using the paraxial approximation [6, 8]. This is tolerable if the scatterer is small and sufficiently far away from the transducer.

Bubble Emitted Pressure Field Equivalently to the scatterers, the bubbles are modelled as point sources that radiate into a homogeneous medium:

$$\nabla^2 p_{\mathrm{b}q}(\boldsymbol{r},t) - \bar{c}^{-2} \ddot{p}_{\mathrm{b}q}(\boldsymbol{r},t) = \left(p_0 + \frac{2\sigma_q}{R_{0q}} - p_\mathrm{v}\right) \left(\frac{R_{0q}}{R_q(t)}\right)^{3\gamma} - \left(p_0 + \frac{2\sigma_q}{R_q(t)} - p_\mathrm{v}\right) \tag{11}$$

The right hand side source term is the pressure just beyond the wall of a gas-bubble q [4]. The time varying bubble radius $R_q(t)$ depends on the pressure $p(\boldsymbol{r}_q,t)$ and can be obtained from the Rayleigh-Plesset equation (5).

Total Pressure Field The incident field in a pulse echo system is travelling outwards and does hence not contribute to the force onto the receiving transducer. The total echo field from all Q scatterers and bubbles is thus obtained by the Green's function solution to (10) and (11) respectively [6, 7]:

$$p(\boldsymbol{r},t) = \sum_{q=1}^{Q} \int_0^t \mathfrak{R}_q\{p(\boldsymbol{r}_q,\tau)\} \frac{\delta(t-\tau-|\boldsymbol{r}-\boldsymbol{r}_q|/\bar{c})}{4\pi|\boldsymbol{r}-\boldsymbol{r}_q|}\,\mathrm{d}\tau \tag{12}$$

The operator $\mathfrak{R}_q\{\cdot\}$ acting onto pressure $p(\boldsymbol{r},t)$ denotes the source terms, i. e. right hand sides in (10) or (11). If the fields $p_\mathrm{s}(\boldsymbol{r},t)$ and $p_\mathrm{b}(\boldsymbol{r},t)$ are weak compared to the incident field $p_\mathrm{i}(\boldsymbol{r},t)$, the latter can replace the total pressure field $p(\boldsymbol{r},t)$ on the right hand side of (12), what is known as Born approximation [6].

Force onto Receiver An ultrasound transducer is sensitive to the force

$$\begin{aligned} f(t) &= \iint_{\mathcal{S}_\mathrm{t}} w(\boldsymbol{s})p(\boldsymbol{r}_\mathrm{t}+\boldsymbol{s},t)\,\mathrm{d}\boldsymbol{s} \\ &= \iint_{\mathcal{S}_\mathrm{t}} w(\boldsymbol{s}) \sum_{q=1}^{Q} \int_0^t \mathfrak{R}_q\{p_\mathrm{i}(\boldsymbol{r}_q,\tau)\} \frac{\delta(t-\tau-|\boldsymbol{r}_\mathrm{t}+\boldsymbol{s}-\boldsymbol{r}_q|/\bar{c})}{4\pi|\boldsymbol{r}_\mathrm{t}+\boldsymbol{s}-\boldsymbol{r}_q|}\,\mathrm{d}\tau\,\mathrm{d}\boldsymbol{s} \end{aligned} \tag{13}$$

that acts onto its surface $\mathcal{S}_\mathrm{t}$. The spatial dependency of the transducer's receive sensitivity is equal to the surface velocity distribution $w(\boldsymbol{s})$ in transmit mode [8]. The spatial impulse response (8) can be used to denote (14) in a short way:

$$f(t) = \sum_{q=1}^{Q} \mathfrak{R}_q\{p_\mathrm{i}(\boldsymbol{r},t)\} * h_\mathrm{spt}(\boldsymbol{r}_q,t) \tag{14}$$

Receive Signal The electromechanical receive dynamics (2) and the models of the subsystems (9), and (14) can be connected to an overall system model:

$$e_\mathrm{rec}(t) = \sum_{q=1}^{Q} \mathfrak{R}_q\left\{2\bar{\rho}e_\mathrm{exc}(t) * h_\mathrm{trm}(t) * \tfrac{\partial}{\partial t}h_\mathrm{spt}(\boldsymbol{r}_q,t)\right\} * h_\mathrm{spt}(\boldsymbol{r}_q,t) * h_\mathrm{rec}(t) \tag{15}$$

2.3 Implementation

A program that computes the signal processing chain from the exciting voltage $e_\mathrm{exc}(t)$ to the receive voltage trace $e_\mathrm{rec}(t)$, as described by (15), has been developed in Matlab (The Mathworks Inc., Natick, MA, USA).

For most transducers, analytic solutions for the spatial impulse responses are unknown. To compute (8) Field II, which provides a powerful numerical method to calculate impulse responses for numerous transducer geometries [1], is used.

The program solves the Rayleigh-Plesset equation (5) numerically by a variable order method for every combination of bubbles and aperture elements. To increase the simulation speed, a critical level for the incident pressure has been introduced below which computation of the bubble oscillation is omitted.

Fig. 1. Simulated B-mode images without (left) and with contrast agent (right)

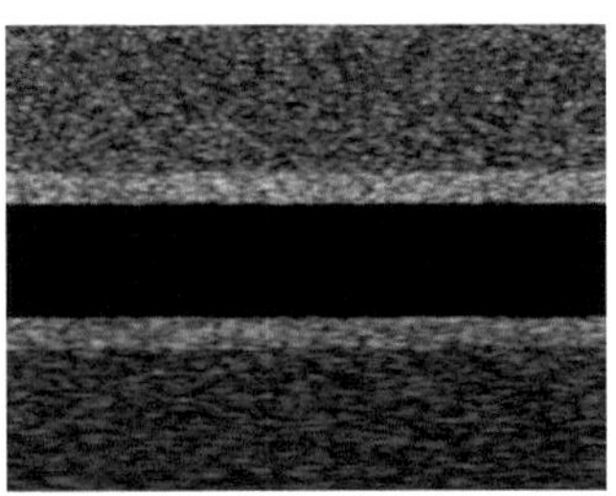

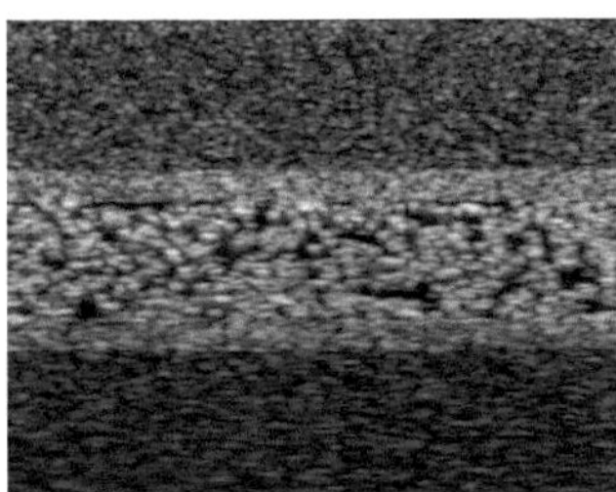

3 Results

To test the simulation program, an ultrasound machine with a 256-element linear array and 3.5 MHz centre frequency has been emulated. In Fig. 1 simulated B-mode images of a blood vessel with 15 mm diameter are shown without and with contrast agent enhancement. The virtual phantom consists of 30 000 randomly distributed scatterers that mimic the vessel walls and surrounding muscular tissue and 1000 air-filled bubbles with normally distributed radii (mean $\bar{R}_0 = 1\,\mu m$, standard deviation $s_{R_0} = 0.3\,\mu m$) as contrast agent.

4 Discussion

Combination of a numerical solver for the Rayleigh-Plesset equation with Field II can consistently simulate contrast agent enhanced ultrasound imaging. The program is useful for the development of novel contrast agent imaging methods.

References

1. Jensen JA. Field: A program for simulating ultrasound systems. In: Proceedings of the 10th Nordic-Baltic Conference on Biomedical Imaging; 1996. p. 351–3.
2. Gerfault L, Cachard C, Gimenez G. Simulation of echographic image of contrast agent. In: IEEE Ultrasonics Symposium; 1998. p. 1815–8.
3. Durning B, Laval J, Rognin N, et al. Ultrasound signals and images simulation of phantoms with contrast agent. In: IEEE International Ultrason Ferroelectr Freq Control Joint 50th Anniversary Conference; 2004. p. 1710–3.
4. Szabo TL. Diagnostic Ultrasound Imaging. Amsterdam: Elsevier; 2004.
5. Insana MF, Brown DG. Acoustic scattering theory applied to soft biological tissues. In: Shung KK, Thieme GA, editors. Ultrasonic scattering in biological tissues. Boca Raton: CRC Press; 2000. p. 75–124.
6. Jensen JA. A model for the propagation and scattering of ultrasound in tissue. IEEE Trans Ultrason Ferroelectr Freq Control. 1991;89(1):182–90.
7. Gehrke T, Cheikhrouhou F, Overhoff HM. A simulation program for ultrasound tomography imaging based on Field II. Proc IFMBE. 2005;11:4393–8.
8. Lhémery A. Impulse-response method to predict echo-responses from targets of complex geometry. Part I: Theory. J Acoust Soc Am. 1991;90(5):2799–807.

Microbubble Oscillation due to Harmonic, Pulsed and Frequency Modulated Excitation with Ultrasound

Tobias Gehrke, Heinrich M. Overhoff

Medical Engineering Laboratory, University of Applied Sciences Gelsenkirchen
tobias.gehrke@fh-gelsenkirchen.de

Abstract. Improved visualization of blood vessels by ultrasound contrast agents requires insonation that is adapted to the dynamics of the contrast agent bubbles. To evaluate the interrelation between parameters of the exciting pressure field and the contrast agent, the dynamics of air filled microbubbles immersed in water are examined by numerical evaluation of the Rayleigh-Plesset equation. Unsymmetrical oscillation is obtained for resonant harmonic excitation, frequency doubling occurs for subresonant excitation and nearly sinusoidal oscillation is exhibited for superresonant excitation. Continuous harmonic and pulsed pressure waves are shown to be unsuitable to excite a mixture of differently sized bubbles due to their non-uniform resonance behaviour. As an alternative, excitation with a linear frequency modulated wave is examined and shown to be a feasible option for adapted contrast agent insonation.

1 Introduction

Segmentation of vessels within an ultrasound image is a prerequisite for automatic image analysis or three dimensional visualization in vascular applications. Small vessels can frequently not clearly been identified in an ultrasound image since they appear buried between stronger echogenic surrounding tissue. Automatic segmentation of those vessels can be simplified by the use of ultrasound contrast agents which significantly enhance the echo amplitudes. Further improvement can be achieved by specifically adapted imaging algorithms such as harmonic imaging or pulse inversion that make use of the contrast agent's nonlinear behaviour [1].

Ultrasound contrast agents are realized as gas-filled microbubbles. The radii of these bubbles oscillate when exposed to sonic waves emitted from an ultrasound transducer [1, 2, 3]. While the bubble's oscillation is nearly linear for small exciting pressures, higher pressures cause asymmetric oscillation and thereby nonlinear bubble dynamics. These asymmetric oscillations are due to a reduced compressibility of the filling gas with decreasing bubble bubble radius.

In order to create oscillation amplitudes large enough to be detected at the body surface by the transducer in receive mode, additionally to a sufficiently high amplitude, the frequency of the exciting wave must be adjusted to the resonance properties of the bubbles [4]. Furthermore, careful adaption of the signal processing i.e. imaging algorithm to the specific nonlinear bubble oscillation can increase the visibility of small vessels. Therefore realistic simulation of the bubble dynamics is a crucial task in the development of contrast agent imaging modalities.

In this paper, the oscillations of air-filled microbubbles in water due to harmonic resonant, subresonant and superresonant forcing as well as due to pulsed and frequency modulated excitation are examined. Real contrast agents consist of a mixture of differently sized bubbles, which hence show non-uniform resonance behaviour. The consequences for parameters of the exciting wave are examined and a proper setting is derived.

2 Materials and Methods

The dynamic behaviour of a single spherically symmetrical gas-bubble immersed in an incompressible fluid can be modelled by a nonlinear differential equation of second order, called Rayleigh-Plesset equation [1, 3]. Properties of the numerical solver and results for defined physical wave propagation and bubble parameters are investigated.

2.1 Rayleigh-Plesset Dynamics

The Rayleigh-Plesset equation

$$\bar{\rho}\left(R(t)\ddot{R}(t)+\tfrac{3}{2}\dot{R}(t)^2\right)= \left(p_0+\frac{2\sigma}{R_0}-p_{\rm v}\right)\left(\frac{R_0}{R(t)}\right)^{3\gamma}-\frac{2\sigma+4\eta\dot{R}(t)}{R(t)}+p_{\rm v}-\left(p_0+\Delta p(t)\right) \quad (1)$$

relates outer pressure changes $\Delta p(t)$ to a time varying bubble radius $R(t)$. Under equilibrium conditions $\Delta p(t) = 0$, the pressure inside the surrounding liquid is p_0. The static bubble radius under equilibrium conditions is $R(t) = R_0$. The surrounding liquid is characterized by its density ρ, dynamic viscosity η, and vapour pressure $p_{\rm v}$. The quantity σ is the surface tension of the liquid-gas interface, and γ denotes the polytropic exponent of the gas inside the bubble.

2.2 Numerical Solver

The Rayleigh-Plesset equation has been implemented in Matlab (The Mathworks Inc., Natick, MA, USA) and numerically solved in the time domain using a variable order BDF (backward differentiation formula) method. The algorithm uses a variable step size Δt that depends on the local rate of change of the solution. This enables detection of quasi-discontinuities as they occur when the bubble radius $R(t)$ approaches zero. Cubic spline interpolation of the solution advances processing steps that require regularly sampled data such as the discrete Fourier transform.

Table 1. Characteristic values of gas (air) and surrounding liquid (water) that have been used for the simulation

Liquid pressure	p_0	100 kPa
Liquid density	ρ	998 kg/m^3
Dynamic liquid viscosity	η	1 mPa
Vapour pressure	p_v	5945 Pa
Surface tension	σ	72.5 mN/m
Polytropic exponent	γ	1

2.3 Simulation Settings

The equation parameters have been set to model an air filled bubble immersed in water at ambient temperature and pressure. Adiabatic gas behaviour $\gamma = 1$ has been assumed. An overview of the simulation settings is given in Tab. 1.

3 Results

The modelled bubble of equilibrium radius $R_0 = 2.26\,\mu m$ exhibits a nonlinear resonance frequency $f_{\text{exc}} = 1260\,\text{kHz}$. In Fig. 2(a) resonant bubble dynamics is visualized in the phase plane for harmonic excitation

$$\Delta p_{\text{har}}(t) = \Delta p_0 \sin(2\pi f_{\text{exc}} t) \tag{2}$$

with $\Delta p_0 = 36\,\text{kPa}$. The steady state phase diagram for excitation of the first and second subharmonic and the first harmonic is shown in Fig. 2(b). The figures reveal that frequency doubling occurs for frequencies below resonance, while excitation with the first harmonic frequency causes nearly sinusoidal oscillation. Simple albeit unsymmetrical oscillation occurs for excitation at resonance. Approaching the minimal bubble radius coincides with a large oscillation velocity. Unsymmetrical oscillation and frequency doubling can also be clearly obtained in the time domain as is shown in Fig. 2, where the varying bubble radius is depicted as a function of time for excitation with the resonance frequency and half the resonance frequency.

Harmonic pressure waves excite only bubbles of distinct size, as can be seen in Fig. 3 where the relative amplitude of oscillation $\Delta R/R_0$ with $\Delta R = \max(R(t)) - \min(R(t))$ is charted as a function of the equilibrium bubble radius R_0 for continuous harmonic excitation with frequency $f_{\text{exc}} = 1260\,\text{kHz}$ (black line). The oscillation amplitude rises very sharply towards its maximum at the resonance radius $R_0 = 2.26\,\mu m$, while the falling edge of the curve is less steep such that considerable oscillation occurs for a small band of radii above the resonance radius. Radii around $R_0 = 4.65\,\mu m$ show harmonic oscillation due to the excitation frequency $f_{\text{exc}} = 1260\,\text{kHz}$. Also subharmonic excitation of bubbles with radii around$R_0 = 1.4\,\mu m$ can be noticed.

Pressure pulses that normally excite bubbles in pulse echo ultrasound imaging have a broader frequency content and are thus capable to excite bubbles of a

Fig. 1. Phase diagrams of bubble oscillations. (a) Oscillation at resonance $f_{\mathrm{exc}} = 1260\,\mathrm{kHz}$. (b) Oscillation for excitation with $f_{\mathrm{exc}} = 420\,\mathrm{kHz}$ (black line), $f_{\mathrm{exc}} = 630\,\mathrm{kHz}$ (dark grey line), $f_{\mathrm{exc}} = 2520\,\mathrm{kHz}$ (light grey line)

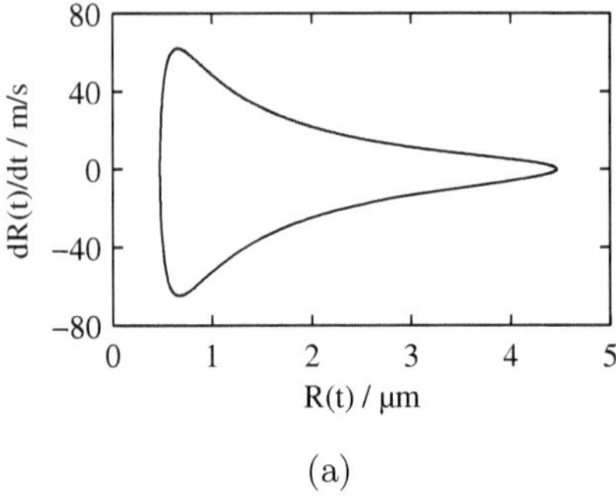

(a) (b)

Fig. 2. Bubble radii $R(t)$ as functions of time t for resonant excitation $f_{\mathrm{exc}} = 1260\,\mathrm{kHz}$ (black line) and subharmonic excitation $f_{\mathrm{exc}} = 630\,\mathrm{kHz}$ (grey line)

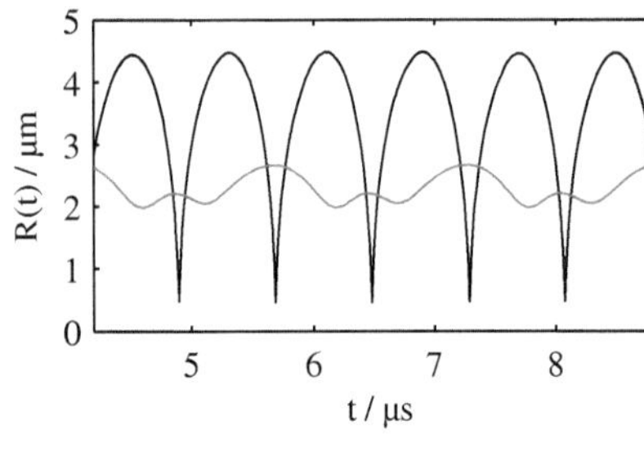

Fig. 3. Relative amplitudes of oscillations $\Delta R/R_0$ as functions of the equilibrium bubble radius R_0 due to continuous harmonic excitation (black line) and pulsed excitation (dark grey line) with frequency $f_{\mathrm{exc}} = 1260\,\mathrm{kHz}$, and due to excitation with a chirp signal whose frequency rises from $f_{\mathrm{exc1}} = 300\,\mathrm{kHz}$ to $f_{\mathrm{exc2}} = 3000\,\mathrm{kHz}$ (light grey line)

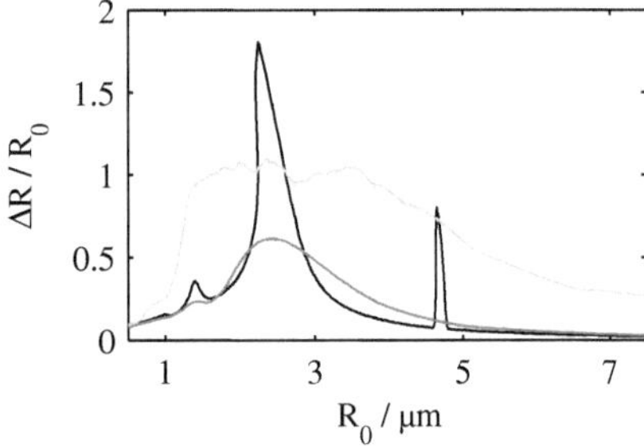

greater radius range than harmonic excitation does. In Fig. 3 the dark grey line shows relative oscillation amplitudes due to excitation with a sinusoidal pulse of $f_{\mathrm{exc}} = 1260\,\mathrm{kHz}$ and three periods length tapered by a Hann window.

The light grey curve in Fig. 3 shows the relative oscillation amplitudes due to excitation with a chirp signal

$$\Delta p_{\mathrm{crp}}(t) = \Delta p_0 \sin\left(2\pi\left(f_{\mathrm{exc1}} + \frac{f_{\mathrm{exc2}} - f_{\mathrm{exc1}}}{2T}t\right)t\right) \tag{3}$$

whose frequency rises linearly from $f_{\mathrm{exc1}} = 300\,\mathrm{kHz}$ to $f_{\mathrm{exc2}} = 3000\,\mathrm{kHz}$. The signal amplitude and duration are $\Delta p_0 = 36\,\mathrm{kPa}$ and $T = 12.1\,\mu s$ respectively.

The signal edges have been tapered to resemble smooth start and ending of signals from real, bandlimited ultrasound systems. Comparison of the three curves in Fig. 3 reveals that - in contrast to harmonic or pulsed excitation - the chirp signal is capable to excite an ensemble of differently sized contrast agent bubbles if its spectrum is adapted to the radius distribution.

4 Discussion

A single microbubble shows distinct resonant behaviour, with moderate excitation pressures causing large oscillation amplitudes. Simulations show that amplitudes at resonance are of the same order as those for subresonant excitation.

In the more realistic case of an ensemble of bubbles with different sizes, harmonic or pulsed pressure waves excite only a small subset of these bubbles. Broadband signals with sufficient energy such as chirp signals proved to excite more bubbles. The application of long duration broadband signals requires pulse compression during the image formation process. For linear pulse echo imaging this task can successfully be accomplished by matched filters [5]. Matched filtering is however not directly adaptable for contrast agent enhanced imaging, since the nonlinear response of the bubbles can not be handled.

The simulations give a general impression about the dynamics of ultrasound contrast agent bubbles. A more realistic model must include the influence of the bubble shells [6, 7], the interrelation between the members of a bubble ensemble, and spherically asymmetric bubbles.

References

1. Szabo TL. Diagnostic Ultrasound Imaging. Elsevier, Amsterdam; 2004.
2. Jong ND, Cornet R, Lancée CT. Higher harmonics of vibrating gas-filled microspheres. Ultrasonics. 1994;32(6):447–53.
3. Hilgenfeldt S, Lohse D, Zomack M. Response of bubbles to diagnostic ultrasound: A unifying approach. Eur Phys J B. 1998;4(2):247–55.
4. Mukdadi OM, Kim HB, Hertzberg J, et al. Numerical modeling of microbubble backscatter to optimize ultrasound particle image velocimetry imaging: Initial studies. Ultrasonics. 2004;42:1111–21.
5. Misaridis T, Jensen JA. Use of modulated excitation signals in medical ultrasound. Part I: basic concepts and expected benefits. IEEE Trans Ultrason Ferroelectr Freq Control. 2005;52(2):177–91.
6. Church CC. The effects of an elastic solid surface layer on the radial pulsations of gas bubbles. J Acoust Soc Am. 1995;97(3):1510–21.
7. Hoff L, Sontum PC, Hovem JM. Oscillations of polymeric microbubbles: effect of the encapsulating shell. J Acoust Soc Am. 2000;107(4):2272–80.

Fluorescence Microscopy Deconvolution Based on Bregman Iteration and Richardson-Lucy Algorithm with TV Regularization

Steffen Remmele, Madeleine Seeland, Jürgen Hesser

Institute for Computational Medicine, University of Heidelberg
remmele@ti.uni-mannheim.de

Abstract. Fluorescence microscopy has become an important tool in biological and medical sciences for imaging thin specimen, even living ones. Due to Out-of-focus blurring and noise the acquired images are degraded and therefore it can be difficult to analyse them. In the last decade many methods have been proposed to restorate these images. One of the most popular methods to restore microscopy images is an iterative Richardson-Lucy Algorithm with Total Variation Regularization. Besides there are some new approaches based on Bregman Iteration to improve the quality of restored images in general. In this paper we formulate a new algorithm for restoring fluorescense microscope images using Bregman Iteration with special attention to the microscopy specific properties. We can proof that the quality of the restored images increases by using the I-divergence and the mean square error criteria.

1 Introduction

1.1 Image Formation Model

Any optical system degrades the acquired images due to the physical properties of the optical aperture and of light itself on the one side and due to the detection process on the other side. These degradations contain two separate parts: the blurring of the image which can be described by a PSF (point spread function) convolution and the additional noise in the image. The type of noise that can be found in the image is dependent on the acquisition process. For fluorescence microscopy it is well-known that there is Poisson noise in the acquired images because it is a low-photon imaginary technique. The Poisson noise will be represented by $\phi(.)$ in this paper. Thus the suitable image formation model where i is the observed image, o the original image, h represents the PSF and $\otimes$ the convolution operator is given by:

$$i = \phi(o \otimes h) \tag{1}$$

In this paper we assume that the PSF is already known. It is possible to use a second image with beads to estimate the PSF in a preceding step or to calculate the PSF due to the physical properties of the used microscope.

1.2 Restoration of Fluorescence Microscope Images

To restore the degradation due to Poisson noise, as mentioned before, it is common to use a Richardson-Lucy (RL) algorithm consisting of an expectation maximization algorithm which calculates the maximum likelihood estimation [1, 2]. Basically the algorithm contains the iterative minimization of the following energy functional H applying the know variables form formula (1):

$$H(o,i) = \int o \otimes h - i \cdot log(o \otimes h) \tag{2}$$

The basic RL algorithm has a huge disadvantage. It amplifies noise after several iterations while first improving the image. In order to overcome this problem one can denoise the image first and use the RL algorithm to deblurr the image afterwards but it is a better solution to add a separate regularization functional. This additional term is weighted with a regularization parameter. A very popular choice for a regularization term is the Tikonov-Miller (TM) regularization which can be combined with the RL energy functional [3].

$$R_{TM}(o) = \int |\nabla o|^2 \tag{3}$$

∇ is the gradient of the image o and $|.|$ decribes the L^2 norm. The TM regularization allows the RL algorithm to converge to a suitable solution but it smoothes the edges. This is a well-known problem and it is possible to use another regularization technique named Total Variation (TV) regularization which preserves the edges. A combined RL and TV algorithm for microscopy contains the TV term [4] which is again weighted with a regularization parameter. This method has another drawback because it rounds corners.

$$R_{TV}(o) = \int |\nabla o| \tag{4}$$

Both techniques are very popular and commonly used. The choice for the regularization term should depend on what one wants to analyse in the reconstructed image.

1.3 Restoration Approach Using the L^2 Norm and the Bregman Iteration

Another modified approach to reconstruct blurred and noisy images is using the Bregman distance introduced in [5]. This distance was added to a blind deconvolution algorithm [6] and later also used to reconstruct a high resolution image on basis of a set of low resolution images [7]. In both approaches a L^2 norm based deblurring functional with TV is used. The blind deconvolution algorithm [6] consists of two independend parts where alternately the image is deblurred and the PSF is estimated. Here it is assumed that the PSF is already known and so only the deblurring of the image is of interest. To reconstruct the image first a common minimization of the combined energy functional containing the deblurring and regularization functional is used. Then the observed image i is modified using $i = i + v_m$ for the $(m+1)$th Bregman iteration with $v_m = i + v_{m-1} - h \otimes o_m$ being a result of the additional Bregman distance in the reconstruction algorithm.

2 Materials and Methods

2.1 New Algorithm for Restoring Fluorescence Microscope Images

The new algorithm is using the bregman distance D [5] which is defined as shown in formula (5).

$$D_\vartheta(x, y) = \vartheta(x) - \vartheta(y) - \langle x - y, \partial\vartheta(y)\rangle \tag{5}$$

In this definition $< ., . >$ denotes the inner product and ∂ the sub-gradient of ϑ. In the new algorithm a RL term H is used for deblurring according to the Poisson noise in the observed image as already described in formula (2). Then the TV regularization term R already known from formula (4) is added in order to get a stable and suitable solution. The TV term is weighted with a regularization parameter λ. The general formula to calculate the result of the reconstruction iteratively using the Bregman distance is then:

$$o_m = argmin_o \left\{H(o, i) + \lambda \cdot D_R(o, o_{m-1})\right\} \tag{6}$$

As mentioned before $H(o, i)$ shall be the RL deblurring term containing the PSF and the functional R used in the Bregman distance D is the TV regularization term. It is necessary to start this approach with an empty image and to do the first step without using the Bregman distance and only apply the regularization term R. In order to formulate the algorithm a new term named *Breg* is introduced which contains an additional image with the same size as the observed image and is supposed to be filled with zeros at the beginning.

The algorithm itself consists of two separate steps which have to be executed in every Bregman iteration. The first step is to reconstruct the image iteratively starting with an empty image and then using the result of the previous step as start image afterwards. This reconstruction is done according to the following formula for $m = 1...n$ with n being the requested amount of Bregman iterations.

$$o_m = argmin_o \left\{H(o, i) + \lambda R_{TV}(o) - \lambda \langle o, Breg\rangle\right\} \tag{7}$$

The formula (7) has its origin in formula (6) with the constant parts being removed and the additional *Breg* term. The second step of the algorithm in each iteration step is the modification of the Breg term according to the Bregman distance in formula (5) and formula (6). This modification is given by the fact that the minimization of the considered functional in formula (7) yields the property that the derivative is zero for a minimum of a functional.

$$Breg = Breg - \frac{1}{\lambda}\partial H(o_m, i) \tag{8}$$

In formula (8) $\partial H(o_m, i)$ describes the gradient of the RL functional $H(o, i)$.

Table 1. Results

	I-div	MSE
Original & Degraded	1.304.030	22.459.100
Original & Reconstructed (RL & TV)	67.671	21.536.600
Original & Reconstructed (New algorithm)	56.951	18.058.600

2.2 Measure the Quality of the Results

To quantify the quality of the restored images it is usual to use the I-divergence and the mean square error (MSE) criteria, as you can see in formulas (9,10), measured between two images A and B (both are 3D and of the same size):

$$I_{A,B} = \sum_{ijk} \left\{ A_{ijk} ln(\frac{A_{ijk}}{B_{ijk}}) - (A_{ijk} - B_{ijk}) \right\} \tag{9}$$

$$MSE_{A,B} = \sum_{ijk} \{A_{ijk} - B_{ijk}\}^2 \tag{10}$$

It is a problem to use these criteria on real images because the original image is not known exactly. However, for simulated data it is a good measurement of the quality of the restoration comparing the original image and the restored one. The original image is degraded according to the physical assumptions of the fluorescence microscopy serving as basis for the restoration algorithm.

3 Results

The results of simulated images can be seen in table 1. In the first row the I-div and the MSE of the original and the degraded image is shown. In the second row the quality measurement of the well-known RL approach with TV is listed and in the last row the results of the new algorithm can be seen.

In figure 1 the result of the algorithms can be seen. In 1a) the original image is shown and in 1b) the noisy and blurry image used for the simulation. Figure 1c) shows the result of the RL with TV algorithm and 1d) the result of the new developed algorithm.

4 Discussion

We have proved that the quality of the reconstructed images can be improved by using the new algorithm compared with RL and TV, as shown in table 1. Both the I-div and the MSE show an approximately 15% better value for the reconstructed images. The new algorithm is able to reconstruct finer structures in the image as well.

The result of the new algorithm is highly dependent on the amount of Bregman iterations. With a very high number of iterations the algorithm would reconstruct the degraded image itself which is not the requested result. To start

Fig. 1. a) original image b) blurry and noisy c) RL & TV d) new algorithm

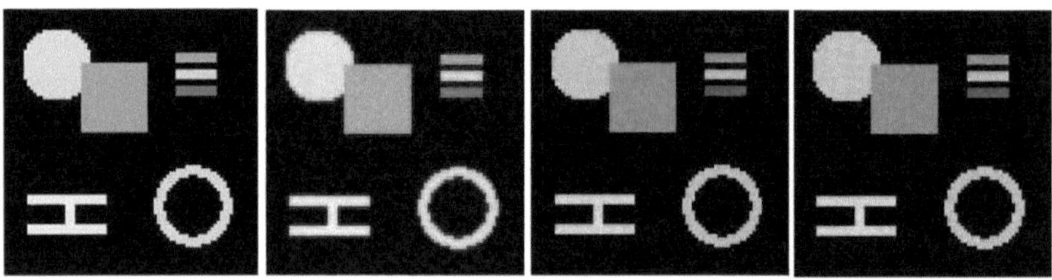

the algorithm an empty image is used which is reconstructed iteratively. In every step finer structures are reconstructed which means that after some iterations the noise is reconstructed as well. During the iterative process before the noise is reconstructed the intermediate result is very close to the original image which is a very good solution for the reconstruction. It is difficult to stop the algorithm in case of real images where the original image is not known. One possibility is to use the discrepancy principle [8] to stop the algorithm and we plan to add that to the new algorithm in future.

References

1. Lucy LB. An iterative technique for rectification of observed distributions. Astronom J 1974;79(6):745–65.
2. Dellard F. The expectation maximization algorithm. Technical Report number GIT-GVU-02-20, 2002.
3. Van Kempen GMP, Van Vliet LJ. The influence of the regularization parameter and the first estimate on the performance of Tikhonov regularized non-linear image restoration algorithms. J Microsc 2000;198(1):63–75.
4. Dey N, et al. Richardson-Lucy algorithm with total Variation regularization for 3D microscope deconvolution. Microsc Res Tech 2006;69:260–6.
5. Bregman L: The relaxation model of finding the common points of convex sets and its application to the solution of problems in convex programming. Comput Math Math Phys 1967;7:200–17.
6. He L, Marquina A, Osher SJ. Blind deconvolution using TV regularization and Bregman iteration. Int J Imaging Syst Tech 2005;15(1):74–83.
7. Marquina A, Osher SJ. Image Super-Resolution by TV-Regularization. 2007.
8. Lie J, Nordbotton J. Inverse scale space for nonlinear regularization. J Math Imaging Vis Arch 2007;27(1):41–50.

Intersection Line Length Normalization in CT Projection Data

Jan Müller, Thorsten M. Buzug

Institute of Medical Engineering, University of Lübeck, 23538 Lübeck, Germany
mueller@imt.uni-luebeck.de

Abstract. We present a method to improve the quality of common sinogram restoration algorithms, which are used for metal-artifact reduction in X-ray CT. The presented approach is based on the idea that the intersection length of all beams through the object of interest can approximately be calculated from a preliminary reconstruction of the object. Incorporating this information to the reconstruction allows significant reduction of streak artifacts. Additionally, it is shown that the information about intersection length may also be used to improve the detection of metal shadows within the sinogram.

1 Introduction

As shown on the left side in Fig. 1, metal objects inside the field of view cause artifacts in the reconstructed CT image. The predominant effect for these artifacts arises from inconsistent sinogram entries, which are a direct consequence of non-linear beam-hardening. One approach to correct for these erroneous values and, therefore, to reduce metal artifacts is to replace all corrupted sinogram entries with artificially generated values. If these surrogate values are chosen for instance by incorporating a priori knowledge, the quality of the reconstructed image is improved. There are several ways to calculate these artificial values. Two methods, which are related to each other are presented in [1] and [2]. A chain of clustering, segmentation and forward/backward projection is used to reconstruct a preliminary image, which represents an approximate distribution of air, soft tissue, and bones. A forward projection of this image is then used to fill the gaps in the original sinogram. A second approach is presented in [3] and [4]. Here, corrupted data is replaced with interpolated values from adjacent detectors. This interpolation is usually done independently for each view. In [5] a method is proposed, which uses data from more than one view to generate new values by means of an directional interpolation scheme.

In the present paper a method is proposed that can generally be incorporated into any interpolation based method. It is shown that a normalization of the sinogram improves both the reduction of metal artifacts and the detection of corrupted data compared to interpolation methods based on the original projection data.

Fig. 1. The uncorrected reconstruction f (left) and the image support supp(f) (right), which is generated from an image which was corrected with a common metal artifact reduction method (Fig. 4)

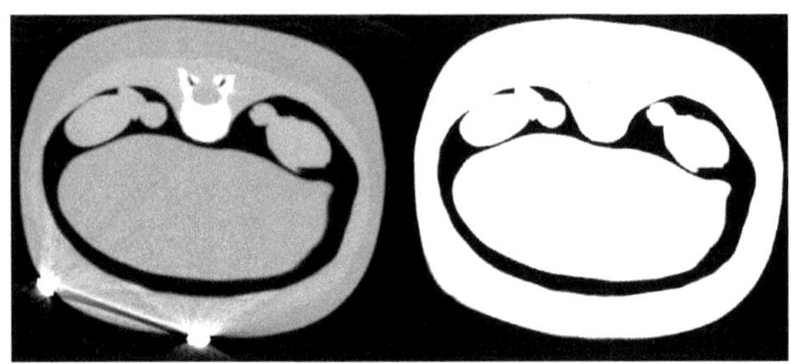

2 Methods

A problem which complicates the interpolation (and also the actual detection of corrupted sinogram entries) is that the value of a particular sinogram entry does not only depend on the material of the object but also on the intersection line length of the corresponding beam through the object: For example, a beam attenuated by a metal object and having a short intersection line with the body may have a smaller attenuation value than a beam, which is only attenuated by soft tissue and bone, but having a long intersection line through the body.

To reduce this influence, a normalization of the sinogram with respect to the intersection line lengths of each beam is proposed. It is based on the idea that the shape of an object can be approximately reconstructed even if the projection data is corrupted by the presence of metal objects. The calculation of the normalized data and its application to metal artifact reduction are as follows:

1. Creation a binary image which separates air and tissue (Fig. 1)
2. Calculation of a forward projection of the image. The values of this data are proportional to the intersection line length of each beam with the object (Fig. 2, middle image)
3. Division of the original sinogram data by the intersection length information. This results in a normalized sinogram, which contains the average attenuation value for each beam (Fig. 2, right image)
4. Detection of metal shadows and/or application interpolation based metal artifact reduction methods
5. Multiplication of the corrected normalized sinogram by the length-sinogram
6. Reconstruction of the image

Since metal artifacts in the uncorrected reconstruction may complicate the binarization process, it is recommend to apply a simple sinogram interpolation scheme as presented in [3] and [4]. Although this preliminary reconstruction still contains artifacts (Fig. 4, top row), it is nevertheless possible to extract shape information with a simple thresholding segmentation. The division in step 3 must

Fig. 2. The original sinogram (left), the forward projection of the mask (center) and the normalized sinogram (right)

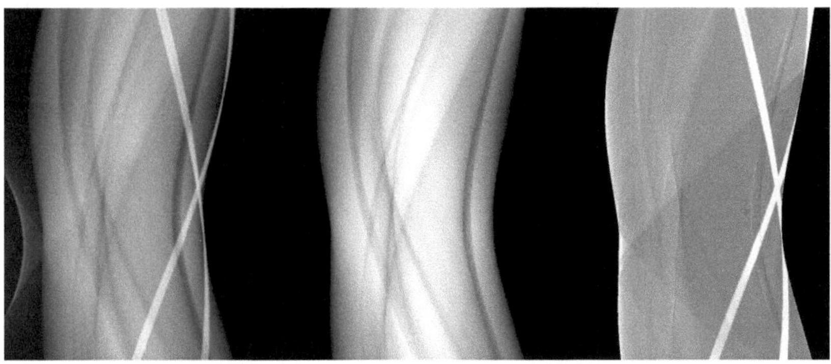

be regularized in order to avoid divisions by very small numbers or zero at the edge of the object.

To demonstrate the influence of the normalization a scan of an abdominal CT-phantom with two externally attached steel markers is used. The corresponding sinogram is shown in Fig. 2. The reconstructed cross section including the metal artifacts can be seen in Fig. 1 and Fig. 4 respectively. The sinogram was restored using the linear and spline based methods as described in [3] and [4]. Additionally, the same interpolation methods were both applied to the normalized sinogram.

3 Results

All three sinogram types are presented in Fig. 2. The profile of one view from the original and the normalized sinogram are plotted in Fig. 3. As it can be seen, the overall appearance of the averaged sinogram is flatter than the original one. Beams through metal objects are more prominent, because of their larger normalized attenuation. This information can be used for more advanced detection schemes of metal shadows. However, the present paper deals only with the improvement of the performance of the interpolation.

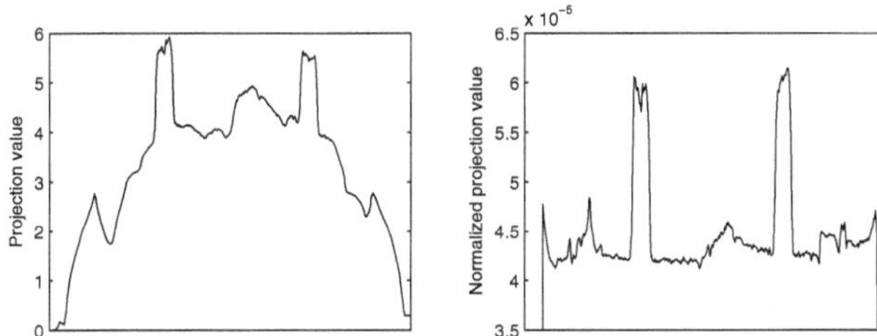

Fig. 3. The same view for both the original and the normalized sinogram

Fig. 4. Upper row: the uncorrected reconstruction of the phantom with (left) and without (right) markers. The second image serves as ground truth. Middle row: traditional linear (left) and spline (right) interpolation. Bottom row: the same interpolation methods, but this time applied to normalized sinogram data

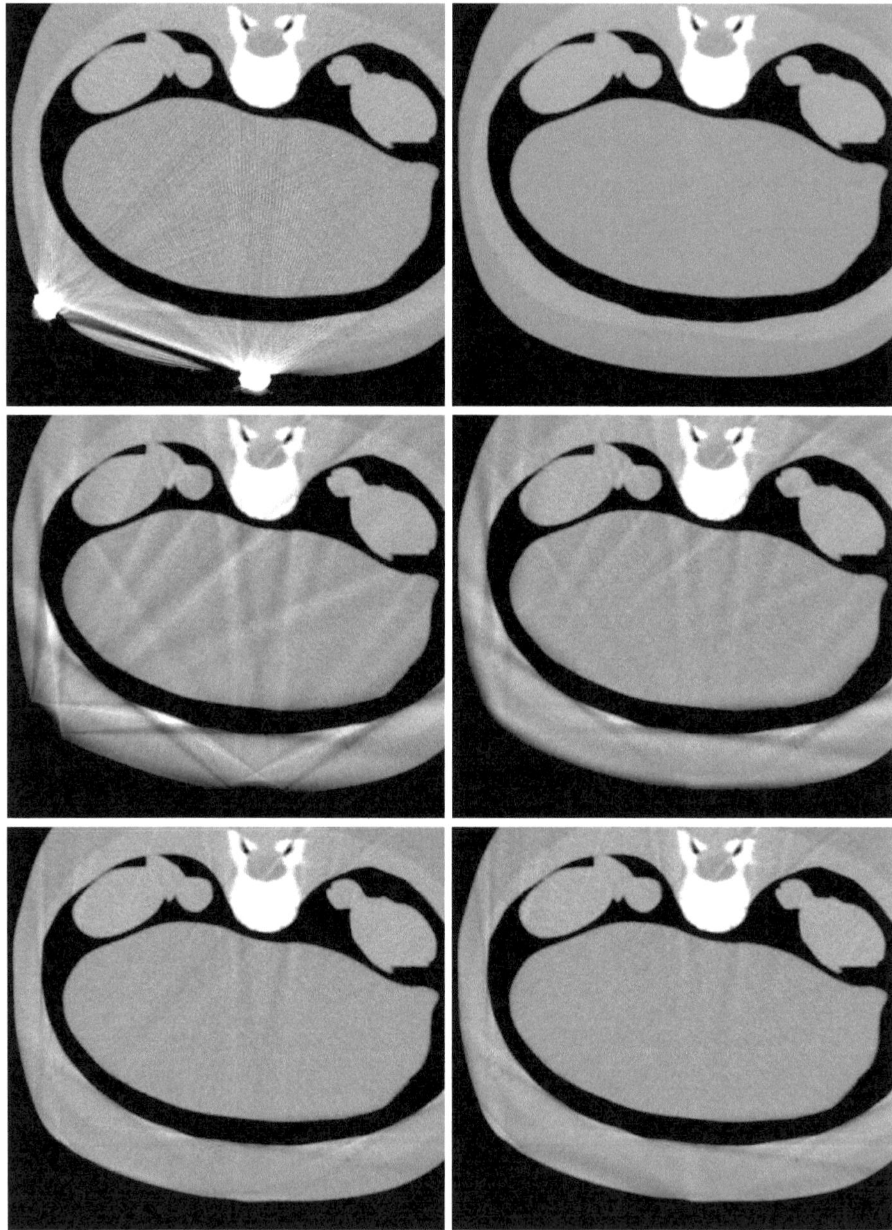

Fig. 5. Top row: Projection data with (left) and without (right) metal markers. The second scan serves as ground truth. Bottom row: Restorated sinograms using linear interpolation on original (left) and normalized (right) data.

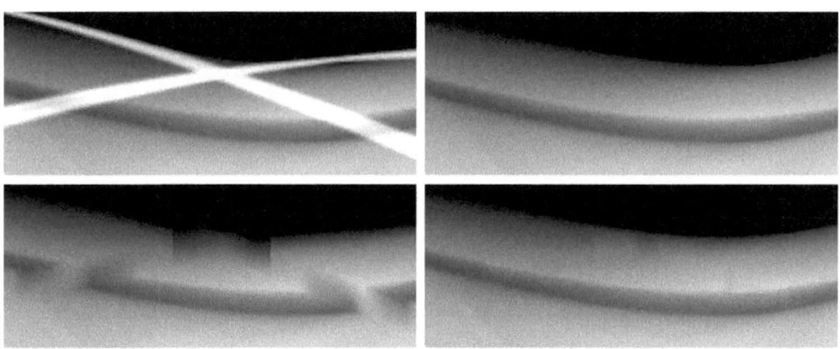

In the lower row of Fig. 5, results of the linear interpolation method applied to original (left) and normalized (right) data are shown. The interpolation result using normalized data resembles the ground truth data (upper right image) more closely, because the sinusoidal traces in the sinogram propagate into the interpolated areas in a natural way. The reconstruction results for linear (left) and spline based (right) interpolation methods applied to both type of datasets are shown in Fig. 4. As it can be seen, the use of normalized data significantly reduces streak artifacts which are characteristic for common interpolation based sinogram restoration methods.

4 Discussion

The results presented in Fig. 5 show that the combination of normalized sinogram data and simple interpolation schemes leads to a more plausible interpolation and, therefore, to a considerable reduction of interpolation artifacts (Fig. 4). The reason for this is, that at least an approximate calculation of the intersection length is possible for all beams. Thus, some information of the discarded projection data is still known and can be used to improve the interpolation.

References

1. Bal M, Spies L. Metal artifact reduction in CT using tissue-class modeling and adaptive prefiltering. Med Phys. 2006;33(8):2852–9.
2. Schmitt H, Timmer J, Koehler T. A three-pass method for metal artifact reduction in computed tomography. Med Phys. 2007;34:2571.
3. Glover GH, Pelc NJ. An algorithm for the reduction of metal clip artifacts in CT reconstructions. Med Phys. 1981;8(6):799–807.
4. Kalender WA, Hebel R, Ebersberger J. Reduction of CT artifacts caused by metallic implants. Radiology. 1987;164(2):576–7.
5. Oehler M, Buzug TM. Statistical image reconstruction for inconsistent CT projection data. Methods Inf Med. 2007;3:261–9.

Validation Metrics for Non-rigid Registration of Medical Images Containing Vessel Trees

Thomas Lange[1], Hans Lamecker[2], Michael Hünerbein[1], Sebastian Eulenstein[1], Siegfried Beller[1], Peter M. Schlag[1]

[1]Department of Surgery and Surgical Oncology, Charité - Universitätsmedizin Berlin
[2]Zuse Institute Berlin
thomas.lange@charite.de

Abstract. Validation of non-rigid registration methods is still a challenging task. Different evaluation criteria were published, yet no widely accepted gold standard exists. The aim of this paper is to provide quantitative evaluation metrics suited for clinical 3D images containing vessel trees, such as liver or brain data. We present a method to identify corresponding points on different vessel trees by extracting consistent graph minors interactively. Four different metrics based on these correspondencies are proposed.

1 Introduction

Validation of non-rigid registration approaches is a difficult problem. While an accepted gold standard exists for validation of rigid registration methods[1] only few papers address this issue for non-rigid registration [2, 3]. The published methods are based on simulated data or physical phantoms [4] on the one hand and a restriction of the validation to some important anatomical structures that can be identified in real clinical data on the other hand. The restricted validation on anatomical structures can be based on richly annotated (labeled, segmented) real images [3] or interactively assigned corresponding anatomical landmarks [5].

Since it is challenging to generate simulated data or physical phantoms, possessing realistic imaging and deformation properties, we focus on restricted validation methods for real clinical data. Often vessel trees are suitable anatomical structures for registration validation in particular in liver and neurosurgery.

In a first step corresponding vessel branchings in both modalities are identified interactively. Then an automatic algorithm determines corresponding substructures (graph minors) of the vessel trees while verifying their consistency. Four evaluation metrics are defined on those substructures. To validate a non-rigid registration result the vessels in the model data are deformed with the computed transformation and the metrics measure how close corresponding vessel parts in the reference data are after the transformation.

2 Methods

It is assumed, that a segmentation and center line extraction (via skeletonization) of the vessel trees from two different data sets (e.g. CT and 3D ultrasound) exists. In our case the center lines consist of linearly interpolated 3D node point sequences. Based on those nodes the vessels can be represented as a tree (Fig 1a). Let $T = (V, E)$ and $\hat{T} = (\hat{V}, \hat{E})$ be directed trees for the reference resp. model data. All edges point in the direction to the given root nodes $r \in V$ and $\hat{r} \in \hat{V}$. The node subsets $B \subseteq V$ and $\hat{B} \subseteq \hat{V}$ contain all branching nodes (node degree $\delta(v) > 2$). Let $P(v, w)$ be the unique path from node v to node w. We call a path between two branching nodes or a branching and an end node ($\delta(v) = 1$) a (vessel) segment path.

The trees $T, \hat{T}$ are not identical and only parts of the underlying anatomical vessel tree (supertree) can be identified in both modalities. There is no subtree isomorphism of $T, \hat{T}$ to a common supertree and even no homeomorphism. Due to missing branches a segment path in T might be represented by several segment paths in $\hat{T}$ and vice versa (Fig. 1a). In addition the order of branching points or other topological changes might occur (Fig.1b) caused by inaccuracies in the image processing pipeline. To get a subtree isomorphism the contraction of some segment paths to one single node is necessary. This means a supertree contains T and $\hat{T}$ as a minor. Intuitively, a graph G is a minor of a graph H, if G can be obtained from H by a series of vertex/edge deletions and edge contractions.

As the consistent assignment of branching nodes and segment paths is only heuristically solvable based on geometric properties [6], we interactively define a subset of corresponding branching points $(b_i, \hat{b}_i)$, $i = 1, \ldots, n$, $b_i \in B, \hat{b}_i \in \hat{B}$. Let $B_{corr}, \hat{B}_{corr}$ contain all b_i resp. $\hat{b}_i$. To ease the interaction, a mouse click can be set onto the vessel surface nearby the branching point and the nearest branching point on the center line graph is determined automatically.

2.1 Determination of Corresponding Segment Paths

Algorithm 1 determines for two given vessel center line trees $T, \hat{T}$ and a subset of corresponding branching node pairs $(b_i, \hat{b}_i), i = 1 \ldots n$ corresponding path pairs

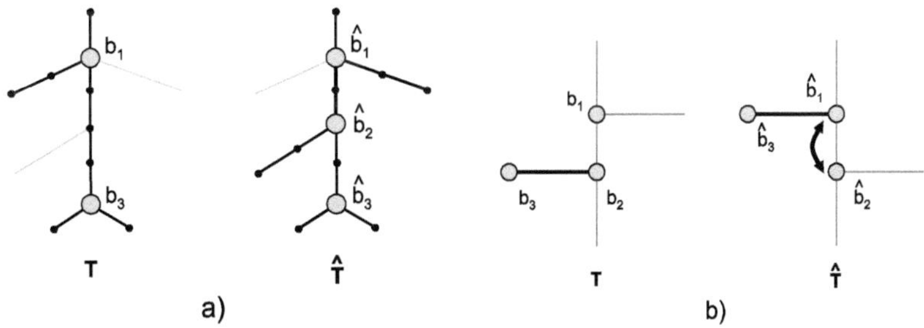

Fig. 1. a) Reference T and model tree $\hat{T}$are minors of the underlying anatomical tree (grey). b) Caused by inaccuracies the order of the branching nodes might be exchanged.

$(P_i, \hat{P}_i)$. As the directed path to the root is unique, the algorithm starts from each corresponding branching point and ends, if another corresponding branching point or a point, which has already been visited, has been reached. The second termination criterion is necessary because not all branching points might have been interactively assigned. It is important to check if the reached points are an assigned branching point pair in order to detect topological or assignment errors. Most of the inconsistencies can be resolved by automatic contraction of very short segment paths. Remaining problems are eliminated interactively. Based on the resulting path pairs each model path $\hat{P}_i$ is reparameterized according to the reference path P_i. This means the relative distances between successive reference nodes are transfered to the length of the model path. Now each node on a reference line corresponds to a point on the model line. Let $(p_j, \hat{p_j}), j = 1, \ldots, m$ be all corresponding point pairs on all segments.

Algorithm 1 *CorrespondingPaths*

All nodes in V and $\hat{V}$ are unmarked.
for $n = 1$ to n **do**
  Let $v := b_i$, $\hat{v} := \hat{b}_i$ {Start with corres. node pair}
  repeat
    Mark v, $v := parent(v)$
  until v is already marked or $v \in B_{corr}$ or v is root r
  repeat
    Mark $\hat{v}$, $\hat{v} := parent(\hat{v})$
  until $\hat{v}$ is already marked or $\hat{v} \in \hat{B}_{corr}$ or $\hat{v}$ is root $\hat{r}$
  if $(v, \hat{v})$ is a corresponding node pair $(b_j, \hat{b}_j)$ **then**
    Set $P_i := P(b_i, v)$ and $\hat{P}_i := P(\hat{b}_i, \hat{v})$
  else
    Set $P_i := \emptyset$ and $\hat{P}_i := \emptyset$
    print Resolve topological inconsistency at paths starting at $(b_i, \hat{b}_i)$
  end if
end for

2.2 Evaluation Metrics

Distance of corresponding points on center lines: The most simple metric is the average distance between corresponding point pairs.

$$M_{dist}(T, \hat{T}) := \frac{1}{m} \sum_{j=1}^{m} \|p_j - \hat{p}_j\| \tag{1}$$

Weighted point distance: The corresponding center line points are generated with some location uncertainties. The uncertainties along the lines are usually higher than perpendicular to the lines. In particular location uncertainties of the branching points lead to translations of the correspondences along the lines. Let Σ_j be an estimated covariance matrix of the anisotropic location uncertainty for the point pair $(p_j, \hat{p}_j)$. Based on these weighting matrices a weighted distance measure can be defined [7]:

$$M_{weighted}(T, \hat{T}) := \frac{1}{m} \sum_{j=1}^{m} (p_j - \hat{p}_j)^T \Sigma_j^{-1} (p_j - \hat{p}_j) \tag{2}$$

Directional deviation metric: From the vessel center lines in each corresponding point pair $(p_j, \hat{p}_j)$ (except in the branching points) a normalized tangential vector pair $(d_j, \hat{d}_j)$ can be computed. The sine of the angle between the direction vectors is a measure for the deviation of the two directions. As the cross product $(\times)$ is related to the sine an evaluation metric can be defined by:

$$M_{dir}(T, \hat{T}) = \frac{1}{m} \sum_{j=1}^{m} \left\| d_j \times \hat{d}_j \right\| \tag{3}$$

Segment-wise relative volume overlap: A metric that is less dependent on the center line extraction is the relative volume overlap of corresponding vessel segments. Each voxel is assigned to the closest segment path point. For all points on corresponding segment paths $P_i, \hat{P}_i$ the assigned voxels define the volumes $V_i, \hat{V}_i$ of the particular segments.

$$M_{vol}(T, \hat{T}) := \frac{1}{n} \sum_{i=1}^{n} \frac{V_i \cap W_i}{V_i \cup W_i} \tag{4}$$

3 Results

The corresponding path algorithm has been exemplarily applied to the portal veins extracted from preoperative contrast-enhanced CT (Fig. 2a) and intraop-

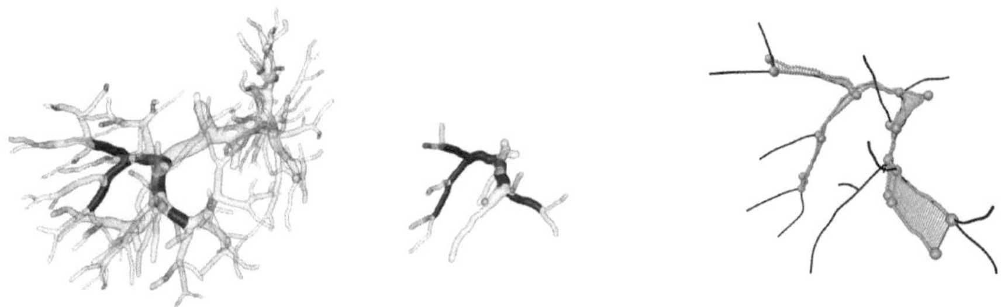

Fig. 2. a) Portal veins extracted from contrast-enhanced CT data and b) from 3D Powerdoppler ultrasound data (black: corresponding vessel segments). c) Vessel center lines from ultrasound data (black) and corresponding points in CT data (small spheres and grey lines) determined from corresp. branching nodes (big spheres).

erative 3D powerdoppler ultrasound data (Fig. 2b). Based on the corresponding center line point pairs a rigid transformation was computed. The remaining deviations of the vessels are illustrated in Fig. 2c) and are on average 4.5 mm.

4 Discussion and Future Work

In computer assisted liver surgery one important task is to non-rigidly register preoperative 3D models of anatomical structures to intraoperative 3D ultrasound data [8, 9] which are the reference data for navigation systems in liver surgery [10]. We introduced validation methods for the accuracy of non-rigid registration approaches on image pairs containing vessel trees. Each validation metric stresses a different aspect of registration accuracy. The metrics can be applied for registration validation of preoperative CT with intraoperative ultrasound data or pre- and postoperative CT data of the liver for follow-up studies. The aim is to generate a database of corresponding segment paths for portal and hepatic veins from 20-25 cases for each of the two applications. One important future task is to improve the precision of the center line extraction and to investigate the remaining uncertainties of the correspondences more rigorously. In particular the segmentation of the vessels might be improved by fitting local vessel models.

References

1. West J, Fitzpatrick JM, Wang MY, et al. Comparison and evaluation of retrospective intermodality brain image registration techniques. J Comput Assist Tomogr. 1997;21(4):554–66.
2. Hellier P, Barillot C, Corouge I, et al. Retrospective evaluation of inter-subject brain registration. Proc MICCAI. 2001; p. 258–65.
3. Christensen G, Geng X, Kuhl J, et al. Introduction to the non-rigid image registration evaluation project (NIREP). Proc WBIR. 2006; p. 128–35.
4. Reinertsen I, Descoteaux M, Siddiqi K, et al. Validation of vessel-based registration for correction of brain shift. Med Image Anal. 2007;11(4):374–88.
5. Reinertsen I, Lindseth F, Unsgaard G, et al. Clinical validation of vessel-based registration for correction of brain-shift. Med Image Anal. 2007;11(6):673–84.
6. Charnoz A, Agnus V, Malandain G, et al. Design of robust vascular tree matching: Validation on liver. Proc IPMI. 2005; p. 443–55.
7. Rohr K, Stiehl H, Sprengel R, et al. Landmark-Based Elastic Registration Using Approximating Thin-Plate Splines. IEEE Trans Med Imaging. 2001;20(6):526–34.
8. Lange T, Eulenstein S, Hünerbein M, et al. Augmenting intraoperative 3D ultrasound with preoperative models for navigation in liver surgery. Lect Notes Comp Sci. 2004;3217:534–41.
9. Lange T, Lamecker H, Hünerbein M, et al. A new class of distance measures for registration of tubular models to image data. Proc BVM. 2007; p. 101–5.
10. Beller S, Hünerbein M, Eulenstein S, et al. Feasibility of navigated resection of liver tumors using multiplanar visualization of intraoperative 3D ultrasound data. Annal Surg. 2007;246(2):288–94.

Effiziente nichtlineare Registrierung mittels diskreter Optimierung

Ben Glocker[1,2], Nikos Komodakis[1,3], Nikos Paragios[1], Georgios Tziritas[3], Nassir Navab[2]

[1]GALEN Group, Mathématiques Appliquées aux Systèmes, Ecole Centrale de Paris
[2]Computer Aided Medical Procedures (CAMP), Technische Universität München
[3]Computer Science Department, University of Crete
glocker@in.tum.de

Kurzfassung. In diesem Beitrag wird eine neuartige Methode für die nichtlineare Bildregistrierung vorgestellt. Dabei wird das klassische Energieminimierungsproblem Intensitäts-basierter Methoden in eine Markov Random Field Formulierung eingebettet. Dieses ermöglicht die Nutzung von effizienten diskreten Optimierungsmethoden, die unabhängig von der tatsächlich verwendeten Kostenfunktion eine quasi-optimale Lösung berechnen. Free Form Deformations werden als Transformationsmodell in Betracht gezogen und die Registrierung wird so auf ein diskretes Labeling-Problem reduziert. Jedem Kontrollpunkt wird eine Verschiebung zugeordnet und so die optimale Konfiguration des Modells errechnet. Das viel versprechende Potential des Frameworks wird klinischen Daten evaluiert.

1 Einleitung

Die nichtlineare Registrierung ist eine der schwierigsten Problemstellungen in der medizinischen Bildverarbeitung. Allgemeines Ziel dabei ist es, eine lokale Transformation zu bestimmen, die zwei Signale zueinander in Beziehung setzt. Obwohl diese Signale gleiche oder zumindest ähnliche Objekte abbilden, unterscheiden sie sich oftmals erheblich in ihrer Form und Intensität, wie zum Beispiel in der Bildregistrierung bei Daten aus unterschiedlichen Bildmodalitäten. Da die abgebildeten Objekte oftmals zusätzlich ihre Form über die Zeit ändern, werden Methoden benötigt, die diese nichtlineare Beziehung berücksichtigen und kompensieren können. Um die entsprechende Transformation zu berechnen, wird häufig ein mathematisches Modell in Form einer Kostenfunktion aufgestellt, die im allgemeinen hochgradig nichtkonvex, und daher schwierig zu optimieren ist. Viele der in der Literatur vorgeschlagenen Methoden können nur suboptimale Lösungen liefern. In diesem Beitrag stellen wir ein neuartiges Framework zur nichtlinearen Bildregistrierung vor. Die hier präsentierte Kombination von kontinuierlichen Deformationsmodellen mit diskreten Optimierungsmethoden hat zwei entscheidende Vorteile:

1. Nutzung von effizienten und diskreten Optimierungsalgorithmen mit quasi-optimalen Lösungen

2. Unabhängigkeit und damit Flexibilität in der Auswahl der Kostenfunktion

Nichtlineare, lokale Bildregistrierung wird oft anhand geometrischer oder photometrischer Kriterien durchgeführt. Landmarken-basierte Verfahren [1, 2] sind klassische Beispiele für Verfahren, die geometrische Merkmale benutzen. Oft werden dafür anatomische Merkmale [3] oder Strukturen extrahiert, die zum Beispiel mittels Minimierung der Euklidischen Distanz registriert werden. Ein Hauptnachteil dabei ist die teilweise schwierige Selektion und Extraktion von geeigneten Landmarken, wo hingegen die Stärke in der Einfachheit des Optimierungsprozesses liegt.

Intensitäts-basierte Verfahren suchen nach visuellen Korrespondenzen zwischen dem Ziel- und Quellbild [4] und versuchen mittels Gradientabstiegsverfahren [5] oder variationellen Methoden [6] eine Kostenfunktion basierend auf einem Ähnlichkeitsmaß zu minimieren. Ähnlichkeitsmaße können dabei zum Beispiel die Summe der quadrierten Differenzen [7], Cross Correlation [7] oder nichtlineare Maße, wie Mutual Information [8], Kullback-Liebler divergence [9] oder Correlation Ratio [10] sein. Die Implementierung des Optimierungsprozesses muss dabei meist speziell auf das verwendete Ähnlichkeitsmaß angepaßt werden.

2 Material und Methoden

In diesem Beitrag präsentieren wir eine neue Methode, die für intra- und intermodale nichtlineare Bildregistrierung genutzt werden kann. Um die Glattheit des zu bestimmenden Deformationsfeldes zu garantieren und den Parameterraum des Problems zu reduzieren repräsentieren wir die Transformation mittels Free Form Deformations (FFD). Das Registrierungsproblem wird in eine Markov Random Field (MRF) Formulierung eingebettet und mit Hilfe effizienter MRF-Algorithmen gelöst, wobei eine Zuordnung von sogenannten Labels zu den Kontrollpunkten berechnet wird, die eine Minimierung der Kostenfunktion zum Ziel hat. Die Optimierung ist dabei unabhängig von der Konstruktion des MRFs und damit unabhängig von der Wahl der Kostenfunktion, da keine Ableitungen bestimmt werden müssen. Unseres Wissens, ist dies die erste Arbeit, in der kontinuierliche Deformationsmodelle, wie FFD, mit effizienter MRF-Optimierung kombiniert werden. Neben der bereits erwähnten Vorteile, die Unabhängigkeit von der Kostenfunktion und den quasi-optimalen Lösungen durch die diskrete Optimierung, wird eine signifikante Verbesserung der Performanz im Vergleich zu herkömmlichen Methoden basierend auf Gradientabstiegs-Verfahren erzielt.

Im Folgenden wird die mathematische Herleitung unseres Frameworks skizziert. Für weitere Details verweisen wir auf [11]. Das Registrierungsproblem kann als Energieminimierungsproblem formuliert werden:

$$E(\mathcal{T}) = \int_{\Omega} \rho(g(\mathbf{x}), f(\mathcal{T}(\mathbf{x})))d\mathbf{x} \tag{1}$$

wobei $\mathcal{T}$ die gesuchte Transformation des Quellbildes f beschreibt, um dieses mit dem Zielbild g zu registrieren. Die optimale Registrierung wird durch Minimierung der Energie E unter Berücksichtigung des Ähnlichkeitsmaßes ρ erreicht.

Das Transformationsmodell und das zugehörige Deformationsfeld $\mathcal{D}$ basierend auf FFD kann wie folgt formuliert werden:

$$\mathcal{T}(\mathbf{x}) = \mathbf{x} + \mathcal{D}(\mathbf{x}) \quad \text{und} \quad \mathcal{D}(\mathbf{x}) = \sum_{p \in G} \eta(|\mathbf{x} - \mathbf{p}|)\, \mathbf{d}_p \tag{2}$$

wobei $\eta(\,\cdot\,)$ die Gewichtungsfunktion ist, die den den Einfluss der einzelnen Kontrollpunkte bestimmt. In unserer Implementierung betrachten wir hierfür kubische B-Splines. Die neutrale Position eines Kontrollpunkts wird als $\mathbf{p}$ definiert und dessen aktuelle Verschiebung durch $\mathbf{d}_p$. Ziel ist die optimale Konfiguration der Kontrollpunkte zu bestimmen, so dass die beiden Bilder bestmöglich registriert sind.

Unser neuartiger Ansatz für die Lösung dieses Problems beruht auf der Idee, das Problem als diskretes Labeling aufzufassen. Dabei agieren die Kontrollpunkte als diskrete Variablen und die möglichen Verschiebungen $\mathbf{d}_p$ werden durch sogenannte Labels u_p ausgedrückt. Jedem Kontrollpunkt wird ein Label zugewiesen, dass die bestmögliche Deformierung beschreibt. Ein solches diskretes Labeling-Problem kann als klassisches MRF-Problem ausgedrückt werden:

$$E_{\text{total}}(u) = \sum_{p \in G} V_p(u_p) + \sum_{p,q \in N} V_{pq}(u_p, u_q) \tag{3}$$

Hierbei steht u für das Labeling. Die sogenannten Singleton Potentials $V_p(u_p)$ beschreiben die Kosten, die eine Zuweisung des Labels u_p zu dem Kontrollpunkt $p \in G$ verursachen. Die Pairwise Potentials dienen als Regularisierungsterm für die Zuweisung der Labels u_p und u_q an die benachbarten Kontrollpunkte $p, q \in N$. Durch eine proportionale Bestrafung der Distanz zwischen zwei Labels wird eine Glättung des resultierenden Labelings erreicht.

Um das Registrierungsproblem in die MRF-Formulierung einzubetten, definieren wir die beiden Potentialfunktionen wie folgt:

$$V_p(u_p) = \frac{1}{|G|} \int_{\Omega} \eta^{-1}(|\mathbf{x} - \mathbf{p}|) \rho(g(\mathbf{x}), f(\mathbf{x} + \mathbf{d}^{u_p})) d\mathbf{x} \tag{4}$$

Diese Datenterme können als lokale Auswertung des Ähnlichkeitsmaßes aufgefasst werden. An jedem Kontrollpunkt wird entsprechend der inversen Gewichtungsfunktion [11], ausgedrückt durch η^{-1}, bestimmt, wie gut die Registrierung lokal im Bereich des Kontrollpunkts ist. Als Regularisierungsterm betrachten wir eine stückweise glatte Distanzfunktion:

$$V_{pq}(u_p, u_q) = \lambda_{pq} \min\left(|\mathbf{d}^{u_p} - \mathbf{d}^{u_q}|, T\right) \tag{5}$$

Da die Menge der Labels endlich definiert wird, jedoch die vorliegende Deformation oftmals unbekannt ist, benutzen wir einen Multi-Level Ansatz. Sowohl die Bild- und FFD-Auflösung wird sukzessive erhöht als auch die Menge der möglichen Kontrollpunktverschiebungen sukzessive verfeinert [11].

Für die Optimierung verwenden wir einen kürzlich entwickelten effizienten MRF-Optimierungsalgorithmus basierend auf linearer Programmierung, Fast-PD [12]. Dessen Stärke liegt insbesondere in der hohen Performanz und den quasi-optimalen Lösungen für MRF-Probleme.

Tabelle 1. Ergebnisse für die graue Gehirnsubstanz bei der MR Registrierung. Die linken Zahlen sind die Ergebnisse nach affiner Registrierung, rechts die Ergebnisse nach nichtlinearer Registrierung. In Klammern ist die prozentuale Verbesserung angegeben

Datensatz	DICE	Sensitivität	Spezifität
1	0.6959 / 0.8752 (26%)	0.7466 / 0.8752 (17%)	0.9650 / 0.9847 (2%)
2	0.7188 / 0.8365 (16%)	0.7082 / 0.8365 (18%)	0.9796 / 0.9894 (1%)
3	0.6964 / 0.8053 (16%)	0.6402 / 0.8053 (26%)	0.9821 / 0.9878 (1%)
4	0.7261 / 0.8927 (23%)	0.7803 / 0.8927 (14%)	0.9718 / 0.9851 (1%)
5	0.6959 / 0.8672 (25%)	0.7252 / 0.8672 (20%)	0.9695 / 0.9828 (1%)
6	0.7001 / 0.8012 (14%)	0.6214 / 0.8012 (29%)	0.9854 / 0.9901 (1%)
7	0.6900 / 0.8601 (25%)	0.6554 / 0.8601 (31%)	0.9779 / 0.9867 (1%)

3 Ergebnisse und Diskussion

Wir evaluieren unsere Registrierungsmethode quantitativ anhand medizinischer Datensätze und können zeigen, dass sub-voxel Genauigkeit mit verschiedensten Kostenfunktionen erreicht wird. Beispielhaft wird hier eines der Experimente präsentiert. Segmentierte 3D MR Gehirndatensätze werden benutzt, um die Registrierungsgenauigkeit zu bestimmen. Die Datensätze inklusive Referenzsegmentierungen wurden vom Center for Morphometric Analysis am Massachusetts General Hospital zur Verfügung gestellt und stehen unter folgender Adresse zum Download bereit: http://www.cma.mgh.harvard.edu/ibsr/. In Tabelle 1 sind die Ergebnisse zu sehen, wenn wir einen der 8 Datensätze als Atlas auswählen und zu den restlichen 7 registrieren. Die übertragene Segmentierung der grauen und

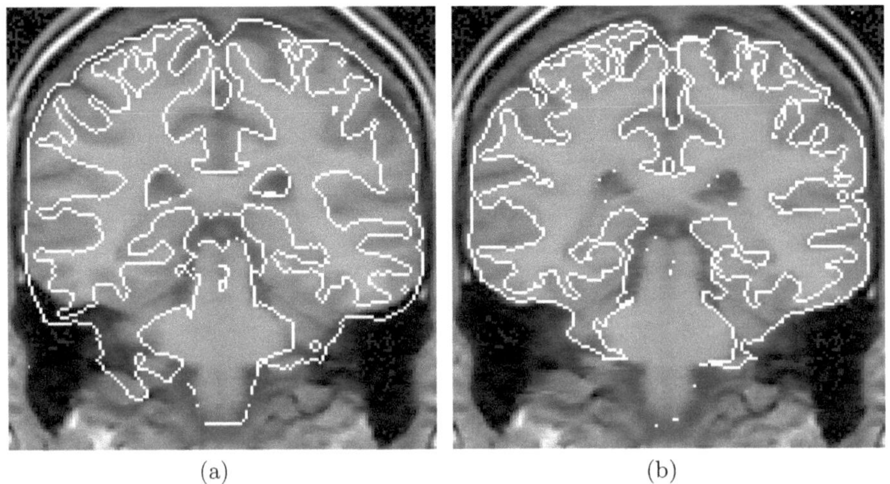

(a) (b)

Abb. 1. Überlagerung des Umrisses der grauen Gehirnsubstanz nach (a) affiner (DICE 0.726) und (b) unserer nichtlinearen Registrierung (DICE 0.893)

weißen Gehirnsubstanz wurde dann mit den entsprechenden manuellen Referenzsegmentierungen verglichen.

Weitere klinische Daten wurden benutzt, um den Vergleich mit dem bisherigen quasi Gold-Standard FFD Registrierer [5] basierend auf Gradientabstiegsverfahren zu ermöglichen. Wir konnten zeigen, dass mit unserem Framework eine 3D-3D Registrierung mit einen immensen Geschwindigkeitsvorteil bei visuell besseren Ergebnissen erzielt werden kann. Die Registrierungszeit der herkömmlichen Gradienten-basierten Methode wurde von ca. 120 Minuten auf 2 Minuten reduziert [11]. Weitere Anwendungsgebiete und Ergebnisse präsentieren wir in [13].

Literaturverzeichnis

1. Hellier P, Barillot C. Coupling dense and landmark-based approaches for nonrigid registration. IEEE Trans Med Imaging. 2003;22(2):217–27.
2. Rohr K, Fornefett M, Stiehl HS. Spline-based elastic image registration: integration of landmark errors and orientation attributes. Comp Vis Image Understand. 2003;90(2):153–68.
3. Pennec X, Ayache N, Thirion JP. Landmark-based registration using features identified through differential geometry. In: Handbook of Medical Imaging; 2000. p. 499–513.
4. Cachier P, Bardinet E, Dormont D, et al. Iconic feature based nonrigid registration: the PASHA algorithm. Comp Vis Image Understand. 2003;89(2-3):272–98.
5. Rueckert D, Sonoda L, Hayes C, et al. Nonrigid registration using free-form deformations: Application to breast MR images. IEEE Transa Med Imaging. 1999;18(8):712–21.
6. Modersitzki J. Numerical Methods for Image Registration. Oxford University Press; 2004.
7. Hajnal J, Hill DLG, Hawkes DJ, editors. Medical Image Registration. CRC Press; 2001.
8. Maes F, Collignon A, Vandermeulen D, et al. Multimodality image registration by maximization of mutual information. IEEE Trans Med Imaging. 1997;16(2):187–98.
9. Zollei L, Fisher J, Wells W. An introduction to statistical methods of medical image registration. In: Paragios N, Chen Y, Faugeras O, editors. Handbook of Mathematical Models in Computer Vision. Springer; 2005.
10. Roche A, Malandain G, Pennec X, et al. The correlation ratio as a new similarity measure for multimodal image registration. Proc MICCAI. 1998.
11. Glocker B, Komodakis N, Paragios N, et al. Inter and intra-modal deformable registration: Continuous deformations meet efficient optimal linear programming. In: Information Processing in Medical Imaging; 2007.
12. Komodakis N, Tziritas G, Paragios N. Fast, Approximately optimal solutions for single and dynamic MRFs. Proc CVPR. 2007.
13. Glocker B, Komodakis N, Paragios N, et al. Primal/Dual linear programming and statistical atlases for cartilage segmentation. Proc MICCAI. 2007.

Fluid Extensions for Optical Flow and Diffusion-Based Image Registration

Jens-Peer Kuska[1], Patrick Scheibe[2], Ulf-Dietrich Braumann[2]

[1]Interdisciplinary Centre for Bioinformatics, University Leipzig, 04107 Leipzig
[2]Translational Centre for Regenerative Medicine, University Leipzig, 04103 Leipzig
kuska@informatik.uni-leipzig.de

Abstract. The present paper derives two new equations for the nonlinear registration of images based on Euler-Lagrange equations. It offers a systematic way to construct fluid extensions to registration equations based on variational principles.

1 Introduction

Nonlinear image registration has various applications in image processing ranging from three-dimensional reconstruction of serial sections over segmentation with help of image atlases to the measurement of changes during the development of a disease.

The goal of image registration is to find a vector transformation $\boldsymbol{u}(\boldsymbol{x})$ so that the sample image $S(\boldsymbol{x})$ under the transformation $S(\boldsymbol{x} - \boldsymbol{u}(\boldsymbol{x}))$ matches the template image $T(\boldsymbol{x})$. Additionally, such transformation $\boldsymbol{u}(\boldsymbol{x})$ is required to satisfy some smoothness condition. One way to obtain such a transformation is to use physically motivated equations, e.g. the Navier-Lamé equation for the deformation $\boldsymbol{u}$ [1] or solving the Navier-Lamé equation for the velocity field $\dot{\boldsymbol{u}}$ and to use the time integral of the velocity as the displacement field [2]. The variant that uses the two fields $\dot{\boldsymbol{u}}(\boldsymbol{x})$ and $\boldsymbol{u}(\boldsymbol{x})$ is called fluid registration.

Another possibility to derive a differential equation for the displacement field is to apply a variational approach [3, 4, 5, 6] that combines various conditions for the displacement field. This approach typically yields a static, time and velocity independent equation for the displacement field $\boldsymbol{u}(\boldsymbol{x})$. To obtain a smooth convergence of the nonlinear equation one introduces an artificial time and solves a diffusion-like equation [7, 8]. Since the displacement field is modified by a diffusion like process, the convergence of the variational equations is rather slow comparing to the fluid registration. The present paper offers a way to construct dynamic equations for the velocity field on the basis of variational equations without the help of fluid dynamics.

2 Materials and Methods

2.1 Undamped Equation of Motion

For the registration of the sample image $S(\boldsymbol{x})$ onto the template image $T(\boldsymbol{x})$ with $\boldsymbol{x} \in \mathbb{R}^2$, a displacement field $\boldsymbol{u}(\boldsymbol{x}, t) = (u_1(\boldsymbol{x}, t), u_2(\boldsymbol{x}, t))^\top$ with $\{\boldsymbol{u} : \mathbb{R}^2 \mapsto \mathbb{R}^2\}$

must be found so that

$$\mathcal{V}[\boldsymbol{u}] = \frac{1}{2}\int_{\Omega} (T(\boldsymbol{x}) - S(\boldsymbol{x} - \boldsymbol{u}(\boldsymbol{x}), t))^2 \, \mathrm{d}^2\boldsymbol{x} \tag{1}$$

should be minimal. The displacement field should obey some smoothness condition. We will use the function $\mathcal{T}[\dot{\boldsymbol{u}}]$ for the smoothness of the Lagrangian. For the case of optical flow-based image registration the smoothness constraint is defined as

$$\mathcal{T}_{\mathrm{F}}[\dot{\boldsymbol{u}}] = \frac{\mu}{2}\int_{\Omega} \sum_{i=1}^{2} (\Delta \dot{u}_i(\boldsymbol{x}, t))^2 \, \mathrm{d}^2\boldsymbol{x} \tag{2}$$

and for the diffusion registration

$$\mathcal{T}_{\mathrm{D}}[\dot{\boldsymbol{u}}] = -\frac{\mu}{2}\int_{\Omega} \sum_{i=1}^{2} (\nabla \dot{u}_i(\boldsymbol{x}, t))^2 \, \mathrm{d}^2\boldsymbol{x} \tag{3}$$

The Euler-Lagrange equation for

$$\mathcal{L}(\dot{\boldsymbol{u}}, \boldsymbol{u}) = \mathcal{T}[\dot{\boldsymbol{u}}] - \mathcal{V}[\boldsymbol{u}] \tag{4}$$

yields

$$\mu\frac{\mathrm{d}^2}{\mathrm{d}t^2}\left(\Delta^2 \boldsymbol{u}\right) + \left[T(\boldsymbol{x}) - S(\boldsymbol{x} - \boldsymbol{u}(\boldsymbol{x}, t))\right] \nabla S(\boldsymbol{x} - \boldsymbol{u}(\boldsymbol{x}, t) = 0 \tag{5}$$

for the optical flow-based image registration and

$$\mu\frac{\mathrm{d}^2}{\mathrm{d}t^2}\left(-\Delta \boldsymbol{u}\right) + \left[T(\boldsymbol{x}) - S(\boldsymbol{x} - \boldsymbol{u}(\boldsymbol{x}, t))\right] \nabla S(\boldsymbol{x} - \boldsymbol{u}(\boldsymbol{x}, t) = 0 \tag{6}$$

for the diffusion registration. Both equations are free from dissipation of the energy $\mathcal{H} = \mathcal{T} + \mathcal{V}$ and the solution will start to oscillate. Since we are interested in the minimum of $\mathcal{V}$ one has to add friction forces.

2.2 Dissipative Forces

Friction forces are not an integral part of the Euler-Lagrange equations but they can be included as additional summand in the force Eqns. (5) and (6), respectively. We will add two kinds of friction forces, one that act independently of the position in space, and a second force that includes the spatial dependence by space derivatives of the velocity field. As position-independent friction force the function $\boldsymbol{f}_{\mathrm{l}} = -\mu\gamma\dot{\boldsymbol{u}}$ will be used. The second dissipative force will depend on the partial derivatives of the velocity field. The Navier-Stokes equation would suggest a term proportional to $\boldsymbol{f}_{\mathrm{v}} = -\mu\nu\Delta\dot{\boldsymbol{u}}$ (the viscosity term), and for the optical flow-based case a term $\boldsymbol{f}_{\mathrm{v}} = -\mu\nu\Delta^2\dot{\boldsymbol{u}}$ will be used.

Adding the two friction forces to the left hand side of the Eqns. (5) and (6), the fluid extension for the optical flow-based registration is given by the solution of the equation

$$\mu\frac{\mathrm{d}^2}{\mathrm{d}t^2}\left(\Delta^2 \boldsymbol{u}\right) + \left[T(\boldsymbol{x}) - S(\boldsymbol{x} - \boldsymbol{u}(\boldsymbol{x}, t))\right] \nabla S(\boldsymbol{x} - \boldsymbol{u}(\boldsymbol{x}, t)) = -\mu\gamma\, \dot{\boldsymbol{u}}(\boldsymbol{x}, t) - \mu\nu\Delta^2\dot{\boldsymbol{u}}(\boldsymbol{x}, t) \tag{7}$$

and for the diffusion-based version one gets

$$\mu \frac{\mathrm{d}^2}{\mathrm{d}t^2}(-\Delta \boldsymbol{u}) + [T(\boldsymbol{x}) - S(\boldsymbol{x} - \boldsymbol{u}(\boldsymbol{x},t))]\, \nabla S(\boldsymbol{x} - \boldsymbol{u}(\boldsymbol{x},t)) = \\ -\mu\gamma\, \dot{\boldsymbol{u}}(\boldsymbol{x},t) - \mu\nu \Delta \dot{\boldsymbol{u}}(\boldsymbol{x},t). \tag{8}$$

The only force free solution of the equations is obtained for the case that the displacement field $\lim_{t\to\infty} \boldsymbol{u}(\boldsymbol{x},t)$ transforms the sample image on the template image. In this case, the force $[T(\boldsymbol{x}) - S(\boldsymbol{x} - \boldsymbol{u}(\boldsymbol{x},t))]\, \nabla S(\boldsymbol{x} - \boldsymbol{u}(\boldsymbol{x},t))$ is zero, and the friction will cause the velocity field also going to zero. The differential constraint to the velocity field may hinder a perfect match in this case, the vector fields will oscillate, but the friction term $\boldsymbol{f}_{\mathrm{v}}$ hinders the creation of waves thus keeping oscillations local. A sufficiently strong damping should restrict the local oscillation amplitude to values smaller than the pixel distance.

With the two Green functions

$$G_{\mathrm{F}}[\Delta^2 g(\boldsymbol{x})] = g(\boldsymbol{x}) \tag{9}$$

$$G_{\mathrm{D}}[(-\Delta) g(\boldsymbol{x})] = g(\boldsymbol{x}) \tag{10}$$

one gets the explicit system of second order equations that can be solved by a standard method for initial value problems. With either $G = G_{\mathrm{F}}$ or $G = G_{\mathrm{D}}$ the explicit version of the equations (7) and (8) can be written as

$$\ddot{\boldsymbol{u}}(\boldsymbol{x},t) = -\frac{1}{\mu} G\left[(T(\boldsymbol{x}) - S(\boldsymbol{x} - \boldsymbol{u}(\boldsymbol{x},t)))\, \nabla S(\boldsymbol{x} - \boldsymbol{u}(\boldsymbol{x},t))\right] \\ -\gamma\, G\left[\dot{\boldsymbol{u}}(\boldsymbol{x},t)\right] - \nu\, \dot{\boldsymbol{u}}(\boldsymbol{x},t). \tag{11}$$

3 Results

Three examples of the fluid extension of diffusion and optical flow-based registration will be shown. The integration of the equations of motion is stopped when the registered image $S(\boldsymbol{x} - \boldsymbol{u}(\boldsymbol{x}))$ does not change more than 1×10^{-5} per pixel. The intensities of sample and template image are all normalized to the interval $[0, 1]$. The step size control typically takes hundred times larger time steps for the diffusion-based registration than for the optical flow-based variant, but also requires longer absolute time intervals to achieve convergence.

The first example maps a circle on a 128×128 grid onto the letter "C" (Fig. 1a). The parameters for the optical flow-based registration are $(\mu, \nu, \gamma) = (0.5, 0.00045, 8)$ and for the diffusion-based equation $(\mu, \nu, \gamma) = (0.125, 0.00045, 8)$.

As a second example we show the transformation of an angry face onto a smiling one (Fig. 1b). This example in particular is challenging for the registration because the vector field must develop several singularities to transform the eyebrows and the mouth. To make the difference between the two displacement fields more illustrative, the distortion of a regular grid as caused by the displacement field is shown as overlay on the registration results. The parameters for the

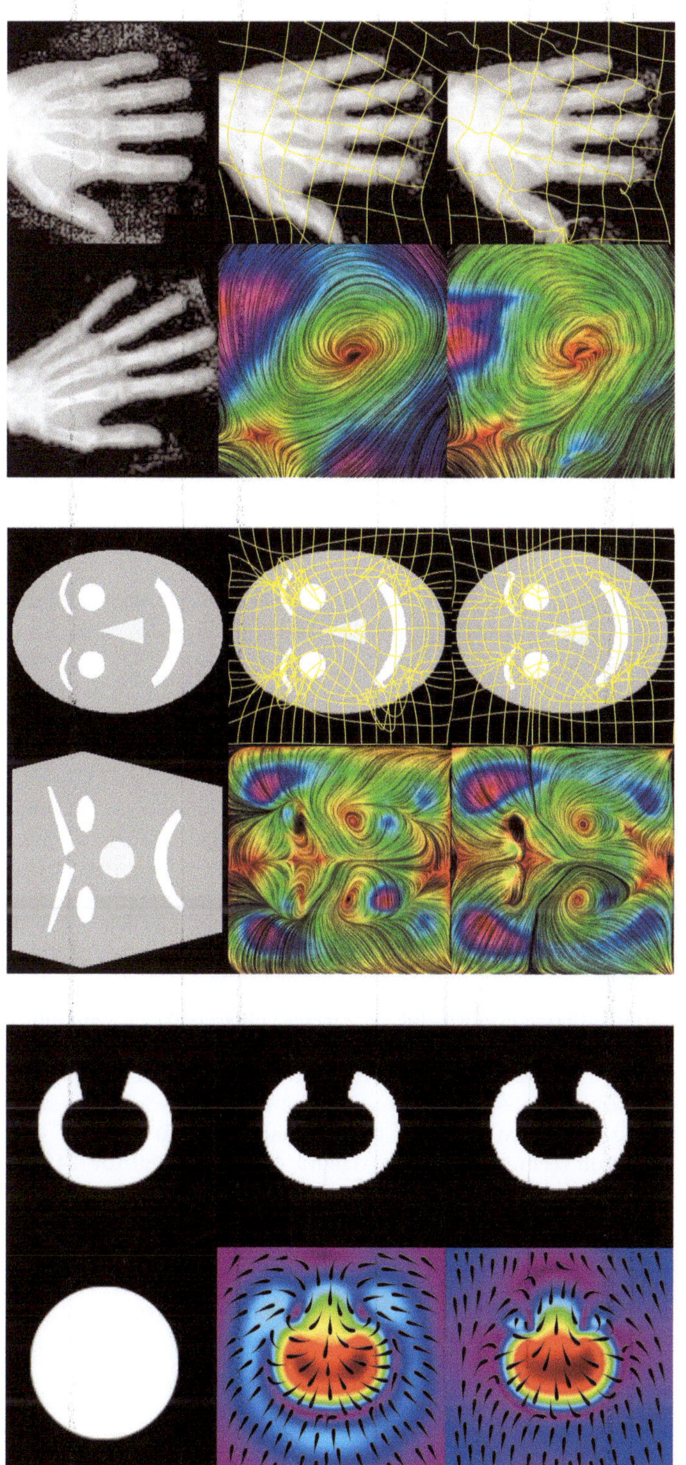

Fig. 1. Overview on three different registration tasks (top row: the image pairs; middle row: results for the fluid extension of the optical flow-based method using Eqn. (7); bottom row: results for the fluid extension of the diffusion-based method using Eqn. (8)). A: Registration of a circle onto the letter "C". B: Registration of an angry "face" onto a smiling one. C: Registration of two radiographs of different hands. The respective displacement vector fields are To underline the structure of the singularities in the respective displacement vector fields $\boldsymbol{u}(\boldsymbol{x})$, a line integral convolution [9] is used to visualize them (a: with flow fishes, b/c: with dot patterns, underlying color codes displacement magnitude)

optical flow-based version are $(\mu, \nu, \gamma) = (0.5, 0.00015, 6)$ and for the diffusion registration $(\mu, \nu, \gamma) = (0.5, 0.0003, 6)$.

The last example maps two radiographs of hands (Fig. 1c). The overlayed displacement of the regular mesh shows the lower smoothness of the diffusion registration compared with the optical flow-based variant.

4 Discussion

We have presented two new equations for nonlinear image registration based on the optical flow and the diffusion registration. Instead of the introduction of an artificial time, the new equations require a smooth velocity field and solve a system of second order differential equations for the displacement field. Both registration methods can be treated in a unified way. Based on the underlying variational approach, the design of special fluid like registration equations is possible by addition of future constrains for the displacement or the velocity field.

Acknowledgement. The project is supported by the Federal Ministry of Education and Research (BMBF), grant PTJ-BIO/31P4282 (MS CartPro) and grant PTJ-BIO/031390 (TRM Leipzig).

References

1. Christensen GE, Rabbit RD, Miller MI. Deformable templates using large deformation kinematics. IEEE Trans Image Process. 1996;10(5):1435–47.
2. Bro-Nielsen M, Gramkow C. Fast fluid registration of medical images. Proc VBC. 1996; p. 267–76.
3. Braumann UD, Kuska JP. A new equation for nonlinear image registration with control over the vortex structure in the displacement field. Proc ICIP. 2006; p. 329–32.
4. Amit Y. A nonlinear variational problem for image matching. SIAM J Sci Comp. 1994;15(1):207–24.
5. Modersitzki J. Numerical Methods for Image Registration. New York, NY: Oxford University Press; 2004.
6. Fischer B, Modersitzki J. A unified approach to fast image registration and a new curvature based registration technique. Linear Algebra Appl. 2004;380:107–24.
7. Fischer B, Modersitzki J. Fast diffusion registration. AMS Contemporary Mathematics, Inverse Problems, Image Analysis, and Medical Imaging. 2002;313:117–29.
8. Fischer B, Modersitzki J. Curvature based image registration. J Math Imaging Vis. 2003;18(1):81–5.
9. Cabral B, Leedom LC. Imaging vector fields using line integral convolution. Proc SIGGRAPH. 1993; p. 263–72.

Geometric Alignment of 2D Gel Electrophoresis Images

Stefan Wörz[1,2], Marie-Luise Winz[1,2], Karl Rohr[1,2]

[1]BIOQUANT, IPMB, University of Heidelberg, Germany
[2]Dept. Bioinformatics & Functional Genomics, DKFZ Heidelberg, Germany
s.woerz@dkfz.de

Abstract. A key technique for protein analysis is the geometric alignment of 2D gel electrophoresis (2-DE) images. We introduce a new hybrid elastic registration approach for 2-DE images, which is based on analytic solutions of the Navier equation. With this approach cross-effects in elastic deformations can be handled, which is important for the registration of 2-DE images. We have successfully applied our approach to register 2-DE gel images of different levels of complexity and have performed a quantitative evaluation of the results. We have also performed a comparison with a previous hybrid elastic registration scheme.

1 Introduction

2D gel electrophoresis (2-DE) is the method of choice for analyzing protein expression in the field of proteomics. By this technique a very large number of proteins can easily and simultaneously be separated, identified, and characterized. This is important for understanding protein function. 2-DE separates proteins based on their electrical charge and molecular mass resulting in a 2D array of dark spots (proteins) on a bright background (Fig. 1). Often a reference population is compared with a test population to analyze the effect of medication.

To accurately and quantitatively compare the generated 2D protein profiles, three main image analysis steps are required, namely, (1) geometric alignment of 2-DE images, (2) detection of spots, and (3) quantification of spots (e.g., shape, contrast). For a general overview we refer to [1]. In this work, we focus on the geometric alignment of 2-DE images. The core task is to find an optimal geometric transformation between image data, which is known as image registration. Due to complex physical and chemical processes the locations of proteins generally vary in different 2-DE images and therefore nonrigid or Elastic registration schemes have to be applied (for a survey see, e.g., [2]). Severe problems in the case of 2-DE images are that the spot shapes are largely different, that certain spots do not appear in corresponding images, and that spots may smear over a larger area as well as overlap each other.

Previous work on 2-DE image registration can be classified into landmark-based and intensity-based schemes. Landmark-based schemes first extract landmarks from the images and then compute a transformation based on these features (e.g., [3]). With intensity-based schemes the image intensities are directly exploited to compute the transformation (e.g., [4]). Moreover, hybrid approaches that combine landmark-based and intensity-based methods have been proposed, which allow to combine advantages of both types of methods (e.g., [5, 6, 7]). However, with these approaches only coarse physical deformation models have been used, for example, based on thin-plate splines [7] or clamped-plate splines [6], or using a Gaussian function for regularization of the deformation field [5].

In this contribution, we introduce an approach for the registration of 2-DE images, which is based on an improved physical deformation model using analytic solutions of the Navier equation. In contrast to previous spline-based approaches for the registration of 2-DE images (e.g., [5, 6, 7]), with this approach cross-effects in elastic deformations can be handled, which is important in the case of 2-DE images. Moreover, our approach allows to include landmark correspondences to aid the registration in regions which are difficult to register using intensity information alone. In contrast to [8] where brain images have been registered, we here use a different energy functional where landmark correspondences are directly incorporated instead of requiring an additional deformation field.

2 Materials and Methods

We have developed a new hybrid approach for elastic registration of 2-DE images. This approach is based on an energy minimizing functional J_{Hybrid}, which comprises three energy terms to incorporate the intensity and landmark information as well as to regularize the deformation field $\mathbf{u}$, and reads

$$J_{Hybrid} = \lambda_I \, J_{\mathrm{Data},I}(g_1, g_2, \mathbf{u}) + J_{\mathrm{Data},L}((\mathbf{p}_i, \mathbf{q}_i), \mathbf{u}) + \lambda_E \, J_{\mathrm{Elastic}}(\mathbf{u}) \quad (1)$$

To constrain the transformation to elastic deformations we chose the elastic energy J_{Elastic} according to the (force-free) Navier equation, which represents the regularization of the deformation field. Since the approach is based on the Navier equation, cross-effects in elastic deformations can be taken into account, i.e., a contraction in one direction leads to a dilation in orthogonal directions, which allows to model local deformations caused by the fixation of the gel.

To register images with minimal user interaction, the idea is to exploit the intensity information as much as possible. Since in our application the images

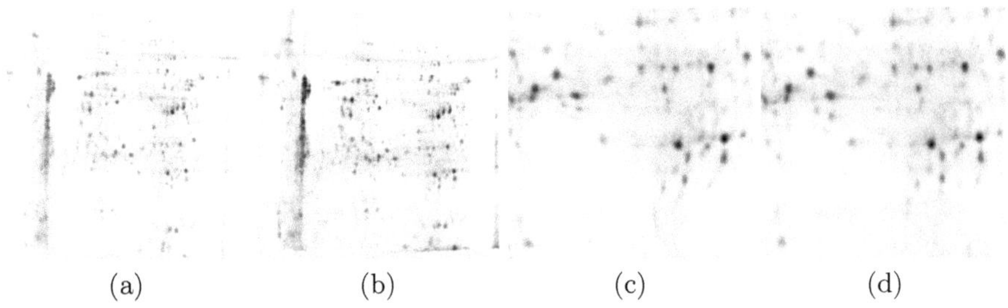

(a) (b) (c) (d)

Fig. 1. Source (a) and target (b) 2-DE images as well as sections of registration results using the previous approach [5] (c) and the new approach (d)

are of the same modality, we use sum-of-squared intensity differences for the intensity similarity measure $J_{\text{Data},I}$. Moreover, our approach allows to also include landmark correspondences $(\mathbf{p}_i, \mathbf{q}_i), i = 1, \ldots, n$, to aid the registration in regions which are difficult to register using intensity information alone. To include the landmarks we define $J_{\text{Data},L}$ based on Gaussian elastic body splines (GEBS), which are analytic solutions of the Navier equation and which have been shown to be superior compared to previously proposed elastic body splines [9]. Note that in contrast to [8], we here directly incorporate the landmark correspondences in J_{Hybrid} instead of requiring an additional deformation field. An advantage is that the landmark and intensity information can be weighted w.r.t. each other more directly and thus the weighting is easier to control.

An efficient way of minimizing J_{Hybrid} is to minimize it alternatingly w.r.t. the intensity information and w.r.t. the remaining functional. For the minimization w.r.t. the intensity information we use the method of Levenberg/Marquardt, which typically converges within few iterations. For the minimization of the overall functional we have derived an analytic solution, which uses matrix-vector convolutions and which is given by

$$\mathbf{u}(\mathbf{x}) = \mathbf{x} + \boldsymbol{\phi}_I(\mathbf{x}) * \left(\mathbf{u}^I(\mathbf{x}) - \mathbf{x}\right) + \boldsymbol{\phi}_L(\mathbf{x}) * \sum\nolimits_{i=1}^{n} \mathbf{G}(\mathbf{x} - \mathbf{p}_i)\ \mathbf{c}_i \qquad (2)$$

where "$*$" denotes the convolution and $\mathbf{G}$ is the matrix-valued GEBS basis function. Furthermore, $\mathbf{u}^I$ is the result of Levenberg/Marquardt minimization and the coefficients $\mathbf{c}_i$ are obtained from the landmark correspondences using GEBS. The matrix-valued functions $\boldsymbol{\phi}_I$ and $\boldsymbol{\phi}_L$ are computed based on the landmark correspondences, the GEBS basis function, as well as the scalar weights λ_I and λ_E. To cope with affine differences in the images, we apply a pure intensity-based affine registration scheme [10] prior to elastic registration.

3 Results

We have applied the new hybrid registration approach to register 2D polyacrylamide gel electrophoresis images of three different levels of complexity (easy, medium, and difficult). The images are courtesy of Prof. G-Z. Yang, Royal Society/Wolfson MIC Laboratory, Dept. of Computing, Imperial College of Science, Technology, and Medicine, London/UK. In each case, gel images are compared from a reference group with those from a test group [4]. All images represent human protein expressions and have a size of 1024×1024 pixels.

To analyze the performance of our approach, we have carried out a quantitative evaluation of the registration results. An obvious measure for the registration accuracy is the number of correctly matched spots. However, note that counting the spots is a non-trivial task in the case of 2-DE images, and also tedious and time consuming. Based on spot counting we obtain the overall number of spots that should ideally match as well as the correctly and incorrectly matched spots. The quantitative evaluation has been performed for images of easy and medium complexity. Tables 1 and 2 show the resulting number of correctly matched spots, the number of incorrectly matched spots, and the fraction of correct matches.

Table 1. Quantitative evaluation results for images of easy complexity (208 ideally matching spots) using affine registration, a previous elastic registration approach [5], and the new approach: Number of correctly (n_{correct}) and incorrectly ($n_{\text{incorrect}}$) matched spots as well as fraction of correct matches

Approach	Information	n_{correct}	$n_{\text{incorrect}}$	Correct
Affine [10]	intensity	128	80	61.5%
Gaussian [5]	intensity	187	21	89.9%
	hybrid	201	7	96.6%
GEBS	intensity	200	8	96.2%
	hybrid	203	5	97.6%

Table 2. Same as Table 1 but for images of medium complexity (158 spots)

Approach	Information	n_{correct}	$n_{\text{incorrect}}$	Correct
Affine [10]	intensity	130	28	82.3%
Gaussian [5]	intensity	137	21	86.7%
	hybrid	149	9	94.3%
GEBS	intensity	150	8	94.9%
	hybrid	153	5	96.8%

4 Discussion

Applying our elastic registration approach without using landmarks, we achieved good overall registration results for all considered 2-DE images. Only in some regions, in particular, regions with a large number of tiny spots or regions located at the image border, the results are worse compared to other regions. However, by inclusion of a relatively small number of landmarks the registration accuracy could be significantly improved in the respective regions. Moreover, we have quantitatively evaluated the registration result. For the images of easy complexity (Table 1) 208 spots should ideally match. Applying the new registration scheme and using only intensity information, we obtain 200 correctly matched spots (8 incorrectly matched) which calculates to 96.2% correct matches. In contrast, the previous approach in [5] yields only 187 correctly matched spots (21 incorrectly matched), and a pure affine approach is much worse (80 incorrectly matched). By additionally incorporating landmarks, the performance of the new approach improves, i.e., only 5 spots are incorrectly matched. Applying the approach in [5] using additional landmarks yields 7 incorrectly matched, i.e., the result is improved but worse compared to the new approach. For the images of medium complexity we obtained comparable results (Table 2). From Tables 1 and 2 it can be seen that both elastic approaches yield quite good results. However, it also turned out that for the previous approach [5] the use of additional landmark information is crucial to achieve satisfactory matching results of 96.6% and 94.3%. In contrast, the new approach achieves this level of accuracy without including landmarks, and yields even better results when landmark information is used (97.6% and 96.8%). Therefore, the new approach is well suited in a fully automatic setting and the performance can further be improved when landmark correspondences are available.

Moreover, by comparing the resulting deformation grids of both elastic approaches we found that the new approach yields more realistic deformations, in particular, distortions leading to spot smearing as in the case of using [5] are reduced. As an example, Fig. 1 shows a section (384 × 384 pixels) of the registered images for both elastic approaches for images of easy complexity. It can be seen that the new approach (d) yields a registration result without significant distortions. In contrast, the previous approach [5] yields distortions leading to significant smearing, for example, see the bottom right in (c).

In summary, we introduced a new hybrid elastic registration approach for the geometric alignment of 2-DE gel images. With this approach cross-effects in elastic deformations can be handled, which is important for the registration of 2-DE images. We have successfully applied our approach to register 2-DE gel images of different levels of complexity and we found that the approach is superior to a previous hybrid scheme.

Acknowledgement. This work has been funded by the Deutsche Forschungsgemeinschaft (DFG) within the project ELASTIR (RO 2471/2).

References

1. Berth M, Moser FM, Kolbe M, et al. The state of the art in the analysis of 2D gel eletcrophoresis images. Appl Microbiol Biotechnol. 2007;76(6):1223–43.
2. Zitova B, Flusser J. Image registration methods: a survey. Image Vis Comput. 2003;24:977–1000.
3. Efrat A, Hoffmann F, Kriegel K, et al. Geometric algorithms for the analysis of 2D-eletrophoresis gels. J Comp Biology. 2002;9(2):299–316.
4. Veeser S, Dunn MJ, Yang GZ. Multiresolution image registration for two-dimensional gel electrophoresis. Proteomics. 2001;1:856–70.
5. Rohr K, Cathier P, Wörz S. Elastic registration of electrophoresis images using intensity information and point landmarks. Pattern Recog. 2004;37(5):1035–48.
6. Rogers M, Graham J, Tonge RP. 2D Electrophoresis gel registration using point matching and local image-based refinement. Proc 15th British Machine Vision Conf. 2004.
7. Wang X, Feng DD. Hybrid registration for 2D gel protein images. Proc 3rd Asia-Pacific Bioinf Conf. 2005 Jan.
8. Wörz S, Rohr K. Hybrid spline-based elastic image registration using analytic solutions of the navier equation. Proc BVM. 2007; p. 151–5.
9. Kohlrausch J, Rohr K, Stiehl HS. A new class of elastic body splines for nonrigid registration of medical images. J Math Imaging Vis. 2005;23(3):253–80.
10. Thévenaz P, Ruttimann UE, Unser M. A pyramid approach to subpixel registration based on intensity. IEEE Trans Image Process. 1998;7(1):27–41.

Detection of Point Scatterers by Regularized Inversion of a Linear Ultrasound System Model

Tobias Gehrke, Heinrich M. Overhoff

Medical Engineering Laboratory, University of Applied Sciences Gelsenkirchen
tobias.gehrke@fh-gelsenkirchen.de

Abstract. Scatterer detection in medical ultrasound imaging can be formulated as an inverse problem concerning a linear system model based on point scatterers. The applicability of different methods of regularized inversion is examined and a novel regularization scheme specifically adapted to ultrasound imaging is introduced. The results show that standard inversion methods fail in ultrasound imaging while the proposed new method is a feasible way to improve axial resolution without amplifying erroneous signal components. The consequences of A-line detection by regularized inversion for B-mode imaging are examined by numerical simulations.

1 Introduction

In medical ultrasound imaging sound waves are emitted from a transducer into body tissue and partially scattered back at inhomogeneously distributed scatterers with individual scattering coefficients. Since scattering takes place at different depths within the tissue, the scattered waves of a single pulse-echo sequence contain a "fingerprint" of the tissue in axial direction, the so called A-line. A complete image is constructed by consecutive side-by-side arrangement of A-lines from repeated pulse-echo sequences. The reconstruction of a single A-line from the scattered data within an ultrasound image can be understood as the spatially sensitive estimation of scattering coefficients from the scattered waves. Conventional ultrasound imaging algorithms employ unspecific methods such as envelope detection and matched filtering for this task. The receive signal is however known to be the sum of blurred, scaled, and time delayed replica of the excitation signal, where the blurring is caused by the transducer's dynamic behaviour, diffraction and absorption. Inclusion of an analytic model for the dynamic system behaviour into the estimation process has the potential to partly reverse the blurring and thereby to improve the resolution of ultrasound images.

A common analytic model for the dynamic behaviour of an ultrasound imaging system is investigated with respect to the properties of image reconstruction by system inversion. Several standard approaches for system inversion are investigated with respect to to their robustness against erroneous receive data and their applicability in B-mode imaging. Furthermore, a novel inversion scheme, that is specifically adapted to ultrasound imaging by combining envelope detection with regularized inversion, is developed and tested.

2 Materials and Methods

2.1 Model for an Ultrasound Imaging System

Ultrasound imaging uses the process chain: emit signal - electromechanical emit transformation - wave propagation and scattering - electromechanical receive transformation - receive signal. A discrete linear model for the calculation of ultrasound B-mode images relates the transducer's electric receive signal $\boldsymbol{y}$ to the scattering behaviour of the tissue [1]:

$$\boldsymbol{y} = \boldsymbol{\Psi} \boldsymbol{s} \tag{1}$$

Considering a single A-line, the column vector $\boldsymbol{s}$ contains the scattering coefficients of scatterers at consecutive distances, with a zero element if no scatterer exists. The lower triangular Toeplitz matrix $\boldsymbol{\Psi}$ contains time shifted pulse-echo-wavelets. A pulse echo wavelet is the receive signal due to a single point scatterer of unit strengths. For brevity it is assumed here that the pulse-echo-wavelet is invariant to the scan direction.

2.2 Model Inversion

By inversion of the model for the ultrasound imaging system (1), the scattering vector

$$\tilde{\boldsymbol{s}} = \boldsymbol{\Psi}^{\#} \boldsymbol{y} \tag{2}$$

can be estimated. Matrix $\boldsymbol{\Psi}^{\#}$ reverses the blurring effect of $\boldsymbol{\Psi}$ and thereby provides an estimate with good axial resolution. In many cases $\boldsymbol{\Psi}^{\#}$ is of the form [2]

$$\boldsymbol{\Psi}^{\#} = \left(\boldsymbol{\Psi}^{\mathrm{T}} \boldsymbol{\Psi} + \lambda^2 \boldsymbol{H}\right)^{-1} \boldsymbol{\Psi}^{\mathrm{T}} \tag{3}$$

with matrix $\boldsymbol{H}$ specific to the inversion method.

Noise in $\boldsymbol{y}$ can cause large undesired oscillations of high frequency in the estimated solution $\tilde{\boldsymbol{s}}$. Thus $\boldsymbol{\Psi}^{\#}$ must ensure that $\tilde{\boldsymbol{s}}$ is insensitive to noise.

Unregularized Inversion The scattering vector can be estimated by solving (1) with the pseudoinverse of the system matrix, i.e. by choosing $\boldsymbol{\Psi}^{\#} = \boldsymbol{\Psi}^{\dagger}$ in (2) or $\boldsymbol{H} = 0$ in (3).

Singular Value Truncation A matrix whose pseudoinverse provides a noise insensitive estimation $\boldsymbol{s}_{\nu}^{\mathrm{tsvd}}$ can be obtained by truncating the ν smallest singular values of $\boldsymbol{\Psi}$. The resulting matrix $\boldsymbol{\Psi}_{\nu}$ is the closest rank-ν approximation to $\boldsymbol{\Psi}$ [2, 3] and thus the system characteristics is largely maintained. The corresponding regularized inverse in (2) becomes $\boldsymbol{\Psi}^{\#} = \boldsymbol{\Psi}_{\nu}^{\dagger}$.

Small Solution Norm Condition Approximately solving the system (1) subject to a small solution norm provides a noise robust estimate [2, 4]:

$$\tilde{\boldsymbol{s}}_{\lambda}^{\text{tik}} = \underset{\boldsymbol{s}\in\mathbb{R}^n}{\operatorname{argmin}} \left\{ \|\boldsymbol{\Psi s} - \boldsymbol{y}\|_2^2 + \lambda^2 \|s\|_2^2 \right\} \tag{4}$$

The regularization parameter λ adjusts the trade-off between a small residual norm and a small solution norm. This method, known as Tikhonov regularization, can be given in terms of a regularized inverse (3) with $\boldsymbol{H}$ being the unity matrix.

Small First Derivative Constraint A smooth and thereby noise insensitive estimate is obtained by minimizing

$$\tilde{\boldsymbol{s}}_{\lambda}^{\text{sfd}} = \underset{\boldsymbol{s}\in\mathbb{R}^n}{\operatorname{argmin}} \left\{ \|\boldsymbol{\Psi s} - \boldsymbol{y}\|_2^2 + \lambda^2 \|\boldsymbol{D s}\|_2^2 \right\} \tag{5}$$

with matrix $\boldsymbol{D}$ being a discrete approximation of the first derivative operator and $\boldsymbol{H} = \boldsymbol{D}^{\mathrm{T}}\boldsymbol{D}$ (3) [2, 3].

Envelope as Solution Norm Weighting Envelope detection is commonly performed for A-line computation. It is computationally simple and relatively insensitive to noise but provides only moderate resolution. To increase the resolution of the A-lines, envelope detection and regularized inverse filtering can be combined, by regarding the envelope of the receive signal $\tilde{\boldsymbol{s}}^{\text{env}} = \text{env}(\boldsymbol{y})$ as a rough pre-estimate, which is refined by a system inversion process. Thereto Tikhonov regularization is generalized such that the estimated solution is weighted before its norm is calculated

$$\tilde{\boldsymbol{x}}_{\beta,\lambda}^{\text{tew}} = \underset{\boldsymbol{x}\in\mathbb{R}^n}{\operatorname{argmin}} \left\{ \|\boldsymbol{\Psi s} - \boldsymbol{y}\|_2^2 + \lambda^2 \|\boldsymbol{L s}\|_2^2 \right\} \tag{6}$$

The weighting matrix

$$\boldsymbol{L} = \text{diag}(\boldsymbol{l}) = \text{diag}\left(1 - \frac{(1-\beta)\tilde{\boldsymbol{s}}^{\text{env}}}{\max(\tilde{\boldsymbol{s}}^{\text{env}})}\right) \tag{7}$$

causes samples $\tilde{\boldsymbol{s}}^{\text{env}} = 0$ to contribute completely to the norm $\|\boldsymbol{L s}\|_2^2$, while samples belonging to large pre-estimated scattering strengths $\tilde{\boldsymbol{s}}^{\text{env}} \approx \max(\tilde{\boldsymbol{s}}^{\text{env}})$ are suppressed by the weighting. Thereby it is ensured that oscillations at positions without scatterers are suppressed without affecting the system inversion in the vicinity of scatterers. The influence of the pre-estimate is controlled by $\beta \in [0, 1]$. Expression as a regularized inverse in terms of (3) yields $\boldsymbol{H} = \boldsymbol{L}^{\mathrm{T}}\boldsymbol{L}$.

2.3 Simulation Settings

The inversion methods are tested with a synthetic example consisting of two point scatterers at $z = 1.2\ mm$ and $z = 2.3\ mm$ of different scattering strengths.

The pulse-echo-wavelet has been determined experimentally. Gaussian noise is added to the simulated receive signal. The optimal regularization parameters are determined empirically.

A-line detection by regularized inversion with envelope solution norm weighting is included into a linear-array ultrasound imaging system, that has been emulated in the simulation software Field II [5]. A virtual phantom consisting of seven axially aligned point scatterers in $5mm$ distance to each other is used to evaluate the feasibility of the reconstruction algorithm for B-mode image reconstruction. As a comparison the same simulation has also been performed with a conventional envelope detection algorithm.

3 Results

Unregularized inversion and regularization by first derivative constraint were not able to produce meaningful results. The estimated scattering strengths obtained by the other three methods are shown in Fig. 1. The achieved axial resolutions, signal to noise ratios (SNR), and peak to sidelobe ratios (PSR) are summarised in Tab. 1.

The simulated B-mode image obtained by inversion with envelope solution norm weighting is displayed in Fig. 2(a). As a comparison the ultrasound image of the same phantom obtained by conventional envelope detection is shown in Fig. 2(b). Note that the grey scale in both images is applied after log-compression. Regarding the central axial image axis reveals that the axial resolution is significantly improved by regularized inversion compared to envelope detection. This however comes at the cost of strong artefacts in vertical direction that appear as white "wings" in image Fig. 2(a).

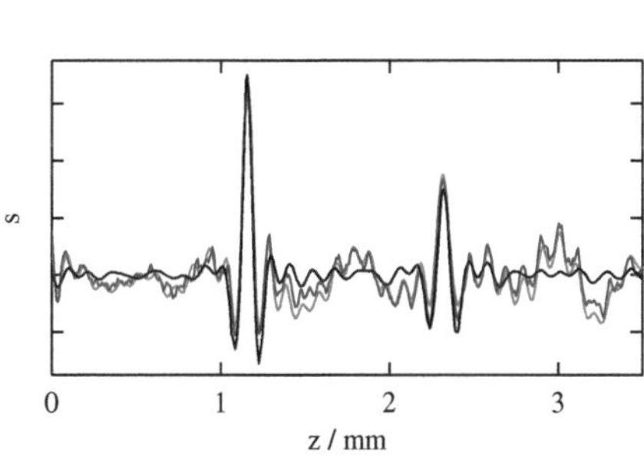

Fig. 1. A-lines estimated from noisy receive signals. Obtained by singular value truncation (light grey), Tikhonov Regularization (dark grey) and by regularized inversion with envelope weighting (black)

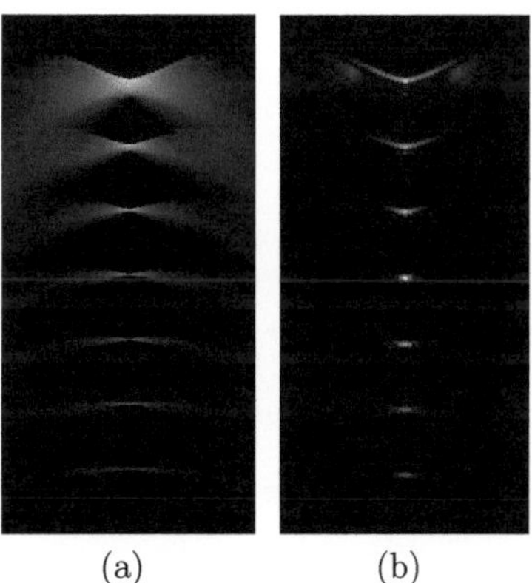

Fig. 2. Simulated ultrasound images of seven point scatterers. Obtained by regularized inversion with envelope weighting (a) and by conventional envelope detection (b)

Table 1. Characteristic values of estimated A-lines

	Resolution [mm]	SNR [dB]	PSR [dB]
Unregularized	0.008	< 0	∞
Truncation	0.054	20.4	22.9
Tikhonov	0.054	21.0	24.8
Derivative	0.054	2.0	17.6
Weighting	0.054	34.4	26.4

4 Discussion

Unregularized inversion and regularization relying on a small first derivative of the solution are not applicable for ultrasound imaging; the first owing to the noise susceptibility of the system matrix's pseudoinverse, the second since the scattering vector consists of sharp peaks, which contradict the specification of a smooth solution. Expectedly singular value truncation and Tikhonov regularization gave similar results due to the close connection between filtering of singular components and solution norm reduction [3, 5]. Both do not provide SNR and PSR sufficient for ultrasound imaging. Regularized inverse filtering with envelope weighting is able to enhance the axial resolution compared to envelope or matched filter detection without degrading SNR and PSR to much and is thus the suitable candidate for an application in medical ultrasound imaging.

The applicability of the envelope weighting algorithm for B-mode imaging is currently limited due to strong artefacts. These artefacts are owed to the fact that the system model is one-dimensional along the individual A-lines, i.e. do not account for diffraction of the wave during its propagation through the tissue. It is expected that inclusion of diffraction into the system model reduces the vertical artefacts significantly.

References

1. Shen J, Ebbini ES. A new coded excitation ultrasound imaging system: Part I: Basic principles. IEEE Trans Ultrason Ferroelectr Freq Control. 1996;43(1):131–40.
2. Hansen PC. Rank-Deficient and Discrete Ill-Posed Problems: Numerical Aspects of Linear Inversion. Philadelphia: SIAM; 1998.
3. Vogel CR. Computational Methods for Inverse Problems. Philadelphia: SIAM; 2002.
4. Hansen PC. The truncated SVD as a method of regularization. BIT Numeric Math. 1987;27(4):534–53.
5. Jensen JA. Field: A program for simulating ultrasound systems. Proc 10th Nordic-Baltic Conf Biomed Imaging. 1996; p. 351–3.

Automatische Lokalisation und hämodynamische Charakterisierung von Gefäßstrukturen bei arteriovenösen Malformationen

Nils Daniel Forkert[1], Dennis Säring[1], Jens Fiehler[2], Till Illies[2], Heinz Handels[1]

[1]Institut für Medizinische Informatik
[2]Klinik und Poliklinik für Neuroradiologische Diagnostik und Intervention
Universitätsklinikum Hamburg-Eppendorf, 20246 Hamburg
n.forkert@uke.uni-hamburg.de

Kurzfassung. Im Beitrag werden Verfahren zur automatischen Detektion des Kerns der Arteriovenösen Malformation (AVM) sowie der zuleitenden (Feeder), ableitenden (Drainagevenen) und „en passge“ Blutgefäße präsentiert. Als Eingabe hierfür dienen hochaufgelöste 3D- sowie zeitlich-räumliche 4D-MRT-Bildsequenzen. Durch eine kombinierte Analyse der Intensität, der Geschwindigkeit und des relativen Einflusszeitpunktes des Blutes werden Gefäßstrukturen automatisch charakterisiert. Die vorgestellte Methode zur Detektion des Kerns wurde anhand von manuellen Segmentierungen validiert und ergab eine mittlere Volumenübereinstimmung von ca. 88%. Drainagevenen und Feeder konnten mit einer Genauigkeit von 95% detektiert werden.

1 Einleitung

Eine zerebrale Arteriovenöse Malformation (AVM) ist eine Gefäßmissbildung im Gehirn, die sich durch das Fehlen eines kapillären Gefäßbettes mit abnormem Kurzschluss zwischen dem arteriellen und dem venösen System auszeichnet (Shunt), dem sog. Kern. Durch die veränderten hämodynamischen Bedingungen resultieren dysplastische Veränderungen der zu- und abführenden Gefäße mit einem erhöhtem Blutungsrisiko, neurologischen Ausfällen und einer Sauerstoffunterversorgung des Gehirns. Das vorrangige Ziel einer invasiven AVM-Behandlung ist die vollständige Ausschaltung der AVM aus dem Blutkreislauf und eine damit einhergehende Verhinderung einer intrakraniellen Blutung. Dafür stehen u.a. endovaskuläre Embolisation, neurochirurgische Operation und stereotaktische Radiochirurgie sowie deren Kombination als Verfahren zur Verfügung [1]. Zur Abschätzung des chirurgischen Behandlungsrisikos sind vor allem die Lokalisation und Quantifizierung der AVM, Detektion von Feeder, Drainagevenen und "en passage" Gefäße sowie die Beurteilung des zeitlichen Einströmverlaufes des Blutes von besonderem Interesse.

Um die Größe und Lage einer AVM zu bestimmen, ist eine genaue Detektion des AVM-Kerns von zentraler Bedeutung. In der Literatur findet sich hierfür lediglich die Arbeit von Nyui et al. [2], die auf Faktoranalyse beruht und ein Vorwissen über arterielle, venöse und Rauschsignale vorraussetzt.

2 Material und Methoden

2.1 Material

Mittels neuer paralleler MRT-Bildgebungstechniken wie beipielsweise GRAPPA (generalized autocalibrating partially parallel acquisition) können zeitaufgelöste kontrastmittelgestützte 4D-TREAT-Sequenzen (time-resolved echo-shared MR-angiography technique) mit einer zeitlichen Auflösung im Sub-Sekundenbereich erzeugt werden. Die visuelle Bildqualität ist bei den 4D-TREAT-Bilddaten mit einer zeitlichen Auflösung von ca. 0,5 s und einer Voxelgröße von $1,875 \times 1,875 \times 5,0$ mm^3 eher gering. Daher werden zusätzlich räumlich hochauflösende 3D TOF-MRA (time-of-flight) aufgenommen, welche durch einen verbesserten Blut-zu-Hintergrund-Kontrast und einer geringen Voxelgröße von $0,469 \times 0,469 \times 0,5$ mm^3 eine detaillierte Segmentierung des Gefäßsystems und eine Quantifizierung von Größe und Lage der AVM ermöglichen [3].

2.2 Analyse der Hämodynamik mittels TREAT

In der 4D-TREAT-Seqeunz wird mittels referenzbasierter Kurvenanpassung voxelweise der Einflusszeitpunkt des Blutes für den dazugehörigen zeitlichen Signalverlauf bestimmt [4]. Hierbei wird zunächst ein normierter, gemittelter patientenindividueller Referenzsignalverlauf aus den Daten extrahiert. In einem weiteren Schritt wird unter Berücksichtung von unterschiedlichen Einflussgeschwindigkeiten für jedes Voxel die zeitliche Verschiebung zwischen dem Signalverlauf und dem Referenzsignalverlauf berechnet, wobei die quadratische Abweichung der Signalkurven minimal wird. Basierend auf dieser Definition werden voxelweise die Einströmzeitpunkte berechnet, wodurch das zeitlich-räumliche Datenvolumen auf einen 3D-Datensatz reduziert wird. Die so berechneten Einflusszeitpunkte können auf Basis eines affinen 3D-3D Registrierungsverfahren [5] auf den TOF-Datensatz übertragen werden.

2.3 Annahmen zur Methodik

Eine Bestimmung des AVM-Kerns ist die Vorraussetzung, um die wichtigen Parameter wie Größe und Lage einer AVM sowie zuleitende und ableitende Gefäße zu bestimmen. Die hier vorgestellte Methode zur Detektion des AVM-Kerns basiert auf zwei Annahmen:

1. Der AVM-Kern stellt sich im 3D-TOF-Datensatz durch eine lokal erhöhte Dichte von hohen Intensitätswerten dar.
2. Das fehlende Kapillarbett im AVM-Kern führt zu einem deutlich verringerten Widerstand im Gefäßsystem und somit zu einer erhöhten Flussgeschwindigkeit und dadurch zu einem relativ frühen Einflusszeitpunkt des Kontrastmittels in der AVM.

Diese Eigenschaften sollen benutzt werden, um den AVM-Nidus aus den vorhandenen Bildsequenzen zu extrahieren und mit manuell segmentierten AVM-Kernen zu vergleichen.

2.4 Extraktion des AVM-Kerns

Zur Extraktion des AVM-Kerns wird ein Parameterdatensatz $P : \Omega \rightarrow W$mit $\Omega \subseteq \mathbb{Z}^3$ und $W \subseteq \{0, 1\}$ berechnet, der unter Berücksichtigung der zuvor gemachten Annahmen die Zugehörigkeit für jedes Voxel zum AVM-Kern charakterisiert. Für jedes Voxel x berechnet sich $P(x)$ durch die Linearkombination der Intensität $I(x)$, der Geschwindigkeit des Blutes $V(x)$ und dem relativen Einflusszeitpunkt $T(x)$ $(I, V, T : \Omega \rightarrow W)$:

$$P(x) = S(x) \cdot (w_1 I(x) + w_2 V(x) + w_3 T(x)) \tag{1}$$

wobei mit

$$S(x) = \begin{cases} 1, \text{wenn } x \in \text{Gefäß} \\ 0, \text{sonst} \end{cases} \tag{2}$$

die Gefäßzugehörigkeit des Voxel beachtet wird. Voxel mit einem großen Wert $P(x)$ werden dem AVM-Kern zugeordnet.

In einem ersten Schritt wird eine Segmentierung S des individuellen Gefäßsystems aus dem 3D-TOF-Datensatz mittels Region-Growing und manueller Korrektur in orthogonalen Sichten generiert.

Als Datensatz I dient der 3D-TOF-Datensatz. Zusätzlich wird im 4D-TREAT-Datensatz die Flussgeschwindigkeit v für jedes Voxel näherungsweise durch das Maximum der diskret approximierten Ableitung des zeitlichen Intensitätsverlaufs bestimmt. Mittels einer Registrierung [5] wird eine voxelweise Übertragung auf den TOF-Datensatz ermöglicht, so dass ein Datensatz V entsteht. Auf Basis der mittels des 4D-TREAT-Datensatz berechneten Einflusszeitpunkte und der Segmentierung wird ein mittlerer Einflusszeitpunkt $\bar{t}$ für das Gefäßsystem bestimmt. Für jeden Voxel wird nun der Einflusszeitpunkt t von dem mittleren Einflusszeitpunkt $\bar{t}$ subtrahiert. So entsteht ein 3D-Datensatz T mit relativen Einflusszeitpunkten.

Der AVM-Kern kann nun über eine lokale Anhäufung hoher P-Werte bestimmt werden. Hierfür werden die auftretenden P-Werte für jede Schicht in axialer Richtung aufsummiert, sowie Mittelwert und Maximum berechnet. Dieses wird analog für die coronare und sagittale Ebenen durchgeführt. Ausgehend von den Mittelwerten kann eine Boundingbox berechnet werden, indem sich der AVM-Kern befindet (Abb. 1). Das so berechnete Volumen wird abschließend mit einem Largest Connected Component Filter bearbeitet um Gefäße auszuschließen, die nicht direkt mit dem AVM-Kern verbunden sind, auszuschließen.

Auf Basis des so bestimmten AVM-Kerns können dann die für den Mediziner wichtigen Informationen wie Größe und Lage des Kerns bestimmt werden.

2.5 Definition Drainagevenen und Feeder und „en passage" Gefäßen

Für den extrahierten AVM-Kern kann nun der mittlere Einflusszeitpunkt im Kern bestimmt werden. In einem weiteren Schritt werden die Gefäßvoxel in der näheren Umgebung zum AVM-Kern analysiert. Gefäßteile, die keine Verbindung zum AVM-Kern aufweisen, werden als „en passage" eingeordnet. Für die verbliebenen Gefäßvoxel werden die dazugehörigen Einflusszeitpunkte des Kontrastmittels analysiert. Voxel, die einen früheren Einflusszeitpunkt aufweisen als der AVM-Kern, werden als Feeder eingeordnet, Voxel die einen späteren Einflusszeitpunkt aufweisen als Drainagevenen.

3 Ergebnisse

Bei der Entwicklung der Analyse standen 10 Datensätze von Patienten mit einer AVM zur Verfügung, in denen von einem erfahrenen Neuroradiologen der AVM-Kern manuell segmentiert wurde. Erste Ergebnisse eines Vergleichs der automatischen Detektion im Vergleich zu der manuellen Segmentierung ergab durchschnittliche Volumenübereinstimmung von 88% und eine Sensitivität von 76%, bei $w_{1,2,3} = \frac{1}{3}$. Die Ergebnisse der automatischen Detektion wurden von den medizinischen Experten als qualitätiv wertvoll eingestuft. Die benötigte Zeit für die automatische Detektion lag bei ca. 5 Minuten, wobei bei der vorgestellten Methode keine Benutzinteraktion von Nöten ist, im Vergleich zu durchschnittlich 30 Minuten, die für die manuelle Segmentierung benötigt wurde.

Für die Beurteilung der automatischen Detektion von Drainagevenen und Feeder wurden diese in einem ersten Schritt durch Experten, auf Basis von medizinischem Wissen, ohne Anzeige der automatischen Detektion, bestimmt und die Ergebnisse mit der automatischen Detektion verglichen. Dabei zeigte sich, dass durch die vorgestellte Methode eine Übereinstimmung von 95% erreicht wurde. Die Ergebnisse der automatischen Detektion von AVM-Kern, Drainagevenen, Feeder und „en passage" Gefäße können farbüberlagert in den 2D-TOF-Schichtbildern und auf einem 3D-Oberflächenmodell des Gefäßsystems dargestellt werden (Abb. 2).

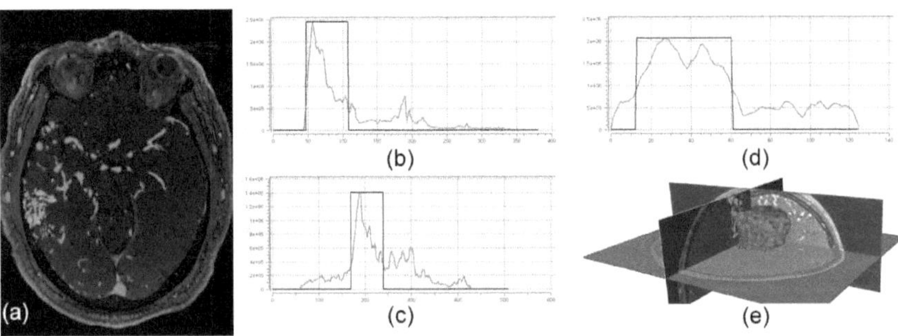

Abb. 1. Farbcodierte Darstellung des AVM-Kern (grün) auf TOF-MRT (a), aufsummierte P-Werte für alle Schichten in axialer, coronaler und sigittaler Ebene (b-d) und 3D-Oberflächenmodell des AVM-Kern (e)

Abb. 2. Farbcodierte Darstellung der Feeder (rot), Drainagevenen (blau) des AVM-Nidus (grün) sowie „en passage“ Gefäße (gelb) auf TOF-MRT-Schicht(a), im 3D-Oberflächenmodell (b) und im geschnittenen Teilvolumen des Oberflächenmodell (c)

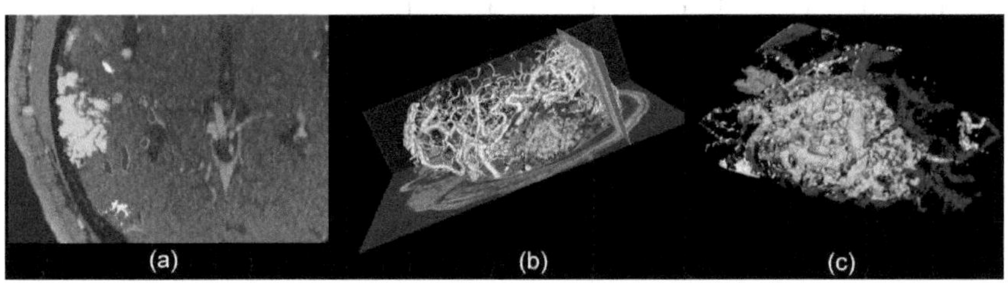

4 Diskussion

Es wurde ein neues Verfahren zur Detektion des AVM-Nidus sowie der zuleitenden, ableitenden und „en passage“ Blutgefäße präsentiert. Eine erste Evaluation der automatischen Detektion des AVM-Kerns ergab eine Übereinstimmung des Zielvolumens von ca. 88% im Vergleich zu der manuellen Segmentierung. Um genauere Aussagen über die Genauigkeit der vorgestellten Methode machen zu können, sind manuelle Segmentierungen von weiteren Experten im Bereich der Neuroradiologie notwendig, da auf Grund der hohen Komplexität der Struktur der AVM mit einer hohen Inter-Observer-Varianz zu rechnen ist. Diese könnte man mit Hilfe dieses Verfahrens optimieren. Die durchschnittliche Zeit von ca. 5 min., die für die automatische Detektion benötigt wird und währenddessen keinerlei Benutzerinteraktion von Nöten ist, stellt im Vergleich zu den 30 min., die im Mittel für die manuelle Segmentierung benötigt wird, eine deutliche Zeitersparnis dar. Die Detektion von zuleitenden und ableitenden Gefäßen wurden von erfahrenen Neuroradiologen als hilfreich insbesondere für die Diagnose und Therapieplanung eingestuft.

Für die nähere Zukunft ist es geplant, die Ergebnisse der Detektion des AVM-Kerns durch eine parameterindividuelle Gewichtung der Gewichte der Linearkombination zu verbessern.

Literaturverzeichnis

1. Grzyska U. Treatment of cerebral arteriovenous malformations. Hamburg Concept Clinical Neurorad. 2004;14(1):41–7.
2. Nyui Y, Ogawa K, Kunieda E. Extraction of arteriovenous malformation with factor analysis. Proc ICIP. 2000;2:621–4.
3. Spetzler RF, Martin NA. A proposed grading system for arteriovenous malformations. J Neurosurg. 1986;65:467–83.
4. Forkert ND, Säring D, Ehrhardt J, et al. Analyse der Hämodynamik von zerebralen arteriovenösen Malformationen in 4D-MR-Bilddaten mittels referenzbasierter Kurvenpassung. Biomed Techn. 2007;52.
5. Säring D, Fiehler J, Forkert ND, et al. Visualization and analysis of cerebral arteriovenous malformation combining 3D and 4D MR image sequences. Int J Comp Assist Radiol Sur. 2007;2:75–9.

Finite-Element-Modellierung von respiratorischen Lungenbewegungen als elastizitätstheoretisches Kontaktproblem zur Bewegungsschätzung in 4D-CT-Daten

René Werner[1], Jan Ehrhardt[1], Rainer Schmidt[2], Heinz Handels[1]

[1]Institut für Medizinische Informatik
[2]Klinik und Poliklinik für Strahlentherapie und Radioonkologie
[1,2]Universitätsklinikum Hamburg-Eppendorf
r.werner@uke.uni-hamburg.de

Kurzfassung. Die Berücksichtigung atmungsbedingter Bewegungen im Rahmen der Strahlentherapie von Lungentumoren bedarf der detaillierten Analyse der Atemdynamik. Ein Hauptproblem ist die realitätsgetreue Schätzung der Bewegungen, die zwischen zu unterschiedlichen Atemphasen aufgezeichneten Bilddaten auftreten. In dieser Studie werden hierzu die Lungenbewegungen in Anlehnung an die Physiologie der Atmung modelliert: Die Lungenventilation wird als elastizitätstheoretisches Kontaktproblem formuliert, das mit Finite-Elemente-Methoden gelöst wird. Zur Modellevaluation werden 4D-CT-Daten herangezogen. Abweichungen zwischen modellbasiert prädiktierten und manuell bestimmten Landmarkenpositionen liegen zumeist innerhalb der Interobserver-Variabilität der manuellen Landmarkenpositionierung. Die Genauigkeit von modellbasierter Prädiktion und manueller Lokalisierung ist somit vergleichbar; der Modellansatz erscheint zur Bewegungsschätzung geeignet.

1 Einleitung

Atembewegungen stellen eines der Hauptprobleme der Strahlentherapie von Lungentumoren dar. Die Bestrahlung wird in der Regel auf einem dreidimensionalen CT-Datensatz des Patienten geplant. Ihr liegt somit ein lediglich statisches Abbild der Patientenanatomie zugrunde. Atembewegungen führen folglich zu Unsicherheiten hinsichtlich der Tumorposition. Die Unsicherheiten werden berücksichtigt, indem Sicherheitssäume entsprechend angepasst werden. Die resultierende Vergrößerung des zu bestrahlenden Volumens geht allerdings zu Lasten des Normalgewebes; die Wahrscheinlichkeit von behandlungsbedingten Nebenwirkungen erhöht sich. Um die Bewegungen im Rahmen der Strahlentherapie explizit berücksichtigen zu können, müssen Atemdynamik und Auswirkungen auf die Bestrahlung detailliert analysiert werden. Werden hierzu räumlich-zeitliche Bilddaten des Patienten eingesetzt, ist eine möglichst realitätsgetreue Schätzung der Bewegungen, die zwischen zu unterschiedlichen Atemphasen aufgezeichneten Bilddaten auftreten, eine Voraussetzung für verlässliche Resultate.

Zur Schätzung dieser Bewegungsfelder werden häufig nicht-lineare Registrierungsverfahren verwendet [1], die jedoch in der Regel keine Modellannahmen über die Atmung selbst beinhalten. In der vorliegenden Studie sollen die Lungenbewegungen auf Basis der Anatomie und Physiologie der Atmung modelliert und der Modellierungsansatz mittels Finite-Elemente-Methoden (FEM) implementiert werden. Auch bestehende Ansätze zur FEM-Modellierung von Lungenbewegungen (z. B. [2, 3]) lassen oftmals einen Bezug zur Physiologie der Atmung vermissen. Zhang et al. schlagen in [4] vor, die Atmung als kontinuumsmechanisches Kontaktproblem aufzufassen. Dieser Ansatz soll weitergeführt werden. In Ergänzung zu [4] wird das zugehörige Randwertproblem hergeleitet. Die Implementierung des Modellierungsansatzes unterscheidet sich deutlich von der in [4] dargestellten Umsetzung.

Ein wesentlicher Schwachpunkt bestehender Ansätze zur Modellierung der Lungenbewegung ist die fehlende Validierung der Modelle. Es werden häufig keine (z. B. [1, 3]) oder nur wenige zugehörige quantitative Kenngrößen ([2]: Validierung auf Basis von grob aufgelösten 2D-MR-Daten) aufgeführt. Erst seit jüngerer Zeit ist eine entsprechende Modellevaluation durch die Einführung von Verfahren zur räumlich-zeitlichen Bildgebung ermöglicht. In diesem Beitrag werden 4D(=3D+t)-CT-Daten von Lungentumorpatienten herangezogen, um patientenspezifische Modelle zu generieren und die Modellgenauigkeit zu validieren.

2 Material und Methoden

2.1 Modellierungsansatz

Das makroskopische Bewegungsverhalten der Lunge wird durch die Lungenventilation bestimmt. In dem zwischen Lungenfell (ist mit der Lungenoberfläche verwachsen) und Brustfell (kleidet den Thoraxinnenraum aus; geht an der Lungenwurzel in das Lungenfell über) befindlichen Pleuraspalt herrscht ein Unterdruck. Kommt es durch Kontraktion der Atemmuskulatur zur Erweiterung des Lungen-Brustkorb-Raumes, erhöht sich der Unterdruck und wirkt als Kraftübertragung auf die Lungenoberfläche. Die Lunge folgt somit der Erweiterung, wobei aufgrund einer im Pleuraspalt befindlichen Flüssigkeit ein reibungsloses Gleiten des Lungenfells entlang des Brustfells stattfindet. Dieser Prozess wird modelliert. Das Prinzip und das zugehörige elastizitätstheoretische Kontaktproblem sind in Abb. 1 aufgeführt; nachstehende Formelverweise beziehen sich auf diese Abbildung. Als treibende Kraft wird ein uniformer Unterdruck auf die Oberfläche der Lungengeometrie zur Phase maximaler Ausatmung ausgeübt. Lediglich der Bereich der Lungenwurzel wird ausgespart und als unbewegt angenommen. Die Ausdehnung der Lunge wird durch eine Zielgeometrie (Lungengeometrie zu maximaler Einatmung) begrenzt. Angestrebt ist ein Zustand, in dem deformierte Initial- und die Zielgeometrie annähernd deckungsgleich sind. Gesucht ist das Verschiebungsvektorfeld, das sich ergibt, wenn lungeninterne Spannungen die äußeren Kräfte kompensieren (Kräftegleichgewicht; Gl. 1, 3, 4). Hierbei wird das Lungengewebe vereinfachend als homogen, isotrop und linear-elastisch angenommen, d. h. es gilt das verallgemeinerte Hooksche Gesetz und das elastische

Abb. 1. Zur Verdeutlichung des Modellierungsansatzes. Links: Struktur der Domäne. Rechts: zu lösendes Randwertproblem (Notationen: σ: Cauchy-Spannungstensor; ε: Green-Lagrange-Verzerrungstensor; $\mathbf{S}$: 2. Piola-Kirchhoff-Spannungstensor; $\mathbf{C}$: Elastizitätstensor; $\mathbf{F}$: Deformationsgradient; $\mathbf{n}$: nach außen gerichteter Normalenvektor; $\bar{p}$: intrapluraler Druck; p_n: Kontaktdruck; g: Abstand zwischen den Geometrien).

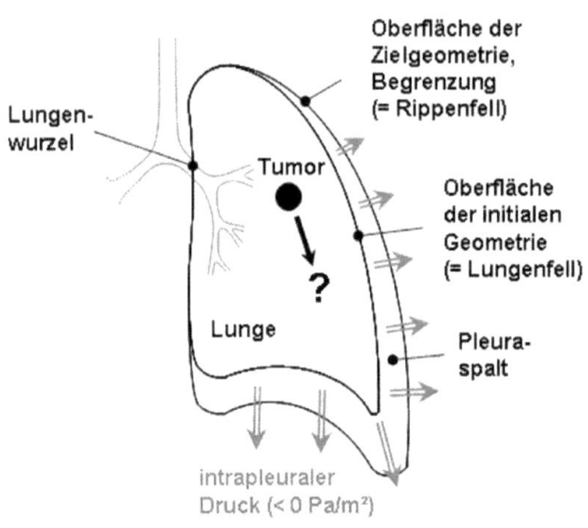

Gesucht: Verschiebungsvektorfeld $\mathbf{u}: \mathbb{R}^3 \rightarrow \mathbb{R}^3$ für die initiale Geometrie

Differentialgleichungssystem:

Gleichgewichtsbedingung:

(1) $\operatorname{div} \sigma = \mathbf{0}$

Zusammenhang Verschiebungsvektorfeld / Verzerrung / Spannung:

(2) $\varepsilon = \frac{1}{2}\left(\nabla \mathbf{u} + \nabla \mathbf{u}^T + \nabla \mathbf{u}^T \nabla \mathbf{u}\right)$
$\mathbf{S} = \mathbf{C}\,\varepsilon$ mit $\mathbf{C} = \mathbf{C}(\nu, E)$
sowie $\sigma = (1/\det \mathbf{F})\,\mathbf{F}\,\mathbf{S}\,\mathbf{F}^T$
mit $\mathbf{F} = \nabla \mathbf{u} + \mathbf{I}$

Randbedingungen:

Lungenwurzel, Zielgeometrie:

(3) $\mathbf{u} = \mathbf{0}$

Lungenfell im deformierten Zustand:

(4) $\sigma\,\mathbf{n} = (\bar{p} + p_n)\,\mathbf{n}$

(5) $\left.\begin{array}{l} g \geq 0 \\ p_n \leq 0 \\ p_n \cdot g = 0 \end{array}\right\}$ Signorini-Bedingungen

Verhalten wird durch Querkontraktionszahl ν und Elastizitätsmodul E festgelegt (siehe Gl. 2). Um den angestrebten Zustand zu erreichen, wird der Druck sukzessive erhöht. Kontakt zwischen deformierter Initial- und Zielgeometrie wird als reibungslos modelliert; ein Durchdringen der Geometrien wird durch Einführung der Signorini-Bedingungen [5] verhindert: Falls der Abstand zwischen den Geometrien kleiner null wird, wird ein Kontaktdruck eingeführt, der einer Durchdringung entgegenwirkt (Gl. 5).

2.2 Implementierung und Modellevaluation

Das Randwertproblem wird unter Verwendung von Finite-Elemente-Methoden gelöst (Software: COMSOL Multiphysics, COMSOL AB, Schweden). Die Kontaktbedingungen werden mittels des Augmented-Lagrange-Verfahrens erfüllt (siehe z. B. [6]). Zur Evaluation des Modellierungsansatzes werden 4D-CT-Daten von vier Lungentumorpatienten mit unterschiedlicher Tumorlokalisation und -beweglichkeit betrachtet (Auflösung: $0.98 \times 0.98 \times 1.5\,\text{mm}^3$,10-14 Atemphasen). Zu den Phasen maximaler Aus- und Einatmung werden die Lungenflügel segmentiert (Regionenwachstumsverfahren, interaktive Korrektur der Segmentierungen durch einen Experten). Auf Basis der Segmentierungen werden mit dem in die FEM-Software integrierten Netzgenerator Tetraeder-Netze erzeugt, auf deren Grundlage das gesuchte Verschiebungsvektorfeld berechnet wird.

Literaturangaben zu den Werten der elastischen Konstanten ν und E für Lungengewebe differieren deutlich. So wählen z. B. Sundaram et al. ν=0.2 und

E=0.1 kPa [3], Zhang et al. hingegen ν=0.35 und E=4 kPa [4]. In dieser Studie wird deshalb der Einfluss der elastischen Konstanten auf das berechnete Verschiebungsfeld für $\nu \in \{0.1; 0.4\}$ und $E \in \{0.25; 1.0\}$ kPa analysiert.

Die Genauigkeit der patientenindividuellen Modelle wird anhand lungeninterner Landmarken (Lungentumoren, Verzweigungen des Bronchialbaums, Lungenspitze und -basis) validiert. Die Landmarken werden durch mehrere Medizinstudenten (zwischen drei und sechs pro Patient) in den CT-Daten zu maximaler Ein- und Ausatmung identifiziert. Es werden die landmarkenspezifischen Interobserver-Variabilitäten der Lokalisierung ermittelt. Ausgehend von der manuellen Landmarkenlokalisierung zu maximaler Ausatmung wird die Landmarkenposition zu maximaler Einatmung modellbasiert prädiktiert, indem zu der originären Position der berechnete Verschiebungsvektor addiert wird. Abweichungen zwischen der manuell zu der Phase maximaler Einatmung bestimmten und der modellbasiert prädiktierten Landmarkenposition werden analysiert.

3 Ergebnisse

Die patientenindividuellen Modelle bestehen aus ca. 40 000 – 70 000 Tetraedern pro Lungenflügel. Die Rechenzeiten belaufen sich auf etwa 1 h (PC mit zwei Intel-Xeon-Dual-Core-Prozessoren, 3.0 GHz, 16 GB RAM; Implementierung bislang nicht laufzeitoptimiert). Der Druck, der erforderlich ist, um Initial- und Zielgeometrie zur Deckung zu bringen, hängt von der Wahl der Werte für die elastischen Konstanten ν und E ab (größere Werte von ν und E bedingen eine höhere Steifigkeit des Materials). So ist für E=0.25 kPa und ν=0.3 kPa z. B. ein Druck $\bar{p} \approx 80\text{N/m}^2$, für E=1.0 kPa und ν=0.3 kPa hingegen ein Druck $\bar{p} \approx 250\text{N/m}^2$ erforderlich. Ein signifikanter Einfluss der Werte der elastischen Konstanten auf das berechnete Bewegungsfeld wird nicht beobachtet.

Die Modellevaluation erbringt, dass Abweichungen zwischen manuell bestimmten und modellbasiert prädiktierten Landmarkenpositionen zumeist innerhalb der beobachteten landmarkenspezifischen Interobserver-Variabilitäten liegen. Für die Lungentumoren wurden Abweichungen von 1.1 bis 4.0 mm beobachtet (Mittelwert: 2.5±1.1 mm), wobei die Tumorbeweglichkeiten zwischen 2 und 20 mm liegen. Eine Abhängigkeit zwischen Abweichung und Tumorbeweglichkeit oder -lokalisation ist nicht zu erkennen. Für die Bifurkationen des Bronchialbaumes sowie Lungenspitze und -basis wurden Abweichungen von 2 bis 7 mm festgestellt (Mittelwert: 4.4±1.6 mm). Die Interobserver-Variabilitäten der manuellen Landmarkenpositionierung reichen von 2 bis zu 14 mm (Mittelwert: 7.0±3.7 mm).

4 Diskussion

Es wurde ein Ansatz zur biophysikalischen Modellierung lungeninterner Atembewegungen dargestellt und mittels Finite-Elemente-Methoden implementiert. Im Gegensatz zu bestehenden FEM-Modellen der Lunge [2, 3, 4] wird das Modell anhand von 4D-Bilddaten von Lungentumorpatienten evaluiert. Im Rahmen

Abb. 2. Schätzung lungeninternen Bewegungsfelder zwischen maximaler Aus- und Einatmung (gleicher Patient, gleiche Schicht; farbkodiert: Bewegungsamplitude). Links: mit dem FEM-Ansatz berechnet (blau: Bewegungen bis zu 25 mm). Rechts: Schätzung mittels dämonenbasierter Registrierung (blau: Bewegungen ≈15 mm; Bild aus [1]).

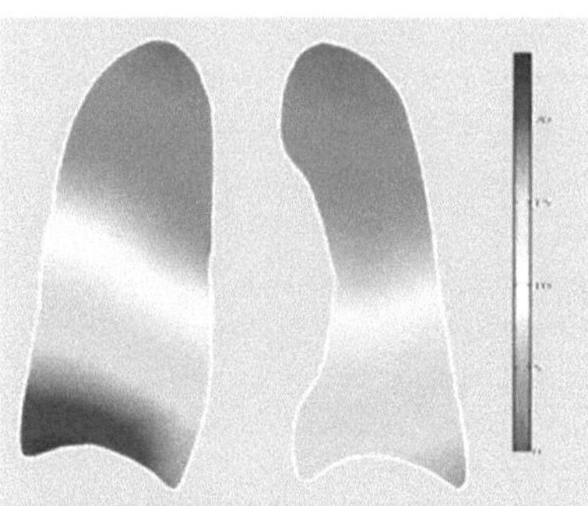

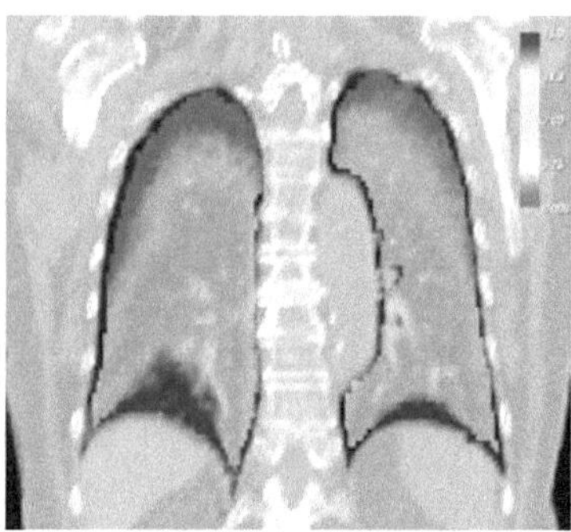

der ermittelten (allerdings recht großen) Interobserver-Variabilität sind Genauigkeit von manueller Landmarkenlokalisierung und modellbasierter Prädiktion der Landmarkenpositionen vergleichbar. Die modellbasierte Bewegungsfeldschätzung erscheint somit – trotz vereinfachender Annahmen wie des linear-elastischen Verhaltens oder der Homogenität des Lungengewebes – plausibel.

Wie beschrieben bestehen neben einer FEM-Modellierung weitere Techniken zur Schätzung atmungsbedingter Bewegungen. In Abb. 2 sind Bewegungsfelder, die mit verschiedenen Methoden berechnet wurden, gegenübergestellt. Sie unterscheiden sich teils deutlich. Es stellt sich sich die Frage, welche Methoden die „Realität" besser abbilden und inwieweit die Unterschiede in Bezug auf klinisch relevante Fragestellungen (Dosisakkumulation) entscheidend sind. Diese Themen werden ein Schwerpunkt unserer weiteren Forschungstätigkeiten sein.

Literaturverzeichnis

1. Handels H, Werner R, Schmidt R, et al. 4D medical image computing and visualization of lung tumor mobility in spatio-temporal CT image data. Int J Med Inform. 2007;76S:S433–S439.
2. Santhanam AP, Fidopiastis CM, Langen K, et al. Visualization of tumor-influenced 3D lung dynamics. Proc SPIE. 2006;6141:0C–1–0C–12.
3. Sundaram TA, Gee JC. Towards a model of lung biomechanics: pulmonary kinematics via registration of serial lung images. Med Image Anal. 2005;9(6):524–37.
4. Zhang T, Orton NP, Mackie TR, et al. Technical note: A novel boundary condition using contact elements for finite element based deformable image registration. Med Phys. 2004;31(9):2412–5.
5. Kikuchi N, Oden JT. Contact Problems in Elasticity: A Study of Variational Inequalities and Finite Element Methods. Philadelphia: SIAM; 1988.
6. Zienkiewicz OC, Taylor RL, Zhu JZ. The Finite Element Method: Its Basis & Fundamentals. 6th ed. Elsevier Butterworth-Heinemann; 2005.

Curvature- and Model-Based Hatching of Patient-Specific Muscle Surfaces

Christian Tietjen, Rocco Gasteiger, Alexandra Baer, Bernhard Preim

Department of Simulation and Graphics, Otto-von-Guericke-University Magdeburg
tietjen@isg.cs.uni-magdeburg.de

Abstract. In this paper, we introduce a new method for hatching patient-specific, anatomic 3D surface models, in particular hatching of muscle surfaces. However, the method is transferable to other structures, *e. g.*, , vessels. Since 3D surface models are extracted from binary segmentation masks, the curvature orientation is rough and noisy and the final hatching direction is falsified. The goal of this work is the correction and the completely automated computation of the hatching direction.

1 Introduction

In medical textbooks, didactically prepared illustrations are used to comprehensively present complex scenarios. Specific visualization goals are a better object discrimination and perception of the object's shape [1]. In this illustrations, muscle fibers are often depicted by using hatches.

There are different approaches to map hatching on surfaces [2, 3, 4]. All approaches depend on a well-defined curvature field for the hatching line alignment. A texture-based approach is most suitable, because it is frame-coherent (the hatching lines are attached on the surface), real-time capable and it is possible to zoom in very closely. This is not achieved by image- or object-based approaches.

Hatching is also helpful to improve interactive 3D visualizations. To uncover hidden objects, primarily transparency is applied. Though, it is challenging to find an adequate degree of transparency. The hiding object's shape is either not recognizable or the hidden objects are barely visible. Therefore, opacity mapping may help when the texture is aligned to the muscle fibers [5].

This work focusses on hatching of muscular structures, namely the automatic generation of correctly aligned hatching lines on surfaces derived from segmented clinical CT/MRI datasets. So far, previous work only relied on curvature information [6]. Since 3D surface models are extracted from binary segmentation masks, the curvature orientation is rough and noisy and the final hatching direction is falsified, even though the surface is smoothed. This fact may also cause singularities (*e. g.*, vortices), which also falsify the final direction.

Furthermore, the mathematically correct curvature does not correspond to the muscle fiber direction in most cases. Additional model-based knowledge is needed to improve the curvature field. Therefore, the muscle fiber direction has to be ascertained. The final direction reflects the shape of the surface and the direction of the muscle fibers.

2 Materials and Methods

Our approach to map hatching textures on muscle surfaces consists of three steps: curvature approximation, determination of the muscle fiber direction and combination with the curvature approximation, as well as surface parameterization to map hatching textures.

Step 1: At first we smooth an instance of the anatomical surface by Laplacian smoothing. On this instance, we estimate the two principle curvature directions used for the original vertices (Fig. 1(a)). We employ quadratic surface fitting at each vertex v for curvature approximation [7]. This method needs only three incident vertices (inclusive v) in contrast to five or nine neighbors for more accurate approximation operators. In practice we found that the results provided by this method are accurate enough [8]. Additional, we apply an optimization method presented in [2] to smooth principle curvature directions at unstable vertex locations.

Step 2: We implemented two methods to approximate the direction of muscle fibers. The first one is performed by a skeletonization in voxel space according to Selle et al. [9]. We extract a 3D skeleton from previous skeletonization which consists of linked skeleton voxels s_i. For each v, we determine the nearest s_i and calculate a vector $\hat{r}_v$ which is perpendicular to the local skeleton direction of s_i. The skeletonization method is only appropriate for almost cylindrical muscles to determine a meaningful centerline. Hence, we implemented a main axis computation and select the longest axes to approximate the direction of fiber (Fig. 1(b)).

After the previous step, two principle curvature directions and a model-based preferential direction $\hat{r}_v$ at each vertex v are available. In the following, we merge these information to a single vector field with one vector for each face. For the initial vector field, we select at each vertex v the principle direction which has the smallest angle to $\hat{r}_v$ and denote this direction as $\hat{f}_v$. We improve the alignment of each $\hat{f}_v$ to the preferential direction $\hat{r}_v$ and to the incident neighborhood. The optimization is processed by rotating $\hat{f}_v$ in direction of $\hat{r}_v$. For each optimization step, we rotate $\hat{f}_v$ into the direction of $\hat{r}_v$ and calculate the average angular deviation to all $\hat{f}_i$ in the incident neighborhood. Rotation stops if the angle between $\hat{f}_v$ and $\hat{r}_v$ as well as the angular deviation becomes larger in comparison to the previous step. This corresponds to a local minimum. Finally, we assign to each face the average vector of its vertices and the resulting vector field is used in the following surface parameterization (Fig. 1(c)).

Step 3: The mapping of 2D textures on 3D surfaces requires a surface parameterization which has a minimum of distortions. Due to the rough and complex surface of the medical volume datasets, common two-pass methods are not appropriate and cause strong texture distortions. We employ *lapped patches* from Praun et al. [10] and extend their approach to a global parameterization. In contrast to Praun et al., we create each patch depending on its neighbored patch and map it relative to its neighbor in a global parameter space. This results in a complete unfolded surface. Finally, we treat patch boundaries to avoid almost all texture seams. In contrast to [10] no texture blending for minimizing visible texture seams is necessary at these vertices.

The entire patch growing is based on the surface geometry and the underlying vector field from step 2. For the first patch, we select an arbitrary face as reference face D_{ref} and define a local basis consisting of the face vector $\hat{f}$, face normal $\hat{n}$ and vector $\hat{s}$ which is perpendicular to both vectors. We employ a change of bases into the xy-plane of the world coordinate system to align $\hat{x}\|\hat{s}$, $\hat{y}\|\hat{f}$ and $\hat{z}\|\hat{n}$. This plane is in the following our global parameter space. Further faces around D_{ref} are rotated in the tangent plane of D_{ref} and transformed into the parameter space according to the local base of D_{ref}. The transformation is performed relative to the reference face to preserve the topology in the parameter space. The patch growing is continued until a projection window W around D_{ref} is covered or a certain stop criteria are satisfied. The projection window is associated to the complete texture. The stop criteria consider the avoiding of strong texture distortions and variations in the direction of the vector field around D_{ref}. Finally, a global outline of all parameterized faces is calculated.

Based on the start patch, further patches are created to cover the surface. For each new patch, an inner face from the global outline list is selected and denoted as new reference face D_{ref} for the current patch. Analog to the start patch, we create a new basis and perform a transformation to the parameter space. In contrast to the start patch, we translate the new D_{ref} to the position in its previous patch to perform a continued unfolding at the current patch boundaries. The further patch growing is similar to the start patch but the rotated patch faces are transformed relative to the new position of D_{ref}. The surface parameterization is finished, if every face belongs to at least one patch which results in a complete unfolded mesh.

Some faces are part of more than one patch and each patch has a slight varying alignment to its neighbored patches. Hence, several vertices in overlapped regions have multiple parameter coordinates. Initially, this results in visible texture seams at patch boundaries. We resolve this seams by averaging correspondent parameter coordinates of affected vertices in the parameter space. This simple approach achieves an continued texture over patch boundaries without strong visible texture distortions. The graphic hardware scales the resulting parameter coordinates between the interval $[0, 1]$ and converts them into texture coordinates for texture access.

3 Results

The method described in this paper makes it possible to render real-time capable and frame-coherent hatching textures on anatomical surfaces (Fig. 1(d)). Since texture rendering is directly supported by the graphics hardware, there are no noticeable runtime-differences in comparison to rendering without texture.

User interaction is reduced to the adjustment of a few parameters, for which default values could by found. For surface smoothing, we select $w = 0.7$ and one iteration for the Laplacian smoothing. The weighting factor w specifies the strength of vertex displacement and is defined between 0.0 and 1.0. The optimization method of [2] has two thresholds

$$\frac{\max(|\kappa_1|, |\kappa_2|)}{\min(|\kappa_1|, |\kappa_2|)} > \delta_{\text{ratio}} \wedge \max(|\kappa_1|, |\kappa_2|) > \delta_{\text{reliable}} \quad (1)$$

to describe parabolic vertices where curvature estimations are assumed as stable. Principle curvature directions of non-parabolic (i. e. unstable) vertices are aligned at these stable directions. We determined the average of each parameter as default value. The values κ_1 and κ_2 in Eq. 1 defines the principle curvatures values. The last parameter affects the maximum allowed angle deviation of the direction vector of a reference triangle D_{ref} to a new triangle candidate for adding it to the given patch. We denote this parameter as $\alpha_{\text{divergence}}$ and select 5° as appropriate value which has a good trade off between texture minimization and memory consumption.

Finally, the parameterization of the surface has to be performed only one time per anatomical structure in a pre-processing step and the time needed for pre-processing is also maintainable.

4 Discussion

The goal of the paper at hand was to develop a fully automatic and real-time capable approach to hatch surfaces derived from clinical 3D-datasets in interactive visualizations. For that purpose, we combined a curvature- and model-based vector field and mapped the final hatching on the surface by using texture. The generated vector field is robust against rough and noisy anatomical surfaces. Only a

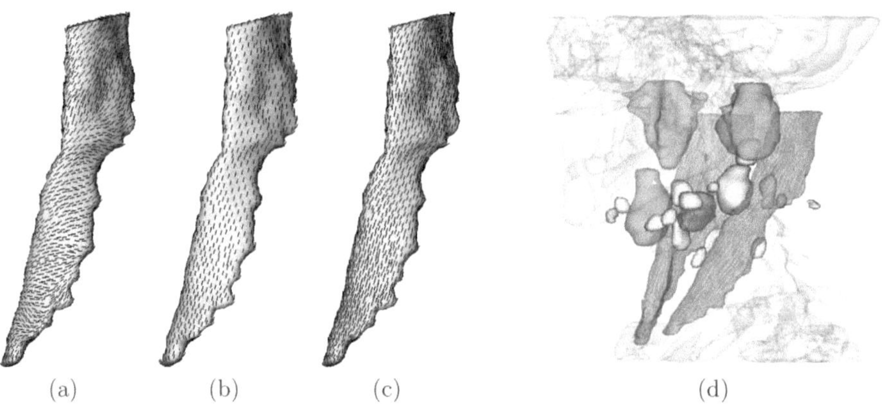

Fig. 1. (a) Visualization of the curvature field. (b) Visualization of the preferential direction. (c) Combination of both fields. (d) Applied texture mapping. Due to the *Opacity Mapping*, the muscle and the lymph nodes lying behind are distinguishable

few singularities and discontinuities were observed. Regarding the parameterization, these critical points caused visible texture distortions. Especially triangles with differing size lead to a strong averaging of the parameter coordinates. These problem may be solved by regularizing the size of the triangles.

For bended muscles, the longest main axes does not approximate the initial fiber direction sufficiently. The creation of geometric centerline by adaptively dividing the main axes and moving the new junctions in the local geometric center of the model should achieve satisfying results.

Furthermore, completely different approaches for defining preferential direction might be helpful for hatching other types of surfaces. It is possible to extract the inner skeleton of structures, *e. g.*, , the middle line of vessels [9], to use it as model-based vector field. The definition by an intermediate surface is also possible.

We also aim at evaluating the usefulness of the generated hatched surfaces for medical visualizations, according to Interrante et al. [1]. We are particularly interested in the impact on the perception of the object's shape and the differentiation of separate structures.

Acknowledgement. We thank MeVis Research for providing advanced MeVisLab features. Christian Schulz we thank for the analysis and implementation of the curvature approximation. This work was carried out in the framework of a project supported by the Deutsche Forschungsgemeinschaft (DFG) (Priority Programme 1124, PR 660/3-1).

References

1. Interrante V, Fuchs H, Pizer SM. Conveying the 3D shape of smoothly curving transparent surfaces via Texture. IEEE Trans Vis Comput Graph. 1997;3(2):98–117.
2. Hertzmann A, Zorin D. Illustrating smooth surfaces. In: SIGGRAPH; 2000. p. 517–26.
3. Zander J, Isenberg T, Schlechtweg S, et al. High quality hatching. Comput Graph Forum. 2004;23(3):421–40.
4. Praun E, Hoppe H, Webb M, et al. Real-time hatching. In: SIGGRAPH; 2001. p. 579–84.
5. Krüger A, Tietjen C, Hintze J, et al. Interactive visualization for neck dissection planning. In: EuroVis; 2005. p. 295–302.
6. Kälberer F, Nieser M, Polthier K. QuadCover: Surface parameterization using branched coverings. Comput Graph Forum. 2007;26(3):375–84.
7. Goldfeather J. Understanding Errors in Approximating Principal Direction Vectors. University of Minnesota, Department of Computer Science and Engineering; 2003.
8. Schulz C. Approximation von Krümmungsinformation für die medizinische Visualisierung. University of Magdeburg: Dept. of Computer Science; 2005.
9. Selle D, Preim B, Schenk A, et al. Analysis of vasculature for liver surgery planning. IEEE Trans Med Imaging. 2002;21(11):1344–57.
10. Praun E, Finkelstein A, Hoppe H. Lapped textures. In: SIGGRAPH; 2000. p. 465–70.

Comparison of Different Metrics for Appearance-Model-Based 2D/3D-registration with X-ray Images

Philipp Steininger[1], Karl D. Fritscher[1], Gregor Kofler[1], Benedikt Schuler[1], Markus Hänni[2], Karsten Schwieger[3], Rainer Schubert[1]

[1]Institute for Biomedical Image Analysis, UMIT Hall in Tirol, Austria
[2]AO Development Institute, AO Foundation Davos, Switzerland
[3]AO Research Institute, AO Foundation Davos, Switzerland
philipp.steininger@umit.at

Abstract. The general idea of the presented work is to overcome known problems with segmentation and analysis of 2D radiographs by registering a 3D appearance-model. Therefore this paper introduces a novel method to register 2D x-rays with 3D appearance-models by optimizing the appearance and pose of the model until a virtual radiograph of the generated model-instance optimally fits the investigated x-ray. The approach was tested on a sample set of 15 human femur specimen using different metrics and optimization techniques to investigate the impact on the resulting implicit 2D-segmentation. The first promising results are presented and discussed in detail.

1 Introduction

2D radiographs suffer from considerable information loss compared to the associated real patient anatomy. This is mainly due to overlaps and summation of organs as a consequence of an x-ray's projective nature. In addition, the missing depth information results in ambiguity concerning the origin of 2D shape variation which is a mixture of pose and 3D shape variation leading to insufficient segmentation results. To overcome these problems registration of radiographs with CT-datasets of the patient can help and methods for this approach have been proposed frequently. For instance, a pre-operative CT-scan of the investigated anatomical region can be aligned with an intra-operative x-ray of the same patient to verify the 3D patient position during interventions [1, 2]. Nevertheless, in many clinical situations a CT-image is not indicated and therefore not available. In these cases, it would be desirable to reconstruct the 3D anatomy based on x-ray images without relying on pre-acquired CT-scans of the same patient by substituting the CT-image with a statistical 3D model. In this context Lamecker et al. [3] presented a semi-automatic approach for extracting the 3D geometry of the pelvis from coronal and sagittal x-rays based on a 3D statistical shape model and a known camera calibration. As a consequence of the usage of a pure shape model in this and similar approaches the 3D intensity-distribution of the modeled region is not reconstructed. Hence it is often desired to derive not only 3D shape information on certain structures of a patient from radiographs, but also 3D intensity reconstruction. This is useful in situations were the intensity values are used, e.g. estimating the local anchorage quality of osteoporotic bone in order to enable efficient surgical planning of femoral fracture fixations.

To overcome these limitations of using shape models an approach to use a 3D appearance-model (AM) [4] of the investigated anatomical region for intensity-based 2D/3D-registration will be proposed in this work. By continuously varying the appearance of the model, the 3D anatomy is successively approximated. This approach is expected to allow analyses directly based on the shape, pose and intensity-distribution of the resulting 3D model-instance. In the following we will focus on the human femur. More precisely, we zoom in on the femur's implicit 2D-segmentation in x-rays which can be achieved by projecting the resulting model-instance onto the x-ray-plane.

In the past, different metrics for intensity-based registration [1, 5] were suggested which significantly influence the registration accuracy. Therefore our goal was to study these metrics regarding their suitability for the described approach.

2 Materials and Methods

The underlying AM is a so-called 'InShape'-model [4] of the human femur. It is a combined shape-intensity model S generated from 15 manually segmented CT-scans S_i of femur specimen. By parameterizing the model $S(\alpha) = \bar{S} \cdot U_k \alpha$ with a k-dimensional coefficient vector α the shape-intensity instances S_i of the training set can be approximated. $\bar{S}$ denotes the mean shape-intensity pair and U_k defines a matrix whose columns represent the first k orthogonal modes of shape-intensity variation within the training set.

In our approach the registration process is divided into two stages: In a first step the spatially initialized mean shape-intensity instance of the 'InShape'-model is projected onto a virtual image-plane using ray-casting. This digitally reconstructed radiograph (DRR) is then rigidly aligned with the investigated x-ray during an intensity-based 2D/2D-registration sub-procedure (e.g. [1, 2]). The DRR's image-plane is pre-configured and does not need any preparative calibration procedures. The resulting 2D transformation of the 2D/2D-registration is used for initializing the model's pose in the next step. In this second step, a 2D/3D-registration process, the model's pose and appearance is optimized until the DRR of the generated model-instance optimally matches the examined x-ray as illustrated in Fig. 1(a). The six degrees of freedom of the involved rigid 3D transformation together with k model parameters used for determining the shape and intensity-distribution of the actual model-instance are optimized. This is done with respect to an intensity-based measure calculated from the overlay of the actual DRR and the investigated radiograph.

In both registration stages different metrics and optimization methods have been applied including powell optimization (P) [6], 1+1 evolutionary optimization (OE) [7], mean reciprocal square difference metric (MD) [8], mattes mutual information metric (MM) [9] and normalized mutual information metric (NM) [5]. The result of the complete registration process is a geometrical 3D transformation (3 rotational and 3 translational components) on the one hand and a specific appearance of the model (k-dimensional vector) on the other hand.

3 Results

The approach described in section 2 was tested on a training set of 15 human femur specimen. Both CT-scans and x-ray images of all specimen have been available at original resolutions of 0.254 mm and 0.1 mm respectively. An 'InShape'-model [4] of the femur with a final resolution of 1.0 mm was generated based on these manually segmented CT-scans. The resulting AM comprised the upper regions of the femur and a short part of the shaft (Fig. 1(a)).

Two study settings were used for evaluation. In the first setting, the spatial position of the mean-shape instance for 2D/2D-registration was manually initialized as accurate as possible using the femoral head midpoint as reference. In the second setting the initial spatial position of the mean-shape instance for the first stage was interactively altered up to 6.0 mm in x- and y-direction in order to simulate manual initialization by an expert. For both settings the introduced two-stage registration process was applied utilizing different combinations of optimization techniques and metrics.

After a total number of 600 optimization-iterations (termination condition) the final output of the presented two-stage strategy is a specific model-instance whereof a DRR is calculated. The x-ray of the investigated femur specimen as

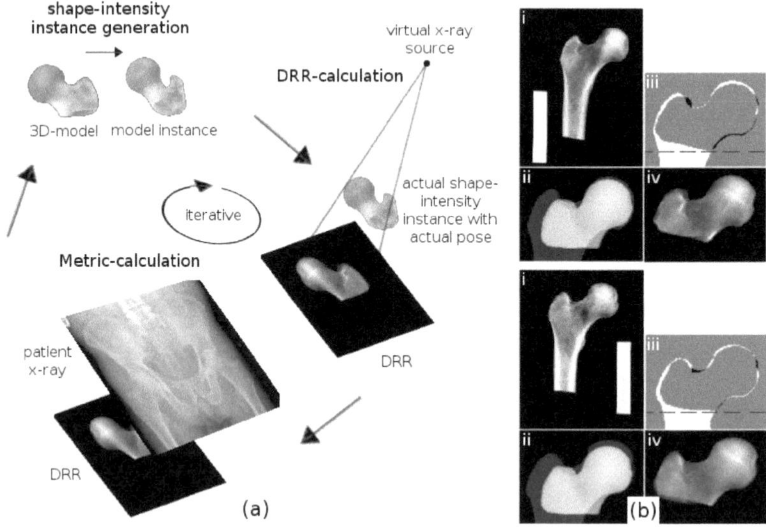

Fig. 1. (a) 2D/3D-registration scheme and (b) two exemplary qualitative results

Table 1. Results of the *first setting* on a set of femur specimen radiographs ($n = 15$)

Registration		SI [1]			HD [mm]			CD [mm]		
2D/2D	2D/3D	mean	SD	max	mean	SD	max	mean	SD	max
MD,OE	MM,OE	0.902	0.038	0.953	7.114	2.655	12.011	3.741	1.351	6.094
MD,OE	MD,OE	0.911	0.036	0.959	5.498	2.197	11.517	3.371	1.405	5.610
MD,OE	NM,OE	0.933	0.024	0.968	4.239	1.502	6.223	2.778	1.000	4.748
NM,OE	MM,OE	0.891	0.041	0.972	6.188	2.548	10.644	4.197	1.519	6.092
NM,OE	MD,OE	0.899	0.042	0.962	4.913	1.465	6.958	3.778	1.450	7.341
NM,OE	NM,OE	0.895	0.046	0.969	5.597	1.891	10.035	4.127	1.758	6.375
MM,P	MM,OE	0.913	0.038	0.961	4.970	1.770	7.685	3.618	1.129	6.105
MM,P	MD,OE	0.839	0.246	0.962	10.057	16.546	67.006	6.888	12.646	50.417
MM,P	NM,OE	0.926	0.031	0.965	4.018	1.203	6.223	3.008	1.365	5.507

well as the generated output DRR can be binarized using a threshold. Furthermore the investigated x-ray must be cropped to the size of the femur's bounding box in the DRR (see dashed lines in images iii in Fig. 1(b)). Three common similarity measures can be calculated from the superimposed cropped binarized x-ray A and the binarized DRR B: the κ-statistic-based similarity index $SI = 2|A \cap B|/(|A| + |B|)$ where $|\cdot|$ denotes the size of a set, the directed hausdorff distance $HD = \max_{a \in A} \min_{b \in B} ||a - b||$ and the contour mean distance $CD = \max(h(A, B), h(B, A))$ where $h(A, B) = \max_{a \in A} \min_{b \in B} ||a - b||$. These measures rate the 2D-segmentation quality of our approach.

Table 1 lists the results of the first study setting. The first two columns show the applied combinations of metrics and optimizers in the two registration stages. Next, the values of arithmetic mean, standard deviation and maximum for each considered similarity measure over the complete set of investigated femur specimen radiographs ($n = 15$) are depicted. The best results were achieved by applying the combinations MD/OE (2D/2D) and NM/OE (2D/3D) resulting in $SI = 0.933 \pm 0.024$, $HD = 4.239 \pm 1.502\,\text{mm}$, and $CD = 2.778 \pm 1.000\,\text{mm}$.

In the second setting with less accurate initialization the combinations MD/OE (2D/2D) and NM/OE (2D/3D) also performed best. Over the specimen training set the investigated measures amounted to $SI = 0.928 \pm 0.026$, $HD = 4.736 \pm 1.959\,\text{mm}$ and $CD = 3.406 \pm 0.693\,\text{mm}$.

Fig. 1(b) shows two exemplary qualitative results (upper images: first setting, lower images: second setting). The investigated femur specimen images (i), logarithmic overlays showing the initial spatial position of the mean shape-intensity instance (ii), the resulting segmentations as binary difference images (iii) and the DRRs of the final model-instances (iv) are depicted.

4 Discussion

The combinations of MD/OE for 2D/2D-registration and NM/OE for 2D/3D-registration perform best in both studies. Furthermore it can be stated that the loss of precision in the second study setting, due to a less accurate initialization, is only marginal. These results show that the described two-stage registration in general is suited for the segmentation of femur structures in radiographs. As seen on Fig. 1(b), the 2D-segmentation quality in the femoral head region tends to be better than in the region of the greater trochanter which may be a consequence of stronger appearance variations in this anatomical area. Behiels et al. [10] compared three different 2D-segmentation approaches based on active shape models (ASM) over a set of proximal femur x-rays. Our segmentation method's performance is comparable to the results presented in [10]. As a consequence of the low number of outliers, the maximum segmentation errors (HD) of our method are relatively small. Therefore our approach appears to be more robust compared to [10]. Another advantage of our approach is that variations in shape (actually appearance) and changes in pose of the investigated anatomical structure are modeled separately. Hence the result also reflects these two aspects explicitly in contrast to ASMs. Currently, the DRR quality is still not optimized. Thus, the next step in this project will be the generation of more realistic DRRs by considering the implicitly modeled electron densities of the investigated anatomical structure. This enhancement of the virtual x-ray is expected to further increase the total reconstruction quality. Since the sample size is too low for validated statements, we currently started to evaluate the presented two-stage registration in the course of a clinical study ($n = 340$). Besides the 2D-segmentation quality we will also evaluate the accuracy and robustness of the reconstructed 3D model appearances compared to the acquired CT-scans of the patients. First results of this study will be available in the near future.

References

1. Maintz JBA, Viergever MA. A survey of medical image registration. Med Image Anal. 1998;2(1):1–36.
2. Birkfellner W, Seemann R, Figl M, et al. Wobbled splatting: A fast perspective volume rendering method for simulation of x-ray images from CT. Comp Prog Med Biol. 2003;50:N73–N84.
3. Lamecker H, Wenckebach T, Hege H. Atlas-based 3D-shape reconstruction from x-ray images. Proc ICPR. 2006; p. 371–4.
4. Fritscher KD, Gruenerbl A, Schubert R. 3D image segmentation using combined shape-intensity prior models. J Comp Assist Rad Surg. 2007;1:341–50.
5. Pluim JPW, Maintz JBA, Viergever MA. Mutual information based registration of medical images: a survey. IEEE Trans Med Imag. 2003;22:986–1004.
6. Press WH, Flannery BP, Teukolsky SA, et al. Numerical Recipes in C. 2nd ed. Cambridge University Press; 2002.
7. Rechenberg I. Evolutionsstrategie. Optimierung technischer Systeme nach Prinzipien der biologischen Evolution. Frommann Holzboog; 1973.
8. Holden M, Hill DLG, Denton ERE, et al. Voxel similarity measures for 3D serial MR brain image registration. Proc IPMI. 1999; p. 472–7.
9. Mattes D, Haynor DR, Vesselle H, et al. PET-CT image registration in the chest using free-form deformations. IEEE Trans Med Imag. 2003;22(1):120–8.
10. Behiels G, Maes F, Vandermeulen D, et al. Evaluation of image features and search strategies for segmentation of bone structures in radiographs using active shape models. Med Imag Anal. 2002;6(1):47–62.

Patient Alignment Estimation in Six Degrees of Freedom Using a CT-scan and a Single X-ray Image

B.P. Selby[1], G. Sakas[1], S. Walter[2], W.-D. Groch[3], U. Stilla[4]

[1]Cognitive Computing and Medical Imaging, Fraunhofer IGD Darmstadt, Germany
[2]Medcom GmbH, Darmstadt, Germany
[3]Fachbereich Informatik, University of Applied Sciences Darmstadt, Germany
[4]Photogrammetry and Remote Sensing, Technische Universitaet Muenchen, Germany
pselby@medcom-online.de

Abstract. Particle beam treatment allows accurate dose delivery onto carcinogen tissue. The reachable accuracy is limited by patient alignment errors relative to the beam source. Errors can be corrected manually or by automatic comparison of two X-ray images to a CT-scan but correction mostly does not cover all degrees of freedom (DoF). In this contribution we present a solution that makes use of one X-ray image and computes full 6 DoF alignment correction by gray value based comparison to a CT. By using regions of interest, we are able to increase performance and reliability.

1 Introduction

A rapid growing number of commercial health centers exploit the advances of particle beams. Particle beam based radiotherapy allows accurate application of the treatment dose onto carcinogen tissue with accuracy less than 1.0 mm and therefore efforts accurate alignment of the patient in the facility [1]. Tracking external markers or patient fixation does not suffice the setup precision requirements. It is common practice in image guided radiotherapy to align patients manually in the device by visual evaluation of X-ray images and digital reconstructed radiographs (DRRs) to estimate misalignments [2]. The CT data recorded during the treatment planning serves as reference position of the relevant body part. X-ray images, acquired before treatment from within the radiation device, reflect the real patient alignment.

During the time consuming and error prone manual procedure, the alignment of the respective body region may change, leading to degradation of the treatment results. Additionally, manual alignment cannot be done for six degrees of freedom (DoF), because rotational misalignments can hardly be detected visually in the 2D images.

To overcome these problems automatic procedures can be used for determination and correction of patient alignment errors. As described in [3, 4], this can be done by registration of two 2D images to a reference CT series. For example

2 kV X-ray images can be registered with the projections of a CT projected to 2D space. However, using two X-ray images implies twice the exposure applied to the patient and is coupled with much higher expenses, than if just a single X-ray image would be used.

To overcome these drawbacks, our approach implements a gray-value distribution based image comparison between a single X-ray image acquired from within the treatment device and digital reconstructed radiographs that we generate on demand from a CT volume for hypothetical patient positions.

2 Methods

The automatic procedure consists of the following steps (Fig. 1 left): Generation of a suitable DRR for an estimated patient position, gray-value based comparison of the DRR to the region of interest (ROI) in the X-ray image, maximization of the similarity measure through repeated DRR generation with 6 free parameters (rigid transformation: 3 shifts, 3 rotations) and finally calculation of correctional values for the patient alignment (Fig. 2 right).

2.1 Projection of the CT

As we have to perform several iterations of DRR renderings, we use a raytracing algorithm optimized for our purpose. We do not intend to generate high quality DRRs, but DRRs that are adapted for fast rendering and comparison with an X-ray image.

When scattering is neglected, the intensity of an X-ray passing through the respective object is given by the Radon transform

$$I = I_0 \cdot \exp\big(- \int_{-\infty}^{\infty} f(x, mx + b)\big) dx \qquad (1)$$

where I_0 is the intensity of the X-ray at the source and the integral is the line integral along the ray. As we do not know the source energy, we just choose I_0 to normalize the expression in (1) to a resulting intensity range of $I \in [0.0, 1.0]$,

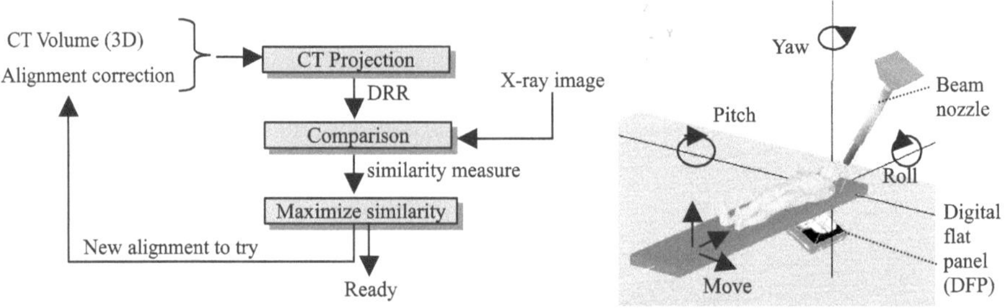

Fig. 1. Correction procedure (left) and treatment geometry (right)

which can be scaled to discrete 12 bit pixel values. In our case, the object the ray runs through is the CT volume. We can increase performance by precalculating and storing f for each voxel. f can be obtained by transformation of the CT's Hounsfield values to their attenuation factors. Computation of I for each pixel resided in a plane corresponding to the geometric setup of the digital flat panel (DFP) for the X-ray image gives the DRR image. For further performance enhancement, we transfer the area of a ROI, if defined in the X-ray image by the radiotherapist, to it's assumed position in the DRR, using the preliminary alignment of the patient. We build-up a bit-mask in the DRR image domain defining the pixels contained in the ROI and perform the rendering only for the respective pixels.

2.2 Comparison of the DRR to the X-ray Image

There exists a wide range of gray value based image comparators. As methods like crosscorrelation or usage of difference images are not suitable for images that differ in much more aspects than contrast and intensity, we decided to use mutual information as similarity measure [4]. The Mutual Information is given by

$$\mathrm{MI}\,(A,B) = \int\!\!\int P\,(a|b)\ln\left(P\,(a|b)\right) - \int P\,(a)\ln P\,(a) - \int P\,(b)\ln\left(b\right) \quad (2)$$

where P is the probability of gray value a from image A (X-ray image) or of gray value b from image B (DRR). The integrals mean integration over all existing gray values. However, we suppress high and low gray values to improve performance and to reduce the influence of features coming from corrupt pixel values or metallic objects, as fixation equipment. Therefore we only integrate over the center of the joint histogram given by $P\,(a|b)$ that consists of 80% of the image pixels. This also assures, that extreme pixels that do rarely match, are not taken into account. If the radiotherapist has defined a ROI, we only use the gray values residing this area to compute the similarity, so only the relevant image parts are used (Fig. 2).

2.3 Maximization of the Similarity Measure and Alignment Correction

To find the rigid transformation T for the current patient pose we minimize the negative similarity value given in (3):

$$\mathrm{OPT} = \min\left(-MI\,(A, B\,(T))\right) \quad (3)$$

where B is the projected CT. The elements of T serve as free parameters in the optimization and for each change of T we need to reproject the CT-scan.

We minimize by the downhill simplex approach [5] for 6 parameters (3 shifts and 3 rotations). The minimization procedure is ready, as soon as the 6D simplex of 7 sextupels becomes smaller than $\sigma_{\mathrm{dist}} = 0.25$ mm or $\sigma_{\mathrm{angle}} = 0.25°$.

Table 1. Correction results for different alignment errors

Dataset	Intended alignment error (Rotation/Shift)	Error after correction (Rotation/Shift)	Calculation time (in seconds)
Skull	1°/1mm	0.4°/0.7mm	53
Skull	2°/5mm	0.4°/0.6mm	42
Skull	3°/10mm	0.4°/0.9mm	61
Pelvis	1°/1mm	0.3°/1.1mm	82
Pelvis	2°/5mm	0.4°/1.0mm	85
Pelvis	3°/10mm	0.6°/1.8mm	97
Skull	2°/5mm (4mm along X-ray)	0.5°/2.9mm	55
Pelvis	2°/5mm (4mm along X-ray)	0.7°/4.3mm	121

The resulting transformation T corresponds to the difference between the current patient alignment as seen by the DFP and the reference alignment given by the simulated spacial position of the CT volume and the Isocenter in CT coordinates in the treatment device. To receive the correction for the alignment parameters of the patient table we finally transfer the inverse transformation $\mathbf{inv}(T)$ to coordinates for the table that realign the patient.

3 Results

Tests have been performed using a CT dataset (295 slices, 0.8 mm slice distance) of a human scull phantom (Fig. 3) and a CT dataset (300 slices, 1.0 mm slice distance) of an anathomic pelvis phantom. We produced intended alignment errors as can be expected in real treatment situations and used respective X-ray images taken from within a tratment device to computed the correction (Tab. 3).

Using a ROI, the results are slightly more inaccurate in general, but the algorithm is able to find a correction in much shorter time (inverse proportional

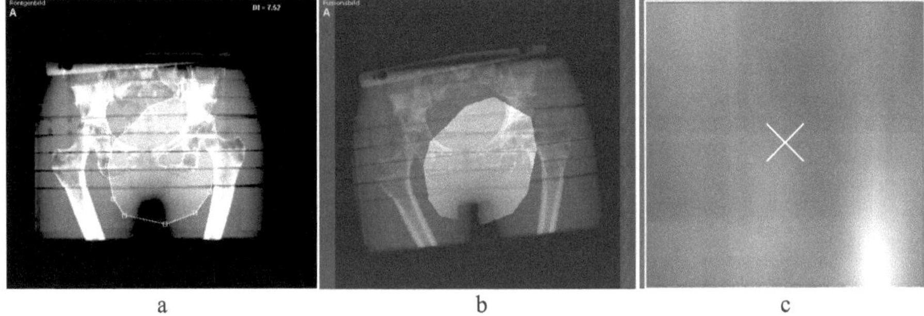

Fig. 2. X-ray image of pelvis phantom with ROI (a); overlaid with respective DRR (b); Mutual Information for 20cm x 20cm transformations (current MI value at center)

to the ROI area) and it shows to be more stable if disturbing features can be excluded.

4 Discussion

Automatic image based position correction is mandatory for efficient operation of a commercial particle beam treatment facility. The results show that our automatic position correction procedure is able to improve or verify the initial patient alignment. The number of X-ray images can be reduced to one X-ray image, whereas manual setup would need several iterations and pairs of X-ray images. In this way the X-ray dose applied onto the patient can be reduced. The acceleration of the setup procedure assures a contemporary radiation treatment with fewer changes of the patient alignment before treatment and additionally allows a higher patient throughput. However, compared to the automatic method proposed in [3], which makes use of 2 images, the single X-ray image approach suffers from lower accuracy if large translations along the X-ray beam axis occur (Tab. 1: 4mm along X-ray). That is because using a single X-ray image this translation value highly depends on correct determination of the image scale,

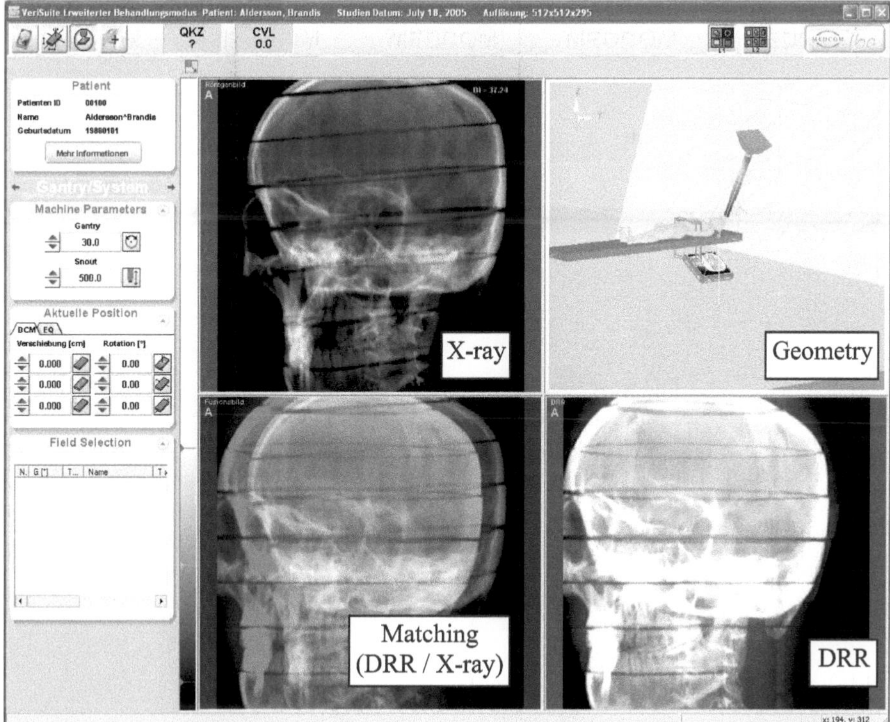

Fig. 3. Alignment correction application with images of a human scull phantom

which is, depending on the geometric setup of the X-ray equipment, not very sensitive to changes in translations of the patient. But, as higher accuracy could be achieved using higher resolution CT-scans and a modified alignment of the X-ray equipment, it should be possible to overcome this problem and to benefit from the advantages using only a single DFP.

References

1. Verhey LJ, Goitein M, McNulty P, et al. Precise positioning of patients for radiation therapy. Int J Radiat Oncol Biol Phys. 1982;8(2):289–94.
2. Thilmann C, Nill S, Tücking T, et al. Correction of patient positioning errors based on in-line cone beam CTs: Clinical implementation and first experiences. Int J Radiat Oncol Biol Phys. 2005;63(1):550–1.
3. Selby B, Sakas G, Walter S, et al. Detection of pose changes for spatial objects from projective images. In: Photogrammetric Image Analysis, The International Archives of the Photogrammetry, Remote Sensing and Spatial Information Sciences; 2007. p. 105–10.
4. Clippe S, Sarrut D, Malet C, et al. Patient setup error measurement using 3D intensity-based image registration techniques. Int J Radiat Oncol Biol Phys. 2003;56(1):259–65.
5. Press WH, Teukolsky SA, Vetterling WT, et al. Numerical Recipes in C. vol. 2. Cambridge: Cambridge University Press; 1992.

Entwicklung und Optimierung eines elastischen Registrierungsverfahrens für CTA und RA Daten

Ralf O. Floca[1], Roland Metzner[1], Christian R. Wirtz[2], Hartmut Dickhaus[1]

[1]Institut für Medizinische Biometrie und Informatik, Universität Heidelberg
[2]Neurochirurgische Klinik, Universitätsklinikum Heidelberg
ralf.floca@med.uni-heidelberg.de

Kurzfassung. Problemspezifische Optimierung von parametrisierten Bildverarbeitungsmethoden ist eine häufig vorkommende Aufgabenstellung. Eine möglichst automatisierte Optimierungsstrategie ist hierbei in vielerlei Hinsicht attraktiv und wünschenswert. Das frei verfügbare F.r.e.e. (flexible registration and evaluation engine) ermöglicht eine solche systematische, maschinelle Optimierung. Diese Möglichkeit wird für die Entwicklung eines elastischen Registrierungsverfahrens für CT Angiographie- und konventionellen Rotationsangiographieaufnahmen genutzt. Beide getrennt vorliegenden Informationsquellen werden dadurch erfolgreich in die OP Navigation integriert und erleichtern so einen komplikationsfreien operativen Eingriff. Dieser Beitrag belegt die Qualität des Registrierungsverfahrens und die Möglichkeit der automatisierten Optimierung.

1 Einleitung

Hohe Leistungsfähigkeit von Bildverarbeitungsverfahren ist im Kontext klinischer Anwendungen wichtig. Sie kann jedoch nur gewährleistet werden, wenn Verfahren auf die entsprechende Problemstellung angepasst sind. Begründet ist dies im „no free lunch“ Theorem von Wolpert [1]. Danach führt gute Performance in einer Problemklasse zu einem Performanceverlust in anderen Klassen. Somit können Verfahren nicht per se auf neue Problemstellungen übertragen werden. Sie müssen erst evaluiert und wenn notwendig angepasst werden. Diese Evaluierung ist gerade im Bereich der klinischen Anwendungen bedeutsam, denn der mangelnder Transfer von Entwicklungen in die klinische Praxis ist oft in unzureichender Evaluierung begründet (Jannin et al. [2] und Lehmann [3]). Das Framework f.r.e.e. [4] behandelt diese Problematik. Es bietet eine Infrastruktur für automatisierte Parameteroptimierung und für die Verfahrensevaluierung.

In diesem Beitrag wird die Registrierung von CT Angiographie- (CTA) und 3D Rotationsangiographieaufnahmen (RA) aus konventioneller Röntgendurchleuchtung [5] behandelt. Beide Modalitäten werden im Rahmen einer Aneurysmadiagnostik und anschließender operativer Therapie erfasst. Bisher lag die RA, trotz ihrer Qualität (hohe Auflösung und guter Kontrast), getrennt von der OP-Navigation vor und musste durch den Operateur während der OP an einem

Schaukasten verglichen werden. Durch die mit f.r.e.e. konzeptionierte und optimierte Registrierung sollen die RA Bilder für eine OP-Navigation integriert zur Verfügung gestellt werden und somit die Durchführung der OP unterstützen. Dies ist wünschenswert, da OP-Eingriffe zum Setzen eines Clips mit Komplikationen behaftet sind; diese können laut einer Studie von McLaughlin et al. [6] sogar bis zu 20,3% der OPs betreffen.

Im Folgenden werden die Evaluierung und Optimierung dieser elastische Registrierung dargelegt, die Ergebnisse erörtert und damit die Effektivität der Parameteroptimierung und die Qualität des Verfahrens belegt.

2 Material und Methode

Bis jetzt ist kein offen zugängliches Werkzeug bekannt, mit dem Registrierungsverfahren automatisiert möglichst optimal eingestellt werden können, obwohl ein großes Spektrum an Standardisierungsvorschlägen für Bildverarbeitungsmethoden für medizinische Anwendungen existiert. Vielmehr ist es häufig ein zeitraubender empirischer Prozess, in dem mittels Versuchsserien oder Erfahrungswerten nach einer brauchbaren Parametereinstellung gesucht wird. Das von uns realisierte System f.r.e.e. erlaubt es u.a. diese Suche systematisch auf die Maschine zu verlagern. Die offene Architektur bietet eine einfache und dynamische Integrationsmöglichkeit für zu optimierende Verfahren, Optimierungsmethoden und individuelle Qualitätsmaße (Metriken). Es ist somit über seinen ursprünglichen Methodensatz hinaus ein allgemeines Optimierungswerkzeug für alle parametrisierbaren Methoden, für die man eine Metrik zur Qualitätsbestimmung definieren kann. Darüber hinaus werden Multiprozessorsysteme unterstützt, da die Optimierung in f.r.e.e. parallelisierbar ist. F.r.e.e. ist in ISO-C++ implementiert und plattformunabhängig. Detailliertere Informationen bezüglich f.r.e.e. und seiner Funktionalität finden sich auf der Projektseite (http://freetk.sourceforge.net) und im zugehörige Artikel [4].

Die RA ist eine Bildgebungsmodalität, mit der kontrastmittelgefüllte Gefäßstrukturen in hoher Auflösung (ca. 0,18×0,18×0,18 mm^3) räumlich abgebildet werden. Das abgebildete Volumen ist meist 256^3 Voxel groß und bildet damit nur einen kleinen Ausschnitt des Kopfes ab. Die CTA deckt mit einer typischen Größe von 512×512×130 Voxel den ganzen Kopf ab, ist jedoch schlechter aufgelöst (ca. 0,42×0,42×1 mm^3), wie in Abb. 1 dargestellt. Die Registrierung der CTA und RA Daten soll möglichst schnell und mit minimaler Nutzerinteraktion durchgeführt werden.

Um diese Registrierung durchzuführen, wurde ein mehrstufiger Prozess mit f.r.e.e konzeptioniert. Die erste Stufe ist eine rigide Vorregistrierung (Rotation/Translation). Zur Initialisierung muss hierfür ein Initialisierungspunktepaar in beiden Bildern grob gewählt werden (Toleranz: ca. 2 mm). Nachdem die Vorstufe abgeschlossen ist, wird das Zwischenergebnis nun elastisch mittels B-Splines registriert. Beide Stufen nutzen als Metrik die Mutual Information nach Mattes (Mattes MI) [7]. Eine intensitätsgetriebene Registrierung wurde nach ersten Untersuchungen gewählt, da die Gefäßsegmentierung in der CTA nicht trivial ist.

Dies liegt vor allem an der Auflösung und dem diffusen Grauwertprofil in dem sich Knochenränder, umliegendes Gewebe und Gefäße überlappen. Die elastische Registrierung ist notwendig, da nicht rigide Deformationen am Gefäßbaum vorliegen, die durch eine rein rigide Registrierung nicht kompensiert werden können.

Es wurden insgesamt 19 Verfahrensparameter optimiert (u.a. Stichprobengröße und Binning der Mattes MI, Auflösung des B-Spline-Grids und Schrittgröße der Registrierung). Die Verfahrensoptimierung wurde mittels einer evolutionären Strategie [8] durchgeführt. Insgesamt dauerte die hier vorgestellte Optimierung des Verfahrens knapp 10 Tage (P4 2GHz, 2 GB RAM).

Neben der Evaluierung der Verfahrensgenauigkeit für das optimierte Verfahren sollte auch die Hypothese H1 „Die automatisierte Optimierung führt zu einer echten Verbesserung der Ergebnisqualität" geprüft werden. Für die Optimierung des Verfahrens wurden 5 Bildpaare an Aneurysmapatienten (Trainingsdaten) genutzt und für die Evaluierung 12 weitere Bildpaare (Testdaten). In all diesen wurden Referenzpunktpaare für die Verfahrensevaluierung /-optimierung festgelegt. Der Registrierungsfehler dieser Bildpaare wurde mit den Testdaten ermittelt und diente als Grundlage für einen einseitigen Test, mit welchem die Hypothese geprüft wurde.

3 Ergebnisse

Der mittlere Registrierungsfehler lag vor der Optimierung des Verfahrens bei 4,8 mm (SEM 0,81 mm) und nach der Optimierung des Verfahrens bei 1,6 mm (SEM

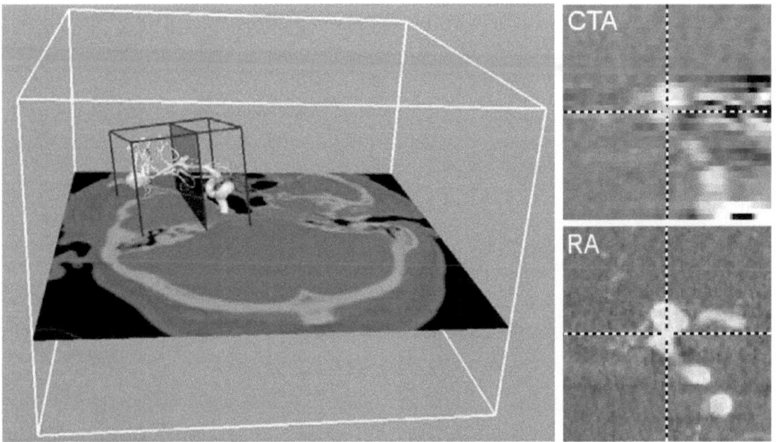

Abb. 1. Links: Verdeutlichung der Größen- und Lagesituation von CTA (weißer Kasten) und RA Volumen (schwarzer Kasten). Die Gefäßrekonstruktion der RA ist weiß eingeblendet, der beispielhafte RA Bildausschnitt (siehe rechts) ist als dunkeler Schnitt angedeutet und von der CTA ist ein horizontaler Schnitt dargestellt. Rechts: Beispiel für Auflösungs- und Qualitätsunterschiede der Ausgangsdaten CTA und RA; mit Initialisierung (gepunktetes Kreuz)

0,153 mm). Typische Bilder einer Registrierung sind in Abb. 2 dargestellt. Da bei Registrierungsfehlerstichprobe keine Normalverteilung angenommen werden kann (laut Kolmogorow-Smirnow-Test), wurde mittels Mann-Whitney-U-Test geprüft. Die Korrektheit der Hypothese H1 wird durch den Test mit einem Fehler von unter 2,5% bestätigt. Auch lässt sich feststellen, dass mit über 95% Wahrscheinlichkeit der maximale Fehler pro Fall minimiert wurde; ohne Optimierung betrug der mittlere maximale Fehler 6,3 mm (SEM 2,1 mm), optimiert hingegen 2,6 mm (SEM 0,4 mm). Im extremsten Fall wurde der Fehler von 25,7 mm auf 4,7 mm gesenkt. Die gesamte Registrierung (mit Dateneinlesen und Ergebnisspeicherung) benötigt im Mittel ca. 5,5 min (Intel Core Duo 1,7 GHz; 2 GB RAM).

4 Diskussion

Der ermittelte mittlere Registrierungsfehler von 1,6 mm kann im Kontext dieser Anwendung als akzeptabel angesehen werden. Dies ist dadurch begründet, dass die Bildauflösung der CTA bis zu 1 mm beträgt und dass das OP-Navigationssystem selbst eine Ungenauigkeit von 1 mm hat. Des Weiteren ist der qualitative Eindruck für den Operateur vorrangig. Die gewonnen Daten werden genutzt, um die Topologie des Gefäßes in der Operationszone zu verdeutlichen (z.B. für den Operateur verdeckte zuführende und abführende Gefäße beim Aneurysma) und so darzustellen, wie sie während des operativen Zugangs tatsächlich ausgerichtet sind. Somit ist eine möglichst genaue Registrierung wünschenswert, jedoch eine plausible visuelle Integration der RA-Daten vorrangig. Insgesamt sind die Ergebnisse sehr vielversprechend und von klinischer Seite als gut befunden. Das System wurde bisher für 3 Operationen im produktiven Einsatz genutzt und in allen Fällen erfolgreich eingesetzt.

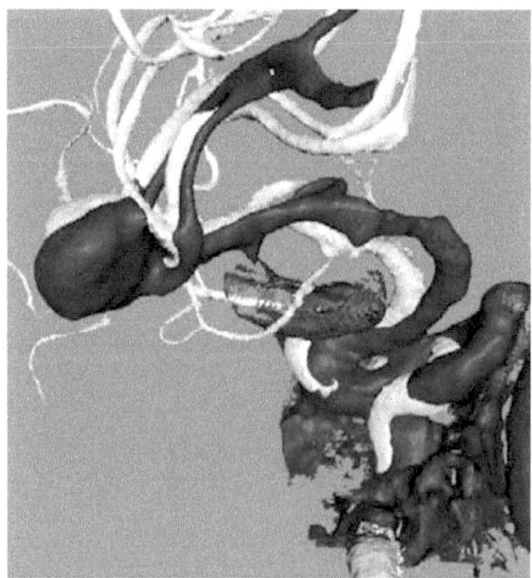
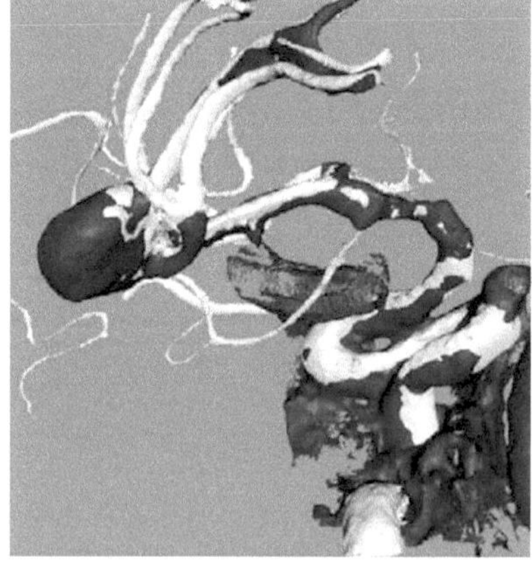

Abb. 2. Effekt der elastischen Registrierung. Links: Überblendung der Gefäßrekonstruktion aus CTA (schwarz) und RA (weiß) vor der elastischen Registrierung. Rechts: Überblendung nach der elastischen Registrierung

Die Hypothese H1 wird gegen einen Fehler von 2,5% geprüft und bestätigt. Somit ist gezeigt, dass die automatisierte Optimierung nicht rigider und mehrstufiger Registrierungsverfahren (rigide+elastisch) erfolgreich möglich ist. Die Genauigkeit des Verfahrens wurde allgemein verbessert. Ebenso wurde die Robustheit des elastischen Verfahrens erhöht, da die Auflösung des Grids und Schrittgröße der Registrierung auf die Datennatur angepasst wurden. Diese Anpassung wird unter anderem an der teilweise extremen Senkung des maximalen Fehlers deutlich.

Da der Trainingsdatensatz recht klein war, besteht die Gefahr des Overfittings. Deshalb könnte die Qualität des Verfahrens unterschätzt worden sein. Aus diesem Grund soll noch einmal mit einem inzwischen größeren Trainings- und Testdatenbestand optimiert und evaluiert werden. Des Weiteren muss noch evaluiert werden wie stark sich der Verfahrenseinsatz letztlich auf den Therapieerfolg auswirkt und hilft das Auftreten von Komplikationen zu vermindern.

Unsere Ergebnisse motivieren f.r.e.e. auch für andere Bereiche zur Verfügung zu stellen. Dies ist, zusammen mit der Entwicklung effizienterer Optimierungsstrategien und der Vergrößerung der Metrikauswahl, unser nächstes wichtiges Ziel. Aufgrund der modularen Struktur von f.r.e.e. ist eine Erweiterung in Form neuer Verfahren, Optimierungsmethoden und Metriken einfach zu realisieren. Dies und die Veröffentlichung des Frameworks (http://freetk.sourceforge.net) unter der GNU GPL motiviert zur Nutzung auch abseits der originären Aufgabenfelder. Wünschenswertes und angestrebtes Langzeitziel ist die Schaffung einer personalisierbaren, also auf die eigene Datensituation und Infrastruktur angepasste, Benchmark für medizinische Bildverarbeitungsmethoden. F.r.e.e. stellt einen ersten wichtigen Schritt in diese Richtung dar.

Literaturverzeichnis

1. Wolpert D, Macready W. No free lunch theorems for optimization. IEEE Trans Evol Comput. 1997;1(1):67–82.
2. Jannin P, Fitzpatrick JM, et al DJH. Validation of medical image processing in image-guided therapy. IEEE Trans Med Imaging. 2002;21:1445–9.
3. Lehmann TM, Bredno J. Strategies to configure image analysis algorithms for clinical usage. J Am Med Inform Assoc. 2005;12(5):497–504.
4. Floca R, Dickhaus H. A flexible registration and evaluation engine (f.r.e.e.). Comp Meth Prog Biomed. 2007;87(2):81–92.
5. Koppe R, Klotz E, et al MG. Die 3-D-Rotationsangiographie (3-D-RA) in der Neuroradiologie. Clin Neuroradiol. 2003;13(2):55–65.
6. McLaughlin N, Bojanowski MW. Early surgery-related complications after aneurysm clip placement: An analysis of causes and patient outcomes. J Neurosurg. 2004;101:600–6.
7. Mattes D, Haynor DR, Vesselle H. Non-rigid multimodality image registration. Proc SPIE. 2001; p. 1609–20.
8. Beyer HG, Schwefel HP. Evolution strategies: A comprehensive introduction. Nat Comput. 2002;1:3–52.

Registrierung im Fokus
Beschleunigung variationeller Methoden für die Bildregistrierung

Nils Papenberg, Jan Modersitzki, Bernd Fischer

Institut für Mathematik, Universität zu Lübeck, Wallstraße 40, 23560 Lübeck
papenber@math.uni-luebeck.de

Kurzfassung. In vielen praktischen Problemstellungen ist der Anwender nur in wenigen ausgezeichneten Bildbereichen an einer hochgenauen Registrierung interessiert. Dieser Umstand wird in der vorliegenden Arbeit konsequent umgesetzt. Es wird eine Multiresolutionsstrategie vorgestellt, die es dem Anwender erstmalig erlaubt, auf ausgewählte Bildbereiche zu fokussieren. Das Verfahren ist in einen variationellen Kontext eingebettet und bietet einen deutlichen Geschwindigkeitsvorteil gegenüber herkömmlichen Methoden. Neben der Herleitung wird die Wirkungsweise des Verfahrens beispielhaft illustriert und die Qualität der Ergebnisse diskutiert. Es zeigt sich, dass dieser neue Ansatz den problemangepassten Einsatz variationeller Methoden in zeitkritischen Anwendungen erlaubt.

1 Einleitung

Im Bereich der Bildregistrierung haben sich variationelle Methoden als erfolgreiches Werkzeug etabliert. Eine Eigenschaft dieser Methoden ist es, dass sie für jeden Voxel des einen Bildes (Referenzbild) seinen korrespondierenden Punkt im anderen Bild (Templatebild) bestimmen. Nachteilig ist dies bei hochaufgelösten drei- (oder höher-) dimensionalen Daten. So müssen im Falle der Registrierung zweier Volumen-Daten mit 512^3 Voxeln mehr als 400 Millionen Unbekannte bestimmt werden, um ein dichtes Deformationsfeld zu erhalten, das in der Auflösung der Daten liegt.

Nachteilig um so mehr, da in vielen Fällen nur die Registrierung bestimmter Bereiche für den Anwender von Interesse sind, beispielsweise für eine Operationsplanung die Umgebung eines Tumors. Registrierungsergebnisse andere Bildbereiche (wie entfernt liegende Organe oder Bildhintergrund) sind nicht benötigt, werden aber mit hohen Zeitkosten bestimmt. In dieser Arbeit stellen wir erstmalig ein Verfahren vor, dass diesen Nachteil behebt.

Wesentlicher Bestandteil ist eine neue Multiresolutionsstrategie. Bisherige variationelle Methoden lösen zuerst ein grob diskretisiertes Registrierungsproblem, dessen Lösung dann als Startwert auf einer feineren Diskretisierung genutzt wird, so iterierend, bis die gewünschte Diskretisierungsauflösung erreicht ist [1, 2]. Das neue Verfahren liefert ein Registrierungsergebnis nur für ein vom Anwender vorher bestimmtes Gebiet. Beginnend mit einem grob diskretisierten Problem strebt die neue Multiresolutionsstrategie auf dieses Zielgebiet zu, in dem sie bei einem Wechsel der Diskretisierungsauflösung das zu registrierende Gebiet verkleinert, bis das Zielgebiet erreicht ist. Aus der Verkleinerung des Gebietes folgt, dass die Anzahl der Diskretisierungspunkte beim Wechsel der Gitter konstant und klein gehalten werden kann bei gleichzeitiger Verfeinerung der realen Auflösung im Zielgebiet.

2 Material und Methoden

Wir beschreiben das neue Verfahren in mehreren Schritten. Als erstes wiederholen wir kurz die Herleitung nicht-linearer Registrieralgorithmen. Im zweiten Schritt beschreiben wir den neuen Gitterwechsel und führen als Drittes diese Bausteine zu einem Algorithmus zusammen.

Der variationelle Ansatz basiert auf der Minimierung eines Funktionals $\mathcal{J}$ bezüglich der gesuchten Transformation y:

$$\mathcal{J}(y) = \mathcal{D}(\mathcal{T}(y), \mathcal{R}) + \alpha \mathcal{S}(y) \xrightarrow{y} \min$$

Hierbei sind $\mathcal{R}, \mathcal{T}$ die gegebenen d-dimensionalen Bilder, $\mathcal{T}(y)$ das transformierte Bild, $\mathcal{D}$ ein Distanzmaß, $\mathcal{S}$ ein Regularisierer und α ein Regulariserungsparameter (vergleiche [1]). Zur Ableitung eines Algorithmus verwenden wir einen Discretize-Optimize Ansatz [2]. Dafür wird das Gebiet $\Sigma \subset \mathbb{R}^d$ der Registrierung mittels eines Gitters $X \in \mathbb{R}^n$ diskretisiert. Gesucht ist nun das transformierte Gitter $y(X) = Y \in \mathbb{R}^n$. Nach Diskretisierung der Maße $\mathcal{D}$ und $\mathcal{S}$ erhalten wir ein diskretes Optimierungsproblem, das mit einem Gauß-Newton-Verfahren gelöst wird.

Wir erklären als nächstes den Kern des neuen Algorithmus: die Fokussierung von einen größeren Gebiet auf ein kleineres. Dazu betrachten wir zwei quaderförmige Gebiete Σ^o (*outer*) und Σ^i (*inner*) mit $\Sigma^i \subset \Sigma^o$, (Abb. 1, links). Beide Gebiete sind durch regelmäßige Gitter $X^o, X^i \in \mathbb{R}^n$ diskretisiert (Abb. 1, mitte). Eine Tranformation $Y^o \in \mathbb{R}^n$ auf dem großen Gebiet wird zur Bestimmung einer

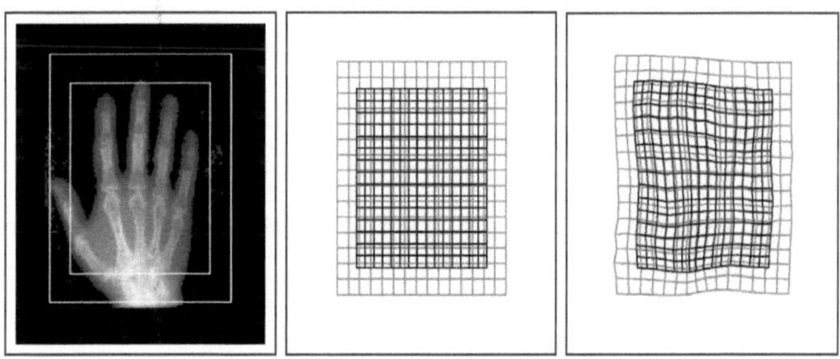

Abb. 1. Illustration des Gitterwechsels. *links:* Beispieldaten mit Gebieten Σ^o (außen) und Σ^i; *mitte:* Diskretierungen der Gebiete X^o (hell) und X^i (dunkel); *rechts:* Deformiertes Gitter Y^o auf Σ^o (hell) und interpoliertes deformiertes Gitter Y^i auf Σ^i (dunkel)

Transformation auf dem kleinen Gebiet Σ^i verwendet, indem wir an den Punkten X^i eine Transformation Y^i bestimmen. Hierzu interpolieren wir die Werte der Transformation auf dem großen Gebiet Y^o. Bei diesem Vorgehen wird das Gebiet und die Diskretisierungsauflösung kleiner, jedoch bleibt die Anzahl der Gitterpunkte konstant und klein (Abb. 1, rechts).

Das eigentliche Verfahren nutzt nun beide Bausteine. Nach Festlegen des Zielgebietes durch den Anwender wird mittels des beschriebenen Registrierungsalgorithmus ein Deformationsfeld auf den grob diskretisierten Bilddaten bestimmt. Dieses Ergebnis wird nun als Startwert einer Registrierung auf einem kleineren Gebiet genutzt, in dem es auf dieses mittels des beschriebenen Gitterwechsels transferiert wird. Dieser Ablauf wiederholt sich, wobei die immer kleiner werdenden Gebiete suksessiv auf das Zielgebiet zustreben. Das Verfahren endet, wenn für das Zielgebiet eine Deformation bestimmt ist.

Zwei Eigenschaften dieses Verfahrens sind hervorzuheben: Zum einen wird deutlich, dass bei der Bestimmung des Deformationsfeldes für das Zielgebiet globale Informationen einfließen, die durch den speziellen Gitterwechsel erhalten bleiben und auf das lokale Zielgebiet transferiert werden. Zum anderen, dass das zu wählende Zielgebiet nur im Referenzbild festgelegt werden muss, da der Algorithmus das hierzu korrespondierende Gebiet im Templatebild automatisch durch den beschriebenen Gitterwechsel bestimmt.

3 Ergebnisse

Zur Darstellung der prinzipiellen Arbetisweise des Algorithmus wählen wir ein 2-dimensionales Beispiel, an 3-dimensionalen Daten illustrieren wir den zu erzielenden Zeitgewinn.

Das Referenzbild des $2d$-Beispiels ist in Abb. 2, oben links, dargestellt, zusammen mit einem vom Anwender gewählten Bereich um den Daumen der dargestellten Hand. Für diesen Bereich ist weiterhin eine Diskretisierung dargestellt, dessen korrespondierendes Gitter im Templatebild automatisch gefunden werden soll. Desweiteren werden die einzelnen Gebiete gezeigt, auf denen der Algorithmus innerhalb der beschriebenen Multiresolutionsstrategie rechnet. Der Bildinhalt des Zielgebietes ist darunter in der Auflösung des Gitters gezeigt. Registrierungsergebnis ist das deformierte Gitter, das in Abb. 2, oben mitte, zusammen mit dem Templatebild gezeigt wird. Der vom Algorithmus gefundene, zum Zielgebiet im Referenzbild korrespondierende Ausschnitt ist darunter gezeigt. In jedem Level des Algorithmuss wurde das aktuelle Gebiet mit 32×32 Punkten diskretisiert. Als Maße verwenden wir SSD und elastische Regularisierung. Als Vergleich sind die Daten mit einem herkömmlichen Verfahren [3] gerechnet worden. Der Zielausschnitt des Ergebnisses ist in gleicher Abbildung unten rechts gezeigt.

Die Stärke des Algorithmus zeigt sich bei 3-dimensionalen Daten. Um zu zeigen, um wie viel schneller der vorgestellte Algorithmus ist, vergleichen wir einen herkömmlichen Algorithmus [3] mit dem neu vorgestellten Verfahren. Wir nutzen als Testvolumen MR-Daten des Knies von Dr. J. Sénégas (Philips Research

Tabelle 1. Vergleich der Laufzeiten zwischen herkömmlicher Multiresolutionsstrategie und neuem Verfahren

Verfahren	gemittelte Laufzeit	relative Laufzeit
Herkömmliches Verfahren	12min 42sec	100.00%
Neuer Algorithmus (Zielgebiet: Gelenkköpfe)	44sec	5.72%
Neuer Algorithmus (Zielgebiet: Gelenkspalt)	10sec	1.31%

Europe - Hamburg) der Größe $128 \times 128 \times 64$ (Abb. 3). Als Zielgebiet wählen wir im Referenzbild den Bereich um den Gelenkspalt. Dies Gebiet wird so diskretisiert, dass es in der gleichen realen Auflösung liegt wie die Daten. Testrechner ist ein Intel Xeon 3Ghz mit 12GB Arbeitsspeicher, die Algorithmen sind in Matlab implementiert. Aus Platzgründen visualisieren wir die Ergebisse nicht.. Der herkömmliche Algorithmus benötigt zur Registrierung der Daten 12min 42sec (gemittelt aus 5 Testläufen), der neu vorgestellte Algorithmus 44sec (ebenfalls gemittelt). Dies bedeutet eine Beschleunigung um Faktor 16. Wählen wir den Zielbereich enger um das Gelenk, bestimmt das neue Verfahren die Deformation in 10sec (5 Testläufe gemittelt), was 1/75 der Ausgangszeit ist (Tabelle 1).

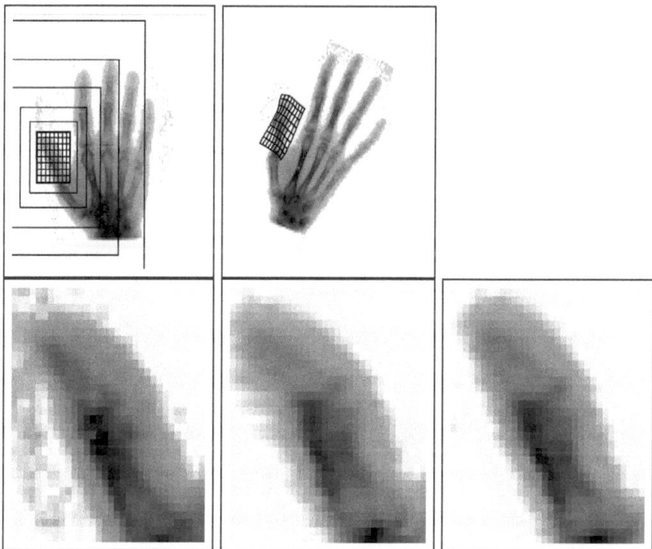

Abb. 2. Ergebnis 2*d*-Beispiel: *oben links:* Referenzbild mit Zielgebiet und Diskretisierungsgitter; *oben mitte:* Templatebild mit automatisch bestimmtem deformierten Gitter; *unten links:* Bildausschnitt im Referenzbild; *unten mitte:* Templatebild, ausgewertet auf deformiertem Gitter; *unten rechts:* Zielausschnitt, bestimmt mit herkömmlichem Verfahren

Abb. 3. Datensatz für $3d$-Beispiel; *links:* Template; *rechts:* Referenz

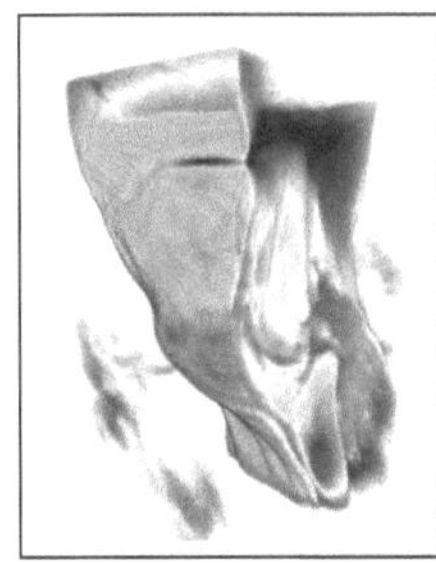

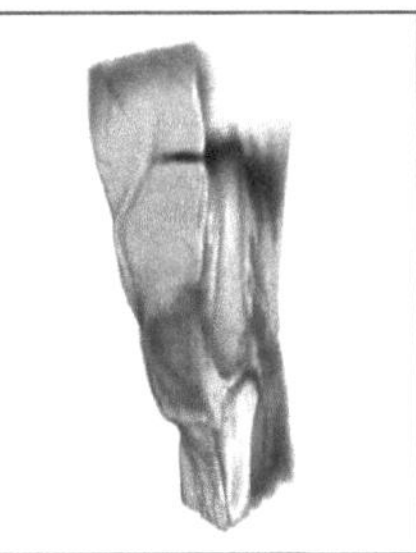

4 Diskussion

Wir haben eine neue Strategie für ein Multiresolutionsverfahren im Bereich der variationellen Bildregistrierung vorgestellt, die es ermöglicht, die Registrierung großer Datenvolumen drastisch schneller als bisher durchzuführen, vorausgesetzt, dass der Anwender zuvor ein Zielgebiet, bsp. die Umgebung eines Tumors, bestimmte Gewebebereiche etc, ausweist. Diese Strategie ist weitaus speicherplatz- und zeiteffizienter als herkömmliche Multiresolutionsstrategien. Dennoch sind die Ergebnisse qualitativ gleichwertig zu den bisher erzielten Resultaten.

In dieser Arbeit haben wir aufgrund der gebotenen Kürze den Algorithmus nur für die Wahl des SSD-Maßes und des elastischen Regularisierers vorgestellt. Das Nutzen anderer Maße, wie *normalized gradient field* [4] oder *mutual information* [5], und anderer Regularisierer ist möglich und bereits umgesetzt.

Wir können als Resümee festhalten, dass in Anwendungen, bei denen die Registrierung bestimmter Teilbereiche von Interesse ist, die vorgestellte Strategie eine deutliche Beschleunigung darstellt und es erstmalig ermöglicht, variationelle Methoden in zeitkritischen Anwendungsgebieten zu nutzen.

Literaturverzeichnis

1. Modersitzki J. Numerical Methods for Image Registration. Oxford University Press; 2004.
2. Haber E, Modersitzki J. A multilevel method for image registration. SIAM J Sci Comput. 2006;27(5):1594–607.
3. Papenberg N, Schumacher H, Heldmann H, et al. A fast and flexible image registration toolbox: Design and implementation of the general approach. Proc BVM. 2007.
4. Haber E, Modersitzki J. Intensity gradient based registration and fusion of multimodal images. Lect Note Comp Sci. 2006;3216:591–98.
5. Viola PA. Alignment by Maximization of Mutual Information. MIT Press; 1995.

Automatische Kamerapositionierung für intra-operative Visualisierungen in der onkologischen Leberchirurgie

Konrad Mühler[1], Christian Hansen[2], Mathias Neugebauer[1], Bernhard Preim[1]

[1]Institut für Simulation und Graphik, Otto-von-Guericke Universität Magdeburg
[2]MeVis Research – Center for Medical Image Computing, Bremen
muehler@isg.cs.uni-magdeburg.de

Kurzfassung. In diesem Beitrag wird ein Verfahren vorgestellt, mit dessen Hilfe automatisch gute Blickpunkte auf dreidimensionale Planungsmodelle für die Leberchirurgie berechnet werden können. Das Verfahren passt die Position der virtuellen Kamera während einer Operation dynamisch an, insbesondere im Falle einer Aktualisierung von onkologischen Planungsdaten durch neue intra-operative Befunde.

1 Einleitung

1.1 Motivation

Zur Navigationsunterstützung während komplexer leberchirurgischer Eingriffe werden dem Chirurgen zunehmend getrackter Ultraschall zusammen mit dreidimensionalen Planungsmodellen auf einem Bildschirm direkt am Situs dargeboten (Abb. 1(a)) [1, 2]. Bei den verwendeten Planungsmodellen handelt es sich um patientenindividuelle Modelle der Organoberfläche, Gefäßsysteme und pathologischen Strukturen, die aus prä-operativen Tomographiedaten rekonstruiert werden. Im Verlauf eines Eingriffes kommt es häufig vor, dass sich die dargestellte Planungsszene durch intra-operativ detektierte Metastasen verändert [3]. Um dem Chirurgen jederzeit eine effektive Sicht auf die Daten zu gewährleisten, ist eine Neupositionierung der virtuellen Kamera in vielen Fällen notwendig. Hierfür musste der Chirurg bisher aufwendig mit einer Maus in der Szene navigieren und wurde so unnötig abgelenkt. Wir haben daher ein Verfahren entwickelt, dass automatisch die günstigste Kameraposition in einer Planungsszene berechnet und diese dem Chirurgen intra-operativ in Echtzeit zur Verfügung stellt.

1.2 Stand der Forschung

Im Bereich der intra-operativen Darstellung von dreidimensionalen Planungsdaten wurden in den letzten Jahren eine Reihe an Arbeiten veröffentlicht [1, 4, 5]. Bisher existiert jedoch kein Ansatz, der eine automatische Neupositionierung der Kamera während eines chirurgischen Eingriffes in Abhängigkeit von klinisch relevanten Parametern erlaubt.

Bei der Bestimmung guter Blickpunkte für 3D-Szenen konzentrierten sich bisherige Arbeiten meist auf eine Erweiterung des *viewpoint entropy* Ansatzes [6]. Dabei geht es um die Maximierung des Informationsgehaltes einer Sicht, bspw. durch ein optimales Verhältnis von sichtbaren Polygonen und sichtbarer Fläche [6] oder die Maximierung der sichtbaren Oberflächenkrümmung [7]. Das Maß der *viewpoint entropy* wurde von [8] und [9] auf Volumerendering-Darstellungen übertragen, jedoch auch hier, ohne einzelne Objekte in einer Szene zu unterscheiden.

In [10] wird ein neuartiges Verfahren vorgestellt, mit dem Kamerapositionen für einzelne Objekte in einer Darstellung für Interventionsplanungen generiert werden können. Dabei fließen unterschiedliche Parameter (sichtbare Fläche, Wichtigkeit verdeckender Strukturen, Vorzugsblickwinkel des Nutzers, Stabilität der Positionen, u.v.m.) in die Berechnung einer optimalen Kameraposition ein, wodurch diese in ihrer Bewertung objektiviert wird. Jeder Parameter wird durch eine so genannte *parameter map* repräsentiert, welche eine Funktion des Parameters über alle möglichen Kamerapositionen[1] darstellt. In einem Vorverarbeitungsschritt werden alle statischen Parameter wie sichtbare Fläche und Verdeckungen berechnet. Zur Ermittlung der optimalen Kameraposition zur Laufzeit werden die einzelnen *parameter maps* gewichtet summiert. Das Maximum des Ergebnisfeldes ist die neue Kameraposition. Eine unterschiedliche Wichtung der Parameter erlaubt es, das Verfahren für bestimmte Anwendungen und verschiedene Fragestellungen zu adaptieren.

2 Methoden

Ziel unseres Verfahrens ist es, einem Chirurgen während einer OP möglichst gute Sichten auf die fusionierten, dreidimensionalen Planungsdaten anzubieten. Eine gute Sicht wird dabei durch mehrere Parameter beeinflusst. So sollen mehrere Strukturen entsprechend ihrer aktuellen Bedeutung in einer Sicht erkennbar sein. Außerdem sollen neu hinzukommende Objekte, die erst intra-operativ in die Planungsdaten eingezeichnet werden, berücksichtigt werden.

Grundlage unseres Verfahrens ist die in [10] vorgestellte Methode zur Generierung von guten Kamerapositionen für einzelne Objekte. Wir haben den Ansatz sowohl um eine Methode, gute Sichten für mehrere Objekte zu generieren, als auch um die Möglichkeit, dynamisch erzeugte Objekte in die Bestimmung guter Kamerapositionen einzubeziehen, erweitert.

2.1 Gute Kamerapositionen für leberchirurgische Darstellungen

Bei der Planung und Durchführung von leberchirugischen Eingriffen spielt die relative Lage von Gefäßstrukturen zu umliegenden Metastasen eine wesentliche Rolle bei der Beurteilung der Resektabilität. Gespräche mit unseren klinischen Partnern haben gezeigt, dass diese relativen Lagebeziehungen am besten beurteilt werden können, wenn möglichst viele Gefäßäste in der Darstellung zu

[1] Die Positionen befinden sich äquidistant auf einer die Szene umgebenden Kugel.

erkennen sind. Daher führen wir als neuen Parameter zur Sichtbewertung die Länge der sichtbaren Silhouette einer Struktur ein. Als Silhouette werden dabei all jene Pixel einer projizierten Fläche betrachtet, die in ihrer 4er-Nachbarschaft ein Hintergrundpixel haben. Der Parameter der Silhouettenlänge geht mit relativ hohem Gewicht gegenüber anderen Parametern wie der sichtbaren Fläche in die Berechnung der optimalen Kameraposition ein. Dies führt zu deutlich besseren Sichten auf Gefäßbäume (Abb. 1(b),1(c)).

Um die Adaption der Darstellung auf den Situs für den Chirurgen zu erleichtern, wählt unser Verfahren eine annähernd gleiche Blickrichtung auf die dargestellten Planungmodelle, wie sie der Chirurg auf den Situs hat. Hierfür haben wir die möglichen Blickpunkte auf einen koronalen Sichtbereich mit einer Rotation von 60° axial und sagittal beschränkt. Die Beschränkung auf einen bestimmten Bereich erreichen wir durch die Änderung des existierenden Parameters des Vorzugsblickwinkels zu einem multiplikativen Faktor. Somit werden alle Kamerapositionen, die außerhalb der gewünschten Region liegen, mit 0 bewertet.

2.2 Gute Kamerapositionen für mehrere Objekte

Das bisherige Verfahren [10] war lediglich dazu ausgelegt, gute Kamerapositionen für einzelne Objekte in einer Szene zu ermitteln. Da aber während eines onkologischen Eingriffes eine gute Sicht sowohl auf alle Metastasen als auch auf die verschiedenen Gefäßbäume und Leberterritorien in gleicher Weise garantiert werden soll, wurde das Verfahren erweitert. Dazu berechnen wir die Ergebnisfelder aller beteiligten Objekte (*object maps*) wie in [10] und summieren diese gewichtet auf. Die Wichtung der einzelnen *object maps* erlaubt es, neu hinzugekommenen Metastasen bei der Ermittlung der Kameraposition ein höheres Gewicht gegenüber bereits prä-operativ segmentierten Strukturen zu geben. Das Maximum des sich ergebenden Feldes ist die gesuchte optimale Kameraposition für eine gute Sicht auf alle beteiligten Strukturen.

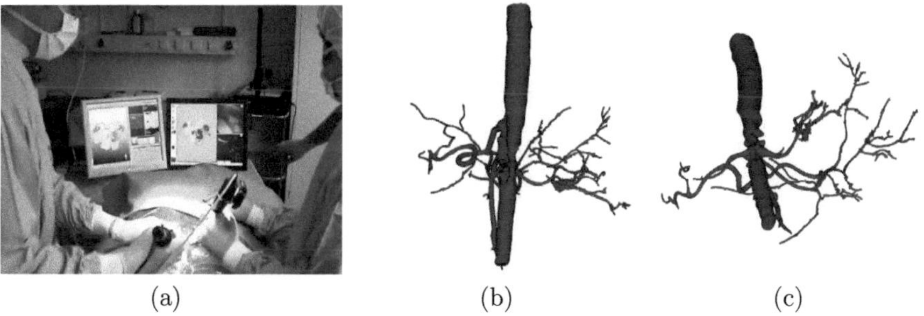

(a) (b) (c)

Abb. 1. (a) Intra-operative Visualisierung von Planungsdaten (UKSH Lübeck). Planungsmodelle und intra-operativer Ultraschall werden dem Chirurgen in einer Darstellung fusioniert präsentiert. Sichten auf eine Leberarterie ohne (b) und mit (c) Berücksichtung des neu eingeführten Silhouettenparameters

Zusätzlich zu dieser Kameraposition werden noch weitere Positionen ermittelt, die jeweils eine gute Sicht auf einzelne Metastasen bieten. Zusammen werden diese Kamerapositionen als Vorschau dem Chirurgen zur Auswahl präsentiert. Dieser kann dann die gewünschte Kameraposition per Touchscreen auswählen und muss nicht mehr aufwendig mit der Maus in der Szene navigieren.

2.3 Einbeziehung dynamischer Objekte in die Kameraberechnung

Das bisher genutzte Verfahren [10] erlaubt es nicht, nach der Vorberechnung neu zur Szene hinzugekommene Objekte in die Berechnung der Kameraposition mit einzubeziehen. Es müssten mit den neuen Objekten wiederum die Vorberechnungen zur Sichtbarkeitsbestimmung durchlaufen werden. Um dies zu vermeiden, aber dennoch die Einbeziehung während der Operation eingezeichneter Metastasen zu ermöglichen, nutzen wir so genannte Stellvertreterobjekte (SO). Dies sind Objekte, die schon zum Zeitpunkt der Vorberechnungen erzeugt werden und so als Vertreter dynamischer Objekte zur Sichtbarkeitsbestimmung herangezogen werden können. Zur Erzeugung der SO wird das Parenchymobjekt der Leber in ca. 30 würfelähnliche Teilobjekte unterteilt.

Anstelle einer neu hinzukommenden Metastase werden die Sichtbarkeitsinformationen der SO in deren Umgebung genutzt. Dabei wird das in Abschnitt 2.2 beschriebene Verfahren zur Sichtpunktberechnung für mehrere Objekte genutzt. Die SO für eine neue Metastase gehen entsprechend gewichtet der Größe ihrer Überlagerung mit der neuen Metastase in die Berechnung ein. So werden nur die SO genutzt, welche die neue Metastase schneiden.

3 Ergebnisse

Mit dem vorgestellten Verfahren ist es möglich, gute Kamerapositionen auf mehrere Objekte in intra-operativen Darstellungen automatisch zu generieren. Au-

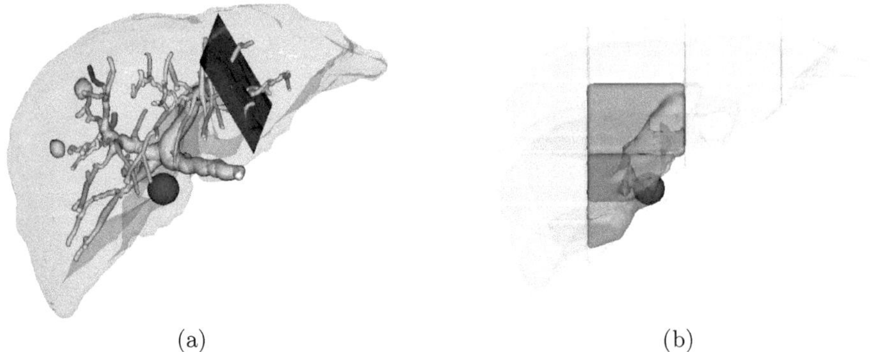

(a) (b)

Abb. 2. (a) Optimale Sicht auf die prä-operativ detektierten Metastasen, den portalvenösen Gefäßbaum und die intra-operativ gefundene Metastase (dunkle Kugel). Ebenfalls zu erkennen ist das fusionierte Ultraschall-Bild. (b) Darstellung der Stellvertreterobjekte für die neue Metastase

ßerdem konnte die Einbeziehung dynamischer Objekte in die Positionsberechnung mittels Stellvertreterobjekten realisiert werden. So können auch neue Befunde in Echtzeit optimal betrachtet werden, ohne dass der Chirurg in der dreidimensionalen Szene navigieren muss. Um verzweigten Strukturen besser gerecht zu werden, wurde als neuer Parameter zur Blickpunktbewertung die Silhouettenlänge eingeführt.

4 Diskussion

Derzeit wird ein Verfahren zur intra-operativen Anpassung der geplanten Resektionsebene entwickelt. Durch automatisch berechnete Kamerapositionen kann der Chirurg bei solchen Anpassungen besonders unterstützt werden. Es ist eine Evaluierung des vorgestellten Verfahrens in Zusammenarbeit mit den klinischen Partnern geplant. Derzeit befindet sich das Verfahren zusammen mit anderen neuen intra-operativen Visualisierungstechniken in der vorklinischen Erprobung.

Danksagung. Dieses Projekt wurde im Zusammenhang mit dem SOMIT-FUSION-Projekt durch das BMBF gefördert (FKZ 01-BE03B und FKZ 01-BE03C). Wir danken Stefan Schlichting (UKSH Lübeck) sowie allen involvierten Chirurgen aus dem FUSION-Projekt.

Literaturverzeichnis

1. Lange T, Eulenstein S, Hünerbein M, et al. Augmenting intraoperative 3D ultrasound with preoperative models for navigation in liver surgery. Proc MICCAI. 2004; p. 543–51.
2. Markert M, Weber S, Kleemann M, et al. Comparison of fundamental requirements for soft tissue navigation with a novel assistance system for open liver surgery. Proc CARS. 2006; p. 498–9.
3. Hansen C, Schlichting S, Markert M, et al. Intraoperative adaptation of preoperative risk analyses for oncologic liver surgery using navigated 2D-ultrasound. Proc CURAC. 2007; p. 155–8.
4. Hansen C, Köhn A, Ritter F, et al. Simultaneous visualization of preoperative planning models and intraoperative 2D ultrasound for liver surgery. Proc Eurographics. 2007; p. 73–6.
5. Nimsky C, Ganslandt O, Enders F, et al. Visualization strategies for major white matter tracts for intraoperative use. Proc CARS. 2005; p. 793–798.
6. Vazquez PP, Feixas M, Sbert M, et al. Viewpoint selection using viewpoint entropy. In: Vision, Modeling, and Visualization; 2001. p. 273–280.
7. Sokolov D, Plemenos D. Viewpoint quality and scene understanding. In: Proc Int EG Symp VR, Archaeology Cultural Heritage; 2005. p. 67–73.
8. Bordoloi U, Shen HW. View selection for volume rendering. In: Proc IEEE Vis; 2005. p. 487–94.
9. Takahashi S, Fujishiro I, Takeshima Y, et al. A feature-driven approach to locating optimal viewpoints for volume visualization. In: Proc IEEE Vis; 2005. p. 495–502.
10. Mühler K, Neugebauer M, Tietjen C, et al. Viewpoint Selection for intervention planning. Proc IEEE EuroVis. 2007; p. 267–74.

Magnetisches Tracking für die Navigation mit dem da Vinci® Surgical System

Felix Nickel[1], Ingmar Wegner[2], Hannes Kenngott[1], Jochen Neuhaus[2], Beat P. Müller-Stich[1], Hans-Peter Meinzer[2], Carsten N. Gutt[1]

[1]Klinik für Allgemein-, Viszeral-, und Transplantationschirurgie, Heidelberg
[2]Abteilung für Medizinische und Biologische Informatik, DKFZ Heidelberg
felix.nickel@med.uni-heidelberg.de

Kurzfassung. In dieser Studie wurde untersucht ob in einem typischen OP-Aufbau mit dem da Vinci® Telemanipulator elektromagnetisches Tracking für die Realisation eines Navigationssystems eingesetzt werden kann. Hierfür wurde in einem realen OP-Aufbau untersucht, wie stark metallische und ferromagnetisch wirksame Objekte wie Operationstisch und Telemanipulator das elektromagnetische Feld des Trackingsystems beeinflussen. Die Ergebnisse zeigen, dass der Telemanipulator nur unwesentlich die Störung des Magnetfeldes durch den OP-Tisch verstärkt. Insbesondere die Bewegung der Instrumente im Trackingvolumen verursachte keine zusätzliche relevante Störung des Magnetfeldes. Bei Begrenzung des Trackingvolumens auf eine Länge von 190 mm, Höhe von 200mm und Breite von 400 mm war der maximale Fehler in diesem Bereich an allen Messpunkten kleiner 10 mm. Der Einsatz von elektromagnetischem Tracking für die Navigation mit dem da Vinci® Surgical System ist somit in einem begrenzten Arbeitsvolumen mit hinreichender Genauigkeit möglich.

1 Einleitung

Navigationssysteme tragen zum Erfolg bei klassischen und telemanipulatorunterstützten minimalinvasiven operativen Eingriffen bei [1, 2]. Die Vorteile und Nachteile der roboterassisstierten und klassischen Minimalinvasiven Chirurgie (MIC) wurden an anderer Stelle diskutiert [3]. Für die Navigation bietet Elektromagnetisches Tracking (EMT) im Vergleich zum Optischen Tracking den Vorteil der Unabhängigkeit von Sichtbehinderungen [1]. Ein Nachteil der EMT-Systeme ist die Anfälligkeit für metallische und ferromagnetische Störquellen, welche im typischen OP-Aufbau vermehrt vorkommen. Solange diese Störquellen statisch sind, kann die Störung der Messung durch Kalibrierung und Softwareabstimmung minimiert werden [4]. Dynamische Störquellen sind schwer zu berücksichtigen. Das Ziel dieser Studie ist es zu untersuchen ob die Aktivität des da Vinci® Telemanipulator und die Bewegung der laparoskopischen Instrumente relevante Störfaktoren für die Genauigkeit des EMT sind und in welchem Bereich innerhalb des Trackingvolumens mit ausreichend hoher Genauigkeit gearbeitet werden kann.

2 Materialien und Methoden

2.1 Aufbau

Der Versuchsaufbau wurde im Hinblick auf die Navigation bei telemanipulatorgestützen, minimalinvasiven Eingriffen im oberen Gastrointestinaltrakt, im Besonderen Ösophagektomien, gewählt. Ein Phantom, welches aus 12 PVC-Röhren mit einer Länge von 50 cm mit einem Innendurchmesser von 5 mm besteht. (Abb.1), wurde so entwickelt, dass sowohl das Messvolumen des EMT in cranio-caudaler Länge mit einem EMT-Sensor kontinuierlich und reproduzierbar abgefahren werden konnte, als auch die beweglichen Instrumente des da Vinci® frei darin agieren konnten. Es wurde ein EMT-System des Typs Aurora® von Northern Digital Inc. (NDI, Toronto, Kanada) verwendet, welches mit einem Messvolumen von 50x50x50 cm angegeben wird [5]. Zur Messung wurde ein 5 DOF (degrees of freedom) Sensor vom Typ Mednetix-5DK und einem dem Innendurchmesser der PVC-Röhren angepassten Außendurchmesser eingesetzt.

2.2 Messungen

Insgesamt drei Messungen wurden als Referenz ohne Metall in einem Umkreis von 2 m erstellt. Dies gab Aufschluss über die Qualität des EMT ohne Störeinflüsse. Danach wurden Messungen im oben beschriebenen OP-Aufbau mit einem handelsüblichem OP-Tisch (Maquet™„Alphamaquet 1150“) durchgeführt. Ein Messversuch bestand aus 12 Einzelmessungen, die jeweils aus dem langsamen, kontinuierlichen Durchziehen des Sensors durch jede der PVC-Röhren bestanden, pro Röhre 200 Messpunkte. Die aus dem EMT System gelesenen Positionen wurden über die Zeit für die spätere Auswertung in einer XML-Datei gespeichert.

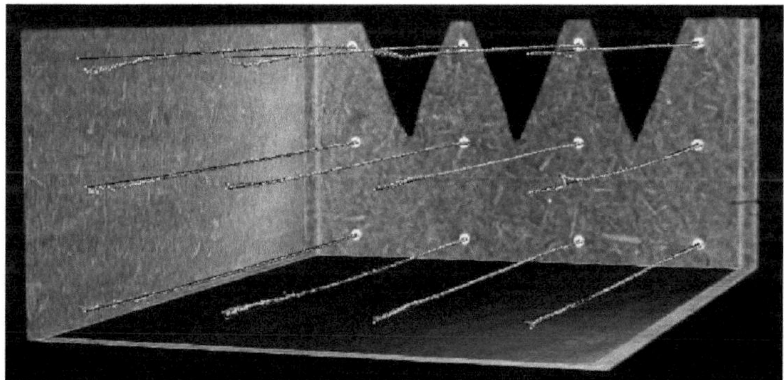

Abb. 1. Schema des Aufbaus: Virtuelle Sicht auf die Innenseite des Phantoms (CT-Datum) und Einblendung der Referenzgeraden (dunkel) welche durch die Mitte der Röhren verlaufen. Die aufgezeichneten Trackingkoordinaten zweier Referenzmessungen in metallfreier Umgebung sind in grau (Messung 1) bzw. und weiß (Messung 2) dargestellt. Die Position des EMT Feldgenerators war auf der rechten Seite

Es wurden Messungen mit dem Phantom direkt auf dem OP-Tisch liegend und mit einem Abstand von 5 cm zwischen Phantom und OP-Tisch durchgeführt, um den Einfluss des OP-Tisches auf die Systemgenauigkeit beurteilen zu können. Hierbei befand sich das da Vinci® Surgical System in 2 m Entfernung. Nach den Messungen wurde das System am Kopfende des Tisches positioniert und die drei Arme des Telemanipulators mit Stereo-Kamera, Schere und Greifwerkzeug im Phantom zentral positioniert. Messungen mit dem da Vinci® im Standby-Modus, in welchem die Motoren mit Strom versorgt werden jedoch die Instrumente sich nicht bewegten, und unter kontinuierlicher Bewegung der Instrumente wurden angefertigt. Zur Überprüfung der Positionstreue über die Zeit wurden an drei unterschiedlichen Positionen innerhalb jeder Röhre (hinteres Ende, Mitte, vorderes Ende) Positionsmessungen über zehn Sekunden aufgezeichnet. Eine Computertomographie des Phantoms ergab die exakten 3D Koordinaten und Bezugspunkte in Form von manuell erstellten Referenzgeraden durch die jeweilige Mitte der Röhren.

2.3 Auswertung

Die Registrierung der CT-Daten des Phantoms mit den gespeicherten Messwerten erfolgte über einen manuellen, punktbasierten Registrierungsprozess. Dadurch wurden CT-Daten und EMT-Daten in ein gemeinsames Koordinatensystem überführt. Die maximalen Fehler der Offset-Vektoren von Bezugsgeraden des CT-Bildes zu tatsächlichen Messpunkten wurden ermittelt. Für die Analyse der aufgezeichneten Messwerte wurde in MATLAB ein Skript erstellt, das alle 12 Teilmessungen einer Messung einliest und jede gemessene Positionskoordinate orthogonal auf die aus dem CT Datum extrahierten Referenzgeraden projiziert. Der absolute Fehler in mm konnte nun durch geometrische Abstandsmessung zwischen dieser, als real angenommenen Position des Sensors, und der Trackingkoordinate errechnet werden. Des Weiteren wurden Mittelwert, Standardabweichung und RMS jeder Teilmessung und Messung errechnet. Mehrfach durchgeführte Messungen validierten die Reproduzierbarkeit des Messaufbaus. Als Voraussetzung für den klinischen Einsatz der Navigation mit EMT zusammen mit dem da Vinci® wurde eine Genauigkeit von unter 10 mm definiert [6]. Deshalb wurde das Trackingvolumen vom Nullpunkt der X-Achse von der Mitte des Messvolumens ausgehend in beide Richtungen begrenzt und der absolute Fehler in diesem Bereich errechnet.

3 Ergebnisse

Tabelle 1 zeigt die maximalen Abweichungen für die Messungen im gesamten Messvolumen sowie durch Begrenzung des Arbeitsvolumens auf eine craniocaudale Länge (X-Achse) von 190 mm, mit Beibehaltung der Höhe von 200mm und der Breite von 400 mm.

Tabelle 1. Ergebnisse: A = Referenz, metallfrei; B = Tisch ohne Abstand; C = Tisch mit Abstand 5 cm vom Op-Tisch; D = da Vinci® Standby; E = da Vinci® bewegt

	A	B	C	D	E
gesamtes Messvolumen	9,9	43,4	32,8	37,9	37,2
begrenztes Arbeitsvolumen	4,0	9,9	8,3	8,5	8,9

4 Diskussion

Die ausgewerteten Größen hängen zusätzlich von Fehlern ab, die durch die punktbasierte Registrierung, Auflösung des CT-Datums, manuelle Definition der Referenzgeraden und orthogonale Projektion der gemessenen Werte auf die Referenzgeraden entstanden. Es wurde jedoch größte Sorgfalt darauf gelegt, diese Fehler so gering wie möglich zu halten. Ferner wird die Variation der einzelnen Navigationsszenarien als wichtiges Kriterium betrachtet. Der maximale Fehler wurde als relevanter Parameter gewählt um die Beachtung von lokal begrenzten Störungen und eine höhere durchschnittliche Genauigkeit im jeweiligen Bereich zu gewährleisten. Eine Genauigkeit von unter 10 mm wurde als hinreichend betrachtet, um die Positionsdaten des elektromagnetischen Trackings in einem Navigationssystem einsetzen zu können [6]. Die Einzelmessungen über die Zeit ergaben, dass im Zentrum des elektromagnetischen Felds eine genauere Positionstreue als im äußeren Bereich vorherrscht (Abb. 2,3). Deshalb wurde das Trackingvolumen vom Nullpunkt der X-Achse von der Mitte des Messvolumens ausgehend in beide Richtungen begrenzt und der maximale Fehler in diesem Bereich errechnet. Im Bereich +/- 96 mm lag der maximale Fehler sämtlicher Messungen unter 10 mm. Die deutlichsten Unterschiede bestanden zwischen der Referenzmessung und der tiefen Einstellung auf dem Operationstisch. Bei Vergrößerung des Abstandes des Messvolumens vom Operationstisch um 5 Zentimeter verkleinerte

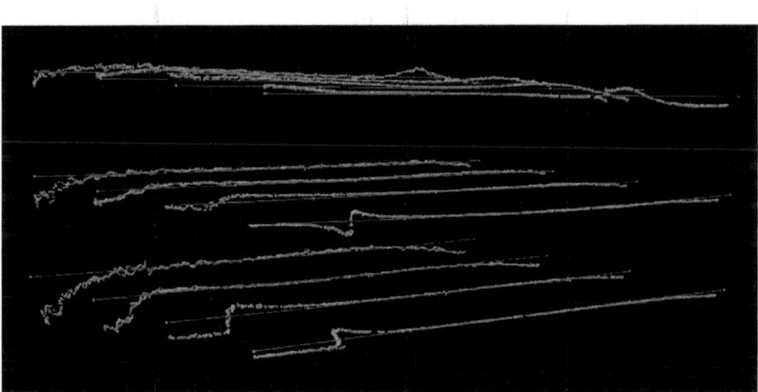

Abb. 2. Messung mit da Vinci in Standby (grau) und bewegt (weiß) mit Referenzgeraden (dunkelgrau). Messungen in Standby und Bewegung zeigen keine relevante Abweichung voneinander. Die Abweichung der Messungen von der aus dem CT-Datum gewonnen Bezugsgeraden, nimmt mit Abstand zur Mitte des Messvolumens zu

Abb. 3. Maximaler Fehler in Abhängigkeit der Position in X-Richtung (cranio-caudale Länge) des Messvolumens gemessen orthogonal zu den Referenzgeraden. Die angezeigten Linien entsprechen den Werten aus den Messversuchen, welche aus jeweils 12 Einzelmessungen bestehen

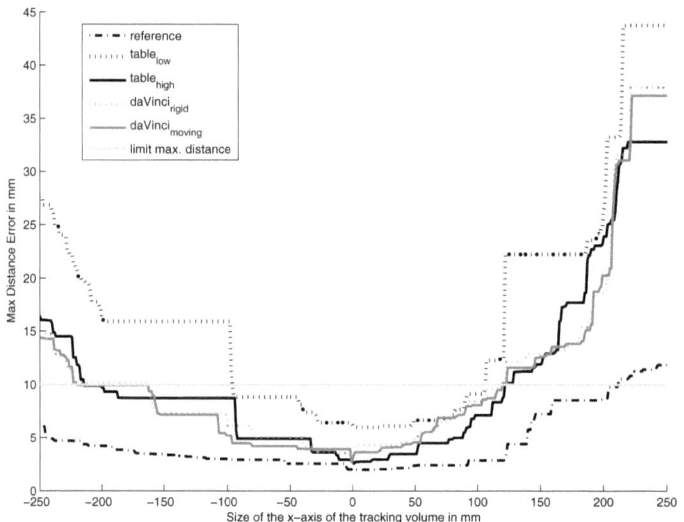

sich der maximale Fehler. Es ist daher anzunehmen, dass die großen Metallflächen des Operationstisches eine starke Verzerrung des magnetischen Feldes verursachen. Sowohl der eingeschaltete als auch bewegte Telemanipulator haben kaum zusätzliche Auswirkungen auf den maximalen Fehler im Vergleich zum höher gesetzten Messvolumen mit OP-Tisch. Die Bewegung der Instrumente im Messvolumen hatte keinen signifikanten zusätzlichen Einfluss auf das EMT und stellt somit keine relevante Störquelle dar.

Literaturverzeichnis

1. Zhang H, Banovac F, Lin R, et al. Electromagnetic tracking for abdominal interventions in computer aided surgery. Comput Aided Surg. 2006;11(3):127–36.
2. Marescaux J, Solerc L. Image-guided robotic surgery. Semin Laparosc Surg. 2004;11(2):113–22.
3. Camarillo D, Krummel T, Jr JS. Robotic technology in surgery: Past, present, and future. Am J Surg. 2004;188(4A suppl):2S–15S.
4. Poulin F, Amiot L. Interference during the use of an electromagnetic tracking system under OR conditions. J Biomech. 2002;35(6):733–7.
5. Frantz D, Wiles A, Leis S, et al. Accuracy assessment protocols for electromagnetic tracking systems. Phys Med Biol. 2003;48(14):2241–51.
6. Kenngott H, Neuhaus J, Gutt C, et al. Entwicklung eines Navigationssystems für die telemanipulatorgestützte Oesophagektomie. BVM. 2006;1(1):331–4.

3D Bildgebung von zerebralen Aneurysmen
Vergleich zwischen CT und MRT

Leonid Goubergrits[1], Jens Pöthke[1], Christoph Petz[2], Hans-Christian Hege[2], Andreas Spuler[3], Ulrich Kertzscher[1]

[1]Labor für Biofluidmechanik, Charité–Universitätsmedizin Berlin
[2]Visualization and Data Analysis, Konrad Zuse Institute Berlin
[3]Neurochirurgie, Helios Klinikum Berlin–Buch
leonid.goubergrits@charite.de

Kurzfassung. Patientenspezifische Strömungs- und die Geometrieanalyse von Aneurysmen basiert auf der 3D-Rekonstruktion aus Daten, die mit modernen Methoden der Bildgebung (z.B. CT und MRT) gewonnen werden. Die unterschiedlichen Charakteristika der Bildgebungsverfahren und die damit verbundenen Unsicherheiten führen zu Variationen der rekonstruierten Geometrien, die sich auf die numerische Berechnung von Strömungsparametern, wie z.B. die Wandschubspannung, auswirken können. Basierend auf CT- und MRT-Aufnahmen eines anatomisch realistischen Referenzmodells eines zerebralen Aneurysmas der Arteria Basilaris vergleichen wir die rekonstruierten Geometrien und die hierin simulierten Blutströmungen. Die Segmentierung und Rekonstruktion des Aneurysmas erfolgte mit Hilfe des Programms AMIRA. Die numerischen Strömungsberechnungen wurden mit dem Strömungslöser FLUENT durchgeführt.

1 Einleitung

Zerebrale Aneurysmen sind lebensgefährlich. Jährlich erleiden etwa 10 von 100.000 Menschen eine akute Blutung infolge der spontanen Ruptur eines Aneurysmas mit einer Sterberate von etwa 50% [1]. Die Abschätzung der Rupturwahrscheinlichkeit und die Entscheidung über die Therapieart sind von der im Aneurysma vorliegenden Blutströmung und von deren Geometrie abhängig. Die modernen Methoden der Bildgebung (z.B. CT, MRT und Rotationsangiographie) zusammen mit den Methoden der 3D-Rekonstruktion ermöglichen uns eine patientenspezifische Analyse der Gefäßgeometrie. Aktuelle Verfahren der numerischen Strömungssimulation erlauben jetzt, die Blutströmung im Aneurysma und in dessen Umgebung zu berücksichtigen. Die Rekonstruktion der Geometrie ist der Schlüssel zur in-vivo Erfassung biofluidmechanischer Parameter der Aneurysmen. Die verschiedenen Methoden der Bildgebung haben jeweils unterschiedliche Vor- und Nachteile, unterschiedliche Auflösungen und eine unterschiedliche Anwendungshäufigkeit in der klinischen Praxis. Keine dieser Methoden kann man als Goldstandard betrachten. Für die Etablierung eines numerischen Modells der Aneurysmenströmung, sowie für das Erfassen geometrischer Parameter müssen die Auswirkungen der verschiedenen Bildgebungsmethoden bei der Geometrierekonstruktion von zerebralen Aneurysmen untersucht werden. Eine weitere Fragestellung ist die Untersuchung der Auswirkungen der Geometrieabweichungen auf die Charakterisierung der Aneurysmen hinsichtlich biofluidmechanischer Parameter. Bis jetzt sind solche Untersuchungen nur für Karotidverzweigungen durchgeführt worden [2, 3]. Ziel dieser Arbeit ist der Vergleich zwischen den rekonstruierten Geometrien und einem relevanten Strömungsparameter, der Wandschubspannung (WSS), basierend auf einer CT- und einer MRT-Aufnahme eines Silikonmodells eines Aneurysmas der Arteria Basilaris.

2 Material und Methoden

2.1 Rekonstruktion und Fertigung des Silikonmodells

Eine 68-jährige Frau wurde für eine chirurgische Operationsplanung mit CT-Angiographie untersucht. Die CT-Aufnahme bestand aus 2 mm dicken Schichten in einem Abstand von 1 mm, bei einer Auflösung von 512x512 Pixel (0,4 mm x 0,4 mm Pixelgröße). In der Aufnahme war ein Aneurysma der Arteria Basilaris erkennbar. Diese Rohdaten wurden mit dem Programm AMIRA [4] segmentiert, und die Geometrie des Aneurysmas wurde rekonstruiert (Abb. 1 links). Der Durchmesser des Muttergefäßes betrug 3,8 mm. Die rekonstruierte Geometrie dient in dieser Arbeit als Goldstandard für unsere vergleichende Untersuchung und wurde für die Herstellung eines dreifach vergrößerten Silikonmodells verwendet. Zuerst wurde das Modell stereolithographisch mit einer Genauigkeit von 0,1 mm erstellt, anschließend wurde daraus ein Hohlmodell aus Zweikomponentensilikon ELASTOSIL® RT 601 (Wacker-Chemie GmbH, München, Deutschland) gefertigt (Abb. 1 rechts).

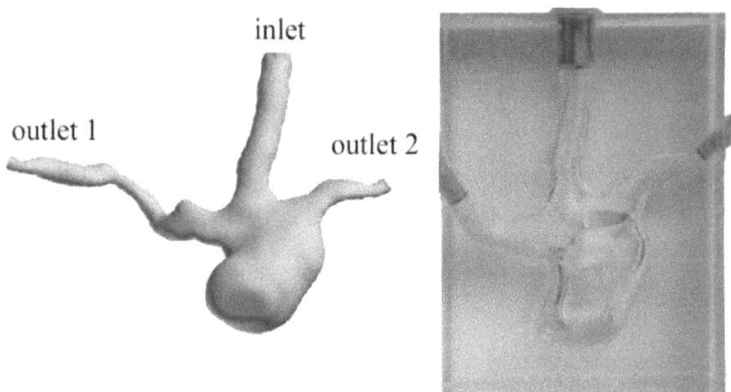

Abb. 1. Computermodell eines rekonstruierten Aneurysmas (links); dreifach vergrößerte Silikonmodell (rechts)

Abb. 2. CT-Schicht des aufgenommenen Aneurysmenmodells (links); Schicht aus der MRT-Aufnahme des Aneurysmenmodells (rechts). Die Aufnahme zeigt das Ringing-Problem der MRT Bildgebung

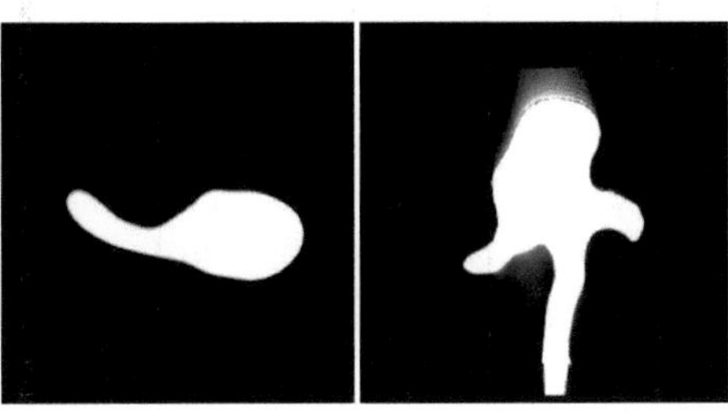

2.2 CT und MRT basierende 3D-Rekonstruktion des Silikonmodells

Das Silikonmodell des Aneurysmas wurde mit CT- und MRT-Bildgebung aufgenommen. Das vergrößerte Modell ermöglichte eine Aufnahme mit hoher räumlicher Auflösung unter idealen Randbedingungen (hoher Kontrast, keine Bewegungsartefakte). Die CT-Aufnahme wurde mit einem Siemens Volume Zoom Scanner (4-Zeiler) durchgeführt (115 Schichten, 1,8 mm Schichtdicke und 0,9 mm Schichtenabstand). Dieses ergab eine Voxelgröße von 0,39 mm x 0,39 mm x 0,9 mm für das Silikonmodell, was einer Voxelgröße von 0,13 mm x 0,13 mm x 0,3 mm der in-vivo Größe des Aneurysmas entspricht. Abb. 2 links zeigt die Aufnahme einer CT-Schicht. Die Rekonstruktion des Aneurysmas erfolgte aufgrund hoher Kontrast halb-automatisch mittels Segmentierungs- und Schwellwertwerkzeugen des Programms AMIRA mit anschließender Glättung (Abb. 3 Mitte).

Die MRT-Aufnahmen wurden mit einem Philips Achiva-3-Tesla Gerät und einer 8 Kanal SENSE Kopfspule und Anwendung der 3D-Spin-Echo-Sequenz durchgeführt. Es ergab eine räumliche Auflösung von 0,48 x 0,48 x 0,48 mm^3, das in-vivo einer räumlichen Auflösung von 0,16 x 0,16 x 0,16 mm^3 entspricht. Abb. 2 rechts zeigt die MRT-Aufnahme eines Schnittes. Abb. 3 rechts zeigt eine mit dem Programm AMIRA rekonstruierte 3D-Geometrie. Auch hierzu wurden Segmentierungs- und Schwellwertwerkzeuge mit anschließender Glättung eingesetzt.

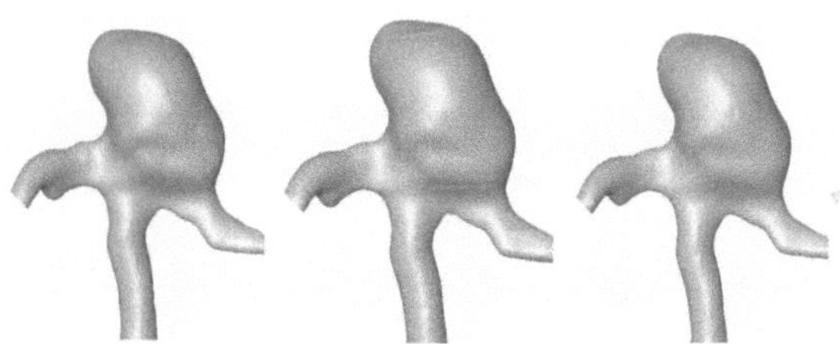

Abb. 3. Ursprüngliche Rekonstruktion als Goldstandard (links); CT-basierte Rekonstruktion (Mitte); MRT-basierte Rekonstruktion (rechts)

2.3 Numerische Strömungsberechnungen

Für die Berechnung des Strömungsverhaltens im Aneurysma mit der Finite Elemente Methode wurde zunächst ein Volumengitter der Geometrie erzeugt. Dazu wurde ein Oberflächengitter mit etwa 50.000 Dreiecken generiert, daran angrenzend ein Grenzschichtgitter bestehend aus drei Schichten Prismen in einer Gesamtdicke von 0,2 mm, wobei die Dicke der ersten Zellschicht nur 0,01 mm beträgt. Diese hohe wandnahe Auflösung wird für die Erfassung der Wandschubspannung (WSS) benötigt. Anschließend wurde das innere Gitter mit etwa 600.000 Tetraedern aufgefüllt. Die Berechnung der 3D Navier-Stokes Gleichungen auf den Gitterpunkten mit einem stationären Volumenstrom von 200 ml/min wurde mit dem Strömungslöser Fluent durchgeführt, aus dessen Ergebnissen die WSS bestimmt wurde.

3 Ergebnisse

3.1 Geometrie

Die rekonstruierten Geometrien aus den CT- und MRT-Aufnahmen wurden mit der Geometrie des Goldstandards verglichen. Dabei wurden die Oberflächenabstände der rekonstruierten Geometrien zu dem Goldstandard berechnet (Hausdorff-Abstand). Abb. 4 zeigt die Verteilungen der Oberflächenabstände. Die linke Abbildung zeigt den Vergleich der CT-basierten Geometrie. Der mittlere Hausdorff-Abstand beträgt, auf Aneurysmengröße skaliert, 0,242 mm. Die rechte Abbildung zeigt die Abstandsverteilung der MRT-basierten Geometrie. Der mittlere auf Aneurysmengröße skalierte Hausdorff-Abstand entspricht hier 0,097 mm.

3.2 Wandschubspannung

Die berechnete mittlere WSS des Goldstandards beträgt 4,02 Pa. Eine um 24% niedrigere mittlere WSS von 3,06 Pa wurde für die CT rekonstruierte Geometrie errechnet. Die MRT-basierte Geometrie ergab eine um 10% geringere mittlere WSS von 3,62 Pa. Die Wandschubspannungsverteilung zeigt sehr ähnliche Muster (Abb. 5).

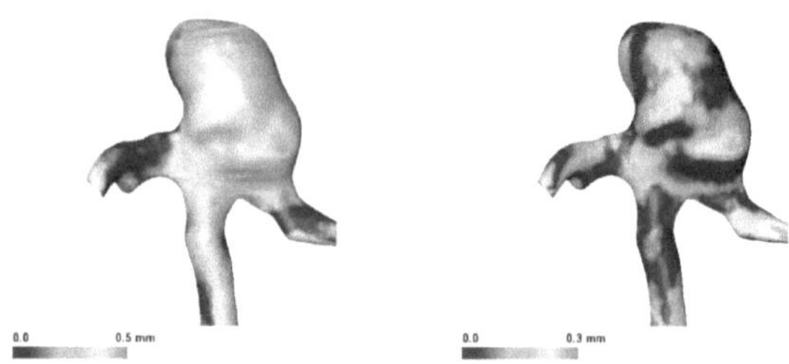

Abb. 4. Farbcodierte Darstellung der Hausdorff Oberflächenabstände zwischen der Ausgangsgeometrie und CT- (links) und MRT-basierten (rechts) Geometrie

Abb. 5. Wandschubspannungsverteilungen über die Oberfläche errechnet aus verschiedenen Geometrien: Ausgangsgeometrie (links); CT-basiert (Mitte); MRT-basiert (rechts)

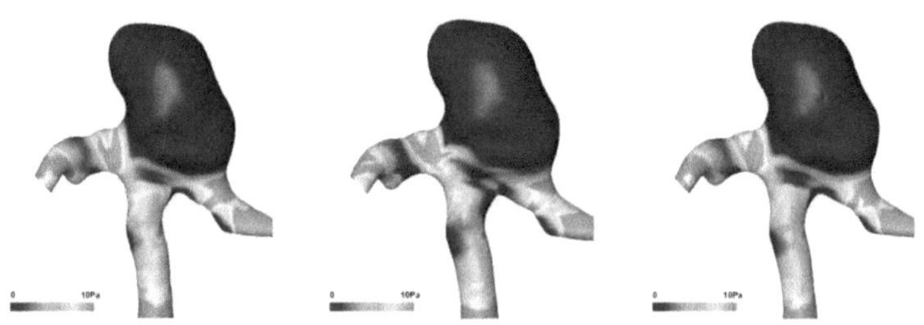

4 Diskussion

Ein dreifach vergrößertes Silikonmodell eines Aneurysmas der Arteria Basilaris wurde mit zwei bildgebenden Verfahren (MRT und CT) aufgenommen und rekonstruiert. Mittels numerischer Strömungssimulationen wurden in beiden Rekonstruktionen und in der Ausgangsgeometrie die Verteilungen der Wandschubspannungen berechnet. Die Ergebnisse zeigen, dass beide Verfahren geeignet sind, um die Form von zerebralen Aneurysmen mit den Gefäßen zu rekonstruieren. Sie können deshalb in klinisch relevanten Studien zur patientenspezifischen Risikoanalyse von Aneurysmen angewendet werden. Bei der gleichen Aufnahmeauflösung weist die MRT-basierte Rekonstruktion einen 2,5-fach niedrigeren Fehler als die CT basierte Rekonstruktion auf. Die CT-basierte Rekonstruktion zeigt bekannte Artefakte in der Form von Stufen, die zu Fehlern der Oberflächenkrümmung führen. Trotz unterschiedlichen Abweichungen von der Originalgeometrie fanden wir für beide Simulationen eine gute Übereinstimmung bei der Ermittlung von Wandschubspannungen. Demnächst soll ein drittes Verfahren, 3D-Rotationsangiographie, mit der gleichen Methode untersucht werden.

Literaturverzeichnis

1. Wiebers DO, Whisnant JP, Huston J, et al. Unruptured intracranial aneurysms: Natural history, clinical outcome, and risks of surgical and endovascular treatment. Lancet. 2003;362(9378):103–10.
2. Glor FP, Ariff B, Hughes AD, et al. Image-based carotid flow reconstruction: A comparison between MRI and ultrasound. Physiol Meas. 2004;25(6):1495–1509.
3. Birchall D, Zaman A, Hacker J, et al. Analysis of haemodynamic disturbance in the atherosclerotic carotid artery using computational fluid dynamics. Eur Radiol. 2006;16(5):1074–83.
4. Stalling D, Westerhoff M, Hege HC. In: Hansen CD, Johnson CR, editors. Amira: A Highly Interactive System for Visual Data Analysis. Elsevier; 2005. p. 749–67.

3D Reconstruction of Neurons from Confocal Image Stacks and Visualization of Computational Modeling Experiments

Susanne Schönknecht[1], Carsten Duch[2], Klaus Obermayer[1], Michael Sibila[1]

[1]Fachgebiet Neuronale Informationsverarbeitung, Fakultät IV, TU-Berlin
[2]School of Life Sciences, Arizona State University, USA
susanne@cs.tu-berlin.de

Abstract. In this study we perform precise geometrical 3D reconstructions of high complex neuronal architectures. First, confocal microscopy was used to scan neurons with submicron resolution. Second, we extracted the center-lines and diameters of the neuron by means of our reconstruction method, and third we used these metric data to generate compartment models that were transported into the proprietary format of modeling software such as NEURON or GENESIS. Fourth, routines were developed in the scripting language of the respective modeling program to perform computational modeling, and finally we transferred the modeling results to the visualization program AMIRA (Indeed Visual Concepts GmbH).

1 Introduction

Precise geometrical reconstructions of neuronal architecture are essential for the investigation of neuronal function. Available commercial reconstruction software tools such as NEUROLUCIDA [1] provide manual tracing methods that are for complex dendritic trees overly tedious and lead to very subjective results. Moreover, by applying the reconstruction layer by layer, this method yields in stepwise structures. Thus, we applied our semi-automatic tracing method [2, 3], we are able to achieve a smoothly fitted geometry.

Compartmental models of neurons for computational purpose can be described using the so called cable equation. Herein the electrical properties of the intracellular fluid and of the neurons passive membrane are assigned to cylindrical compartments of the dendritic tree. The overall parameters Ra (axial resistance), Rm (membrane resistance) and Cm (membrane capacity) describe the specific electrical properties of the neuron, and as a first approximation they are assumed to be equal for each compartment. The time constant τ, the electrotonic length λ, are values for the delay and decay of the voltage signal and were measured by biological experiments as well as the input resistance R_{in}.

The state-of-the art visualization routines for modeling experiments in NEURON and GENESIS are not convenient for highly detailed reconstructions with about 80.000 compartments as in our case. Thus, for the purpose of rough modeling results we reduced the number of compartments. On the other hand, in order to avoid lack of precision, we transformed the visualization of voltage spread (e.g.) into color-coded time-stretched animations. As model we used the moth motoneuron MN5 at different stages of development, which changes from a slow motoneuron that is involved in larval crawling behaviour into a fast adult flight motoneuron. This metamorphosis is accompanied by changes in dendritic shape and electrophysiological properties of the neuron [4]. We addressed the question, how changes in dendritic structure can affect changes in functional behavior.

Highly detailed neuron models enhance the computational cost of neural modeling. Common routines to reduce the number of compartments with low loss of are optimized for neurons with less branching dendritic trees, and do not fulfill requrements of precise and fast modeling tasks with multi compartments as in our dimension.

2 Materials and Methods

2.1 Imaging

The imaging was performed on a Leica SP2 laser scanning confocal microscope by using a 40x oil immersion lens (NA1.25). The excitation maximum of the laser was at 543 nm and the detection range was 565-600 nm. The voxel size was $(0.1x0.1x0.3)\mu m^3$ [2]. The complete 3D datasets were obtained sequentially at three different orientations as axial, sagittal and horizontal.

2.2 Segmentation and Reconstruction of Dendritic Geometry

The reconstruction starts with an initial coarse representation of the neuron, where all branching points (nodes) and their connectivity have to be defined by the user. With the tracing algorithm [2], a “snake” model was generated which consists of points (“snaxels”) defined by their location, radii and edges that connect the nodes. The model is then fitted to the data, thus spanning the 3d graph called skeleton, yielding precise shape and diameter of all dendrites.

2.3 Reducing the Number of Compartments via Cylinder Fit

The skeleton was transformed to cylindrical compartments into NEURON and GENESIS by means of our automated parsers [5]. This is useful because we can apply the cable equation. Herein the signal transmission is calculated by solving a simple differential equation for each time step in each cylinder segment. However, to enhance computational speed, several methods of cylinder fitting were investigated to reduce the number of compartments with a minimal loss of accuracy (Fig. 1). We have investigated three methods of reduction by evalating the same neuron model: first a systematic connection of a special amount of neighboring compartments, sececond the “radii-difference-method”, and third a geometric optimization which constists of adding up the cylindrical lenghtes of a number of compartments, and subtituting the average of the radii for the resulting cylinder.

However, the optimal ratio of reduction in compartments to a minimal deviation in voltage transfer (compared to simulations with full number of compartments) resulted in our "radii-difference-method" (Fig. 1a). Here a cylinder is merged with its neighboring compartment, if the difference of their radii is less then a user defined range. The difference of the first and second cylinder (Fig. 1a, left) is within the range, so that the first cylinder was connected directly with the third one. The difference of the third and fourth cylinder was too large and cylinder four remains in the reconstruction. We have investigated to set the range to $0.1\%, 0.5\%, 1\%, 5\%$, and 10% of deviation.

The loss in computational accuracy was determined by computational simulations, and we compared the results with results of the not reduced model.

2.4 Modeling

In order to provide the model neuron with realistic passive membrane properties, three specific parameters (Ra, Rm and Cm) were estimated from measurable values as time constant (τ), electronic length (λ) and input resistance (R_{in}). For this purpose we explored the parameter space of Ra, Rm and Cm by simulating voltage transfer inside the neuron, and compared the results for R_{in} and λ with the experimental measured values, see [6] for detailes.

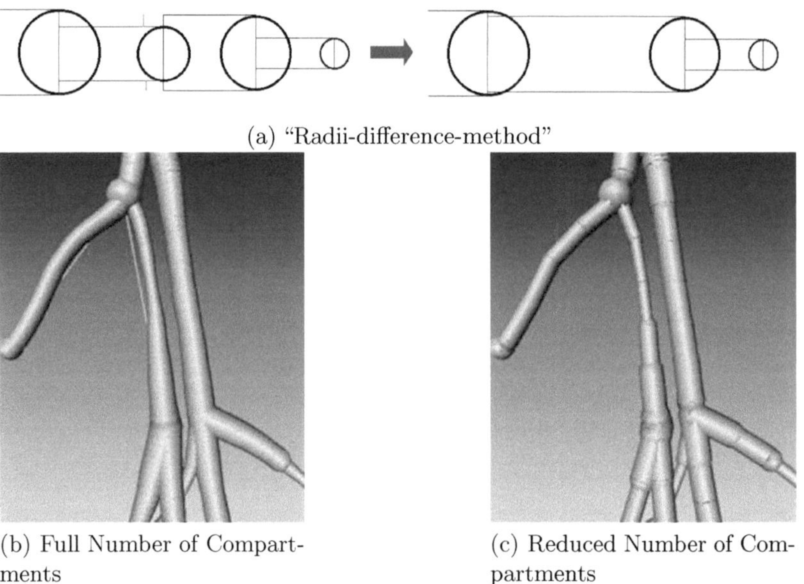

(a) "Radii-difference-method"

(b) Full Number of Compartments

(c) Reduced Number of Compartments

Fig. 1. Results of the zylinder fit method

We performed computational experiments, such as the voltage spread of an action potential (outward, Fig. 2a), and as postsynaptic signal transmission (inward, Fig. 2b), and addressed the following questions: a) Is an action potential capable to affect dendritic outgrowth by being back propagated into distal dendritic subtrees with only passive membrane properties? b) How can distal dendritic inputs affect the putative spike generation zone with passive membrane properties? c) Do depolarizing inputs to growth-cones affect the membrane potential of neighboring growth-cones?

3 Results

The joining of neighboring compartments with radius difference of less then 1% leads to a reduction of 58% of compartments with a voltage error of less then 0,18%. Fig. 2 displays exemplary a specific time point of the spread of action potential. Equipotential regions in the dendritic tree are depicted by equivalent colors. The decrease of membrane potential from spike generation zone to distal dendritic subtrees is about 93%. Vice versa, the voltage attenuation from distal dendritic tips to the root of the tree is about 99,8%. Neighboring growth-cones affect each other with a voltage decay of 99,9%.

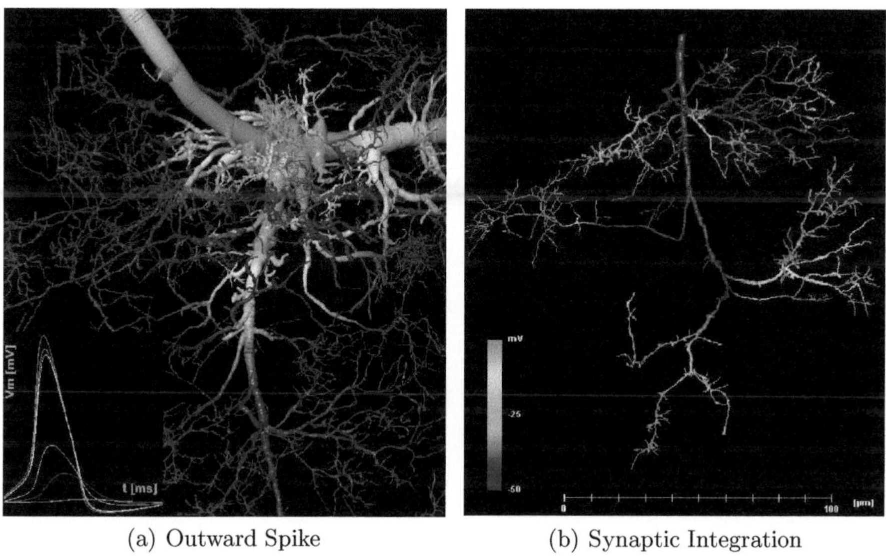

(a) Outward Spike (b) Synaptic Integration

Fig. 2. Color-coded visualization of modeling results Both pictures display the part of the dendritic tree of the same reconstruction of themoth motoneuron MN5. Left: an outward spike was simulated. The voltage spread is depicted colorcoded throughout the dendritic tree. Inset: The time course of the voltage vor selected compartments. Red is close, blue is distal to the spike generation zone. Right: Inward signal integration. Tonic firing inputs to dendritic tips are integrated and processed to the dendritic root. The color bar is valid for both figures

4 Discussion

We have used our semi-automatic reconstruction method and transformation routines to build highly detailed multi-compartmental models of the motoneuron MN5. To enhance computational speed we have successfully developed a method to reduce the number of cylindrical compartments within an acceptable error measure. Computational simulations were performed and imported in AMIRA for visualization.

In order to understand the processes in neurons with highly complex dendritic structure, it is essential to have also an intuitional impression of the modeling results. Thus, the voltage spreads, visualized in color-coded images reveal a most intuitively readable result that can be quantified by means of color bars (e.g). Moreover, our movie animations deliver intuitively the time course of signal transmission for each compartment throughout the dendritic tree, here depicted in terms of voltage-plots (Fig. 2a, inset).

Currently, our simulations focus on refining our model using recent experimental findings: A triangulated surface reconstruction of the neuron gives the possibility to extract a measure for synaptic localization from the second channel confocal data of immuno-labelled synapsin and to map this synaptotagmin distribution upon the skeleton [7]. We aim to include these data into our modeling experiments, and address the functional role of the structural changes for the observed lower excitability of the adult as compared to the larval motoneuron.

References

1. MicroBrightField, Inc, Williston, et al. Neurolucida.
2. Schmitt S, Evers J, Duch C, et al. New methods for the computer-assisted 3D reconstruction of neurons from confocal image stacks. NeuroImage. 2005;23:1283–98.
3. Evers J, Schmitt S, Scholz M, et al. New frontiers in functional neuroanatomy: Precise automatic reconstruction from confocal image stacks. J Neurophys. 2005;93:2331–42.
4. Duch C, Levine R. Remodeling of membrane properties and dendritic architecture accompanies the postembryonic conversion of a slow into a fast motoneuron. J Neurosci. 2001;20(18):6950–61.
5. Schönknecht S, Scholz M, Duch C, et al. Multi compartment model of developmental changes in dendritic shape during postembryonic motoneuron development. Proc Göttingen Neurobiol Conf. 2003.
6. Evers J, Maye A, Schönknecht S, et al. Are changing behavioural demands supported by postembryonic remodeling of neuronal structure? Proc Göttingen Neurobiol Conf. 2005;(55).
7. Evers J, Muench D, Duch C. Developmental relocation of presynaptic terminals along distinct types of dendritic filopodia. Developmental Biology. 2006;(297):241–227.

Vollautomatische Segmentierung der Prostata aus 3D-Ultraschallbildern

Tobias Heimann, Tobias Simpfendörfer, Matthias Baumhauer, Hans-Peter Meinzer

Abteilung für Medizinische und Biologische Informatik, DKFZ Heidelberg
t.heimann@dkfz.de

Kurzfassung. Diese Arbeit beschreibt ein modellbasiertes Verfahren zur Segmentierung der Prostata aus 3D-Ultraschalldaten. Kern der Methode ist ein statistisches Formmodell, das auf Beispieldaten der Prostata trainiert wird. Erster Schritt der Segmentierung ist ein evolutionärer Algorithmus, mit dem das Modell grob im zu segmentierenden Bild positioniert wird. Für die darauf folgende lokale Suche wurden mehrere Varianten des Algorithmus evaluiert, unter anderem Ausreißer-Unterdrückung, freie Deformation und Gewichtung der verwendeten Erscheinungsmodelle nach ihrer Zuverlässigkeit. Alle Varianten wurden auf 35 Ultraschallbildern getestet und mit manuellen Referenzsegmentierungen verglichen. Die beste Variante erreichte eine durchschnittliche Oberflächenabweichung von 1.1 mm.

1 Einleitung

Bei Tumorerkrankungen der Prostata ist die vollständige Entfernung des Organs (Prostatektomie) die erfolgversprechendste Therapie. Eine minimalinvasive Operationsstrategie verringert hierbei das Risiko für Folgeerscheinungen wie Inkontinenz und Impotenz, ist ohne Unterstützung durch OP-Planungs- und Navigationssysteme aber schwieriger durchzuführen. Um den Chirurgen bei diesem Eingriff zu unterstützen, entwickeln wir in unser Gruppe ein Navigationssystem, das Risikostrukturen wie Tumor und Harnleiter in das Kamerabild aus dem Endoskop einblenden kann. Dafür müssen die präoperativen Planungsdaten aus dem CT mit intraoperativen transrektalen Ultraschalldaten (TRUS) registriert werden. Anstatt CT und TRUS Bilder direkt zu registrieren, schlagen wir vor, die Prostataoberfläche aus den TRUS-Daten zu extrahieren und auf die entsprechende Oberfläche aus den CT-Daten abzubilden. Während die Segmentierung der Prostata aus den CT-Daten präoperativ erfolgt und zeitlich unkritisch ist, muss die Segmentierung aus den TRUS-Daten im OP erfolgen und sollte so schnell und automatisch wie möglich vonstatten gehen. Zu diesem Zweck stellen wir in dieser Arbeit ein System zur vollautomatischen Segmentierung der Prostata mit Hilfe statistischer Formmodelle vor, welche sich durch ihre Robustheit besonders gut zur Analyse der verrauschten TRUS-Bilder eignen.

Während für die Segmentierung der Prostata aus CT-Bildern teilweise einfache Techniken wie Regionenwachstumsverfahren angewendet werden können [1], müssen für Ultraschallbilder mit ihrem niedrigen Signal-Rausch-Verhältnis robustere Verfahren verwendet werden. So nutzen sowohl Hodge et al. [2] als auch Zhan und Shen [3] statistische Formmodelle für diese Aufgabe. Eine große Rolle spielen dabei die verwendeten Erscheinungsmodelle, die das Formmodell an die Bilddaten anpassen. In [2] wird die Prostata mit einem ad-hoc Ansatz (dunkle Grauwerte innerhalb, helle außerhalb) vom Hintergrund unterschieden, ein Training findet nicht statt. In [3] dagegen wird eine Gabor Filterbank zur Merkmalsberechnung genutzt und die Ergebnisse an eine Support Vector Machine zur Klassifizierung weiter geleitet.

Während die erste Variante ohne Training das Problem sehr vereinfacht, erscheint die zweite Methode relativ komplex. In dieser Arbeit gehen wir einen Mittelweg zwischen beiden Methoden, indem wir bewährte Grauwertprofile in Verbindung mit einem kNN-Klassifkator nutzen. Bei der Modellsuche in neuen Bilddaten evaluieren wir sowohl Algorithmen mit harten Formbeschränkungen (wie in [2] verwendet) als auch Methoden mit freier Deformation (wie in [3] genutzt).

2 Material und Methoden

Für diese Arbeit wurden 35 TRUS Volumen verwendet, die eine Auflösung von 430x280x200 bis 480x430x250 Voxeln aufweisen. Die Auflösung variiert zwischen 0.15 und 0.2 mm in einer Schicht bei 0.2 bis 0.25 mm Schichtabstand. Zur Glättung der Bilder wurde ein 7x7x7 Median Filter benutzt. Zum Training der Formmodelle und zur Validierung der Ergebnisse hat ein Medizinstudent alle Bilder mit einem interaktiven Oberflächenverfahren segmentiert.

Der erste Schritt zur Erstellung des Formmodells ist die Bestimmung von korrespondierenden Landmarken auf den so erstellten Oberflächen. Hierzu setzen wir ein automatisches Verfahren ein, das auf der Minimierung der Beschreibungslänge (MDL) des Formmodells basiert [4]. Eine Hauptkomponenten-Analyse der so bestimmten Landmarkenpositionen zeigt die größten Variationsrichtungen der Trainingsmenge, die für das statistische Formmodell verwendet werden (Abb. 1).

Zur Beschreibung der Erscheinung wurden an jeder Landmarke in allen Trainingsbildern Grauwert-Profile senkrecht zur Oberfläche eingelesen. Diese Profile wurden abgeleitet und die entstandenen Gradienten auf eine absolute Summe von 1 normalisiert. Die 9 Werte langen Profile wurden in zwei unterschiedlichen Modellen verwendet. Für das erste Modell wurden alle Trainingsprofile mit einer Kovarianzmatrix modelliert. Während der Modellsuche können Kandidatenprofile somit über die entsprechende Mahalanobisdistanz auf ihre Ähnlichkeit zu den trainierten Profilen überprüft werden. Für das zweite Modell wurden zusätzlich zu den Profilen an den korrekten Landmarkenpositionen auch Profile an nach innen und außen verschobenen Positionen eingelesen. Beide Gruppen wurden für das Training eines kNN-Klassifikators genutzt, der während der Modellsuche die Kandidatenprofile so als „Prostatakontur“ oder „Verschoben“ klassifizieren kann. Um das Formmodell auf ein neues Ultraschallbild anzupassen, wurde zuerst eine grobe Initialisierung durchgeführt. Hierzu wurde ein evolutionärer Algorithmus verwendet, der Position, Skalierung und die 5 größten Variationsrichtungen des Modells optimiert. Die Güte einer Einzellösung wurde durch Kombination der Antworten von allen Erscheinungsmodellen bestimmt. Nach einer konstanten Anzahl von 20 Iterationen (über 500 Einzellösungen) wurde das bis dahin beste Ergebnis als Ausgangspunkt für eine lokale Suche verwendet.

Die lokale Suche wurde in den folgenden Variationen ausgeführt:

– *Def*: Eine deformierbare Oberfläche ist an das statistische Formmodell gekoppelt. Die Oberfläche versucht zu jedem Zeitpunkt eine ähnliche Form wie vom Modell vorgegeben anzunehmen, gleichzeitig ziehen die Erscheinungsmodelle ihre Landmarken zu den bestpassenden Positionen in den Bilddaten [5]. Durch dieses System wird eine freie Deformation (zusätzlich zu den vorgegebenen Variationen des Formmodells) ermöglicht. Um die Oberfläche zu stabilisieren, werden Ausreißer in den Kräften der Erscheinungsmodelle durch eine optimale Oberflächensuche mit festen Randbedingungen unterbunden. Diese Randbedingungen setzen fest, dass die Bewegung benachbarter Landmarken nur einen festgelegten Betrag voneinander abweichen darf.

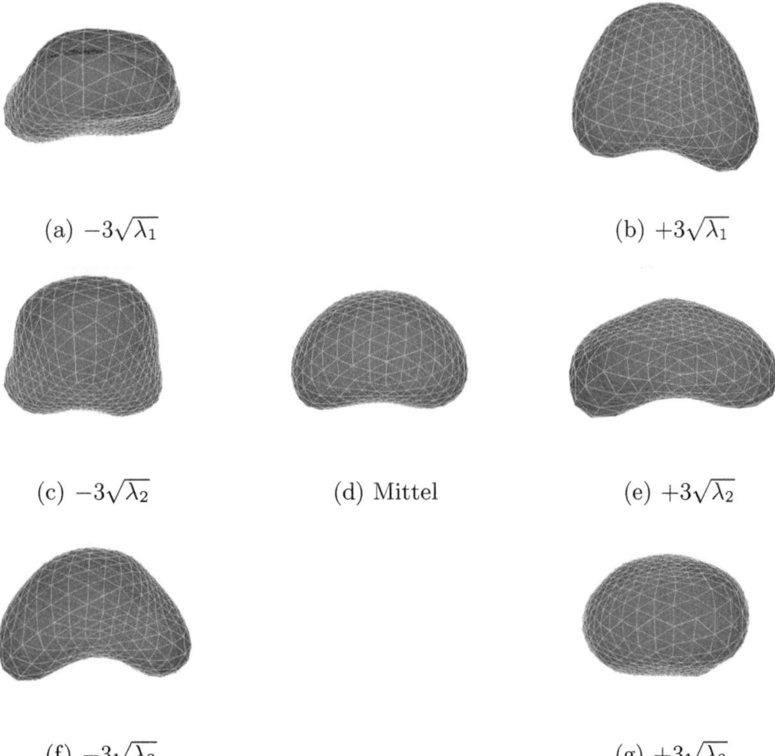

(a) $-3\sqrt{\lambda_1}$ (b) $+3\sqrt{\lambda_1}$

(c) $-3\sqrt{\lambda_2}$ (d) Mittel (e) $+3\sqrt{\lambda_2}$

(f) $-3\sqrt{\lambda_3}$ (g) $+3\sqrt{\lambda_3}$

Abb. 1. Haupt-Variationsrichtungen des Formmodells der Prostata. Bild (d) zeigt die mittlere Form, die anderen Bilder jeweils eine Variation um drei Standardabweichungen

- *App-PW*: Wie *Def*, aber die Kräfte der Erscheinungsmodelle werden mit ihrer Zuverlässigkeit gewichtet, so dass unzuverlässige Erscheinungsmodelle die Oberfläche nicht viel verformen können. Die Zuverlässigkeit eines Erscheinungsmodells wird dabei durch einen Testlauf auf den Trainingsdaten festgestellt.
- *No-OS*: Wie *Def*, aber die Ausreißer-Unterdrückung durch optimale Oberflächensuche wird nicht angewendet.
- *No-FD*: Wie *Def*, aber die deformierbare Oberfläche muss sich immer genau an das Formmodell halten. Es gibt somit keine freie Deformation.
- *App-Std*: Wie *Def*, aber das Standard-Erscheinungsmodell mit Kovarianzmatrix wurde verwendet. Alle anderen Varianten verwenden das nicht-lineare kNN-Modell.

3 Ergebnisse

Die beschriebenen Suchvarianten wurden mit einem „Leave-5-out" Verfahren auf den zur Verfügung stehenden Datensätzen getestet. Dabei wurden sowohl Form- als auch Erscheinungsmodell immer auf 30 Datensätzen trainiert und auf den ausgelassenen 5 getestet. Die erzielten Segmentierungen wurden mit den manuellen Referenzsegmentierungen verglichen und die durchschnittliche Oberflächenabweichung bestimmt. Für die unterschiedlichen Suchvarianten beträgt diese:

Def: 1.2 mm, *App-PW*: 1.1 mm, *No-OS*: 1.7 mm, *No-FD*: 1.2 mm, *App-Std* 1.6 mm. Abbildung 3 zeigt die entsprechenden Boxplots, Abbildung 3 ein repräsentatives Ergebnis. Um die Ergebnisse besser interpretieren zu können, hat der Medizinstudent, der die Referenzsegmentierungen erstellt hat, dieselben Daten zu einem späteren Zeitpunkt noch einmal segmentiert. Ein Vergleich mit den ersten Ergebnissen ergab eine durchschnittliche Oberflächenabweichung von 0.9 mm.

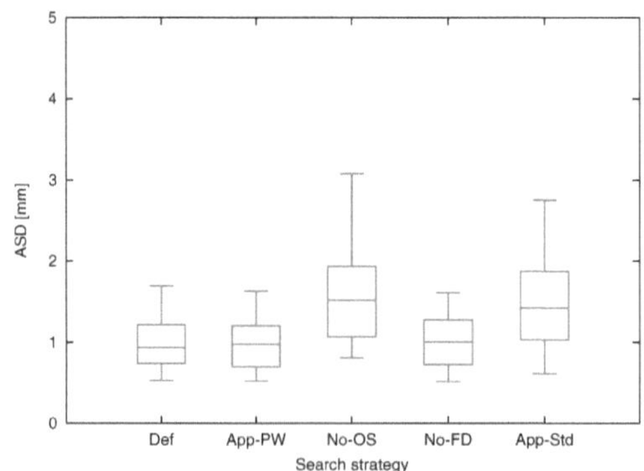

Abb. 2. Durchschnittliche Oberflächenabweichung zwischen den erzielten Ergebnissen und Referenzsegmentierungen für alle getesteten Suchvarianten

Abb. 3. Repräsentatives Segmentierungsergebnis (Median aller Ergebnisse) für Suchvariante *Def* (helle Kontur). Die manuelle Referenzsegmentierung ist zum Vergleich als dunkle Kontur angegeben

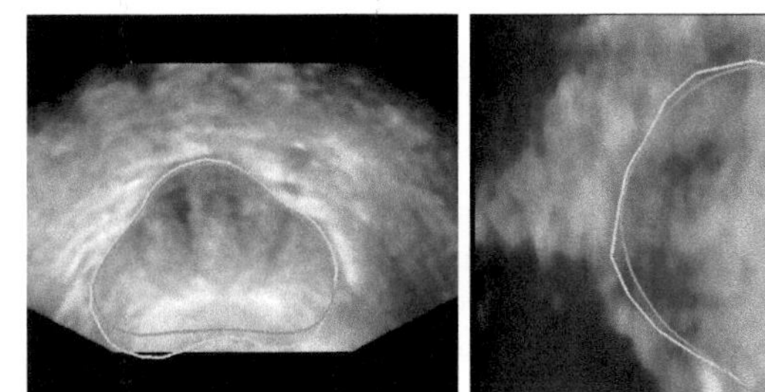
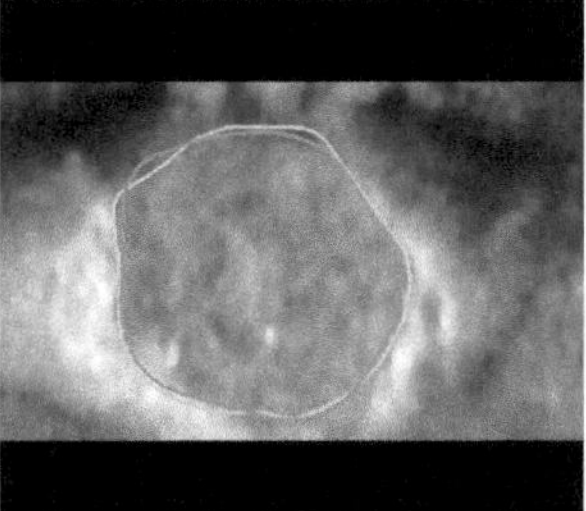

4 Diskussion

Die Ergebnisse zeigen, dass eine robuste Ausreißer-Unterdrückung und ein zuverlässiges Erscheinungsmodell die Qualität der Segmentierung auf Ultraschallbildern deutlich steigern können, was auf das schlechte Signal-Rausch-Verhältnis der Daten zurückzuführen ist. Zusätzliche freie Deformation brachte in diesen Experimenten keinen Vorteil, da die Prostata nur eine relativ geringe Formvariation aufweist und durch das Formmodell ausreichend gut modelliert werden kann. Die Gewichtung der Erscheinungsmodelle konnte die Ergebnisse noch leicht verbessern.

Die Segmentierung eines 3D-Volumens dauerte mit dem vorgestellten Verfahren weniger als zwei Minuten, was für die geplante Anwendung zur initialen Registrierung ausreichend schnell ist. Ein Vorteil des modellbasierten Ansatzes ist, dass die Segmentierung in einem Live-Ultraschallbild sehr schnell aktualisiert werden kann (da wenige Iterationen der lokalen Suche ausreichen) und somit die Prostata praktisch in Echtzeit verfolgt werden kann.

Literaturverzeichnis

1. Mazonakis M, Damilakis J, Varveris H, et al. Image segmentation in treatment planning for prostate cancer using the region growing technique. Br J Radiol. 2001;74(879):243–8.
2. Hodge AC, Fenster A, Downey DB, et al. Prostate boundary segmentation from ultrasound images using 2D active shape models: Optimisation and extension to 3D. Comput Methods Programs Biomed. 2006;84(2-3):99–113.
3. Zhan Y, Shen D. Deformable segmentation of 3-D ultrasound prostate images using statistical texture matching method. IEEE Trans Med Imaging. 2006;25:256–72.
4. Heimann T, Wolf I, Williams TG, et al. 3D Active shape models using gradient descent optimization of description length. Inf Process Med Imaging. 2005;19:566–77.
5. Heimann T, Münzing S, Meinzer HP, et al. A shape-guided deformable model with evolutionary algorithm initialization for 3D soft tissue segmentation. Inf Process Med Imaging. 2007;20:1–12.

Filtering, Segmentation and Feature Extraction in Ultrasound Evaluation of Breast Lesions

Miguel Alemán-Flores[1], Patricia Alemán-Flores[2], Luis Álvarez-León[1], Rafael Fuentes-Pavón[2], José M. Santana-Montesdeoca[2]

[1]Departamento de Informática y Sistemas, Universidad de Las Palmas de Gran Canaria, 35017, Las Palmas, Spain
[2]Sección de Ecografía, Servicio de Radiodiagnóstico, Hospital Universitario Insular de Gran Canaria, 35016, Las Palmas, Spain
maleman@dis.ulpgc.es

Abstract. The early diagnosis of breast cancer depends in many cases on the analysis of medical imaging, mainly mammography, ultrasonography and MRI. This work deals with ultrasound images in order to reduce speckle noise, identify the contour of the nodules and analyze a wide range of criteria which allow distinguishing between benign and malignant tumors. We try to automatize the different phases of the process and extract some objective parameters for a robust and reproducible diagnosis. We provide the physicians with both graphical as well as numerical results for the features which have been analyzed.

1 Introduction

Although mammography is the most widely used modality in breast cancer detection, ultrasonography is a very useful complementary imaging technique which not only provides a different assessment of the lesion, but also allows detecting very small lesions and analyze dense breasts, which is quite difficult using mammography. Radiologists have proved the importance of the information supplied by analyzing a series of criteria on ultrasound images. These include some aspects related to the general shape of the tumor, the relative echogenicity of the different regions and the regularity of the contour [1].

Due to the presence of the characteristic speckle noise, it is quite difficult to perform an accurate automatic segmentation. Therefore, a previous filtering stage is necessary. The information of the contrast as well as the texture of the different regions allow a precise delimitation of the contours. Finally, the automatic analysis of the diagnostic criteria by means of different shape and histogram analysis techniques supplies a deep characterization of the nodules.

Some previous works try to segment the tissues [2] or detect the lesions [3]. Some systems for automatic lesion classification using different features have been proposed [4, 5]. We intend to carry out a whole process to assess the lesions and support the decision making process.

2 Materials and Methods

We have developed a three-stage process to analyze the ultrasound images. The first phase aims at reducing speckle noise, the second one consists in the segmentation of the nodules and the third one is the analysis of the diagnostic criteria. In order to test the accuracy of the results that we obtain with our techniques, we have used a set of 32 nodules in ultrasound images. Each nodule has been delimited and assessed by 3 experienced specialists. The delimitation has been manually performed twice by each specialist and the evaluation consists in the assessment of a set of diagnostic criteria for each nodule. Furthermore, the biopsy has been performed to determine the malignancy or benignancy of the nodules.

2.1 Filtering and Segmentation

Due to the characteristic speckle noise of ultrasound images, a noise reducing filter must be first applied before the segmentation. We have tested different filters, including statistical, morphological, iterative or anisotropic filters. The best results have been obtained using a variation of Perona-Malik filter [6] in which we have included texture information obtained from Gabor filters response. From an inner point, a gradient-guided front-propagation algorithm is used to extract an initial pre-segmentation. This can be used as initial contour for the active contour technique [7], for which we apply a level set approach. We have added Gabor-based texture information also in this phase in order to improve the results of the segmentation. Similar approaches are found in [8, 9]. This allows dealing with heterogeneous edges, diffused contours or gradual transitions. Once the segmentation is obtained, we proceed to analyze the features of the nodule.

2.2 Feature Extraction

The main features which allow discriminating benign from malignant tumors are related to the shape of the nodules, the echogenicity of the different regions and the regularity of their contours. An ellipsoid shape or the presence of two or three gentle and well circumscribed lobulations are considered as benign findings. On the other hand, ramifications or a taller-than-wide shape are considered as malignant findings. Moreover, when examining the smoothness of the contour, if it presents microlobulations, angular margins or spiculation, they are interpreted as malignant findings, as opposite to a rounded and well defined contour. Finally, hyperechogenicity and the presence of a thin echogenic capsule increase the probability of benignancy, whereas calcifications and hypoechogenicity are associated to malignant nodules [1]. In this work, we analyze the global and the local features of the contours as well as the echogenicity histograms, so that some robust, reproducible and accurate measurements can be provided to the specialists in order to perform a more reliable distinction between benign and malignant nodules.

In order to measure how gentle and well circumscribed the contour is, we try to fit to one, two or three overlapping ellipses by means of a gradient descent method. The accuracy of the fitting indicates how smooth the contour is and how many lobulations it consists of. Afterwards, we analyze the shape to locate the eventual ramifications of the nodule. Their relative size with respect to the total size indicate their relevance. The local variations of the contour require a detailed analysis of its regularity. We have developed some techniques which involve the search for pseudo-corners, elliptical arcs or high gradient orientation variance and allow locating angular margins, microlobulations or spiculation.

3 Results

Figure 1 illustrates some of the graphical results which are provided to the specialists. Table 1 shows the values for the sensitivity, specificity, positive predictive value and negative predictive value for the different criteria. Table 2 presents the corresponding values for the area under the ROC (receiver operating characteristic) curve, which combines sensitivity, specificity and discrimination threshold to provide a more general value.

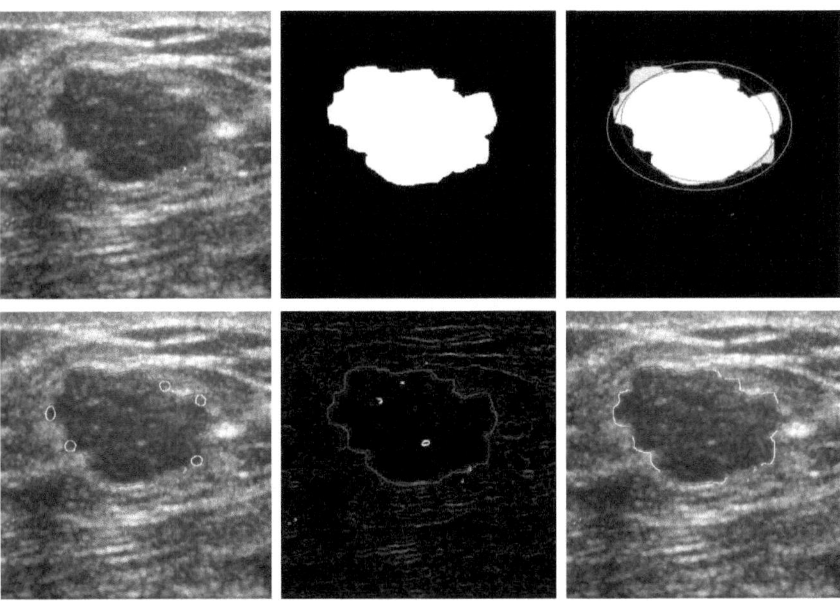

Fig. 1. From top to bottom and left to right: example of a breast nodule, its segmentation and some graphical results for the examination of general shape, microlobulations, calcifications and angular margins

Table 1. Results: PV = predictive value; man = assessment of physicians; auto = automatic assessment

criteria	sensitivity		specificity		positive PV		negative PV	
	man	auto	man	auto	man	auto	man	auto
ellipsoid shape	92	100	45	37	38	37	94	100
gentle lobulations	100	92	48	37	41	35	100	92
capsule	92	30	54	80	42	42	95	75
hyperechogenicity	100	100	2	2	27	27	100	100
hypoechogenicity	92	92	20	20	30	30	87	87
ramifications	76	92	82	37	62	35	90	92
microlobulations	92	100	37	45	35	40	92	100
angular margins	100	92	48	60	41	46	100	95
spiculation	46	53	94	74	75	43	82	81
calcifications	46	30	80	62	46	23	80	70
acoustic shadowing	23	15	71	80	23	14	71	70

Table 2. Results for the area under the ROC curve for the different criteria

criteria	area under the ROC curve
ellipsoid shape	0.79
gentle lobulations	0.79
capsule	0.50
hyperechogenicity	0.98
hypoechogenicity	0.99
ramifications	0.67
microlobulations	0.51
angular margins	0.82
spiculation	0.82
calcifications	0.50
acoustic shadowing	0.75

4 Discussion

We have presented an automatic process to filter, segment and analyze the features of breast nodules in ultrasound images. The results regarding the sensitivity, specificity, positive predicted value and negative predicted value for single features are comparable to those obtained through the examination of the specialists. The area under the ROC curve shows the importance and robustness of every single feature in the final diagnosis and their relation to the result of the biopsy. We can observe that some automatically extracted parameters are individually precise as well as robust. Since the diagnosis is performed by combining the different criteria and interpreting their relevance, degree and coincidence, we are currently working on a further stage, i.e. a pseudo-expert system which can provide much further information to the radiologists. The results are quite satisfactory and encourage the future work in this research field.

References

1. Stavros AT, Thickman D, Rapp CL, et al. Solid breast nodules: Use of sonography to distinguish between benign and malignant lesions. Radiology. 1995;196(1):123–34.
2. Kaufhold J, Chan R, Karl WC, et al. Ultrasound tissue analysis and characterization. Proc SPIE. 1999; p. 73–83.
3. Drukker K, Giger ML, Horsch K, et al. Computerized lesion detection on breast ultrasound. Med Phys. 2002;29(7):1438–46.
4. Rodrigues P, Giraldi G, Provenzano M, et al. A new methodology based on q-entropy for breast lesion classification in 3-D ultrasound images. Proc IEEE Eng Ned Biol Soc. 2006; p. 1048–51.
5. Chang RF, Wu WJ, Woo KM, et al. Automatic ultrasound segmentation and morphology based diagnosis of solid breast tumors. Breast Cancer Res Treat. 2005;89(2):179–85.
6. Perona P, Malik J. Scale space and edge detection using anisotropic diffusion. IEEE Trans Pattern Anal Mach Intell. 1990;12(1):629–39.
7. Caselles V, Kimmel R, Sapiro G. Geodesic active contours. Int J Comp Vis. 1997;22(1):61–79.
8. Sagiv C, Sochen N, Zeevi Y. Integrated active contours for texture segmentation. IEEE Trans Image Process. 2006;15(6):1633–46.
9. Chan TF, Vese LA. Active contours and segmentation models using geometric PDE's for medical imaging. In Malladi, R (ed) Geometric Methods in Bio-Medical Image Processing. 2002; p. 63–75.

Segmentierung pleuraständiger Lungenrundherde in CT-Bildern mittels Ellipsoidapproximation

Jan Hendrik Moltz, Jan-Martin Kuhnigk, Lars Bornemann, Heinz-Otto Peitgen

MeVis Research GmbH – Center for Medical Image Computing
Universitätsallee 29, 28359 Bremen
jan.moltz@mevis.de

Kurzfassung. In diesem Artikel wird ein neuer Algorithmus zur Segmentierung pleuraständiger Lungenrundherde in CT-Aufnahmen vorgestellt. Lungenrundherde mit großflächigem Kontakt zur Brustwand oder anderen gleichdichten Strukturen sind eine besondere Herausforderung für Segmentierungsverfahren. Wir verwenden einen Ray-Casting-Ansatz, um Punkte am sichtbaren Rand der Läsion zu finden, und berechnen aus diesen Punkten ein Ellipsoid, das die Läsionsform approximiert. Innerhalb dieses Ellipsoids werden durch morphologische Operationen die angrenzenden Strukturen abgetrennt. Eine Evaluation mit 333 Rundherden zeigte, dass diese Methode gute Ergebnisse liefert und praktisch ohne Erhöhung des Rechenaufwands in einen allgemeinen Segmentierungsalgorithmus für Lungenrundherde integriert werden kann.

1 Einführung

In der onkologischen Verlaufskontrolle ist die Schätzung des Tumorwachstums aus aufeinanderfolgenden CT-Aufnahmen wichtig für die Beurteilung des Behandlungserfolgs. Bisher geschieht dies durch manuelle Messung der größten axialen Durchmesser der Läsionen. Dabei wird jedoch implizit vorausgesetzt, dass Tumoren kugelförmig sind und symmetrisch wachsen, was im allgemeinen nicht der Fall ist. Außerdem sind solche Messungen subjektiv, fehleranfällig und aufwändig. Ein Software-Assistent erlaubt eine exaktere und reproduzierbarere Schätzung durch volumetrische Messungen in 3D. Eine wichtige Teilaufgabe ist die Läsionssegmentierung. Da der klinische Arbeitsablauf durch den Computereinsatz nicht verlangsamt werden darf, ist Effizienz hier ein wichtiger Aspekt. Daher wurden spezielle Algorithmen für verschiedene Tumorarten entwickelt.

Diese Arbeit beschäftigt sich mit der Segmentierung von Lungenrundherden. Gegeben ist eine Region of Interest, die manuell oder automatisch bestimmt wurde. Diese ROI soll die Läsion vollständig enthalten, und ihr Mittelpunkt soll nahe dem Läsionsmittelpunkt liegen. Außerdem setzen wir nahezu isotrope Voxel voraus. In CT-Aufnahmen der Lunge lassen sich im Wesentlichen zwei Dichteklassen unterscheiden: Während das Parenchym dunkel erscheint, werden Lungenrundherde, aber auch Blutgefäße oder Nachbarstrukturen der Lunge wie die Brustwand, das Herz oder das Zwerchfell hell dargestellt (Abb. 1(a)). Zur Segmentierung von Rundherden mit Kontakt zu einer dieser Strukturen reicht eine reine Schwellwertmethode daher nicht aus.

Von Reeves et al. [1] wurde ein Algorithmus vorgeschlagen, der morphologisches Opening zur Segmentierung von Lungenrundherden verwendet, aber speziell auf kleine Läsionen zugeschnitten ist. Okada *et al.* [2] stellten einen Ansatz vor, der wie unser Verfahren eine Ellipsoidapproximation verwendet, aber diese durch Anpassung eines Gauss'schen Modells berechnet. Dieses Verfahren benötigt für pleuraständige Rundherde jedoch einen zusätzlichen Korrekturschritt.

Die in diesem Artikel beschriebenen Methoden basieren auf dem Algorithmus von Kuhnigk *et al.* [3], der für die Segmentierung kleiner und großer Lungenrundherde mit potenziell starker Vaskularisierung entworfen wurde. Bei pleuraständigen Rundherden wird dort die Tatsache genutzt, dass die Lunge weitgehend konvex ist und dass die Läsionen Konkavitäten erzeugen. Die Idee besteht darin, die ursprüngliche Form zu rekonstruieren, indem die konvexe Hülle des Lungenparenchyms innerhalb der ROI berechnet und die Läsionsmaske am Rand dieser Hülle abgeschnitten wird. In nicht konvexen Teilen der Lunge, z. B. an der Grenze zum Herzen oder zum Zwerchfell, wird die angrenzende Struktur jedoch nicht vollständig entfernt (Abb. 2 (d)-(f)). In dieser Arbeit stellen wir eine Erweiterung des Algorithmus vor, die auch diesen Fall berücksichtigt.

2 Material und Methoden

Unsere Erweiterung von Kuhnigks Algorithmus [3] besteht aus drei Schritten, die im Folgenden erläutert und in Abb. 1 illustriert werden:

1. Identifikation von Punkten am Läsionsrand durch Region Growing und anschließendes Ray Casting vom Saatpunkt aus;
2. Berechnung eines Ellipsoids, das die Form der Läsion approximiert;
3. konvexe Hülle wie oben [3], aber beschränkt auf das dilatierte Ellipsoid.

2.1 Region Growing und Ray Casting

Zu Beginn wird ein Region Growing mit dem ROI-Zentrum als Saatpunkt durchgeführt. Dabei kann der untere Schwellwert fest gewählt werden, z. B. -400 HU, da nur der Tumor und andere hochdichte Strukturen vom Parenchym getrennt werden sollen. Um Punkte an der Grenze zwischen dem Tumor und dem Parenchym zu finden, verwenden wir einen Ray-Casting-Ansatz. Vom Saatpunkt ausgehend werden 98 Strahlen ausgesandt. Dies entspricht einem Strahl durch jedes Oberflächenvoxel eines $5 \times 5 \times 5$-Würfels um den Saatpunkt. Dadurch wird eine symmetrische Verteilung und eine Ausrichtung an das Voxelgitter gewährleistet. Die Strahlen werden verfolgt, bis sie entweder das Parenchym oder den Rand der ROI erreichen (Abb. 1(a)). Im ersten Fall werden die Endpunkte gespeichert und sonst verworfen (Abb. 1(b)). Um den Einfluss anderer Strukturen am Rand der ROI zu verringern, sollten Endpunkte ab einer bestimmten Distanz vom Saatpunkt ebenfalls verworfen werden. Das 95%-Quantil der Distanzen aller Endpunkte erwies sich als guter Schwellwert.

2.2 Ellipsoidapproximation

Typischerweise decken die durch das Ray Casting gefundenen Punkte einen Großteil der tatsächlichen Läsionsoberfläche ab. Unter der Annahme, dass die Läsion näherungsweise ellipsoidförmig ist, versuchen wir, ihre Form zu rekonstruieren, indem wir ein Ellipsoid an diese Punkte anpassen (Abb. 1(c)).

Ein 3D-Ellipsoid ist definiert als Kegelschnitt

$$\{\mathbf{x} \in \mathbb{R}^3 \mid \mathbf{x}^T \mathbf{A} \mathbf{x} + \mathbf{b}^T \mathbf{x} + c = 0\}, \tag{1}$$

für den die symmetrische Matrix $\mathbf{A} \in \mathbb{R}^{3 \times 3}$ positiv oder negativ definit ist. Wegen der Symmetrie hat $\mathbf{A}$ nur sechs Freiheitsgrade, zu denen für $\mathbf{b} \in \mathbb{R}^3$ und $c \in \mathbb{R}$ noch insgesamt vier hinzukommen. Aus den gültigen Endpunkten der 98 Strahlen sollen nun die im Least-Squares-Sinne optimalen Ellipsoidparameter bestimmt werden. Dabei entsteht ein nichtlineares Gleichungssystem, das jedoch mit einem Verfahren von Grammalidis und Strintzis [4] auf ein verallgemeinertes Eigenwertproblem reduziert und effizient gelöst werden kann. Die Definitheit von $\mathbf{A}$ kann dabei zwar nicht garantiert werden, aber unsere Experimente zeigten, dass sie fast immer gegeben ist. Falls die Verteilung der Punkte eine Ellipsoidanpassung unmöglich macht, z. B. weil der Tumor unregelmäßig geformt oder stark mit anderen Strukturen verbunden ist, kann stattdessen eine Kugel berechnet werden. Obwohl dies eine gröbere Approximation ist, erhält man auch in diesen seltenen Fällen zumeist akzeptable Ergebnisse.

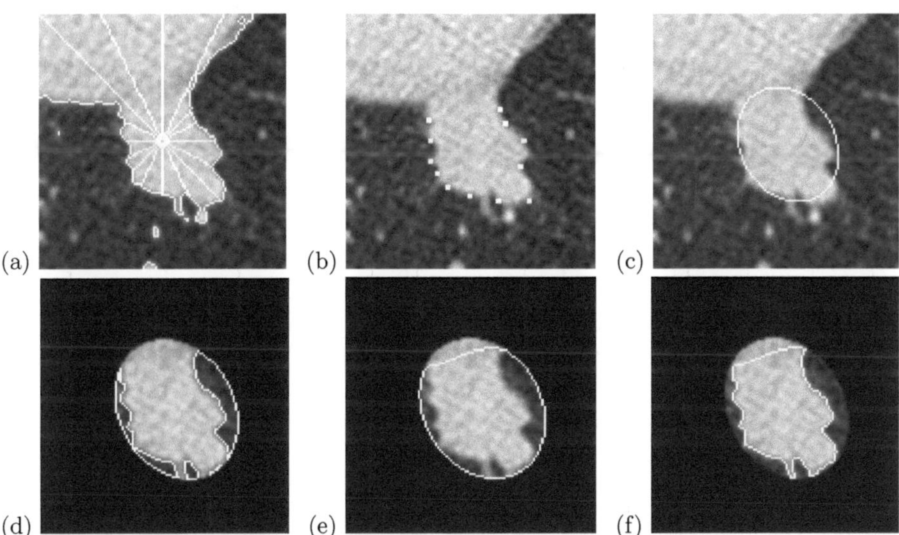

Abb. 1. Schrittweise Illustration des 3D-Algorithmus, veranschaulicht durch die zentrale axiale Schicht. (a) Ergebnismaske des initialen Region Growing und Strahlen zum Rand der Maske. (b) Gültige Strahlenendpunkte am Tumorrand. (c) An die Punkte angepasstes Ellipsoid. (d) Teil der Maske innerhalb des dilatierten Ellipsoids. (e) Konvexe Hülle der inversen Maske innerhalb des dilatierten Ellipsoids. (f) Differenz von konvexer Hülle und inverser Maske

2.3 Konvexe Hülle

Für alle weiteren Berechnungen wird die ROI mit einer leicht dilatierten Version des Ellipsoids maskiert (Abb. 1(d)). Die Dilatation soll sicherstellen, dass der Tumor vollständig enthalten ist. Am Rand enthält das Ellipsoid auch einige Parenchymvoxel, so dass die Idee des Originalalgorithmus, die Parenchymgrenze vor der Entstehung des Tumors durch eine konvexe Hülle zu rekonstruieren, weiterhin anwendbar ist (Abb. 1(e)). Dies funktioniert nun auch in konkaven Bereichen des Parenchyms, denn die Konkavitäten sind innerhalb des Ellipsoids nicht mehr sichtbar und das Ergebnis ist unabhängig von der Größe der ROI (Abb. 1(f)). Aus Performanzgründen wurde die konvexe Hülle als Vereinigung der schichtweisen konvexen Hüllen in den axialen, sagittalen und koronalen Ansichten implementiert. Anschließend werden wie im Originalalgorithmus [3] angrenzende Blutgefäße durch adaptives Opening entfernt.

3 Ergebnisse

In unseren Experimenten nutzten wir eine Datenbank von 333 ROIs mit pleuraständigen Lungenrundherden von verschiedenen Patienten, Kliniken und CT-Geräten. Die Saatpunkte wurden manuell von Radiologen gesetzt. Da bereits umfangreiche Experimente für die Originalversion [3] durchgeführt worden waren, konzentrierten wir uns auf die Effekte der oben beschriebenen Erweiterungen. Es ist oft unmöglich, die genaue Grenze zwischen dem Tumor und einer angrenzenden Struktur zu bestimmen. Daher wurden die Segmentierungsergebnisse visuell begutachtet und daraufhin untersucht, ob unser Ziel, den Tumor entlang der ursprünglichen Parenchymgrenze abzutrennen, erreicht wurde.

Während mit dem Originalalgorithmus in 71% der Fälle das Segmentierungsergebnis als gut bewertet wurde, konnten wir diesen Anteil auf 89% erhöhen. Für weitere 5% wurde ein gutes Ergebnis durch Anwendung des interaktiven Korrekturverfahrens aus [3] erreicht. Die meisten Rundherde, die nicht segmentiert werden konnten, hatten komplexe Formen oder sehr großflächigen Kontakt zu hochdichten Strukturen, so dass eine Ellipsoidapproximation nicht möglich war. Abb. 2 zeigt einige Beispiele erfolgreicher Segmentierungen und lässt im Vergleich mit den vorherigen Ergebnissen eine deutliche Verbesserung erkennen.

4 Diskussion

Wie unsere Experimente zeigen, haben wir einen Algorithmus entwickelt, der die meisten pleuraständigen Lungenrundherde segmentiert, auch wenn das umgebende Parenchym nicht konvex ist. Dies schließt eine Lücke in Kuhnigks Algorithmus [3], der hier systematische Probleme hatte. Unser Verfahren kann dort einfach integriert werden und hat keine Auswirkungen auf isolierte Rundherde. Eine signifikante Erhöhung der Laufzeit konnte trotz einiger zusätzlicher Ope-

Abb. 2. (a)-(c) Beispiele erfolgreicher Segmentierungen mit dem neuen Algorithmus. (d)-(f) Entsprechende Ergebnisse mit der Originalversion

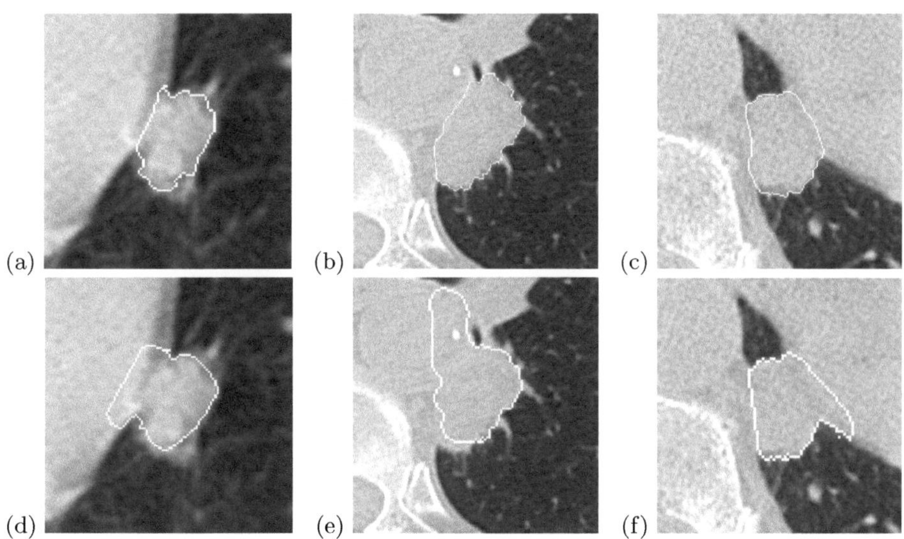

rationen nicht festgestellt werden, da die anschließenden Berechnungen auf das Ellipsoid beschränkt werden können. Die Rechenzeit für eine vollständige Segmentierung beträgt etwa 2 s für große und oft unter 1 s für kleine Tumoren auf einem PC mit einem 2 GHz-Dual-Core-Prozessor.

Unsere Grundidee lässt sich verallgemeinern auf die Segmentierung von Objekten mit einer nur teilweise sichtbaren Grenze, die durch eine einfache geometrische Struktur angenähert werden kann. Wir untersuchen zur Zeit die Anwendbarkeit auf Lebermetastasen und vergrößerte Lymphknoten, um die Fähigkeiten onkologischer Software-Assistenten zu erweitern.

Danksagung. Wir danken Siemens Medical Solutions für die Förderung dieser Arbeit im Rahmen des VICORA-Projekts.

Literaturverzeichnis

1. Reeves AP, Chan AB, Yankelevitz DF, et al. On measuring the change in size of pulmonary nodules. IEEE Trans Med Imaging. 2006;25(4):435–50.
2. Okada K, Ramesh V, Krishnan A, et al. Robust pulmonary nodule segmentation in CT: Improving performance for juxtapleural cases. Proc MICCAI. 2005; p. 781–9.
3. Kuhnigk JM, Dicken V, Bornemann L, et al. Morphological segmentation and partial volume analysis for volumetry of solid pulmonary lesions in thoracic CT scans. IEEE Trans Med Imaging. 2006;25(4):417–34.
4. Grammalidis N, Strintzis MG. Head detection and tracking by 2-D and 3-D ellipsoid fitting. Proc CGI. 2000; p. 221–226.

Segmentation of Axonal Fibres in Tissue Slices

Nico Scherf[1], Jens-Peer Kuska[2], Claudia Heine[1], Ulf-Dietrich Braumann[1], Heike Franke[3]

[1]Translational Centre for Regenerative Medicine, University Leipzig, 04103 Leipzig
[2]Interdisciplinary Centre for Bioinformatics, University Leipzig, 04107 Leipzig
[3]Rudolf Boehm Institute of Pharmacology & Toxicology, Univ. Leipzig, 04107 Leipzig
nscherf@trm.uni-leipzig.de

Abstract. This work focuses on the segmentation of axonal structures in digital images of organotypic slice co-cultures. An image processing chain is presented, which relies on anisotropic diffusion for preprocessing of the images and the intelligent scissors method for segmentation. This method requires manual user interaction to set the starting points. To overcome this drawback, the initial parameters for the intelligent scissors are automatically extracted from the images by a graph-based approach.

1 Introduction

The purpose of this work is to present an image processing chain for the segmentation of biocytin-traced axonal fibres in digital images of organotypic dopaminergic co-cultures of the rat brain. The segmentation step is crucial in order to be able to analyse the properties of axonal outgrowth depending on different factors (for the biological motivation behind this we refer the reader to [1]). A similar question was investigated by [2]. But whereas Pakura et al. were interested in the overall structure of the neural tissue, we like to analyse and compare the properties of single fibres. So we need a segmentation method able to track single fibres as exact as possible. The segmentation of line-like structures is a common problem in medical image processing (e.g. [3] or [4]). Most approaches base on global methods such as thresholding with additional local constraints depending on e.g. morphological features or curvature. We decided to use an anisotropic diffusion filter to enhance the line-like structures as well as to close small gaps along the fibres. The segmentation itself is obtained by the intelligent scissors approach [5] which leads to single spatially connected contours representing the axonal fibres. This method requires manual interaction. To overcome this disadvantage we propose a way to automatically extract the initial parameters for this segmentation from the image itself.

2 Materials and Methods

2.1 Preprocessing

The original images (an example is shown in Fig. 1(a)) are preprocessed to enhance the axonal structures for further segmentation. Since there is no useful colour information in the original images, we use a greyscale version instead. We are interested in the line-like structures, so at first a Laplacian of Gaussian (LoG) filter is applied to enhance the edges. This is shown in Fig. 1(b). The distribution of the grey-values along a single fibre is not homogeneous. This is due to the three-dimensional structure of the specimen under consideration (some parts of a fibre simply lie outside of the focal plane), and on the other hand the staining of the fibres itself might be inhomogeneous. We use a filter that enhances line-like structures and is able to close small gaps along a single axonal fibre. This is achieved by an anisotropic diffusion filter described in [6] that smoothes the image along the edges and therewith enhances the spatial coherence of the fibres. The resulting image is shown in Fig. 1(c). By this step, some structures of the background are also increased, so a further smoothing step is needed. Since we are interested in removing the background noise while preserving the important structures, a total-variation filter [7] is used. This filter only requires the standard deviation of the background noise as parameter. The TV-filtered image is depicted in Fig. 1(d).

2.2 Segmentation

As mentioned in the introduction, there is a great range of different segmentation strategies and none is superior to others in all possible contexts. When tracking the structure of a single fibre, on ideally wants a single spatially connected

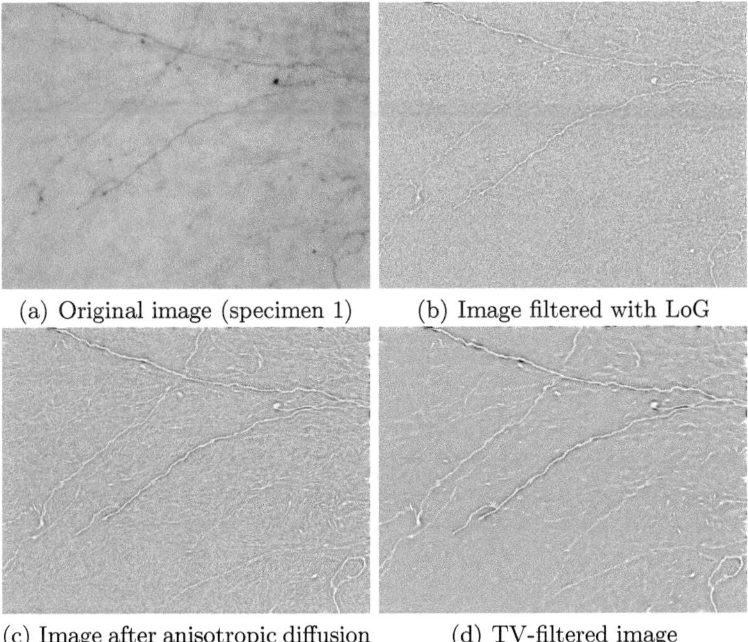

(a) Original image (specimen 1)

(b) Image filtered with LoG

(c) Image after anisotropic diffusion

(d) TV-filtered image

Fig. 1. Preprocessing

structure. When using morphological operators and thresholding, the resulting segmentation also consists of small structures that are not connected to a single fibre. In principle, this can be handled by removing structures that are too small (e.g. [2]). But this approach also removes small parts along the fibres, if there are between two gaps. An appropriate method for extracting the axons are the intelligent scissors proposed by [5]. By choosing two points on the fibre the intelligent scissors segmentation is able to track the path between them. The resulting contour is connected, so it is possible to interpolate gaps that occur. The segmentation result seems to be appropriate for analysing the properties of the axonal outgrowth, but this method has one great disadvantage: it is semi-automatic. User interaction is needed to place the initial points on the fibres. To overcome this problem, an automatic initialisation method, i.e. the extraction of reasonable starting points from the image itself is used.

2.3 Parameter Extraction

The quantification method presented by [8] is able to extract a graph structure from images of astrocytes. Based on this approach we are able to extract points in the image, that lie on the ends of the fibres and therewith are ideal as initial points for the intelligent scissors segmentation. At first the preprocessed image is binarised by simple thresholding (Fig. 2(a)). No other thresholding method is used, since the grey-values in the filtered images nearly follow an ideal Gaussian distribution. From the binarised image, a graph structure of connected parts of the foreground is constructed (for details see [8]). Here, all structures with a number of vertices that is too small, are removed. The result is depicted in Fig. 2(b). Now the vertices of the graph (shown in red in Fig. 2(b)) are taken as initial points for the intelligent scissors. Two points are selected as initial pair, if their distance is above a given threshold. Then all combinations of such points are used as initialisation, leading to a bundle of possible fibre-tracks.

3 Results

An example of the results of the segmentation are shown in Fig. 3. One can see from this images, that the main fibre tracks can be segmented. A single fibre from the detected bundles is depicted in Fig. 3(b). The structure of the axonal outgrowth is well captured by the segmentation results. Fig. 3(c) and Fig. 3(d) show two further segmentation results from different specimens. One way of analysing the structure of a single extracted axon is to take the fibre as a one-dimensional signal and to look at the frequency distribution of this signal. As an example in Fig. 4 the structure of the fibre in Fig. 3(b) is plotted together with a log-log plot of the coefficients of the Fourier transform.

4 Discussion

While the segmentation method yields adequate results on the example images, extensive testing in laboratory practice will follow to demonstrate the method's

Fig. 2. Feature Extraction

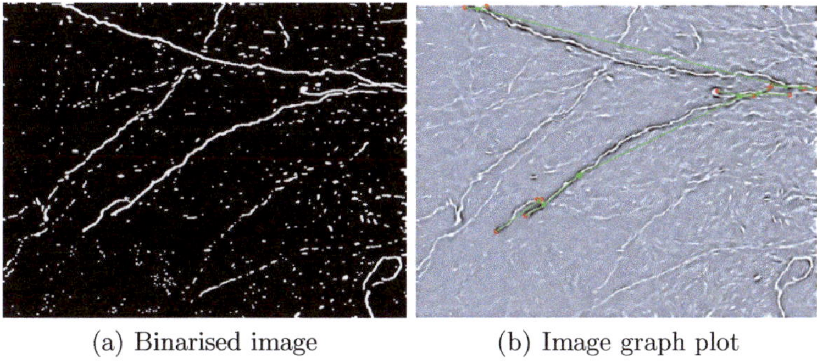

(a) Binarised image (b) Image graph plot

reliability. It is of great advantage that the resulting structures are connected lines, which can be used to analyse the different forms of growth of the axon fibres. One remaining point is the selection of single fibres from the bundles that are segmented. Since most combinations of start points lead to nearly the same structures (as can be seen from Fig. 3(a)) a simple way is to select the longest fibre from all the overlapping results as a representative. The aim of further work is the evaluation of other criteria for selecting a single representative fibre from the result as well as extracting additional features from the segmented fibres.

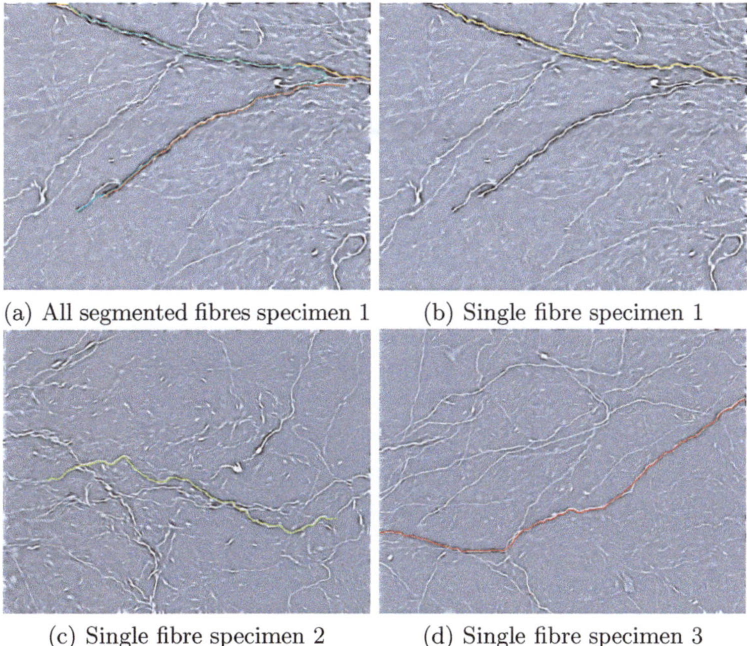

(a) All segmented fibres specimen 1 (b) Single fibre specimen 1

(c) Single fibre specimen 2 (d) Single fibre specimen 3

Fig. 3. Result of the intelligent scissors segmentation

Fig. 4. Analysis of a single fibre

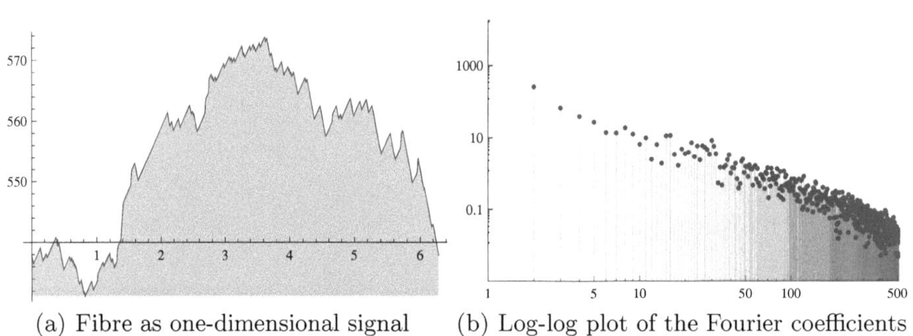

(a) Fibre as one-dimensional signal (b) Log-log plot of the Fourier coefficients

Acknowledgement. The project is supported by the Federal Ministry of Education and Research (BMBF), grant PTJ-BIO/31P4282 (MS CartPro) and grant PTJ-BIO/031390 (TRM Leipzig).

References

1. Heine C, Wegner A, Grosche J, et al. P2 receptor expression in the dopaminergic system of the rat brain during development. Neuroscience. 2007;149(1):165–81.
2. Pakura M, Schmitt O, Aach T. Segmentation and analysis of nerve fibers in histologic sections of the cerebral human cortex. Proc SSIAI. 2002; p. 62–6.
3. Zana F, Klein JC. Segmentation of vessel-like patterns using mathematical morphology and curvature evaluation. IEEE Trans Image Process. 2001;10(7):1010–9.
4. Jelinek HF, Cree MJ, Leandroa JJG, et al. Automated segmentation of retinal blood vessels and identification of proliferative diabetic retinopathy. J Opt Soc Am A. 2007;24(5):1448–56.
5. Mortensen EN, Barrett WA. Intelligent scissors for image composition. Proc SIGGRAPH. 1995; p. 191–8.
6. Weickert J. Anisotropic Diffusion in Image Processing. Teubner; 1998.
7. Chan TF, Osher S, Shen J. The digital TV filter and nonlinear denoising. IEEE Trans Image Process. 2001;10(2):231–41.
8. Braumann UD, Franke H, Hengstler J, et al. Graph-based quantification of astrocytes. Proc BVM. 2006; p. 379–83.

Einfache Grauwert-Transferfunktion für die Berechnung von digital rekonstruierten Röntgenbildern

Axel Newe[1], Richard Rascher-Friesenhausen[1,2], Heinz-Otto Peitgen[2]

[1]Hochschule Bremerhaven
[2]Mevis Research GmbH, Bremen
axl@axelnewe.de

Kurzfassung. Das Raycasting ist ein etabliertes Verfahren zur Berechnung von Digital Rekonstruierten Röntgenbildern (DRRs), also auf Basis von CT-Daten approximierten Radiographien, welche die Projektion eines Summationsbilds des 3D-CT-Volumens auf eine zweidimensionale Bildebene darstellen. Die Wirkung eines von einem Raycasting-Strahl durchquerten Voxels auf das Ergebnispixel im DRR kann unter anderem mit Hilfe von Transferfunktionen berechnet werden, die den Grauwert des Voxels in einen Schwächungskoeffizienten für den Strahl umrechnen. Es wird ein einfaches mathematisches Modell für eine solche Transferfunktion vorgestellt, dessen Parametrisierung eng an die klinische Praxis angelehnt ist.

1 Einleitung

Die Projektion eines dreidimensionalen CT-Volumens auf eine zweidimensionale Bildebene, bei der aus den Schichtbildern des CTs ein Summationsbild mit allen in Projektionsrichtung hintereinander gelegenen Strukturen entsteht, wird als Digital Rekonstruiertes Röntgenbild (DRR) bezeichnet.

Das ursprüngliche und naivste Verfahren zur Berechnung von DRRs ist das Raycasting, also die Verfolgung einer Anzahl von virtuellen Röntgenstrahlen durch einen virtuellen Patienten hindurch. Dabei wird die Wirkung eines jeden durchquerten Voxels des 3D-Datensatzes auf die Strahlen berechnet:

a) Bei der „Maximum Intensity“-Projektion (MIP) wird nur das Voxel mit dem größten Grauwert berücksichtigt und dieser direkt für das Ergebnispixel übernommen [1].
b) Die „Mean Extinction“-Projektion gewichtet alle durchquerten Voxel gleich und bildet deren arithmetisches Mittel [1].
c) Andere Vorgehensweise versuchen, die tatsächlichen physikalischen Verhältnisse zu simulieren, indem sie die Voxelgrauwerte mit Hilfe einer Transferfunktion in einen Schwächungskoeffizienten umrechnen und davon ausgehend die Abschwächung der Strahlen kalkulieren [2, 3].

Mit dieser Arbeit wird ein einfaches mathematisches Modell für eine Transferfunktion gemäß c) vorgestellt, die über wenige, die klinische Erfahrung widerspiegelnde Variablen parametrisierbar ist.

Abb. 2. Verschiedene Dropfenster-Einstellungen und daraus berechnete DRRs. Einstellung a zeigt eine Kurve mit schmalem, aber hohem Dropfenster; das resultierende DRRs ist sehr kontrastreich. Die Einstellungen b und c weisen Kurven mit zunehmend breiterem und flacherem Dropfenster auf. Die resultierenden DRRs sind dementsprechend weniger kontrastreich

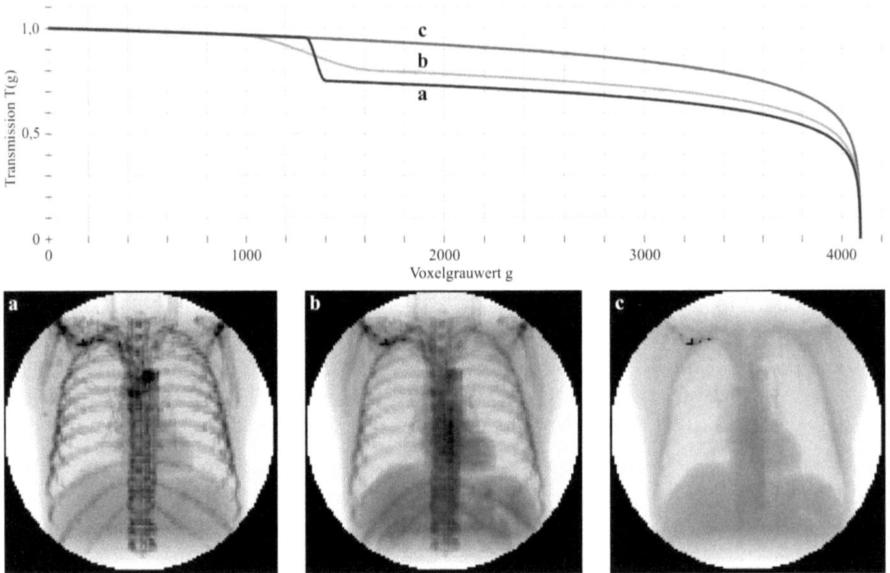

die für die Erzeugung eines DRRs angenommene Strahlenenergie gesteuert werden, indem z.B. bei einer angenommenen hohen Strahlenenergie ein niedriges, breites Dropfenster zum Einsatz kommt (Abb. 2, Einstellung c), bei einer angenommenen niedrigen Strahlenenergie hingegen ein hohes, schmales Dropfenster (Abb. 2, Einstellung a).

Die Mitte des Dropfensters sollte im niedrigen Voxelgrauwertbereich von Knochengewebe liegen, da Röntgenstrahlen mit in der medizinischen Anwendung (ohne Mammographien) üblichen Energien von 60 keV bis 160 keV besonders bei Knochengewebe die oben beschriebene überproportionale Abschwächung aufweisen.

Literaturverzeichnis

1. Löbbert S. Visualisation of Two-Dimensional Volumes. [Dissertation]. TU Berlin; 2004.
2. Sherouse GW. Computation of digitally reconstructed radiographs for use in radiotherapy treatment design. Int J Radiat Oncol Biol Phys. 1990;18(3):651–8.
3. Li X. Digitally reconstructed radiograph generation by an adaptive Monte Carlo method. Phys Med Biol. 2006;51:2745–52.

Haptic Pulse Simulation for Virtual Palpation

Sebastian Ullrich[1], Joel Mendoza[1], Alexandre Ntouba[2], Rolf Rossaint[2], Torsten Kuhlen[1]

[1]Virtual Reality Group, RWTH Aachen University
[2]Anaesthesia Clinic, University Hospital Aachen
s.ullrich@rz.rwth-aachen.de

Abstract. In this paper we propose a software-based approach to simulate the haptics of the human pulse. This effect can then be interactively explored by virtual palpation. The algorithm features a flexible, user-defined setup. In addition the simulation takes dynamic parameters into account and allows for many different use cases.

1 Introduction

The pulse is one of the most essential sources of information for medical diagnosis. It is primarily used for measuring blood pressure or monitoring the circulatory system. In addition, the pulse is a palpable landmark that allows to determine the position of arteries. This knowledge is regularly applied to locate insertion sites for needle penetration in regional anaesthesia. Until now, there is no software-based trainer that simulates this effect for palpation procedure.

Two selected examples are a mechanical-based skill trainer that simulates the pulse with pneumatic tubes in a corpse [1] and a software-based endoscopic simulator, that visualizes hemodynamics without haptics [2]. Instead of these, our focus lies on the haptic simulation of a pulse. Also, our goal is to provide feasible results in real-time and not create an accurate bloodflow simulation.

Our approach is a flexible software-based haptic simulation of the pulse. This allows for different scenarios (i.e., patient data-sets and various body regions) and is also meant to be used as a component in other simulators (e.g., [3]).

2 Materials and Methods

Because the pulse can be only detected in specific areas of the human body we propose a local simulation scheme. First we give a description of the setup and algorithm. Afterwards, the different components are explained in more detail.

2.1 Model and Setup

To model a pulse region we construct it out of one or multiple particles. These particles are then defined as emitting sources for the local pulse (cp. Fig. 1). Usually, the particles reside within an artery and are close to a prominent surface point where the pulse can be palpated. Some typical regions are: carotid pulse (located in the neck), brachial pulse (between biceps and triceps, femoral pulse (located at the thigh), etc. Thus one can define multiple regions.

Then we setup a virtual proxy that is coupled to a haptic input device for palpation [4]. The proxy is used for collision detection and contains, the position and orientation of the tooltip of the device.

2.2 Algorithm of Pulse Simulation

Our algorithm is divided into a two-phase collision detection and the actual simulation:

1) broad phase

```
for all pulse_regions do
  cd_pair = collision_detection(region, proxy)
  if (cd_pair) then narrow_test(cd_pair)
```

2) narrow phase

```
for all pulse_particles of region do
  cd_pair = collision_detection(particle, proxy)
  if (cd_pair) then pulse_simulation
```

3) pulse simulation

```
magnitude = calculate_pulsewave(t, parameters)
force = project(magnitude, distance, collision normal)
send_to_hapticrenderloop(force)
```

2.3 Properties of Pulse Simulation

The particles that define a pulse region contain several specific configurable parameters.

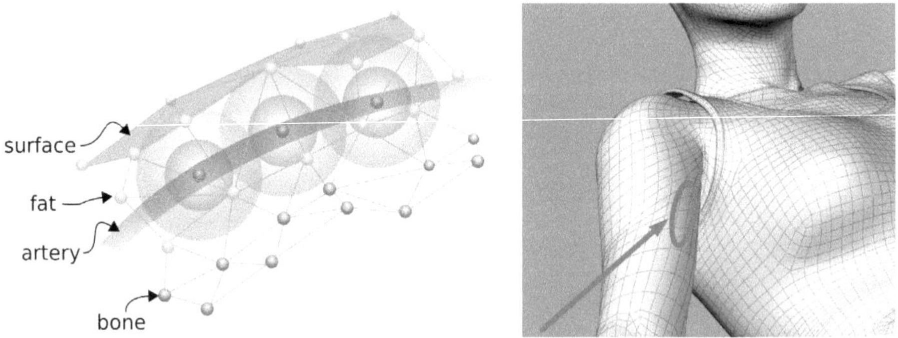

Fig. 1. Setup of several pulse particles to model a pulse region (here: brachial pulse)

- *Pulse range*: One set of parameters that is associated with a particle describes the effective *pulse range*. This determines the space or radial extent relative to the point of the particle's position (cf. Fig. 2) and allows to use a fast point-to-sphere collision detection scheme. If the haptic probe interferes this proximity range, a pulsating force feedback is rendered. Depending on the layer or distance the intensity of the force can be attenuated.
- *Pulse wave*: The human *pulse wave* can have different shapes depending on the current constitution of the patient and on the pulse region. As a first approximation we use the rectangular waveform model. It consists of the pulse's *duty cycle* (D) as the ratio between the pulse *duration* (τ) with the wave *amplitude* and the *period* (T). According to findings from psychophysics this approximation should be sufficient in most cases, because of the just noticable difference in human haptics perception [5] and the limited resolution of the haptics devices. In case a more accurate model is needed, the algorithm supports the use of lookup tables that can be sampled from the readout of medical sensory instruments [6].
- *Pulse rate*: The *pulse rate* of a normal human ranges from 60 to 100 beats per minute (BPM), although this can vary depending on different circumstances (e.g., sports etc.). This corresponds to the length of the pulse period T. In the simulation it can be varied during runtime.

2.4 Haptic Rendering

For the haptic rendering a force and a direction must be computed. The direction is defined by the vector that connects the particle position with the collision point of the particle's sphere with the haptic probe. The force is proportional to the

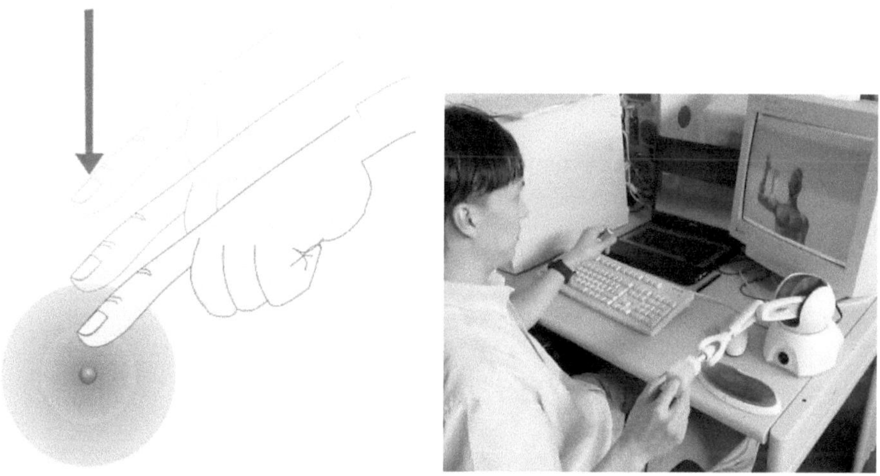

Fig. 2. Two-layered pulse range and desktop setup of the haptic palpation

current pulse wave reading. It can be relatively adjusted to the devices output range. To achieve a consistent pulse frequency (BPM), rendering is maintained by using a haptic timestamp. The timestamp is used to verify delays in the control information of the haptic media. The output of the pulse period is then adjusted as a function of the haptic rate. The haptic surface rendering is done by the virtual proxy as described in section 2.1.

3 Results

As an example we describe the use case of searching for a pulse landmark. A virtual patient is visualized on a VR desktop system. The haptic device is controlled by one or multiple fingers of the user and the current position and orientation is displayed by a virtual hand (cf. Fig. 2). This allows the user to explore the skin surface intuitively in real-time. As soon as the haptic proxy reaches within the effective range of a pulse particle a pulsating effect can be haptically perceived. Depending on the region and penetration depth, the feedback ranges from faint to strong. Furthermore, preliminary evaluations have shown that usually one to three pulse particles are sufficient to represent a pulse region.

4 Discussion

As described by the example in the results, the simulation allows for an intuitive exploration of the human pulse. Through the usage of particles with bounding spheres the collision detection works efficiently. It is very flexible due to the many parameters and the support of lookup tables for different pulse wave forms. In summary, the haptic pulse simulation algorithm contributes to virtual palpation and enables dynamic, pulsating landmarks in real-time. Purely mechanical solutions are more specialized and realistic, but they are also less flexible. In our scenario we emphasize on reusability. Hence, effortless changes are essential. This is covered by our software-based approach and further supported by the individual setup.

Future work could focus on fine tuning the parameters and adding more realism. The collision detection could be extended to support a deformable skin. The parameters can be modified by medical experts and will be evaluated in a user study.

Acknowledgement. This work was funded by a grant from the German Research Foundation (DFG, KU 1132, LE 1108, RO 2000) and also supported by the START program (UK Aachen).

References

1. Schwarz G, Feigl G, Kleinert R, et al. Pneumatic pulse simulation for teaching peripheral plexus blocks in cadavers. Anesth Analg. 2002;95:1822–3.

2. Cakmak H, Kuhnapfel U. Animation and simulation techniques for vrtraining systems in endoscopic surgery. In: Eurographics Workshop on Animation and Simulation; 2000. p. 173–85.
3. Ullrich S, Fischer B, Ntouba A, et al. Subject-based regional anaesthesia simulator combining image processing and virtual reality. Proc BVM. 2007; p. 202–6.
4. Ruspini D, Khatib O. Dynamic models for haptic rendering systems. In: Advances in Robot Kinematics: ARK'98; 1998. p. 523–32.
5. Allin S, Matsuoka Y, Klatzky R. Measuring just noticeable differences for haptic force feedback: A tool for rehabilitation. In: Proc 10th IEEE Symposium on Haptic Interfaces for Virtual and Teleoperator Systems; 2002. p. 299–302.
6. Hlimonenko I, Meigas K, Vahisalu R. Waveform analysis of peripheral pulse wave detected in the fingertip waveform analysis of peripheral pulse wave detected in the fingertip with photoplethysmograph. Measurement Science Review. 2003;3(2):49–52.

Ruler-Based Automatic Stitching of Spatially Overlapping Radiographs

André Gooßen[1], Mathias Schlüter[2], Marc Hensel[2], Thomas Pralow[2], Rolf-Rainer Grigat[1]

[1]Vision Systems, Hamburg University of Technology, D-21079 Hamburg
[2]General X-Ray, Philips Medical Systems, D-22335 Hamburg
andre.goossen@tu-harburg.de

Abstract. We present an algorithm for fast automatic registration of spatially overlapping radiographs. It possesses strong robustness against noise, feature masking and feature displacement. Pivotal for this algorithm is an actual interpretation of the stitching feature instead of a simple detection. The proposed method has been evaluated on 3000 clinical radiographs and proved to be a powerful enhancement of established automatic registration algorithms.

1 Introduction

When imaging long parts of the human body, e.g. legs or spine, in conventional screen-film technique, special cassettes and films of extended length are utilized. Migration to digital radiography limits the image size due to the sensitive area of flat-panel detectors. In order to reproduce the behavior of conventional radiography a large image is assembled from multiple exposures with a small spatial overlap. As the detector has to be moved to the next position between subsequent exposures there is a risk that patient movement or breathing might produce inconsistent content. Refer to Figure 1 for a depiction of the acquisition.

Known algorithms for automatic registration either apply feature-based registration [1], landmark-based registration [2] or plain image-similarity measures [3]. Although proven in computed radiography (CR), feature-based algorithms are not applicable for digital radiography (DR) as the patient may have moved against the feature in subsequent exposures and hence matching the feature is not sufficient in DR. Image-similarity has to deal with ambiguities of the similarity measurement, e.g. recurring structure of the spine, within the region of possible solutions and thus requires a qualified a priori estimation within the large possible overlap spanned by DR images. Landmark-based registration performs well for known content, but since modeling the content of arbitrary medical images is considered extremely difficult or impossible [4], it fails for digital radiographs.

The proposed method overcomes these problems by combining feature-based registration and similarity measurement. However instead of computing inter-image correspondences our method derives correspondences between image coordinates and real world coordinates by not only detecting but also interpreting the feature, metering its information.

Fig. 1. Multiple radiograph acquisition. The patient stands in front of the flat-panel detector. While the detector moves up and down to reach the different exposure positions, the X-ray tube is panned around its rotational axis to expose the detector. An X-ray ruler brought between patient and detector serves as the feature for later composition and distortion removal.

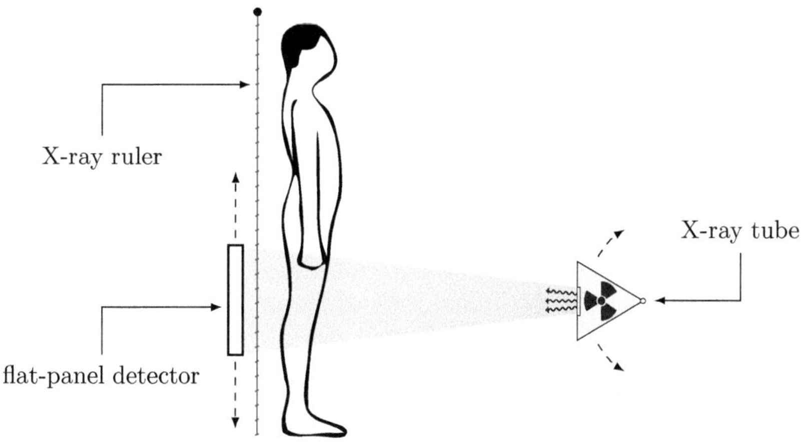

2 Methods and Materials

The proposed method consists of two steps complementing one another. The ruler recognition algorithm locates the feature, i.e. the X-ray ruler and interprets markers and digits on this feature to extract the global meaning. The automatic stitching computes an estimated translation for subsequent images featuring the ruler recognition and refines the translation to match anatomy.

2.1 Ruler Recognition

The algorithm consists of four basic stages executed in a sequential manner:

1. Localization of the ruler line,
2. Binarization of the ruler part,
3. Marker and digit localization,
4. Digit recognition and interpretation.

The first stage utilizes a discrete Radon transform on the source image to locate and parameterize the ruler line. With the line angle and distance to the origin known, the ruler sub-part is deskewed and cropped out of the source image. Finally the crop is binarized using a local-adaptive technique with a threshold that varies along a sliding window over the ruler height. This introduces invariance against translation and rotation of the ruler as well as against spatially varying image intensity or contrast. The resulting image forms the input for subsequent processing stages.

With the ruler line detected, a profile along the line is generated by projection onto the vertical axis. Due to the recurring scale markers and numbers, this profile shows periodicity and hence the marker period and phase can be determined by autocorrelating the profile. Detected marker positions have to be corrected in a hit-or-miss transformation and markers missing due to coverages or bad signal-to-noise ratio are interpolated by linear regression. This interpolation allows the assembling of images with no visible feature within the overlapping region.

To detect numbers at the refined marker locations, a search for connected pixels is performed in each row containing a marker. The resulting groups of connected pixels serve as candidates for digit recognition. The bounding box size of these candidates forms a criterion for filtering out noise (e.g. very small boxes) and artifacts (e.g. very large boxes, wrong aspect ratios, etc.) and for picking the selection to perform the optical character recognition on.

The final stage performs optical character recognition using a dedicated template matching algorithm [5]. In order to correct missing digits or numbers and false recognitions, a virtual ruler is moved along the detected digits. Matching digits increase the score for a certain position, mismatched digits degrade it. Due to the high redundancy, the displacement of maximum congruency determines the positioning of the ruler, i.e. the ruler "snaps in"at the correct position yielding a set of global correspondences of image coordinates to real-world coordinates.

Figure 2 depicts the detected ruler geometry for a selection of clinical images to point out the capabilities of the proposed method. The algorithm is invariant against ruler type and scale font as well as ruler translations, rotations and scaling. Missing geometry is extrapolated automatically to restore information in covered overlap areas.

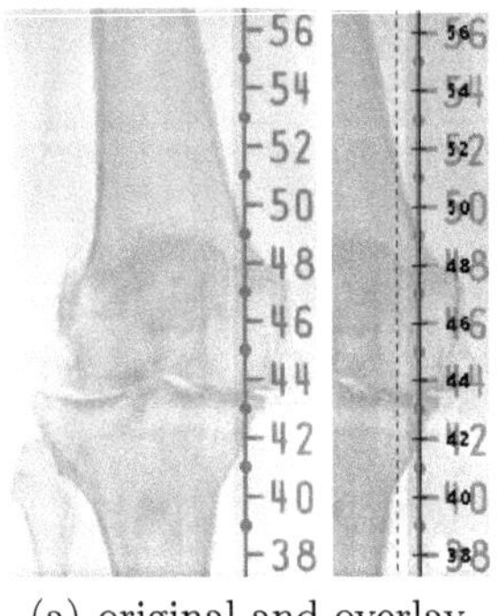

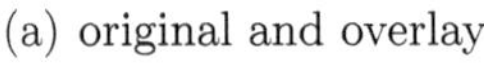
(a) original and overlay

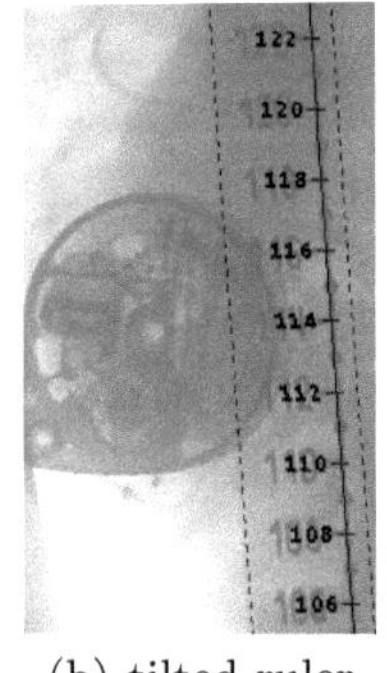

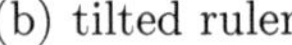
(b) tilted ruler

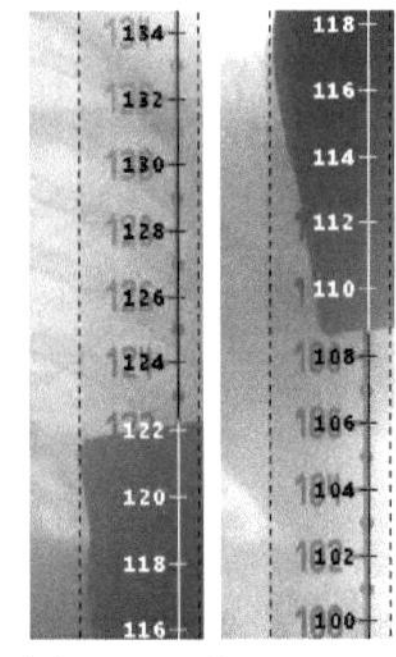

(c) partial coverage

Fig. 2. Detected ruler geometry within four crops of clinical radiographs. The results of the recognition have been overlaid onto the original radiograph. (a) Comparison of original radiograph and detected ruler geometry within an examination of a leg. (b) Detected geometry for a tilted ruler. (c) Detected (black) and extrapolated (white) geometry of a partially covered ruler within a pair of thoracic images.

2.2 Automatic Stitching

Repeating the ruler recognition algorithm for two subsequent images and taking their correspondences yields an initial estimation for the translation between these images. Since the estimation maps ruler coordinates of both images onto each other, the translations have to be refined to map corresponding parts of the anatomy. This is done by performing a correlation of the images in a small window of half the ruler period around the calculated estimation, avoiding ambiguities of the similarity measure. In order to introduce invariance against local intensity, a gradient correlation [6, 7] is used to match image content. For this purpose we project the anatomy fraction and differentiate the derived profile. To deal with noise a low pass filter smooths the profile. Maximizing the normalized cross correlation yields the final vertical and horizontal offset.

2.3 Experiments

An image pool of 3000 radiographs has been used to evaluate the proposed method. The image pool has been acquired on two clinical sites and contains all kinds of anatomies and geometries in two or three single exposures, i.e. one or two stitches per images.

As there is no true optimum for the translation between two subsequent images, the major difficulty for evaluation is the creation of a valid reference. For the evaluation of our method, reference translations have been acquired from manual stitching of the test images by 6 observers. To eliminate influences due to inter-observer variability in manual stitching, we performed a study on a representative subset of 42 image pairs. Each observer had to perform stitching on all of these images and the deviation between stitching translations for the same image derived by different observers was measured in Euclidean distance. The distribution of deviations (cp. histogram in Table 1) determined the failure threshold for automatic stitching to 3 mm.

Images where the deviation between automatically computed translation and manual reference exceeded the threshold are therefore considered as failures.

3 Results

Experiments have shown that the proposed algorithm locates the correct translation in respect to the manual reference within a very small window around the desired reference for the majority of tests. 67 radiographs have been rejected by the algorithm due to operational errors of the acquisition staff, e.g. missing rulers or wrong apertures. This results in 1814 pairs of subsequent images forming the evaluation set.

1611 out of these 1814 image pairs containing valid rulers are registered with a deviation of less than 1 mm. The translations for 99.3% of all valid image pairs lie in the range of less than 3 mm devation. Thus the failure rate is 0.7% for the proposed algorithm. Table 1 lists the results of the evaluation for the proposed method. The average processing time is 158 ms per computed translation for an image pair on an Intel Pentium D 2.8 GHz.

Table 1. Results of automatic stitching for 1814 valid image pairs. Δ represents the measured Euclidean distance of the calculated translation to the reference translation. Deviations > 3 mm sum up to a failure rate of 0.7%. The histogram contrasts the results of the inter-observer study and the proposed method.

Δ	*occurrence*	*fraction*
0-1 mm	1611	88.8%
1-2 mm	147	8.1%
2-3 mm	43	2.4%
3-4 mm	7	0.4%
4-5 mm	4	0.2%
> 5 mm	2	0.1%

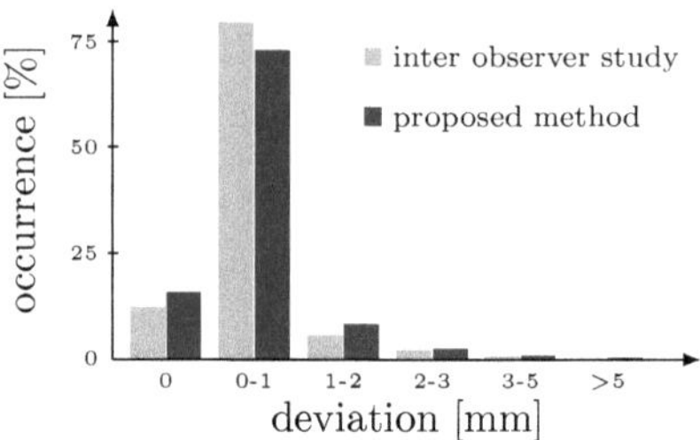

4 Discussion

The proposed method decreases the failure rate of automatic stitches to 0.7%. As is apparent from the results, the performance of the proposed method comes close to the lower boundary formed by the accuracy of manual stitching references. The low processing time results in minimum costs for ruler recognition within the image processing chain.

The high robustness has been proved by processing a large number of clinical images. Manual interaction is strongly reduced by the proposed algorithm and the risk of false automatic stitches, possibly resulting in unnecessary treatment, is minimized.

References

1. Čapek M, Wegenkittl R, Felkel P. A fully automatic stitching of 2D medical data sets. BIOSIGNAL. 2002;16:326–8.
2. Johnson HJ, Christensen GE, Little JA, et al. Consistent landmark and intensity-based image registration. IEEE Trans Med Imaging. 2002;21(5):450–61.
3. Gramer M, Bohlken W, Lundt B, et al. An algorithm for automatic stitching of CR X-ray images. Advances in Medical Engineering. 2007;114:193–8.
4. Lehmann T. Medizinische Bildverarbeitung. In: Kramme R, editor. Medizintechnik: Verfahren, Systeme, Informationsverarbeitung. 2nd ed. Springer; 1997. p. 588–612.
5. Harmon LD. Automatic recognition of print and script. Proc IEEE. 1972;60(10):1165–76.
6. Heipke C. Overview of image matching techniques. OEEPE Official Publications. 1996;33:173–89.
7. Zitová B, Flusser J. Image registration methods: A survey. Image Vis Comput. 2003;21(11):977–1000.

Molecular Surface Decomposition Using Graphical Modeling

Maharavo Randrianarivony[1], Guido Brunnett[2]

[1]Institut für Informatik, Christian-Albrechts-Universität Kiel
[2]Fakultät für Informatik, Technische Universität Chemnitz
maharavo@informatik.tu-chemnitz.de

Abstract. We aim at decomposing molecular surfaces which are in the form of Van der Waals model into a structure adapted for mesh-free modeling. We focus on the generation of spherical patches by using rational Bézier surfaces and homogeneous coordinates. We can achieve exact global continuity by using generalized stereographic projection. We support the theoretical descriptions by practical decompositions of a few molecular surfaces.

1 Introduction

A lot of efforts have been done for mesh-based methods [1] in chemical modeling [2]. In contrast, mesh-free molecular structure is not yet well developed. Having patch representation is advantageous for both visualization and simulation tasks. Among others, OpenGL and ACIS have built-in functions for treating rational spline patches by providing only the required parameters as arguments. Further, NURBS primitives are available in many rendering softwares like POV-RAY. Additionally, generating a multiresolution setting is immediate when a four-sided splitting as we present below is available. Multiresolution structure is well known of being efficient for both fast graphical tasks and numerical simulations. Hence, we want to contribute in the development of algorithms for treatments of mesh-free molecular geometries. Each atom in a molecule is represented as an imaginary sphere whose radius corresponds to the Van der Walls radius [2, 3]. Let us denote by $\mathcal{B}(\omega, \rho)$ the ball of center ω and radius ρ. Consider N balls $\mathcal{B}_k := \mathcal{B}(\Omega_k, \rho_k)$ whose union is connected. The molecular surface is described by $S := \partial \left[\bigcup_{k=1}^{N} \mathcal{B}_k \right]$ which represents a closed surface. We want to tessellate S into m four-sided patches F_i such that the splitting $S = \bigcup_{i=1}^{m} F_i$ is conforming: every two nondisjoint patches F_i and F_j share either a complete edge or a single corner. Our goal is to create functions γ_i such that $F_i = \gamma_i([0,1]^2)$. Additionally, we require global continuity meaning that for two adjacent patches F_i and F_j, there is an affine mapping A such that $\gamma_i(s) = \gamma_j(A(s))$ for all $s \in \partial[0,1]^2$ (Fig. 1).

Relevant works are as follows. From a list of intersecting spheres, one generates the B-rep structures as in [1]. Generation of trimmed surfaces has been treated in [4] with application in mesh. For mesh-free methods, we have used transfinite interpolations in [5] but the mappings are not necessarily globally continuous.

2 Materials and Methods

The description of the molecular surface S as in section 1 is good for CSG where the only geometric primitives are spheres. Since B-Rep structure with parametrizations is more convenient for the surface decompositions, we first convert that CSG representation into B-rep structure. Since the method of doing that is almost standard, we do not present it here. After that conversion, we have trimmed surfaces $\Gamma_k = \sigma_k(\mathcal{D}_k)$ where $\mathcal{D}_k$ is a multiply connected planar domain and $\sigma_k : \mathcal{D}_k \subset \mathbf{R}^2 \longrightarrow \mathcal{B}_k$ represents the stereographic projection with respect to $\mathcal{B}_k$. Since we have now a set of parametric trimmed surfaces [6], we can split them into four-sided patches. The detail of such a decomposition task can be found in [5]. Hence, we focus on the creation of the mappings from the unit square to the spherical patches while achieving global continuity. Although most methods here are described for the unit sphere $\mathbf{U}$, they can be generalized to any sphere. An element of the projective space $\mathbf{E}^3$ with homogeneous coordinates $[w : x : y : z]$ will have the cartesian coordinates $(x/w, y/w, z/w)$. We will need $\mathbf{P} := \{[w : x : y : 0] \in \mathbf{E}^3 \quad \text{with} \quad w, x, y \in \mathbf{R}\}$ which corresponds to the plane $z = 0$ in cartesian coordinates. The creation γ_i uses the next projections from [3]. First, the hyperbolic projection ϑ transforms a point $[e_0 : e_1 : e_2 : e_3]$ to a point in $\mathbf{P}$ given by $\vartheta(\mathbf{e}) := \left[e_0^2 + e_3^2 : e_0e_1 - e_2e_3 : e_1e_3 + e_0e_2 : 0\right]$. Second, the stereographic projection is defined from $\mathbf{P}$ to $\mathbf{U}$ by $\sigma(\mathbf{e}) := \left[e_0^2 + e_1^2 + e_2^2 : 2e_0e_1 : 2e_0e_2 : e_1^2 + e_2^2 - e_0^2\right]$. Finally, the generalized stereographic projection is $\delta = \sigma \circ \vartheta$. For a point $\mathbf{q} = [q_0 : q_1 : q_2 : q_3]$, we define $\bar{\mathbf{q}} := [q_2 : q_3 : -q_0 : -q_1]$ and $\mathbf{q}^{\perp} := [-q_3 : q_2 : -q_1 : -q_0]$. Our approach is based on the fact that the image by δ of a rational Bézier [7] of degree n is a rational Bézier of degree $2n$ which is drawn on $\mathbf{U}$. Note that the converse holds true [3].

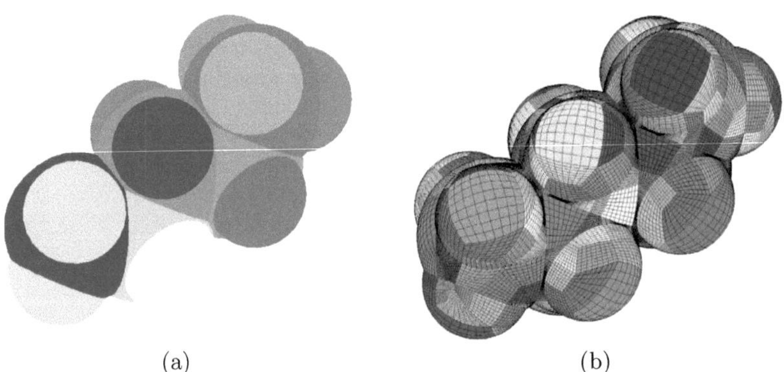

(a) (b)

Fig. 1. Molecular surface (a) and decomposition into foursided patches (b)

2.1 Circular Boundary Parametrization

We want to parametrize a circular arc $\mathcal{C}$ with fixed endpoints as an image of δ. There are already plenty of methods for representing a circular arc as rational Bézier but we explicitly need that it is an image of δ because we intend to obtain global continuity. We suppose that we have four equispaced points $\mathbf{Q}_i$ belonging to $\mathcal{C}$ which is contained in the unit sphere $\mathbf{U}$. We are given also two points $\mathbf{b}_0 \in \mathbf{E}^3$ and $\mathbf{b}_2 \in \mathbf{E}^3$ which are transformed by δ to the first and the last points: $\delta(\mathbf{b}_0) = \mathbf{Q}_0$ and $\delta(\mathbf{b}_2) = \mathbf{Q}_3$. We search a conic $\mathbf{x}$ which maps by δ to the circle $\mathcal{C}$. In other words, we need the internal node $\mathbf{b}_1 \in \mathbf{E}^3$ such that $\mathcal{C}$ is the image of the quadratic Bézier curve $\mathbf{x}(t) = \mathbf{b}_0 B_0^2(t) + \mathbf{b}_1 B_1^2(t) + \mathbf{b}_2 B_2^2(t)$ with $\mathbf{b}_i = [w_i : x_i : y_i : z_i]$. The internal points $\mathbf{Q}_1$ and $\mathbf{Q}_2$ should correspond to the parameter values $t_1 := 1/3$ and $t_2 := 2/3$ as $\delta[\mathbf{x}(t_i)] = \mathbf{Q}_i$. Toward that end, we choose a preimage $\mathbf{q}_i$ of $\mathbf{Q}_i$ by δ. Since $\delta^{-1}(\mathbf{Q}_i) = \{\lambda \mathbf{q}_i + \mu \mathbf{q}_i^{\perp} : \lambda, \mu \in \mathbf{R}\}$, we have $< \bar{\mathbf{q}}_i, \mathbf{x}(t_i) >= 0$ and $< \bar{\mathbf{q}}_i^{\perp}, \mathbf{x}(t_i) >= 0$ which imply:

$$< \bar{\mathbf{q}}_i, \mathbf{b}_1 >= K(\bar{\mathbf{q}}_i, t_i) \qquad < \bar{\mathbf{q}}_i^{\perp}, \mathbf{b}_1 >= K(\bar{\mathbf{q}}_i^{\perp}, t_i) \qquad \text{for} \quad i = 1, 2 \tag{1}$$

where $K(\mathbf{q}, t) := -\frac{1}{B_1^2(t)} \left[< \mathbf{q}, \mathbf{b}_0 > B_0^2(t) + < \mathbf{q}, \mathbf{b}_2 > B_2^2(t) \right]$. The four homogeneous coordinates of $\mathbf{b}_1$ are the solution of the linear system given by (1).

2.2 Spherical Transfinite Interpolation

Let us consider four circular arcs C_k represented as rational Bézier curves which are drawn on the unit sphere $\mathbf{U}$ and which enclose a four-sided spherical surface $\mathcal{H}$ such that $C_k(t) = \sum_{i=0}^{2n} \mathbf{c}_i^k B_i^{2n}(t)$ with $\mathbf{c}_i^k = [w_i^k : x_i^k : y_i^k : z_i^k]$. We assume that C_k are the images of four Bézier curves D_k of degree n by δ. That is, we have $C_k(t) = \delta[D_k(t)]$ with $D_k(t) = \sum_{i=0}^{n} \mathbf{d}_i^k B_i^n(t)$ such that there is coincidence at the corners as $\mathbf{d}_0^1 = \mathbf{d}_0^4$, $\mathbf{d}_n^1 = \mathbf{d}_0^2$,$\mathbf{d}_n^2 = \mathbf{d}_n^3$, $\mathbf{d}_0^3 = \mathbf{d}_n^4$.

What we are searching is not simply a rational Bézier surface which interpolates those curves but a spherical transfinite interpolant $\mathbf{X}$ residing on $\mathbf{U}$:

$$\begin{array}{lll} \mathbf{X}(u,0) = C_1(u), & \mathbf{X}(u,1) = C_3(u) & \forall u \in [0,1] \\ \mathbf{X}(0,v) = C_4(v), & \mathbf{X}(1,v) = C_2(v) & \forall v \in [0,1] \\ \mathbf{X}(u,v) \in \mathbf{U} & \forall\, (u,v) \in [0,1]^2 & \end{array} \tag{2}$$

The desired patch $\mathbf{X}$ will be represented as a rational Bézier surface $\mathbf{X}(u,v) = \sum_{i=0}^{2n} \sum_{j=0}^{2n} \mathbf{b}_{ij} B_i^{2n}(u) B_j^{2n}(v)$ with $\mathbf{b}_{ij} = [w_{ij} : x_{ij} : y_{ij} : z_{ij}]$. That problem amounts to searching for some rational Bézier $\mathbf{Y}$ of degree n which maps by δ to $\mathbf{X}$ as $\mathbf{X}(u,v) = \delta[\mathbf{Y}(u,v)]$ with $\mathbf{Y}(u,v) = \sum_{i=0}^{n} \sum_{j=0}^{n} \mathbf{a}_{ij} B_i^n(u) B_j^n(v)$. On account of the boundary conditions (2), the problem is reduced to the determination of the internal homogeneous control points $\mathbf{a}_{ij}$ of $\mathbf{Y}$. They are found by specifying that the image rational Bézier $\mathbf{X}$ interpolates some given internal points $Q_k \in \mathcal{H} \subset \mathbf{U}$ at $(u_k, v_k) \in [0,1]^2$: $\mathbf{X}(u_k, v_k) = \delta[\mathbf{Y}(u_k, v_k)] = Q_k$ for all $k = 1, ..., m := 2(n-1)^2$. Let $\mathbf{q}_k$ be a preimage of Q_k by the mapping δ. Since we want to achieve $\mathbf{Y}(u_k, v_k) = \mathbf{q}_k$ for all $k = 1, ..., m$, we have two equalities: $\langle \bar{\mathbf{q}}_k, \mathbf{Y}(u_k, v_k) \rangle = 0$, $\langle \bar{\mathbf{q}}_k^{\perp}, \mathbf{Y}(u_k, v_k) \rangle = 0$, $\forall\, k = 1, ..., m$. By denoting the set of indices (i,j) for internal and boundary control points of $\mathbf{Y}$ by $\mathcal{J}$ and $\mathcal{B}$ respectively, we obtain

$$\sum_{(i,j)\in\mathcal{J}} \langle \bar{\mathbf{q}}_k, \mathbf{a}_{ij} \rangle B_i^n(u_k) B_j^n(v_k) = -\langle \bar{\mathbf{q}}_k, \sum_{(i,j)\in\mathcal{B}} \mathbf{a}_{ij} B_i^n(u_k) B_j^n(v_k) \rangle \qquad (3)$$

Similar computations yield relations for $\bar{\mathbf{q}}_k^{\perp}$. Since $\mathbf{a}_{ij}$ for $(i,j) \in \mathcal{B}$ are known, the right hand side of (3) is completely specified. Therefore, this leads to some linear system of equations having $\mathbf{a}_{ij}$ with $(i,j) \in \mathcal{J}$ as unknowns.

3 Results

We have implemented routines in C/C++ and OpenGL in order to decompose some molecular surfaces. The numerical results can be found in Table 1 where the input was taken from PDB files. Note that the runtime measurement has been performed on a machine with processor Intel Core 2.16GHz running Windows Vista. For a triangle having vertices $T := [\mathbf{x}_p, \mathbf{x}_q, \mathbf{x}_r]$ belonging to the sphere $\mathcal{B}(\Omega_k, \rho_k)$, we introduce $\varepsilon(T) := \left|\text{dist}\left(\frac{1}{3}[\mathbf{x}_p + \mathbf{x}_q + \mathbf{x}_r], \Omega_k\right) - \rho_k\right|$. The criterion that quantifies the surface invariability of a mesh $\mathcal{M}$ is $\varepsilon(\mathcal{M}) := \frac{1}{\text{card}(\mathcal{M})} \sum_{T\in\mathcal{M}} \varepsilon(T)$. The patches which are obtained by the mappings from the unit squares are illustrated in Fig. 2.

4 Discussion

The main advantage of our mesh-free method is that it requires few patches in comparison to mesh-based methods. For a surface invariance $\varepsilon(\mathcal{M})$ of order

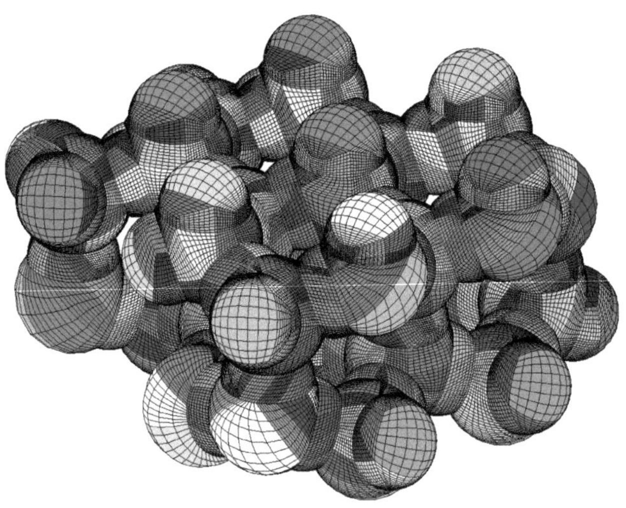

Fig. 2. Decomposition with 1284 four-sided patches

Table 1. Decomposing molecular surfaces: comparison with meshes

Molecule	Nb atoms	Nb patches	Time (patch)	Nb triangles	$\varepsilon(\mathcal{M})$	Time (mesh)
Benzene	12	160	2.26 sec	18615	5.56e-004	4.40 sec
Fullerene	60	360	2.45 sec	102380	6.88e-004	9.09 sec
Propane	11	231	9.65 sec	21927	3.53e-004	11.73 sec
Petane	17	388	11.77 sec	38764	3.31e-004	15.67 sec
Ice	84	1284	71.97 sec	290732	4.96e-004	77.22 sec

10^{-4}, several thousands of triangles are required. Further, only 9 control points for each patch are necessary to completely store the results. Additionally, the patches are exact as opposed to meshes where piecewise linear approximation is required. The runtime depends in fact on the molecular models. In general, the runtime for mesh-free geometric preparation is slightly faster than mesh-based one. But sometimes, the difference is tangible as in the case of fullerene where the surface structure is almost uniform. On the other hand, for every two neighboring patches, the lines incident upon the interface match very well as illustrated in Fig. 2. That is, the global continuity that we discussed in the above theory is obtained. As for the simulation side, there are efficient numerical solvers which accept mesh-free models directly. Those solvers do not require the patch representation to be converted to meshes. A concrete example is the Wavelet-Galerkin solver which needs only the control points for the generation of multiscale bases.

References

1. Laug P, Borouchaki H. Surface grid generation on intersecting spheres. Proc 6th International Conference Numerical Grid Generation. 1998; p. 717–26.
2. Cances E, Mennucci B. New applications of integral equations methods for solvation continuum models: ionic solutions and liquid crystals. J Math Chemistry. 1998;23:309–26.
3. Dietz R, Hoschek J, Jüttler B. An algebraic approach to curves and surfaces on the sphere and on other quadrics. Comput Aided Geom Des. 1993;10(3):211–29.
4. Laug P, Borouchaki H. Molecular surface modeling and meshing. Proc 10th International Meshing Round Table of Sandia National Laboratory. 2001; p. 31–41.
5. Randrianarivony M. Geometric processing of CAD data and meshes as input of integral equation solvers, PhD thesis. Chemnitz: Technische Universität Chemnitz; 2006.
6. Brunnett G. Geometric design with trimmed surfaces. Comput Suppl. 1995;10:101–15.
7. Albrecht G. An algorithm for parametric quadric patch construction. Comput. 2004;72:1–12.

Segmentierung der Knochenoberfläche einzelner Lendenwirbel für die ultraschallbasierte Navigation

Claudia Dekomien, Susanne Winter

Institut für Neuroinformatik, Ruhr-Universität Bochum, 44780 Bochum
Claudia.Dekomien@neuroinformatik.rub.de

Kurzfassung. Für die klinische Umsetzung computerunterstützter Verfahren ist es wichtig, die Datenverarbeitungsschritte so weit wie möglich zu automatisieren. Wir stellen eine Verarbeitungskette vor, die nach modellbasierter Segmentierung eines Wirbels, in CT-Daten, automatisch Knochenoberflächenpunkte einem einzelnen Wirbel zuordnet. Diese Knochenoberfläche dient im nächsten Schritt zur Registrierung der CT-Daten mit dreidimensionalen Ultraschalldaten. Zur Extraktion der Knochenoberflächenpunkte wurde in den CT-Daten ein Ultraschallscan simuliert, während zur Segmentierung einzelner Wirbel ein modifizierter Shape-based Level Set Ansatz eingesetzt wurde. Die Koppelung der beiden Verfahren lieferte die, für die Registrierung relevante, Knochenoberfläche in den CT-Daten, anhand derer die CT-Daten mit dreidimensionalen Ultraschalldaten registriert werden konnten.

1 Einleitung

Die präzise und schnelle Registrierung präoperativer Bilddaten ist eines der Hauptprobleme in der bildbasierten navigierten Chirurgie [1, 2]. Wir haben einen Oberflächen-Volumen-Registrierungsalgorithmus entwickelt, der intraoperativen, dreidimensionalen Ultraschall mit präoperativen CT- oder MRT-Daten registriert. Das Verfahren arbeitet robust [3] und die Prozedur kann jederzeit wiederholt werden. Für Details sei auf die Vorarbeiten verwiesen [4, 5].

Die Knochenoberfläche wird aus den präoperativen Daten extrahiert und in die Ultraschalldaten projiziert. Mit einem Optimierungsverfahren wird diese Knochenoberfläche in den Ultraschalldaten an die richtige Position transformiert. Als Fitnesskriterium dient die Summe der Grauwerte im Ultraschallvolumen, die von den Punkten der Oberfläche abgedeckt werden.

Die Basis für die rigide Registrierung bilden die Knochenoberflächenpunkte, die sich mit dem Ultraschall darstellen lassen. Da sich die einzelnen Wirbel relativ zueinander verschieben, ist es notwendig diese einzeln zu registrieren. Bisher wurde ein manuelles Verfahren verwendet um die einzelnen Knochen voneinander zu separieren. Für eine klinische Umsetzung der Methode ist es allerdings von großem Interesse die präoperativen Benutzeraktionen so gering wie möglich zu halten. Das Ziel unserer Arbeit ist eine möglichst vollständige Automatisierung der präoperativen Datenverarbeitung.

Ein Schritt der Verarbeitungskette besteht aus der Segmentierung der einzelnen Knochen. Schwellwert- oder Region Growing Verfahren haben hier den Nachteil, dass die Segmentierung häufig von einem Knochen in den anderen überläuft. Dieses Problem kann mit dem Einsatz modellbasierter Verfahren [6, 7] gelöst werden. Die Segmentierung mittels eines Shape-based Level Set Ansatzes wurde mit einer schwellwertbasierten Extraktion von Knochenoberflächenpunkten gekoppelt. Damit kann die Oberflächenpunktmenge eines einzelnen Wirbels, die für die Registrierung notwendig ist, automatisch segmentiert werden.

2 Material und Methode

Für die Versuche wurden Spiral-CT-Daten der Lendenwirbelsäule von 16 Patienten und einem Kunststoffphantom verwendet. Die Ultraschalldatensätze wurden mit einem Siemens Sonoline Omnia und einem 5 MHz Curved-Array Ultraschallwandler akquiriert. Die 3D-Rekonstruktion erfolgte durch magnetisches Tracking mit dem 3D Echotech System. Zur einfacheren Handhabbarkeit wurden alle Datensätze in isotrope Daten der Auflösung 0,5 mm x 0,5 mm x 0,5 mm umgewandelt.

Die automatische Segmentierung der Knochenoberfläche eines Wirbels besteht aus drei Schritten: Als erstes wird ein Ultraschallscan in den CT-Daten simuliert. Mit diesem Scan wird von einem Wirbelsäulenabschnitt der Teil der Knochenoberfläche extrahiert, der sich in einer solchen Ultraschallaufnahme abbilden würde. Anschließend wird ein einzelner Wirbel in den CT-Daten segmentiert. Im dritten Schritt werden die extrahierten Oberflächenpunkte dem segmentierten Wirbel zugeordnet. Das Ergebnis sind die Oberflächenpunkte eines einzelnen Wirbels, die sich in einer Ultraschallaufnahmen abbilden. Anhand dieser Punktmenge kann die Registrierung mit dem dreidimensionalen Ultraschall erfolgen.

Die Simulation des Ultraschallscans ist ein halbautomatischer Prozess. Vom Benutzer werden einige Landmarken in den CT-Daten markiert, die den Scan-

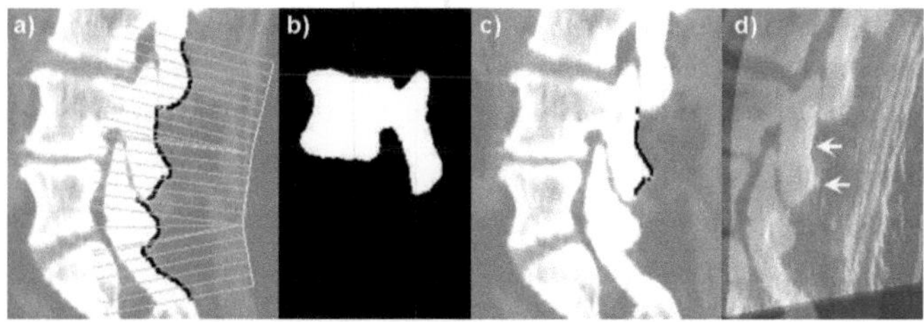

Abb. 1. Verarbeitungskette für die Registrierung einzelner Wirbel in CT- und Ultraschalldaten; a) Simulation eines Ultraschallscanpfades in CT-Daten; b) Ergebnis einer Shape-based Level Set Segmentierung; c) Die segmentierten Oberflächenpunkte eines Wirbels; d) Überlagerung von CT- und Ultraschalldaten nach der Registrierung mittels extrahierter Wirbeloberfläche (die Pfeile markieren die Oberfläche des registrierten Wirbels)

pfad aufspannen, der sich dem intraoperativem Scanpfad annähert. Bei bekannter Schallrichtung werden anhand dieses Scanpfades die Schallstrahlen des Ultraschalls im CT simuliert. Mittels eines Schwellwertes werden diejenigen Knochenoberflächenpunkte extrahiert, die als erstes vom Schallstrahl getroffen werden (Abb. 1a).

Für die Segmentierung der einzelnen Wirbel wurde ein Shape-based Level Set Ansatz gewählt. Das Verfahren ist modellbasiert und kann durch seine Flexibilität komplexe Formen, wie die der Wirbelknochen, darstellen. Der in dieser Arbeit implementierte Algorithmus basiert auf dem von Tsai [6] vorgestellten Verfahren, welches in zwei Punkten modifiziert wurde [8]. Der Algorithmus besteht aus zwei Phasen, der Modellerstellung und der Segmentierungsphase. Dabei wird sowohl die Registrierung der verschiedenen Einzelwirbel zur Modellerstellung, als auch die Anpassung der Segmentierungsfunktion als Optimierungsproblem formuliert. Aufgrund der Robustheit und der großen Reichweite der CMA-Evolutionsstrategie [9] wurde die Lösung der Optimierungen mit diesem Verfahren umgesetzt.

Zur Modellerstellung wurden 20 dreidimensionale Wirbel (Lendenwirbel 3 und 4) von 14 Patienten verwendet.

Im dritten Schritt wurden aus den in Schritt 1 extrahierten Oberflächenpunkten diejenigen Punkte identifiziert, die eine Distanz von weniger als einem Pixel (kleiner 0,5 mm), zur Kontur des Segmentierungsergebnisses aus Schritt 2, aufwiesen. Die so gewonnene Oberfläche wurde dann zur Registrierung mit dreidimensionalen Ultraschalldaten genutzt.

Die Ergebnisse der Registrierung anhand der automatisch segmentierten Oberfläche wurden mit den Ergebnissen einer Registrierung anhand einer manuell segmentierten Oberfläche verglichen. Als Fehlermaß diente der *Target Registration Error*, wobei die Targets definierten anatomischen Regionen entsprachen, die für eine Pedikelverschraubung wichtig sind (Abb. 3). In diesen Regionen wurden Punktsets definiert, für welche nach unterschiedlicher Registrierung die Distanzen bestimmt wurden. Wichtige Regionen der Pedikelverschraubung sind die Schraubeneintrittspunkte in den Wirbel, die Pedikel durch die die Schraube geführt werden und die Corpusvorderkante, die von der Schraube nicht durchbohrt werden darf.

Die Evaluierung wurde mit drei Patienten- und zwei Phantomwirbeln durchgeführt, die nicht zur Erstellung des Modells verwendet wurden.

3 Ergebnisse

Abbildung 1a zeigt die Simulation des Ultraschallscans in einem Patientendatensatz. In Abbildung 1b ist das Ergebnis der modellbasierten Segmentierung und in Abbildung 1c die segmentierte Oberfläche eines einzelnen Wirbels dargestellt. Nach Zuordnung der Oberflächenpunkte zu dem segmentierten Wirbel konnten die CT-Daten anhand der Oberfläche mit den Ultraschalldaten registriert werden (Abb. 1d).

Tabelle 1. Target Registration Error zwischen dem Registrierungsergebnis mit der manuell ausgeschnittenen Oberfläche und dem Registrierungsergebnis mit der automatisch segmentierten Oberfläche. Berechnet wurde für vier definierte anatomische Wirbelregionen der RMS, der mittlere und der maximale Fehler zwischen den beiden Registrierungen

Daten	Pedikel links			Pedikel rechts		
	RMS	Mean	Max	RMS	Mean	Max
Patient1 L3	0,56	0,55	0,56	0,49	0,48	0,57
Patient1 L4	0,22	0,22	0,27	0,38	0,38	0,44
Patient2 L4	0,38	0,38	0,48	0,49	0,48	0,59
Phantom L3	0,00	0,00	0,00	0,00	0,00	0,00
Phantom L4	0,14	0,14	0,17	0,22	0,22	0,26
Daten	Wirbelköpervorderkante			Schraubeneintrittspunkt		
	RMS	Mean	Max	RMS	Mean	Max
Patient1 L3	0,54	0,54	0,64	0,33	0,33	0,38
Patient1 L4	1,06	1,06	1,14	0,23	0,23	0,30
Patient2 L4	1,09	1,09	1,23	0,43	0,43	0,50
Phantom L3	0,00	0,00	0,00	0,00	0,00	0,00
Phantom L4	0,20	0,19	0,28	0,26	0,26	0,29

Im Bereich der Schraubeneintrittspunkte zeigte sich bei Registrierung der Patientendaten ein RMS-Fehler von bis zu 0,43 mm. Die Zielpunkte im Bereich der Pedikel wiesen abweichende Registrierungen von bis zu 0,56 mm RMS-Fehler auf, während sich an der Wirbelkörpervorderkante RMS-Fehler von bis zu 1,09 mm ergaben. Die maximale Abweichung lag hier bei 1,23 mm. Die Phantomdaten konnten mit einem maximalen RMS-Fehler von 0,26 mm, bei maximaler Abweichung von 0,29 mm, im Bereich der Schraubeneintrittspunkte registriert werden. Die Einzelergebnisse aller Wirbel sind in Tabelle 1 aufgelistet. Dabei wurde für jede definierte anatomische Region der RMS-, der durschnittliche und der maximale Fehler berechnet. Die Rechenzeit für die Segmentierung betrug ca. 6 Minuten. Die nachfolgende Registrierung benötigte etwa 3 Sekunden.

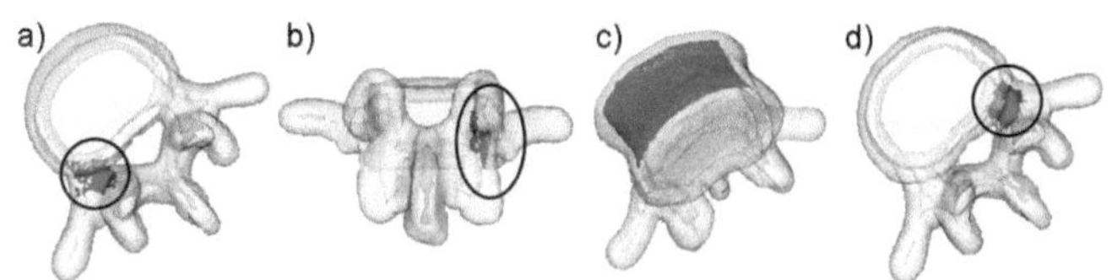

Abb. 2. Punktsets zur Bestimmung des Target Registration Errors a) Pedikel links b) Schraubeneintrittspunkt c) Wirbelköpervorderkante d) Pedikel rechts

4 Diskussion

Zur klinischen Umsetzung computerunterstützter Verfahren ist es wünschenswert die Bearbeitungsschritte so weit wie möglich zu automatisieren. Der in dieser Arbeit vorgestellte Prozess beinhaltet einen Teil der Schritte, die zur präoperativen Vorbereitung von CT-Daten für die intraoperative Registrierung mittels Ultraschall notwendig sind. So ist es gelungen, nach einer halbautomatischen Extraktion der Oberflächenpunkte, die sich im Ultraschall darstellen lassen, automatisch die Punkte zu segmentieren, die zu einem einzelnen Wirbel gehören. Anhand dieser Punktmenge konnten die CT-Daten einzelner Wirbel mit dreidimensionalen Ultraschalldaten registriert werden. Das Verfahren war sowohl auf Phantomdaten, als auch auf Patientendaten erfolgreich.

Der *Target Registration Error* der Schraubeneintrittspunkte und der Pedikel lag bei maximal 0,6 mm Abweichung deutlich unter 1 mm, was in etwa der geforderten Genauigkeit eines Navigationssystems bei der Pedikelverschraubung entspricht. Die Abweichungen von bis zu 1,34 mm im Bereich der Wirbelkörpervorderkante kam in erster Linie durch eine Winkelabweichung zustande. Diese Abweichung erfolgte somit nicht in der für eine Wirbelköperperforation kritischen Richtung bei der Pedikelverschraubung.

Danksagung. Diese Arbeit ist im Rahmen des OrthoMIT-Projekts entstanden und wurde gefördert vom BMBF (Az. 01EQ0424).

Literaturverzeichnis

1. Maintz JBA, Viergever MA. A survey of medical image registration. Med Image Anal. 1998;2(1):1–36.
2. Langlotz F, Nolte LP. Technical approaches to computer assisted orthopaedic surgery. Eur J Trauma. 2004;30(1):1–11.
3. Winter S, Brendel B, et al. Registration of CT and intraoperative 3D ultrasound images of the spine using evolutionary and gradient-based methods. IEEE Trans Evol Comput. 2007;(In Press).
4. Brendel B, Winter S, et al. Registration of 3D CT- and ultrasound-datasets of the spine using bone structures. Comp Aid Surg. 2002;7:146–55.
5. Winter S, Dekomien C, et al. Registrierung von intraoperativem 3D-Ultraschall mit präoperativen MRT-Daten für die computergestützte orthopädische Chirurgie. Z Orthopädie Unfallchirurg. 2007;145:586–90.
6. Tsai A, Yezzi A, et al. A shape-based approach to the segmentation of medical imagery using level sets. IEEE Trans Med Imaging. 2003;22(2):137–54.
7. Benameur S, Mignotte M, et al. 3D/2D registration and segmentation of scoliotic vertebrae using statistical models. Comput Med Imaging Graph. 2003;27:321–37.
8. Dekomien C, Winter S. Segmentierung einzelner Wirbel in dreidimensionalen CT-Daten mit einem modelbasierten Level Set Ansatz. Biomed Technik. 2007;52.
9. Hansen N, Ostermeier A. Completely derandomized self-adaptation in evolution strategies. Evol Comput. 2001;9(2):159–95.

Segmentation of Bony Structures with Ligament Attachment Sites

Heiko Seim[1], Hans Lamecker[1], Markus Heller[2], Stefan Zachow[1]

[1]Visualisierung und Datenanalyse, Zuse-Institut Berlin (ZIB), 14195 Berlin
[2]Centrum für Muskuloskeletale Chirurgie, Charité-Berlin, 13353 Berlin
seim@zib.de

Abstract. This work presents an approach towards reconstructing ligament and tendon attachment sites from 3D medical image data. We apply statistical shape models with an additional free form step to reconstruct the anatomical shape of the distal femur from CT data. After the shape fitting process the locations of ligament attachment sites, which are incorporated in the geometric model, are extracted and their positions optimized via an image based approach. To show the potential of our method we manually extracted the surface of 11 distal femora and their corresponding ligament attachment sites in clinical CT data and compared them to the results of our method.

1 Introduction

Pre-operative functional simulations of the human lower limbs promise, due to optimized surgery parameters, a reduced number of follow-up surgeries and improved functionality in case of total knee arthroplasty. The prerequisites for such simulations are patient individual geometric models of the anatomy of interest reconstructed from medical image data (i.e. CT, MRI), including for example bone and muscle geometry, muscle centerlines or ligament and tendon attachment sites [1]. The latter ones play an important role in computing the transfer of forces during the simulation. In today's biomechanical models those attachment sites are mostly reduced to points in 3D space, which is a strong simplification, because surface like structures have to be assumed to model forces properly. To overcome this problem Kaptein et al. [2] to our knowledge were the first who presented an approach suited for attachment site reconstruction: geometric models of the human shoulder bones with assigned contours of muscle insertions were fitted to surface models of unknown subjects to predict attachments sites. The method is purely based on geometry information.

2 Materials and Methods

By using deformable model segmentation as presented in [3, 4] as initialization, our work extends the idea of Kaptein et al. and introduces an additional attachment site fitting step, based on local image features of individual patient's data.

Fig. 1. Statistical shape model of the knee with outlined attachments sites (left). Shape model fitted to patient data including lateral collateral ligament insertion area (right)

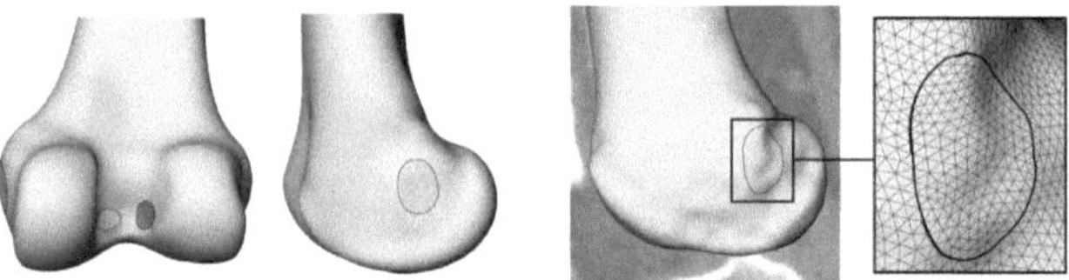

2.1 Deformable Model Generation and Fitting

For the creation of the statistical shape model 11 clinical CT data sets of the distal femur with no or very few pathological changes to the bone structure were manually segmented and their surfaces reconstructed. With the assistance of a radiologist we identified the attachment sites of the collateral (MCL, LCL) and cruciate ligaments (PCL, ACL).

Following the approach by [3] a statistical shape model of the distal femur was generated including direct point-to-point correspondences for the attachment sites of all subjects. The result of this process is a statistical atlas describing the average shape of our training set and its geometric variation as well as the location of the included attachment sites (Fig.1).

The alignment of the shape model to CT data follows the idea presented in [4]: First the statistical shape is fitted by adjusting the available degrees of freedom (transformation, rotation, uniform scaling and statistical shape modes). To overcome the restrictive character of statistical shape models, we add a second free-form step: surface vertices are allowed to move in the direction of strong gradients in a user-defined narrow band around the result of the first step.

2.2 Attachment Site Adaptation

With the geometric model as initialization (Fig. 2), the attachment site will now be moved to a more patient specific position, analyzing the patient's image data. In CT data of the knee ligaments and tendons are hard to distinguish from

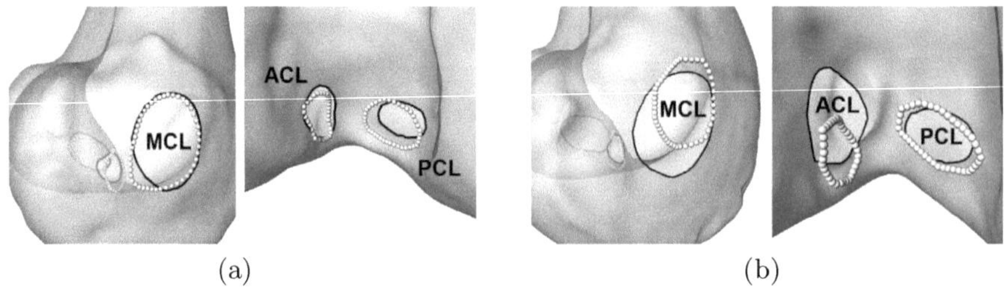

Fig. 2. Manually (black contour) and geometrically reconstructed attachment sites (spheres). Whereas statistical shape reconstruction often provides good initializations (a), patient individual variations may lead to larger spatial deviations (b)

other soft tissues structures, even for a trained radiologist. However, there exist certain characteristics that indicate the presence of such structures. Two features seem promising in CT data: Collagen typical intensity values that can be found on the outside of the bone for incoming ligaments (Fig. 3(a)) and areas with increased thickness and density of cortical bone (Fig. 3(b)) created by strong forces working on the bone surface.

By mapping those features onto the bone surface, the problem of finding a patient specific attachment site can be regarded as a 2D segmentation problem: collagen as well as dense bone tissue create regions of relatively homogeneous intensity on the surface, which can be distinguished from their neighboring structures by intensity differences. The goal is now to move the initial attachment site's contour that comes from the statistical shape model on the surface to match the described image features.

As a first approximate solution to the above mentioned problem and a feasibility study our approach is to tangentially move the initialized contour of the attachment site in a local neighborhood on the extracted bone surface by a globally applied displacement vector $\overrightarrow{v}$. This way we are going to suppress unwanted local shape variations caused by prominent but unwanted image features (i.e. very high bone densities at the femoral shaft and notch). We expect the result to be closer to the patient's attachment site than the geometrically initialized contour.

The practical approach is composed of the following steps: First we sample the gray value data along the surface normal of the evenly distributed triangle vertices of the initialized attachment sites. Only the median intensity value along a profile is projected to suppress noise in the CT data. This results in a scalar field on the surface nodes. We found a sampling with a range of 3mm inwards for the cruciate ligaments (bone density feature) and 3mm outwards for the PCL (collagen feature) suitable for extracting distinct regions fulfilling the above mentioned criteria. The ACL gave no clear results for both methods, because of the general high bone density in its attachment region and its very acute attachment angle. Considering only the nodes on the initialized attachment sites the following assumption holds for the two extracted features: Nodes with higher

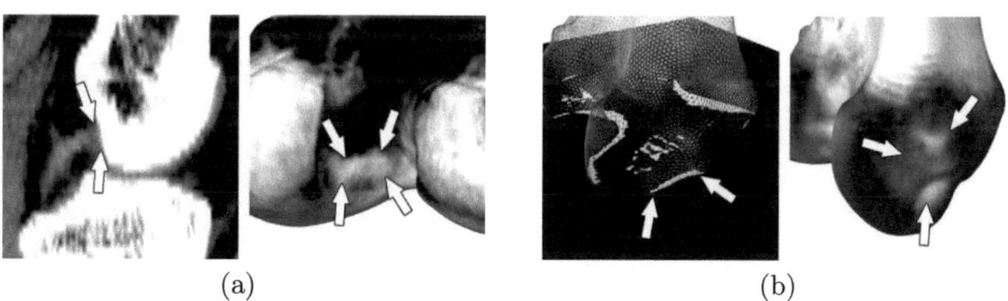

(a) (b)

Fig. 3. Intensity values mapped on the bone surface that indicate an attachment site: Projection of the surrounding soft tissue onto the bone surface creates areas with increased intensity for the PCL (a). By sampling inwards, areas of increased bone density become visible on the surface scalar field (b)

Fig. 4. Displacement of contour: A displacement vector is computed by evaluating the projected scalar values on every vertex (*left*). This vector is applied to every contour control point and tangentially projected onto the surface (*middle*), which yields the new adapted contour (*right*)

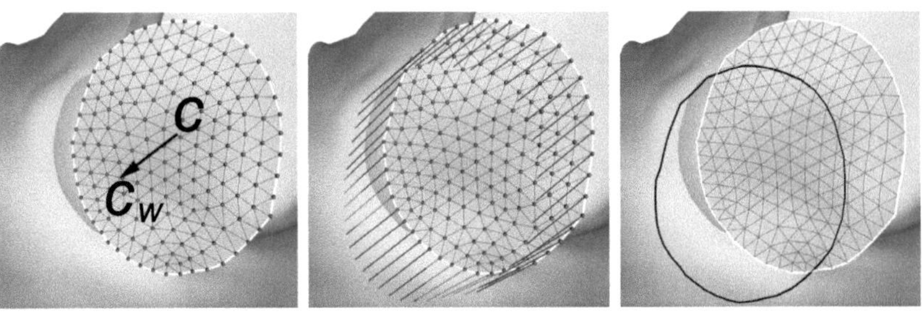

scalar values are more likely to lie on an attachment site. This assumption and the planar character of the structures of interest allow us to compute the displacement vector $\overrightarrow{v}$ as the translation of the geometric center of mass $\overrightarrow{c}$ and the weighted center of mass $\overrightarrow{c_w}$ on the attachment sites triangle vertices using the nodal scalar values as weights (Fig. 4). In a final step the displacement is applied to the contour, by adding the tangentially projected direction and magnitude of $\overrightarrow{v}$ to every contour control point. The resulting 3D coordinate is then projected back onto the surface, creating the new adapted contour.

To prove the potential of our method we validated the results in two stages: First the outputs of the geometric model fitting were compared to the manual segmentations by calculating a two sided surface distance. This was repeated for the locally adapted attachment sites.

3 Results

The average surface distance measures after the statistical shape fitting are presented in table 1. The maximum distances varied in a range from 1.25 mm (ACL) to 13.79 mm (LCL). The dimension of the attachment sites lay between 10 mm to 35 mm. All the geometrical reconstructed insertion sites were at least partly overlapping with their corresponding manual segmentations (surface projections), which is an important precondition for the following local adaptation. Comparing the results before and after image based adaptation from table 1 exposes no significant changes. In some cases the adaptation step even lead to an increase in the measured surface distances. Especially the ACL was prone to misalignment, due to the problems mentioned in section 2.2. For the PCL the results after image based adaptation improved in all data sets.

4 Discussion

We presented a method to segment bony structures including surface representations of ligament attachment sites from unknown CT data sets. This is done

Table 1. Average surface distances of reconstructed attachment sites to manually segmented attachment sites before and after image based adaptation (in mm)

Name	Stage	Mean	Deviation	RMS	Max	Median
PCL	before	0.797	0.756	1.120	3.315	0.420
	after	0.750	0.689	1.040	3.045	0.404
ACL	before	1.055	1.034	1.488	4.223	0.650
	after	1.099	1.013	1.511	4.149	0.729
LCL	before	1.018	1.176	1.560	5.091	0.592
	after	1.069	1.253	1.650	5.122	0.550
MCL	before	0.494	0.658	0.828	3.456	0.236
	after	0.548	0.697	0.891	3.389	0.256

by adjusting a geometric model and performing an image based adaptation on the surface of the extracted model.

The results show that low-level methods, like our adaptation step, are not sufficient for attachment site reconstruction in CT data. The reasons can be found in the data itself (the weak soft tissue contrast) and the basic character of our displacement strategy. To overcome the first problem we are going to apply our method to other image modalities with higher soft tissue contrast like MRI. The improvement of the method itself will be our primary objective. This includes a more sophisticated gray value analysis and a more complex representation of the attachment site (e.g. a 3D model of the ligaments), to include more model knowledge into the reconstruction process. However, looking at the results for the PCL, there is a potential and a demand for an improved image based adaption step. Even if this step fails, we could show that the fitting of the geometric model provides a good guess for the location of the attachment sites.

All the results presented in this work are subject to a bigger clinical study with more data sets and exact knowledge of the patient's attachment site extracted from specialized MRI sequences or Image-Guided Surgery systems.

Acknowledgement. This work is partly funded by the European Commission (FP6 IST Project DeSSOS (027252) and the DFG Research Center Matheon.

References

1. Blemker SS, Asakawa DS, Gold GE, et al. Image-based musculoskeletal modeling: Applications, advances, and future opportunities. J Magn Reson Imaging. 2007;25(2):441–51.
2. Kaptein BL, van der Helm FCT. Estimating muscle attachment contours by transforming geometrical bone models. J Biomech. 2004 Mar;37(3):263–73.
3. Lamecker H, Seebaß M, Hege HC, et al. A 3D statistical shape model of the pelvic bone for segmentation. Proc SPIE. 2004;5370:1341–51.
4. Kainmüller D, Lange T, Lamecker H. Shape constrained automatic aegmentation of the liver based on a heuristic intensity model. Proc MICCAI Workshop 3D Segmentation in the Clinic: A Grand Challenge. 2007; p. 109–16.

Segmentierung der Papille in Fundusaufnahmen
Aktives Kreisbogen-Modell

Torsten Schmidt[1], Axel Doering[2]

[1]Fachbereich Technische Informatik, Fachhochschule Jena
[2]R&D Software, Carl Zeiss Meditec AG, Jena
torsten.schmidt.ts@googlemail.com

Kurzfassung. In der vorliegenden Arbeit präsentieren wir einen praxistauglichen Algorithmus zur automatischen Segmentierung der Disc-Grenze der Papille in Fundusaufnahmen. Ausgehend von einem lokalisierten Papillenpunkt werden Grauwertverläufe in horizontaler und vertikaler Richtung mittels einer Energiefunktion ausgewertet. In einem iterativen Prozess wird die Ellipse der tatsächlichen Disc-Grenze angenähert. Der Papillenrand konnte im Testdatensatz in 88% der Aufnahmen erfolgreich segmentiert werden. Der Algorithmus ist robust gegenüber der Lage des Startpunktes innerhalb der Papille und soll als Unterstützung bei der Glaukombefundung eingesetzt werden.

1 Einleitung

In entwickelten Ländern wird eine Erblindung in ca. 15-20% der Fälle durch degenerative Veränderungen des Sehnervs (Glaukom) verursacht. Die Papille (Sehnervenkopf, Disc) weist bei fortschreitender Erkrankung eine zunehmende Exkavation (Vertiefung, Cup) auf. Nach [1] wird die Größe der Exkavation durch das Verhältnis der horizontalen bzw. vertikalen Durchmesser des Disc- und Cup-Bereiches (Cup/Disc-Ratio) bestimmt, wofür eine Segmentierung mit Ellipsen ausreichend erscheint. Für diese Aufgabe wurden in der Literatur unterschiedliche Verfahren beschrieben, welche sich in die Lokalisierung des Papillenbereiches, Segmentierung des Disc- und Cup-Bereiches unterteilen lassen. Durch die unterschiedlichen Erscheinungsformen und die durch Blutgefäße hervorgerufenen Störungen der Papillenkontur wird diese Aufgabe erschwert.

Die Grundlagen der Lokalisierung des Papillenbereiches bilden unterschiedliche Eigenschaften der Papille bzw. des Papillenumfeldes. In der Literatur wurden Verfahren zur Detektion des Bildbereiches mit der höchsten Intensität [2] bzw. der höchsten Intensitätsänderungen [3] beschrieben. Weiterhin kann Template Matching [4, 5], Principal Component Analysis (PCA) [6] bzw. die Auswertung des Gefäßbaumes [7] verwendet werden.

Für die Segmentierung des Disc-Bereiches existieren unterschiedliche Verfahren. Als erstes kann die Hough-Transformation für Kreise [2] genannt werden. Der Nachteil dieses Verfahrens besteht in der Störanfälligkeit des dazu notwendigen Kantenbildes sowie in dem sehr hohen Rechenaufwand der Hough-Transformation. In [6] wird eine Segmentierungsmethode mit dem Active Shape

Tabelle 1. Statistische Papillenparameter Arbeitsdatensatz

Parameter	Minimum	Mittelwert	Maximum
horizontale Achslänge d_h in Pixel	220	298 (29,5)	400
vertikale Achslänge d_v in Pixel	234	311 (30,9)	400
Achslängenverhältnis $\nu = \frac{d_h}{d_v}$	0,82	0,96 (0,07)	1,17

Model und in [5, 8] mit aktiven Konturen beschrieben. Eigene experimentelle Untersuchungen haben gezeigt, dass die Qualität der Ergebnisse dieser Verfahren sehr stark von der geeigneten Wahl einer initialen Kontur abhängt.

Das hier vorgestellte aktive Kreisbogen-Modell basiert ebenfalls auf aktiven Konturen, wobei Parameter einer nicht rotierten Ellipse (Halbachsen in x- und y-Richtung) angepasst werden. Im Gegensatz zu anderen aktiven Konturmodellen wird keine initiale Kontur benötigt.

Die Segmentierung des Cup-Bereiches ist ohne die Verwendung von 3D-Informationen [8] in der Praxis nicht anwendbar und wird hier nicht weiter untersucht.

2 Material und Methoden

Die Parametrisierung des Verfahrens erfolgt auf der Basis von 190 zufällig ausgewählten Fundusaufnahmen (Arbeitsdatensatz) mit einer einheitlichen Größe von 2196x1958 Pixeln und einem Aufnahmewinkel von 45°. Durch die manuelle Segmentierung des Disc-Bereiches der Papillen mit Ellipsen konnten die erforderlichen Parameter ermittelt werden (Tabelle 1).

Voraussetzung für die Anwendung des aktiven Kreisbogen-Modells ist die Lokalisierung eines Startpunktes M_0 innerhalb der Papille. Für diesen Schritt wurde die Auswertung eines Binärbildes und die Lokalisierung mittels Template Matching untersucht. Die Binarisierung erfolgt, aufgrund der differenzierten Darstellung der Papille, im Grün-Kanal mit einer dynamischen Schranke bei 98% des höchsten Grauwertes. Der Schwerpunkt des größten Binärobjektes bildet den Startpunkt. Über die Objektparameter Formfaktor und Fläche wird ein Vertrauensmaß für die Lokalisierung berechnet. Das erforderliche Template der Papille wurde aus dem Arbeitsdatensatz durch Mittelwertbildung der Papillenbereiche [4] erstellt. Zusätzlich wurde ein Template wie in [5] beschrieben untersucht.

Das aktive Kreisbogen-Modell basiert auf der iterativen Anpassung der vier Scheitelpunkte einer Ellipse an den Randbereich der Papille. Die Segmentierung erfolgt, aufgrund der sehr guten Abbildung des Papillenrandes, im Rot-Kanal bei voller Auflösung. Der Bereich um den Startpunkt wird in vier Sektoren ($\gamma = [1, 2, 3, 4]$) eingeteilt (Abb. 1a). In horizontaler (Sektoren 1, 3) und vertikaler Richtung (Sektoren 2, 4) werden, ausgehend von dem Startpunkt M_n, Grauwertverläufe f_γ auf Suchstrahlen δ erstellt (Abb. 1b). Die Grauwerte auf den Suchstrahlen werden durch den Mittelwert der Grauwerte auf den dazugehörigen konzentrischen Kreisbögen gebildet. Dadurch wird der Einfluss der vom jeweiligen Kreisbogen geschnittenen Blutgefäße minimiert. Die Radien der Kreisbögen sind gleich dem Abstand vom aktuellen Startpunkt.

Die Papille weist höhere Grauwerte als der Augenhintergrund auf. Dadurch beschreibt jeweils ein Minimum des Gradientenverlaufes $g_\gamma = \text{grad}(f_\gamma)$ den Rand der Papille entlang des Suchstrahls. Durch Störungen innerhalb und außerhalb der Papille treten pro Sektor mehrere lokale Minima auf. Das betragsmäßig größte Minimum pro Sektor spiegelt nicht immer den Papillenrand wider. Jede Kombination i der lokalen Minima untereinander muss dabei als mögliche Lösung betrachtet werden. Kombinationen mit Achslängen bzw. Achslängenverhältnissen außerhalb der statistisch ermittelten Randbedingungen (Tabelle 1) werden verworfen und nicht weiter betrachtet. Von den verbleibenden Kombinationen wird diejenige mit der geringsten Energie nach Gleichung 1 bestimmt.

$$E_i = \alpha_1 E_{g_h,i} + \alpha_2 E_{g_v,i} + \alpha_3 E_{d_h,i} + \alpha_4 E_{d_v,i} + \alpha_5 E_{\nu,i} \quad (1)$$

Die Summe der horizontalen bzw. vertikalen Gradienten bildet einen zuverlässigen Indikator für den Papillenrand (Gl. 2,3).

$$E_{g_h,i} = g_{1,i} + g_{3,i} \quad (2)$$

$$E_{g_v,i} = g_{2,i} + g_{4,i} \quad (3)$$

Die Abstände $l_{g_{\gamma,i}}$ der lokalen Minima jedes Sektors vom aktuellen Startpunkt M_n bilden die Achslängen der resultierenden Ellipse. Die Abweichung von den durchschnittlichen Achslängen $\overline{d_h}$ und $\overline{d_v}$ wird durch zwei weitere Terme der Energiefunktion (Gl. 4, 5) über lineare Strafterme berücksichtigt.

$$E_{d_h,i} = \left|\overline{d_h} - (l_{g_{1,i}} + l_{g_{3,i}})\right| \quad (4)$$

$$E_{d_v,i} = \left|\overline{d_v} - (l_{g_{2,i}} + l_{g_{4,i}})\right| \quad (5)$$

Die Abweichung der Achslängenverhältnisse vom durchschnittlichen Achslängenverhältnis $\overline{\nu}$ sowie die Orientierung der Ellipse ist ebenfalls über einen linearen Strafterm (Gl. 6) definiert.

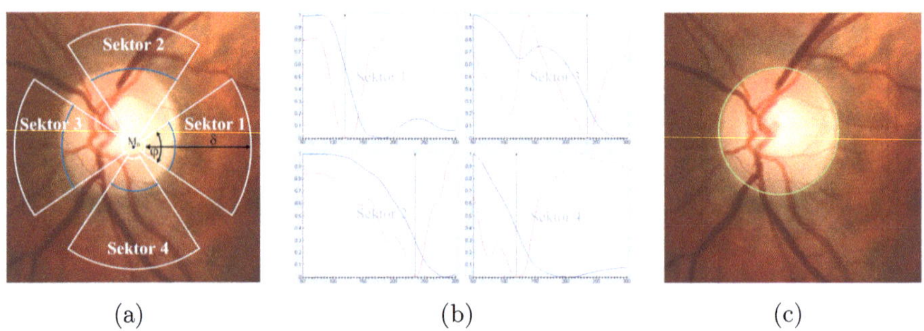

Abb. 1. Segmentierung: (a): Startpunkt M_n, berechnete Scheitelpunkte (blau); (b): f_γ (blau), g_γ (rot), Position Papillenrand (schwarz); (c): Segmentierungsergebnis

Tabelle 2. Lokalisierungsergebnisse

Verfahren	Erfolgsquote (%)	Bearbeitungszeit (ms)
Binärbildauswertung	94,5	530
Template Matching [4]	96,7	1775
Template Matching [5]	74,7	3011

$$E_{\nu,i} = \left| \overline{\nu} - \frac{l_{g_{1,i}} + l_{g_{3,i}}}{l_{g_{2,i}} + l_{g_{4,i}}} \right| \quad (6)$$

Voraussetzung für die Definition eines statischen Parametersatzes $\alpha_1 \ldots \alpha_5$ ist, dass alle Terme der Energiefunktion die gleiche Menge Energie beschreiben. Um dies zu erreichen, wird jeder Term auf den Bereich [0..1] normiert. Die Positionen der Minima der Kombination mit der geringsten Gesamtenergie bilden die vier Scheitelpunkte der resultierenden Ellipse. Der Mittelpunkt dieser Ellipse bildet den Startpunkt für die nächste Iteration.

Der Prozess wird beendet, wenn für den Abstand τ der Mittelpunkte (Gl. 7) in zwei aufeinander folgenden Iterationen $\tau \leq \tau_e$ gilt.

$$\tau = \sqrt{(x_{n-1} - x_n)^2 + (y_{n-1} - y_n)^2} \quad (7)$$

Bei Auftreten eines Zyklus sich wiederholender Koordinaten wird der Mittelwert der beteiligten Koordinaten als neuer Startpunkt verwendet.

3 Ergebnisse

Die Überprüfung der Leistungsfähigkeit der Algorithmen erfolgte auf einem repräsentativen, vom Arbeitsdatensatz unabhängigen Datensatz mit 91 Fundusaufnahmen. Eine positive Lokalisierung liegt vor (Tabelle 2), wenn der detektierte Punkt innerhalb der manuell segmentierten Papille liegt.

Das Segmentierungsergebnis (Tabelle 3) wurde positiv gewertet, wenn die Abweichung der berechneten von den manuell ermittelten Ellipsenparametern innerhalb der Toleranzen bei der manuellen Segmentierung lag. Die Standardabweichung gibt die Abhängigkeit vom Startpunkt, bei einer systematischen Manipulation des Startpunktes relativ zum manuellen Segmentierungsergebnis, an. Zusätzlich wurde der Einfuss des Zentriwinkels φ der Kreisbögen sowie der Wichtungsparameter $\alpha_1 \ldots \alpha_5$ der Energiefunktion untersucht. Ein positives Segmentierungsergebnis ist in Abbildung 1c dargestellt. Die durchschnittliche Bearbeitungszeit pro Bild beträgt $2,1$ Sekunden bei durchschnittlich 9 Iterationen.

Mittels der Hough-Transformation nach [2] konnte in 67,0% der Aufnahmen die Papille mit einer durchschnittlichen Bearbeitungszeit von $11,2$ Sekunden pro Bild erfolgreich segmentiert werden.

Tabelle 3. Segmentierungsergebnisse (Erfolgsquote in % mit Standardabweichung)

α_1:α_2:α_3:α_4:α_5	45°	90°	135°	180°
1,0:1,0:1,5:1,5:1,5	$73,4\ (2,68)$	$82,9\ (1,99)$	$84,4\ (2,50)$	$74,5\ (4,72)$
1,0:1,0:1,0:1,0:1,0	$76,1\ (1,72)$	$87,9\ (1,65)$	$86,0\ (2,50)$	$77,0\ (3,13)$
1,0:1,0:0,2:0,2:1,0	$72,8\ (1,89)$	$85,7\ (2,69)$	$84,5\ (3,32)$	$75,6\ (4,32)$
1,0:1,0:0,2:0,2:0,5	$72,0\ (1,24)$	$81,7\ (1,74)$	$85,1\ (2,81)$	$76,8\ (4,61)$

4 Diskussion

Die Untersuchungen zur Lokalisierung eines Punktes innerhalb der Papille haben gezeigt, dass die Binärbildauswertung ein schnelles Verfahren darstellt. Die Lokalisierung mittels Template Matching nach [4] kann ebenfalls verwendet werden. Die Tauglichkeit des dem Template nach [5] zugrunde liegenden Modells konnte nicht bestätigt werden.

Das entwickelte aktive Kreisbogen-Modell stellt ein schnelles und robustes Verfahren zur Segmentierung der Disc-Grenze der Papille in Fundusbildern dar. Der Einfluss der Blutgefäße konnte durch die Erstellung der Grauwertverläufe basierend auf konzentrischen Kreisbögen sowie der Einbeziehung statistischer Papillenparameter minimiert werden. Im Vergleich zu anderen Verfahren wird beim aktiven Kreisbogen-Modell keine initiale Kontur benötigt. Das Verfahren versagt, wenn der Papillenrand im Rot-Kanal unzureichend abgebildet wird oder der Startpunkt außerhalb der Papille liegt.

Durch die Nutzung von 3D-Informationen kann der entwickelte Algorithmus auf die Segmentierung des Cup-Bereiches angewendet werden. Eine Erweiterung des Verfahrens auf Bilder anderer Auflösung wird ebenfalls entwickelt.

Literaturverzeichnis

1. Niggemeier S. Verlaufsbeobachtung morphologischer und funktioneller Parameter bei verschiedenen Glaukomformen. RWTH Aachen; 2005.
2. Chrástek R, Wolf M, et al. Optic disc segmentation in retinal images. Proc BVM. 2002; p. 263–66.
3. Sinthanayothin C, Boyce JF, Cook HL, et al. Automated localisation of the optic disc, fovea, and retinal blood vessels from digital colour fundus images. Br J Ophthalmol. 1999;83(8):902–10.
4. Osareh A, Mirmehdi M, et al. Colour morphology and snakes for optic disc localisation. In: 6th Med Image Underst Anal Conf. BMVA Press; 2002. p. 21–4.
5. Lowell J, Hunter A, Steel D, et al. Optic nerve head segmentation. IEEE Trans Med Imaging. 2004;23(2):256–64.
6. Li H, Chutatape O. Automated feature extraction in color retinal images by a model based approach. IEEE Trans Med Imaging. 2004;51(2):246–54.
7. ter Haar F. Automatic localization of the optic disc in digital colour images of the human retina. Utrecht University; 2005.
8. Xu J, Chutatape O, et al. Optic disk feature extraction via modified deformable model technique for glaucoma analysis. Pattern Recogn. 2007;40(7):2063–76.

Optimierte Segmentierung der Papille in HRT-Retinaaufnahmen

Oliver Arold[1], Rüdiger Bock[1], Jörg Meier[1], Georg Michelson[2], Joachim Hornegger[1]

[1]Lehrstuhl für Mustererkennung, Universität Erlangen-Nürnberg
[2]Augenklinik Erlangen, Universität Erlangen-Nürnberg
oarold@optik.uni-erlangen.de

Kurzfassung. Der Papillenrand ist ein entscheidendes Merkmal zur Erkennung von krankhaften Veränderungen am Augenhintergrund. Zur Auswertung ist eine Segmentierung nötig, die meist manuell durch den Augenarzt vorgenommen werden muss. Eine robuste, automatische Segmentierung der Papille kann den Arzt unterstützen, die Reliabilität der Segmentierung erhöhen und eine Basis für eine automatische Diagnose schaffen. Die vorgestellte Methode optimiert ein Segmentierungsverfahren mittels Ausreißerdetektion und Spline-Interpolation auf radial abgetasteten binarisierten Reflektionsbildern des Heidelberg Retina Tomographen (HRT). Der Vergleich mit bestehenden Verfahren zeigt, dass der Segmentierungsfehler um 9% reduziert werden konnte und das Verfahren stabiler gegen Artefakte ist.

1 Einleitung

Eine der häufigsten Ursachen für die Erblindung des Menschen ist das Glaukom, bei dem Sehnerven im Bereich der Papille absterben und dadurch das Sichtfeld des Patienten stetig abnimmt. Zur frühzeitigen Diagnose wird häufig die Papillekontur auf HRT-Bildern untersucht. Dazu ist eine manuelle Segmentierung notwendig. Ein zuverlässiges, automatisches Verfahren soll als objektives Bewertungskriterium dienen, die Reliabilität der Papillenvermessung erhöhen und die zeitaufwändigen, manuellen Schritte im Diagnoseverfahren reduzieren.

Lowell stellt in [1] ein Verfahren zur Lokalisierung und Segmentierung der Papille in Fundusbildern vor, bei dem zuerst eine elliptische Kontur um die Papille gelegt und diese dann lokal verformt wird. Bei Tamura wird in [2] mit einer Hough-Tranformation die Kontur der Papille in einem Fundusbild durch einen Kreis approximiert. Chrásteks Verfahren zur automatischen Segmentierung der Papille arbeitet auf HRT-Bildern. Nach einer geeigneten Binarisierung wird zuerst eine Kreiskontur berechnet und diese dann mittels Aktiver Konturen lokal verfeinert [3].

Das in diesem Beitrag vorgestellte Verfahren basiert auf Chrásteks Methoden der Binarisierung von HRT-Bildern. Die Methode verbessert die Bestimmung der Kreiskontur sowie die anschließende Verfeinerung der Konturlinie. Der Algorithmus passt sich besser verschieden großen Papillen an und wird weniger stark von Gefäßen und Artefakten im Binärbild gestört.

2 Material und Methoden

Der hier beschriebene Algorithmus besteht aus einer groben Segmentierung, bei der die Papille durch eine Kreiskontur approximiert wird, und einer feinen Segmentierung, bei der die Kreiskontur lokal angepasst wird. In beiden Schritten wird zuerst das HRT-Bild mittels eines globalen Schwellwertes binarisiert und anschließend Artefakte reduziert, indem kleinere zusammenhängende Strukturen entfernt werden. [3].

2.1 Bestimmung einer Kreiskontur mittels Ringmasken

Das aus dem HRT-Bild berechnete Binärbild wird mit B bezeichnet. Eine Ringmaske $R_b^a = [r^{(a,b)}(x,y)]$ beschreibt einen Ring mit den Radien a und b ($a > b$) und ist folgendermaßen definiert:

$$r^{(a,b)}(x,y) = \begin{cases} 1, & \text{falls } a^2 \geq x^2 + y^2 \geq b^2 \\ 0, & \text{andernsfalls} \end{cases} \tag{1}$$

A_b^a beschreibe die Fläche des entsprechenden Ringes R_b^a, also die Anzahl der gesetzten Punkte in der Ringmaske. Legt man den Mittelpunkt der Maske R_b^a an der Position (x, y) über das Binärbild B, kann man den prozentualen Anteil p_{xy} der gesetzten Punkte in R berechnen:

$$p_{xy} = \frac{\sum_{i=-a}^{i=a} \sum_{j=-a}^{j=a} b_{x+i,y+j} \cdot r^{(a,b)}(i,j)}{A_b^a} \tag{2}$$

Die Radien a und b des Ringes R_b^a werden in jedem Schritt reduziert. Für jede Ringmaske wird dann die Position $(x_{\text{best}}, y_{\text{best}})$ mit maximalem Wert $p_{x_{\text{best}},y_{\text{best}}}$ bestimmt. Der Algorithmus stoppt sobald $p_{x_{\text{best}},y_{\text{best}}}$ größer oder gleich einer Schranke θ ist oder die Radien eine festgelegte Schranke unterschreiten. Im letzteren Fall werden die Werte $(x_{\text{best}}, y_{\text{best}})$ und a mit maximalem $p_{x_{\text{best}},y_{\text{best}}}$ als Kreiskontur verwendet.

2.2 Bestimmung der feinen Konturlinie

Da die tatsächliche Konturlinie der Papille in der Regel kein exakter Kreis ist, wird die gefundene Kreiskontur weiter verfeinert.

Zuerst wird ein Binärbild B berechnet, so dass kleinere Artefakte eliminiert werden, aber die Papille erhalten bleibt (Abb. 1(a)). Als nächstes wird in B ein ringförmiger Bereich um den gefundenen Kreismittelpunkt $(x_{\text{best}}, y_{\text{best}})$ radial von innen nach außen abgetastet (Abb. 1(b)). Im resultierenden Bild $B^{(\text{rad})}$ werden anschließend spaltenweise Konturpunkte detektiert. Da der äußere Rand der Papille segmentiert werden soll, wird dazu jede Spalte α von unten nach oben durchsucht. Für jeden Pixel (α, τ) wird der Anteil $N_n(\alpha, \tau)$ der gesetzten Pixel in einer kleinen Umgebung berechnet:

$$N_n(\alpha, \tau) = \frac{\sum_{i=-n}^{n} \sum_{j=-n}^{n} B^{(rad)}(\alpha + i, \tau + j)}{(2n+1)^2} \tag{3}$$

Ist der Anteil $N_n(\alpha, \tau)$ größer als eine festgelegte Schranke ϕ_{con}, wird der Pixel als Konturpunkt $c_\alpha = \tau$ deklariert. Andernfalls wird der nächst höhere Pixel $(\alpha, \tau - 1)$ getestet. Übersteigt der Wert für keinen Pixel die Schranke ϕ_{con}, wird der Pixel mit dem maximalen Anteil N_n als Konturpunkt festgelegt. Abb. 1(c) veranschaulicht das Vorgehen. Aufgrund von Artefakten und Gefäßen liegen in der Regel nicht alle detektierten Konturpunkte c_α auf dem tatsächlichen Rand der Papille. Daher wird für jeden Konturpunkt c_α der Median m_α in einer kleinen Nachbarschaft berechnet. Weicht dieser um mehr als eine festgelegte

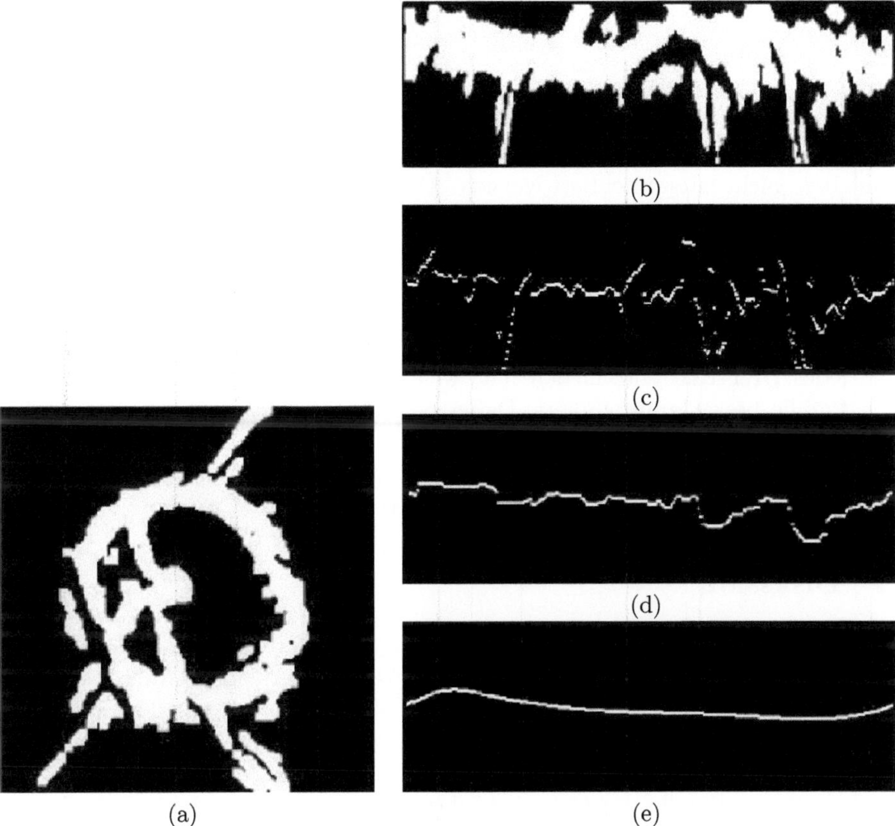

Abb. 1. Radiale Abtastung: (a) binarisiertes und verbessertes Bild B, (b) radial abgetastetes Bild $B^{(\text{rad})}$ (Zentrum: $(x_{\text{best}}, y_{\text{best}})$); Ausreißereliminierung und Spline-Interpolation: (c) detektierte Konturpunkte c_α, (d) Konturpunkte nach adaptivem Medianfilter, (e) Konturpunkte nach RANSAC-Algorithmus und Spline-Interpolation

Tabelle 1. Statistische Ergebnisse der Segmentierungsverfahren in 100 HRT-Bildern

Algorithmus	fehlende Fläche	zusätzliche Fläche	Gesamtfehler
Segmentierung aus [3]	7.2%	19.0%	26.2%
Neue Segmentierung	6.8%	10.6%	17.4%

Schranke ϕ_{med} von c_α ab, wird der Konturpunkt als Ausreißer deklariert und in den folgenden Schritten nicht mehr berücksichtigt (Abb. 1(d)).

Die finale Konturlinie wird mit Hilfe einer Spline-Interpolation durch k ausgewählte Konturpunkte bestimmt. Zur Auswahl der k Stützstellen wird ein RANSAC-Verfahren [4] verwendet, so dass möglichst viele Konturpunkte approximiert werden (Abb. 1(e)).

3 Ergebnisse

Zur quantitativen Bewertung der Ergebnisse hat ein Augenarzt die Papille in 100 zufällig gewählten HRT-Bildern manuell segmentiert. Anschließend wurde die Konturlinie der automatischen Segmentierung mit der Musterlösung des Arztes verglichen, indem die Größen der Flächen berechnet wurden, die fälschlicherweise mit- bzw. nicht mitsegmentiert wurden. Als Referenz wurden die Papillenflächen der manuellen Segmentierung auf eins normiert. Tabelle 1 zeigt die statistischen Werte gemittelt über 100 HRT-Bilder sowohl für das Verfahren aus [3] als auch für die hier vorgestellte Segmentierungsmethode. Abb. 2 zeigt drei Beispiele für die berechneten Konturlinien, die die Verbesserung veranschaulichen.

Zusätzlich wurde eine direkte Evaluation durchgeführt, bei der ein Augenarzt für jedes HRT-Bild entschieden hat, welche der eingezeichneten Konturlinien die Papille besser approximiert. Dabei befand der Arzt in 62 von 100 Fällen das Segmentierungsergebnis des neuen Verfahrens als besser. Die Laufzeit des neuen Verfahrens ist im Vergleich zur Methode aus [3] von 26 auf 63 Sekunden gestiegen (AMD Athlon(TM) XP 2600, 2 GB RAM).

4 Diskssion

Bei beiden verglichenen Methoden werden ca. 7% der eigentlichen Papillenfläche nicht detektiert. Die Konturlinien umschließen also einen Großteil der tatsächlichen Papille. Unterschiede zeigen sich bei der Betrachtung der Fläche, die von der automatischen Segmentierung fälschlicherweise mitsegmentiert wird. Die Konturlinien des Verfahrens aus [3] sind oft zu groß und umschließen Bereiche außerhalb der Papille. Im Gegensatz dazu passt sich die grobe Segmentierung der vorgestellten Methode besser an unterschiedlich große Papillen an. Zudem bewirkt Ausreißereliminierung der feinen Segmentierung, dass die resultierenden Konturlinien der natürlichen Form der Papille entsprechen. Damit reduziert sich die fälschlicherweise segmentierte Fläche von 19.0% auf 10.6%. Das Verfahren verringert den Gesamtfehler um 9%. Die verbesserte automatische Segmentierung erlaubt im klinischen Alltag eine zuverlässigere Diagnoseunterstüzung.

Abb. 2. Segmentierungsergebnisse: gestrichelte Linie: Kontur des Arztes, durchgezogene Linie: berechnete Kontur. Oben: Verfahren aus [3]. Unten: Neues Verfahren

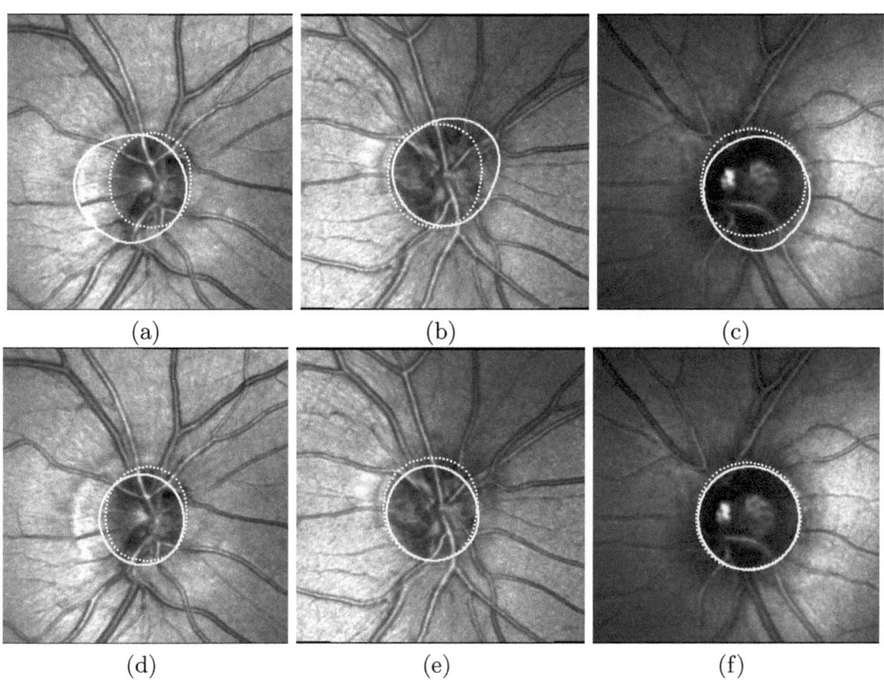

(a) (b) (c)

(d) (e) (f)

Literaturverzeichnis

1. Lowell J, Hunter A, Steel D, et al. Optic nerve head segmentation. IEEE Trans Med Imaging. 2004;23(2):256–64.
2. Tamura S, Okamoto Y, Yanashima K. Zero-crossing interval correction in tracing eye-fundus blood vessels. Pattern Recogn. 1988;21(3):227–33.
3. Chrástek R, Wolf M, Donath K, et al. Automated segmentation of the optic nerve head for diagnosis of glaucoma. Med Image Anal. 2005;9(4):297–314.
4. Fischler MA, Bolles RC. Random sample consensus: A paradigm for model fitting with applications to image analysis and automated cartography. Commun ACM. 1981;24(6):381–95.

Ein routine-integrierbares Planungswerkzeug zur operativen Rekonstruktion der Orbita

Melanie Kleiner[1], Dirk Schulze[2], Pit Jakob Voss[2], Thomas M. Deserno[1]

[1]Institut für Medizinische Informatik, RWTH Aachen
[2]Universitätsklinik für Zahn-, Mund- und Kieferheilkunde (ZMK), Freiburg
Melanie.Kleiner@rwth-aachen.de

Kurzfassung. Bei Frakturen des Orbitabodens kann ein Titangitter zur Rekonstruktion operativ eingesetzt werden. In dieser Arbeit wird ein Planungswerkzeug entwickelt, welches mit Hilfe eines aktiven Konturmodells die Orbita in CT Daten segmentiert, ihr Volumen berechnet und visualisiert. Neben den technischen Integrationsstufen der Funktions- und Präsentationsintegration, welche durch den Einsatz des Medical Imaging Interaction Toolkit (MITK) erreicht werden, sowie der Daten-, und Kontextintegration ist vor allem die Stabilität der eingesetzten Algorithmik für die Routine-Integrierbarkeit wichtig. Erste Stabilitätsuntersuchungen basieren auf 3 von 100 zufällig ausgewählten CT-Datensätzen, wobei das Volumen mit je 50 verschiedenen Startpunkten berechnet wurde. Die so ermittelten Variationskoeffizienten liegen deutlich unterhalb der kritischen 5 % Schwelle.

1 Einleitung

Frakturen des Orbitabodens sind eine der häufigsten Frakturen in der Gesichts- und Kieferchirurgie [1]. Um die Sehfähigkeit weitestgehend wiederherzustellen, wird bei einer in der klinischen Erprobung befindlichen Methode operativ ein Titangitter eingesetzt. Es wird davon ausgegangen, dass das rekonstruierte Volumen dabei eine entscheidende Rolle spielt. Die Operationsplanung kann also durch eine robuste prä- und postoperative Volumenberechnung anhand von Computer Tomographie (CT) Daten sowie einer geeigneten Visualisierung entscheidend und effizient unterstützt werden.

Für die Segmentierung dreidimensionaler CT-Daten existieren viele Methoden. Regionenbasierte Verfahren, wie das Watershed-Verfahren, sind aber nicht in der Lage, Lücken in der Kontur zu schließen. Aktive Formmodelle würden die Form der Orbita in Bezug auf Frakturen zu weit einschränken. Aktive Konturmodelle hingegen liefern immer eine geschlossene Kontur und können sehr unterschiedliche Formvarianten erkennen. Die Segmentierung der Orbita wird daher mit einem diskreten, aktiven Konturmodell durchgeführt [2]. Robuste Parametrierung, Stabilität und Korrektheit sind weitere Grundvoraussetzungen für die Integrierbarkeit des Planungswerkzeugs in die medizinische Routine [3]. Hierzu gehört auch die Möglichkeit des Anwenders, das Segmentierungsergebnis zu kontrollieren. In diesem Beitrag wird dargestellt, wie mit Hilfe des Medical Imaging Interaction Toolkits (MITK), das am Deutschen Krebsforschungszentrum (DKZ) in Heidelberg entwickelt wird, ein routine-integrierbares Planungswerkzeug zur operativen Rekonstruktion der Orbita erstellt wird.

2 Material und Methoden

Von dem Werkzeug müssen die Arbeitsschritte 1. Einlesen der Bilddaten, 2. Initialisierung, 3. Segmentierung, 4. Visualisierung, 5. Volumenbestimmung, 6. Spiegelung und Seitenvergleich, 7. Berechnung des Implantates und 8. Ausgabe der Modellparameter abgebildet werden. Diese Funktionen wurden mit MITK realisiert. MITK verbindet das Insight Segmentation and Registration Toolkit (ITK), mit dem Visualization Toolkit (VTK) [4] und ist besonders für Endanwendungen in der klinischen Praxis geeignet [5]. Zusätzlich bietet das MITK eine Standard-Applikation, in die auf einfache Weise eigene Module eingebettet werden können, sowie Klassen zur Interaktion des Benutzers mit den Bilddaten. Durch die Verwaltung in einer Baumstruktur, können unterschiedliche Strukturen in Relation zu einander dynamisch verwaltet und gleichzeitig in verschiedenen Ansichten konsistent angezeigt werden.

Für die Routine-Integrierbarkeit ist neben der eigentlichen Verfügbarmachung der Bildverarbeitungsalgorithmen sowie den Kontrollmöglichkeiten für den Anwender, welche durch eine geeignete Interaktion realisiert werden können, vor allem die Stabilität des Verfahrens wichtig, was methodisch sauber untersucht werden muss [3]. Hierzu stehen CT-Datensätze von 100 Probanden ohne Frakturen der Orbita zur Verfügung.

2.1 Integrationsstufen

Zunächst lässt sich die Integration einzelner Module zu einem System auf verschiedenen Ebenen untersuchen [6]:

1. *Datenintegration* bedeutet, dass das Planungswerkzeug auf die Daten im PACS Archiv direkt zugreifen kann. Dies ist über das Digital Imaging and Communication in Medicine (DICOM) Protokoll prinzipiell möglich und soll zu einem späteren Zeitpunkt realisiert werden.
2. *Funktionsintegration* bedeutet, dass das Werkzeug von der Arbeitstation des Anwenders aufrufbar ist. Da MITK auf plattformunabhängigen Komponenten aufsetzt, kann das Programm sowohl auf Windows- als auch auf Linux/Unix-Rechnern betrieben werden.
3. *Präsentationsintegration* bedeutet, dass Oberfläche und Bedienung vergleichbar zu Standardmodulen auf dem Computer des Anwenders ist. Auch dies ist durch den Einsatz von MITK gegeben.
4. *Kontextintegration* bedeutet, dass der Zusammenhang (z.B. Patient) zwischen den Applikationen (z.B. Befundungssoftware und Planungswerkzeug) automatisch ausgetauscht wird. Hierfür stehen proprietäre Schnittstellen der Befundungssoftware zur Verfügung.

2.2 Stabilität

Stabilität bedeutet, dass für eine klinische Situation immer der gleiche Messwert ermittelt wird, unabhängig von (tolerierbaren) Variationen in der Verfahrensparametrierung und den (manuellen) Komponenten bei der Initialisierung. Das Planungswerkzeug muss zum einen die Stabilität in Bezug zum gewählten Startpunkt, zum anderen die stabile Schließung der Orbita, und zuletzt die stabile Segmentierung bei unterschiedlichem Bildmaterial gewährleisten. Um die Auswirkungen von schwankenden Startpunkten zu minimieren, ist ein semiautomatisches Verfahren, welches den manuellen Startpunkt noch einmal verschiebt, integriert. In der Umgebung des manuell gewählten Startpunktes wird auf einen Bereich von 40-50 Hounsfield Einheiten eine dreidimensionale Hough-Transformation mit Radius 12mm angewendet, welche den Bulbus Oculi (Augapfel) als Kugel lokalisiert. Der Startpunkt wird auf den Mittelpunkt des Bulbus verschoben. Die Stabilität wird mit folgendem Experiment überprüft:

1. *Hypothese*: Das Verfahren ist unabhängig von der manuellen Wahl des Startpunktes.
2. *Durchführung*: In 3 zufällig ausgewählten Datensätzen wird die Initialisierung an jeweils 50 zufällig bestimmten Voxeln innerhalb der Orbita durchgeführt und das Volumen bestimmt.
3. *Ergebnis*: Das Verfahren wird als hinreichend stabil angesehen, wenn der Variationskoeffizient $< 5\%$ ist [3].

3 Ergebnisse

In dem entwickelten Planungswerkzeug wurden die ersten Arbeitsschritte zur Planung der operativen Rekonstruktion der Orbita bereits realisiert. CT-Daten können vom Benutzer geladen und betrachtet werden. Eine manuelle Startpunktwahl wie auch eine semi-automatische Initialisierung durch automatische Verschiebung auf die Bulbusmitte sind implementiert, sodass der Segmentierungsprozess gestartet, und die Segmentierung als Oberfläche betrachtet werden kann. Das Volumen wird auf beiden Seiten berechnet und gegenübergestellt (Abb. 1). Mit Standard-Komponenten des MITK lassen sich die Daten auch als Volumen visualisieren, Distanzen messen, sowie einzelne Achsen/Teilsegmentierungen oder Ähnliches ein- und ausblenden (Abb. 2). Die Mittelwerte, Standardabweichungen und Variationskoeffizienten der Stabilitätstests sind in Tabelle 1 dargestellt.

4 Diskussion

Die ersten Arbeitschritte zur Planung der operativen Rekonstruktion der Orbita konnten erfolgreich in ein Planungswerkzeug integriert werden, welches nun bereits wertvolle Informationen und Möglichkeiten bietet, um das Orbitavolumen von Patienten zu messen und zu beurteilen. Die Stabilität des Verfahrens konnte

Tabelle 1. Standardabweichung (cm^3), Mittelwert(cm^3) und Variationskoeffizient (%) des Volumens von Segmentierungen mit je 50 zufällig gewählten Startpunkten

Patient	σ	$\bar{x}$	$\sigma/\bar{x}$
1	0,8081	31,0066	2,6063 %
2	0,2118	22,5309	0,9399 %
3	0,1064	27,3546	0,3889 %

in einer kleinen Validierungsstudie belegt werden, da der Variationskoeffizient in allen Fällen deutlich unter 5% lag. Diese Zahlen bestätigen die Ergebnisse einer ersten nicht repräsentativen Untersuchung [7].

Eine Erweiterung des Planungswerkzeuges um die virtuelle Modellierung und Anpassung eines Gitters ist bereits in Arbeit und wird das Planungswerkzeug in seiner Funktionalität abschließen. Für den Einsatz in der klinischen Routine ist auch die Korrektheit (das gemessene Orbitavolumen entspricht dem tatsächlichen Volumen) entscheidend, welche bisher noch nicht überprüft wurde. Da wie in der medizinischen Bildverarbeitung häufig auch in dieser Anwendung keine gesicherten Ground-Truth-Informationen verfügbar sind, kann die Korrektheit nur indirekt mit einem Vergleich des Orbitavolumens rechts und links bei Patienten ohne Orbitafrakturen unter der Annahme, dass diese Volumina gleich sind, erfolgen.

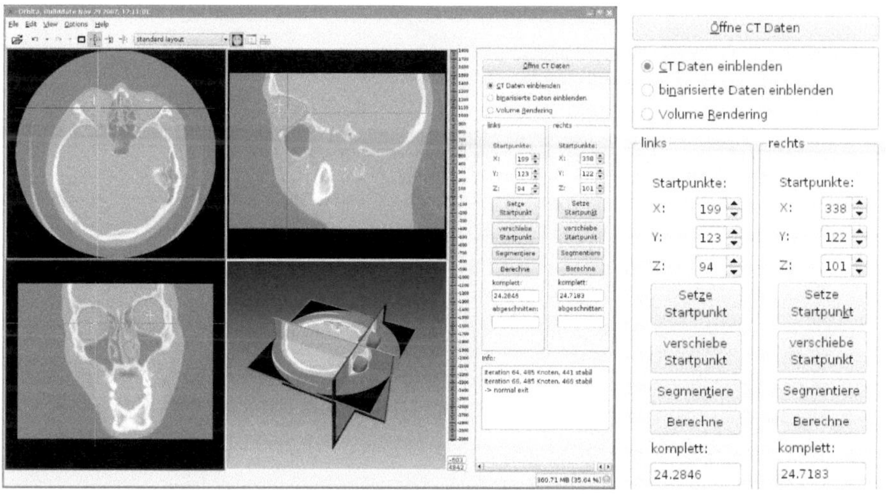

Abb. 1. MITK-basiertes Planungswerkzeug. Die übersichtlichen Funktionstasten sind im rechten Teil der Abbildung vergrößert dargestellt. Für linke und rechte Seite können die Arbeitsschritte: Setzen und Korrigieren der Startpunkte, Segmentierung und Volumenberechnung einzeln durchgeführt werden

Abb. 2. Verschiedene mit MITK generierte 3D Ansichten der segmentierten Orbita

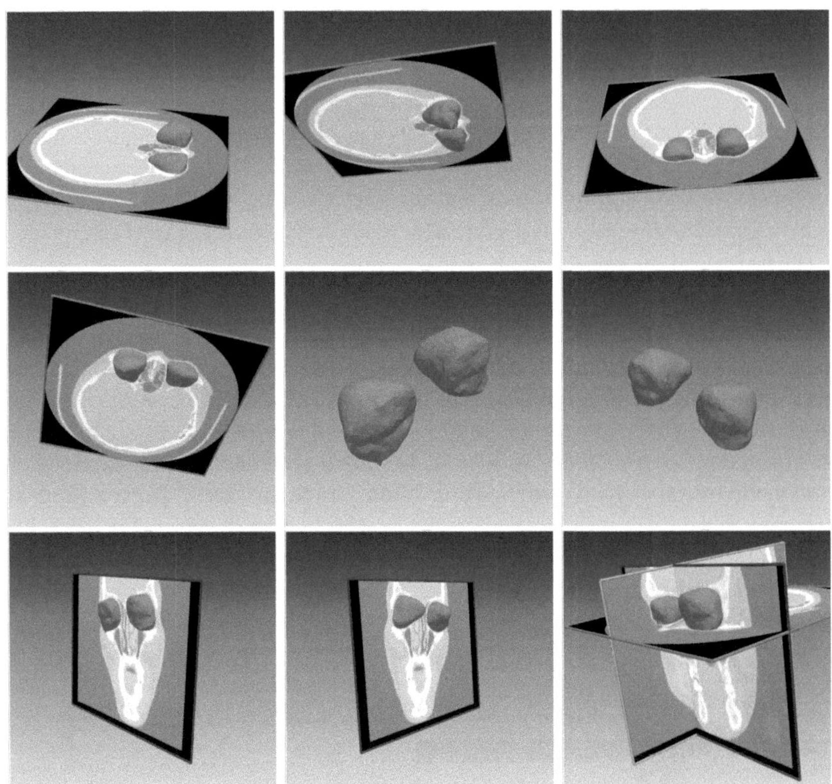

Literaturverzeichnis

1. Shere JL, Boole JR, Holtel MR, et al. An analysis of 3599 midfacial and 1141 orbital blow out fractures among 4426 United States Army Soldiers, 1980-2000. Otolaryngology;130(2):164–70.
2. Bredno J, Lehmann TM, Spitzer K. A general discrete contour model in 2, 3 and 4 dimensions for topology-adaptive multi-channel segmentation. IEEE Trans Pattern Anal Mach Intell. 2003;25(5):550–63.
3. Lehmann TM. Digitale Bildverarbeitung für Routineanwendungen. Deutscher Universitätsverlag, Wiesbaden; 2005.
4. Wolf I, Vetter M, Wegner I, et al. The Medical Imaging Interaction Toolkit (MITK): A toolkit facilitating the creation of interactive software by extending VTK and ITK. Proc SPIE. 2004;5367:16–27.
5. Bitter I, Uitert RV, Wolf I, et al. Comparison of four freely available frameworks for image processing and visualization that use ITK. IEEE Trans Vis Comput Graph. 2007;13(3):483–93.
6. Winter A, Ammenwerth E, Brigl B, et al. Krankenhausinformationssysteme; 2005. In: Handbuch der Medizinischen Informatik, München: Hanser Verlag.
7. Deserno TM, Kleiner MEH, Schulze D, et al. Automatic volumetry for surgical reconstruction of the orbit; 2007. Poster presented at MedInfo2007, Brisbane.

In-Vivo Targeting of Liver Lesions with a Navigation System Based on Fiducial Needles

L. Maier-Hein[1], A. Tekbas[2], A. Seitel[1], F. Pianka[2], S.A. Müller[2], S. Schawo[3], B. Radeleff[3], R. Tetzlaff[1,4], A. Franz[1], A.-M. Rau[1,4], I. Wolf[1], H.-U. Kauczor[4], B.M. Schmied[2], H.-P. Meinzer[1]

[1]German Cancer Research Center, Div. of Medical and Biological Informatics
[2]University of Heidelberg, Dept. of General, Abdominal and Transplant Surgery
[3]University of Heidelberg, Dept. of Diagnostic Radiology
[4]German Cancer Research Center, Dept. of Radiology
l.maier-hein@dkfz-heidelberg.de

Abstract. We assessed the targeting precision of a previously reported needle-based soft tissue navigation system in-vivo. Eight 2 ml agar nodules were implanted into the livers of two swine as tumor models. One medical expert with experience in punctures and one non-expert used the navigation system to target each nodule twice. The targeting error, which includes the system error and the user error, was defined as the distance between the applicator tip and the center of gravity of the lesions in computed tomography (CT) control scans and was 5.3 ± 2.2 mm ($n = 16$) for the expert, 3.2 ± 1.3 mm ($n = 16$) for the non-expert, and 4.2 ± 2.1 mm ($n = 32$) averaged over both subjects. A robust targeting precision of the order of magnitude of 4 mm could improve the treatment standard for CT-guided minimally invasive interventions in the liver dramatically.

1 Introduction

Computed tomography (CT) guided minimally invasive procedures in the liver such as tumor biopsy and thermal ablation therapy frequently require the targeting of hepatic structures that are subject to breathing motion. Unfortunately, commercially available navigation systems are still restricted to applications for rigid structures, such as the skull or the spine. To address this issue, several research groups (e.g. [1, 2, 3, 4]) are investigating methods for compensating organ motion during soft tissue interventions. Different approaches for assessing the accuracy of the navigation systems developed in this context have been applied in the published studies. Zhang et al. [2] implanted tumor models containing radio-opaque CT contrast medium into a silicon liver model mounted on a motion simulator and also conducted experiments in swine with agar injections as nodular targets. Kahn et al. [3] evaluated their navigation system in human cadavers, with three different targets: a predefined position within the ascending aorta, a calcified plaque in an artery, and the tip of a port catheter. Fichtinger et al. [1] conducted experiments in ventilated swine cadavers and used stainless-steel staples as targets.

In a previous report [4], we introduced a needle-based navigation system for minimally invasive interventions in the liver, in which a real-time deformation model is used to estimate the position of a navigation target point continuously from a set of optically tracked navigation aids (Fig. 1). The overall targeting accuracy of the system was assessed ex-vivo with a respiratory liver motion simulator and was 3.5 ± 1.1 mm on average. In this study, we assess the accuracy of our system in-vivo by performing 32 needle punctures in two swine.

2 Materials und Methods

2.1 Navigation System

Our navigation concept, which has been presented and discussed in detail in previous works (e.g. [4]), is illustrated in Figure 2.1: Prior to the intervention, a set of fiducial needles (*navigation aids*) is placed in the vicinity of the lesion (i). Next, a planning CT scan is acquired (ii), which is used to plan a trajectory from the skin towards the target (iii). The navigation aids are localized in the CT image and the registration of the CT coordinate system with the tracking coordinate system is performed based on the positions of the fiducial needles (iv). During the intervention, a real-time deformation model is used to continuously estimate the position of the target point from the current positions of the optically tracked navigation aids (v).

2.2 Accuracy Assessment

This study was approved by the committee on animal care and research of the Regierungspräsidium Karlsruhe. We injected eight 2 ml agar nodules into the livers of two ventilated swine as tumor models (5% agar dilution mixed with contrast agent 1:15 v/v dilution). Note that a volume of 2 ml corresponds to a diameter of approximately 1.5 cm for spherical lesions. One medical expert with experience in punctures (E) and one fourth-year medical student (NE)

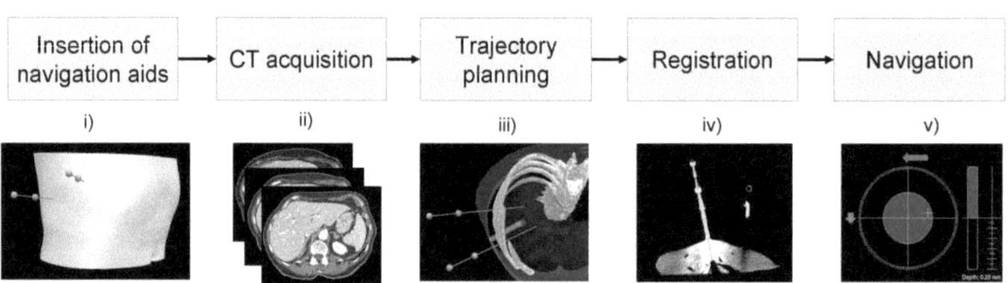

Fig. 1. Soft tissue navigation concept

with no experience in punctures used the navigation system to target each lesion twice (two *passes*). For each pass, an ultrasound (US) device was used to insert the navigation aids such that they were arranged along the cranio-caudal axis of the animal and did not pass a lesion. Silicon patches were utilized to attach the needles firmly to the skin. Both subjects then targeted the set of four lesions according to the following procedure: In an initial preparation step, a planning CT scan was acquired (Toshiba Aquilion 16 slice multidetector CT scanner (Toshiba, Tokyo, Japan); 1 mm slice thickness) showing the entire set of lesions and both navigation aids. Next, the navigation aid models were registered with the planning CT image. For each lesion, the following workflow was then applied:

1. *Trajectory planning*: The lesion was segmented semi-automatically on the basis of the graph-cut algorithm [5] and the navigation target point was set to the center of gravity of the segmented lesion. Next, an insertion point was chosen on the skin such that the trajectory to the target point did not pass any risk structures.
2. *Registration*: In order to register the tracking coordinate system with the CT coordinate system, we monitored the movement of the fiducial needles over two breathing cycles. For each recorded sample k (i.e., eight times per second), we computed the landmark-based rigid transformation Φ_k yielding the smallest fiducial registration error (FRE) according to the least square method. A set of corresponding control points distributed along the registered and tracked navigation aids served as landmarks for this purpose. The transformation $\tilde{\Phi}$ yielding the smallest FRE within the two breathing cycles was then chosen as coordinate transformation.
3. *Navigation*: We used an optically tracked instrument to target the agar nodule with the navigation system. The targeting procedure was conducted at end-expiration in 20 sec intervals, i.e., the intervention was interrupted every

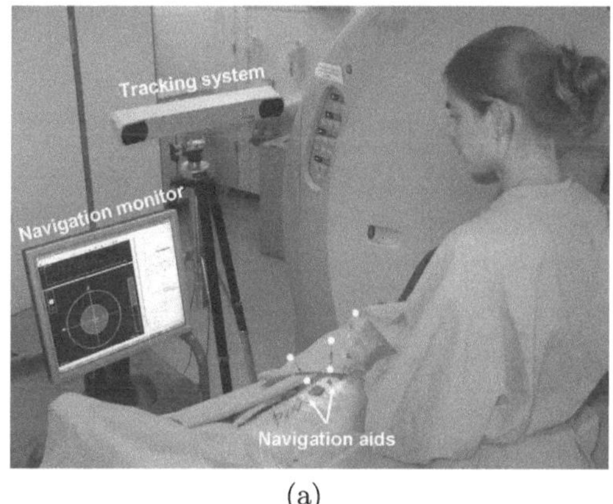

(a)

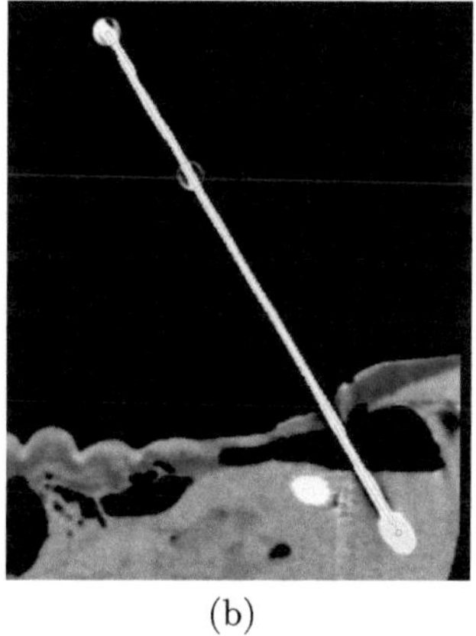

(b)

Fig. 2. Experimental setup (a) and control CT scan (b) showing the registered instrument, the segmented lesion within the liver and the center of gravity of the lesion (circle)

Table 1. CT targeting error (in mm) for the individual trials of the expert (E) and the non-expert (NE).

Lesion	*E, pass 1*	*E, pass 2*	*NE, pass 1*	*NE, pass 2*
Swine 1				
L1	3.7	5.6	2.0	2.0
L2	6.2	3.9	5.1	2.1
L3	7.8	4.4	2.9	3.5
L4	3.1	2.4	2.3	2.3
Swine 2				
L1	5.8	5.2	1.0	3.2
L2	6.1	11.6	6.1	3.8
L3	3.8	6.3	3.3	3.4
L4	3.4	5.0	4.4	2.9

20 sec to ventilate the swine. A navigation monitor provided the visualization for the targeting process (Fig. 2a).

4. *Post-processing*: A CT scan was acquired with the same settings as for the planning CT. The lesion in the control CT image was segmented semi-automatically with the graph-cut algorithm [5], and the reference target position was set to the center of gravity of the segmented lesion (Fig. 2b). The instrument model was then registered with the control CT image and the distance between the computed target point and the position of the instrument tip was recorded as the CT targeting error.

3 Results

Our navigation system was successfully applied for 32 needle punctures according to the workflow described above. The lesions were successfully hit in 97% of all trials (31 out of 32) with a mean fiducial registration error (FRE) of 0.9 ± 0.3 mm (max: 1.7 mm) for computation of the coordinate transformation. The mean final distance between the instrument tip and the center of gravity of the segmented agar nodule was 5.3 ± 2.2 mm (n = 16) for the expert, 3.2 ± 1.3 mm (n = 16) for the non-expert, and 4.2 ± 2.1 mm (n = 32) averaged over both subjects. The results for the individual trials are shown in Table 1. According to the Wilcoxon test, the non-expert obtained significantly better results than the medical expert.

4 Discussion

We assessed the targeting precision of a previously reported soft tissue navigation system and obtained a mean targeting error of 4.2 ± 2.1 mm for 32 needle punctures. The measured error incorporates the *system error*, whose main sources are the CT registration error, the needle tracking error, and the error of the deformation model, and the *user error* which results from an inaccurate needle insertion. It is worth mentioning in this context, that both participants in this study reported a shift of the instrument once they released it to allow for the control CT scan acquisition. Despite the fact that they were allowed to adjust the position until they were satisfied with the targeting error given by the tracking system, optimal positioning was not always possible due to the weight of the instrument and the relatively small layer of tissue between the skin and some of the lesions. One of the lesions shown in Figure 2b, for instance, was located very close to the liver capsule. The non-expert was more successful in inserting the instrument such that it did not move considerably upon release and thus achieved a better user error and therewith CT targeting error.

The main drawback of our navigation concept is the fact that the insertion of two fiducial needles initially increases the invasiveness of an intervention. On the other hand, tracking points *inside* the target organ for motion compensation potentially leads to high accuracy and can thus eliminate the requirement for repeated needle insertions. In fact, our targeting accuracy is higher than that published in related work. Zhang et al. [2] reported a success rate of 87.5% (n = 16) in a silicon liver mounted onto a motion simulator and a mean targeting error of 8.3 ± 3.7 mm (n = 32) in swine. Other groups obtained mean errors of 8.4 ± 1.8 mm (n = 42) in human cadavers [3] and 6.4 ± 1.8 (n = 22) in ventilated swine [1].

From a clinical point of view, a robust targeting precision of the order of magnitude of 4 mm would improve the treatment standard for CT-guided minimally invasive interventions in the liver dramatically. To advance clinical application of our method we are currently conducting a study for comparing the conventional method for CT-guided needle insertions with our approach with respect to accuracy, time, and radiation exposure to the patient.

References

1. Fichtinger G, Deguet A, Fischer G, et al. Image overlay for CT-guided needle insertions. Comp Aid Surg. 2005;10(4):241–55.
2. Banovac HZF, Lin R, et al. Electromagnetic tracking for abdominal interventions in computer aided surgery. Comp Aid Surg. 2006;11(3):127–36.
3. Khan MF, Dogan S, Maataoui A, et al. Navigation-based needle puncture of a cadaver using a hybrid tracking navigational system. Invest Radiol. 2006;41(10):713–20.
4. Maier-Hein L, Pianka F, Seitel A, et al. Precision targeting of liver lesions with a needle-based soft tissue navigation system. Proc MICCAI. 2007;4792(2):42–9.
5. Boykov Y, Kolmogorov V. An experimental comparison of min-cut/max-flow algorithms for energy minimization in vision. IEEE Trans Pattern Anal Mach Intell. 2004;26(9):1124–137.

Planungsunterstützung für Pankreasoperationen bei Hyperinsulinismus von Kindern

J. Dornheim[1], B. Preim[1], U. Preim[1], K. Mohnike[1], O. Blankenstein[2], F. Füchtner[2], W. Mohnike[3], S. Empting[1], K. Mohnike[1]

[1]Otto-von-Guericke-Universität Magdeburg
[2]Charite Universitätsmedizin Berlin
[3]Diagnostisch Therapeutisches Zentrum am Frankfurter Tor, Berlin
jana.dornheim@isg.cs.uni-magdeburg.de

Kurzfassung. Auf Basis von sechs PET/CT-Datensätzen des Pankreas wird eine Computerunterstützung für die Teilresektion der Bauchspeicheldrüse (Pankreas) bei fokalem Hyperinsulinismus von Kindern entwickelt. Ziel ist es, die Lokalisation des krankhaften Fokus im Pankreasgewebe präoperativ dreidimensional zu visualisieren, um so die Sicherheit des Eingriffs zu erhöhen. Die relevanten anatomischen Strukturen werden im CT segmentiert und anschließend dreidimensional visualisiert. Der im PET erkennbare Fokus wird in diese anatomische 3D-Visualisierung eingeblendet. Es zeigt sich eine klare Erkennbarkeit des Fokus in allen sechs Fällen.

1 Einleitung

Der kongenitale Hyperinsulinismus ist eine schwerwiegende Erkrankung der Bauchspeicheldrüse (Pankreas), die meist im ersten Lebensjahr diagnostiziert wird (ca. 15–20 Fälle p.a. in Deutschland). Aufgrund der andauernden Produktion von Insulin erleiden die Patienten häufig schwere Hypoglykämien, die zu statomotorischen und geistigen Entwicklungsstörungen führen können. Zur Vermeidung von Hirnschäden ist die schnelle differentialdiagnostische Abklärung mit entsprechender Therapieeinleitung notwendig. Hierbei ist die Unterscheidung zwischen fokaler und diffuser Form entscheidend: Bei der *fokalen* Form (30–40 % aller Fälle) ist das erkrankte Pankreasgewebe herdförmig abgrenzbar und daher einer Teilresektion zugänglich, d.h. nur der erkrankte Fokus im Pankreasgewebe wird entfernt.

Der Fokus ist für den Operateur nicht sichtbar und nur durch eine begleitende Gewebeuntersuchung darzustellen. Daher hängt die Therapieentscheidung sowie der Erfolg des Eingriffs maßgeblich davon ab, wie gut der Chirurg im Vorfeld der Operation die Lage des Fokus einschätzen kann. Liegt der Fokus beispielsweise ventral auf dem Pankreasschwanz auf, so kann ein schonender endoskopischer Zugang gewählt werden. Liegt er hingegen im Pankreaskopf in unmittelbarere Nähe empfindlicher anatomischer Strukturen (Gallengang, Pankreasgang, versorgende Gefäße) muss die Operationsplanung dies berücksichtigen (z.B. Y-Roux-Plastik).

Die neueste Entwicklung kombinierter PET/CT-Geräte ermöglicht die Identifizierung des Fokus und seine anatomische Lokalisation [1, 2]. Ziel dieser Arbeit war es, auf dieser Basis die Lage des Fokus im Pankreas zu visualisieren, um so die präoperative Planung zu unterstützen. Hierzu sollten die für die Operationsplanung relevanten anatomischen Strukturen aus den CT-Aufnahmen segmentiert und räumlich visualisiert werden. Anschließend erfolgte die Lokalisation des Fokus anhand der PET-Daten und seine Einblendung in die anatomische Visualisierung.

Die hier vorgestellte Methode der Fallaufbereitung und Visualisierung der segmentierten Strukturen wurde in ähnlicher Form erfolgreich zur Planung von Halsoperationen eingesetzt [3]. Für die Visualisierung von PET-Datensätzen wird (z.B. auf radiologischen Workstations) üblicherweise ein Volumenrendering eingesetzt. Eine gemischte Darstellung aus Volumenrendering und segmentierten Strukturen in Oberflächendarstellung wird in [4] untersucht.

2 Material und Methoden

2.1 Datenmaterial

Zur Untersuchung standen 6 PET/CT-Datensätze von Patienten mit fokaler Form des kongenitalen Hyperinsulinismus zur Verfügung. Diese Datensätze enthielten jeweils einen PET-Scan des Patienten, sowie zwei CT-Datensätze in derselben Tischposition, jeweils in portalvenöser und arterieller Phase (Abb. 2.1).

Tabelle 1 zeigt die Größe und Auflösung der verwendeten Datensätze. Eine Registrierung der PET-Daten mit den CT-Datensätzen war nicht erforderlich, da durch das kombinierte PET/CT-Aufnahmeverfahren beide Aufnahmen in derselben Tischposition angefertigt wurden. Es erfolgte daher nur noch eine lineare Interpolation des PET-Datensatzes, so dass hier die Voxelanzahl mit der des CT-Datensatzes übereinstimmte.

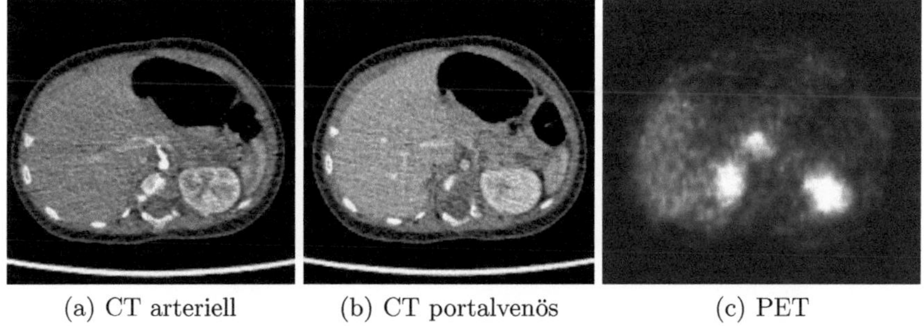

(a) CT arteriell (b) CT portalvenös (c) PET

Abb. 1. Verwendete Datensätze: kombinierter PET/CT-Scan

Tabelle 1. Übersicht der verwendeten Datensätze

	Datensatzgröße		Auflösung (mm)	
	X/Y	Z	X/Y	Z
CT-Datensätze der Patienten 1, 3, 4, 5	512	56	1.367	3.0
CT-Datensätze des Patienten 2	512	126	0.977	1.3
CT-Datensätze des Patienten 6	512	367	0.977	0.5
PET-Datensätze aller Patienten	336	55	2.036	3.0

2.2 Segmentierung

Zunächst mussten die relevanten Strukturen im CT-Datensatz segmentiert werden. Die Zielstrukturen für die Segmentierung waren das Pankreas, die V. mesenterica superior, V. hepatica, V. lienalis aus dem portalvenösen CT-Datensatz, sowie die Aorta, Tr. coeliacus, A. mesenterica superior, Pfortader und A. lienalis aus dem arteriellen CT-Datensatz.

Zur Segmentierung der Blutgefäße war es möglich, diese in jeder dritten Schicht grob durch eine Kontur abzugrenzen und innerhalb dieser Kontur mit einem Schwellenwert die Feinsegmentierung vorzunehmen. Die Segmentierung des Pankreas musste aufgrund der geringen Kontrastierung von der segmentierenden Radiologin manuell durchgeführt werden. Pro Datensatz waren auf diese Weise ca. 20 Minuten zur Segmentierung erforderlich, die Segmentierung des Pankreas nahm dabei den größten Anteil ein (ca. 15 Minuten).

2.3 Visualisierung

Aus den Segmentierungsmasken der Blutgefäße und des Pankreas wurde mit Marching Cubes jeweils eine Iso-Oberfläche erstellt, die dreidimensional visualisiert wurde. Die Farbgebung erfolgte in Anlehnung an schematische Visualisierungen in medizinischen Atlanten. Die Blutgefäße wurden ohne Transparenz dargestellt. Für die Visualisierung des Pankreas war zur Erkennung des intrapankreatischen Gefäßverlaufs und des im Pankreasgewebe befindlichen Fokus ein hoher Transparenzgrad erforderlich. Um die hohe Transparenz auszugleichen, wurde diese Darstellung mit einer Silhouette kombiniert.

Für die Einblendung des Fokus in die anatomische Visualisierung erschien ein Volumenrendering des PET-Datensatzes (Abb. 2.3(a), (b)) naheliegend. Hierzu

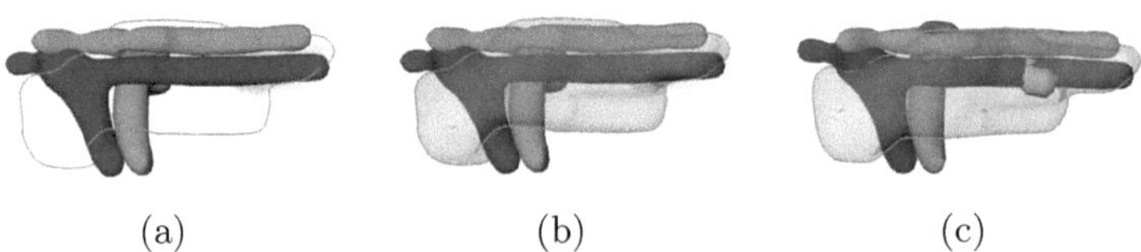

(a) (b) (c)

Abb. 2. Einblendung des Fokus: (a) Volumenrendering des Fokus (rechts oben im Bild) bei transparentem Pankreas, (b) Volumenrendering des Fokus bei semi-transparentem Pankreas (nicht erkennbar), (c) Fokus in der Oberflächendarstellung (gut erkennbar)

wurde dieser anhand des segmentierten Pankreas maskiert, so dass alle Voxel im PET-Datensatz, die außerhalb des Pankreas lagen, den Grauwert 0 erhielten. So liess sich der Fokus aus dem PET-Datensatz isolieren, während die anderen kontrastreichen Strukturen (z.B. Nieren, Blase) ausgeblendet wurden. Zur Darstellung wurde eine lineare Transferfunktion mit den Parametern *center* und *width* verwendet.

Alternativ zum Volumenrendering wurde eine Darstellung des Fokus mit einem manuell eingestellten Schwellenwert und einer daraus generierten Iso-Oberfläche des Fokus erprobt (Abb. 2.3(c)). Nach Aussage der beteiligten klinischen Partner (1 Kinderarzt, 1 Endokrinologe, 2 Kinderchirurgen) beträgt die Größe des Fokus i.A. 5 bis 6 mm; der Schwellenwert kann anhand dieser Maßgabe manuell eingestellt werden. Beide Visualisierungsoptionen wurden den klinischen Partnern zum Vergleich präsentiert.

3 Ergebnisse

Alle Datensätze konnten erfolgreich segmentiert werden. Die Segmentierungsgüte hing dabei vom Signal-Rausch-Verhältnis des Datensatzes ab und variierte stark. Aufgrund der geringen Größe der segmentierten Strukturen wirkt sich hier auch kleineres Rauschen erheblich auf die scharfe Begrenzung der Ränder aus.

Eine weitere Limitierung stellte die sehr schwache Kontrastierung des Pankreas im CT dar, aufgrund derer die Segmentierung des Pankreas selbst für einen Radiologen sehr schwierig und mit großer Unsicherheit behaftet ist. Dies wurde erschwert durch das mangelnde Fettgewebe der jungen Patienten, welches die Strukturgrenzen bei älteren Patienten klar kennzeichnet.

Hinsichtlich der Visualisierung des Pankreas wurde die semi-transparente Darstellung mit Silhouette von den klinischen Partnern befürwortet, da hier sowohl die Oberflächenform als auch die Begrenzung des Pankreas sichtbar ist.

Zur Einblendung des Fokus wurde das Volumenrendering als nicht geeignet empfunden. Gründe hierfür sind die unscharfe Begrenzung und der schwache Kontrast des Fokus im Vergleich zur Oberflächendarstellung der segmentierten Strukturen, auch bei sorgfältiger Einstellung der Parameter *center* und *width*. Als sehr zufriedenstellend wurde hingegen die Einblendung des Fokus als Iso-Oberfläche empfunden, so dass diese Darstellungsform für alle Fälle ausgewählt wurde.

Auf diese Weise konnten alle Fälle erfolgreich visualisiert werden. Abbildung 3 zeigt exemplarisch an drei Fällen die sehr gute visuelle Erkennbarkeit der Fo-

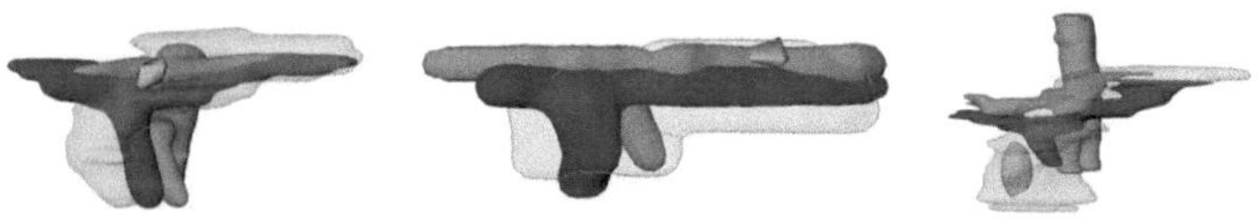

Abb. 3. Ergebnisse der Segmentierung und Visualisierung für die Patienten 2, 4 und 6

kuslokalisation, sowie der Lage zu den relevanten Blutgefäßen und zum restlichen Pankreasgewebe.

4 Diskussion

Es wurde im Rahmen dieser Arbeit erstmals ein Prozess entwickelt, der es ermöglicht, aus PET/CT-Scans der Bauchspeicheldrüse von Kindern mit einer fokalen Form des kongenitalen Hyperinsulinismus eine Visualisierung der pathologischen Situation und des Operationsgebietes zu erstellen. Die Ergebnisse zeigen, dass die Lokalisation der Läsion klar erkennbar ist und somit bereits im Vorfeld der Operation durch den Operateur eingeschätzt werden kann. Dies ermöglicht eine sicherere Operationsplanung und bessere Heilungschancen für die Patienten.

Dies bestätigt auch das Beispiel des Patienten 5, bei dem ein während der ersten Operation nicht gefundener Fokus im Pankreasschwanz erst in einer zweiten Nachoperation erfolgreich lokalisiert und entfernt werden konnte. Anhand des hier vorgestellten Prozesses konnte die Lokalisation des Fokus visualisiert werden und wäre so auch im Vorfeld der Operation klar erkennbar gewesen.

Eine Einschränkung ist aus medizinischer Sicht derzeit noch die Subjektivität der gewonnenen Darstellungen aufgrund der mit Unsicherheit behafteten Segmentierung des Pankreas. Diese Subjektivität existiert jedoch ebenso in der gegenwärtigen Planung anhand von 2D-Schnittbildern, die dem Chirurgen vom Radiologen erläutert werden. Die hier vorgestellte Computerunterstützung kann als Kommunikationsmittel des Radiologen mit dem Chirurgen betrachtet werden, welches die Subjektivität in der Beurteilung des Bildmaterials zwar nicht aufheben kann, jedoch eine bessere Visualisierung der Fokuslokalisation bietet. Eine zunehmende Objektivierung des Planungsprozesses wird angestrebt und hängt von einer besseren Kontrastierung des Pankreasgewebes im CT ab.

Weitere Arbeiten in näherer Zukunft sollen sich auf die Interaktion des Chirurgen mit dem dreidimensionalen Patientenmodell fokussieren, um direkt den Planungsprozess zu unterstützen. Dazu gehören die Einführung von Vermessungswerkzeugen, aber auch die Planung von Resektionsebenen und die automatische Bestimmung von Restvolumina.

Literaturverzeichnis

1. Mohnike, et al. Proposal for a standardized protocol for 18F-DOPA-PET (PET/CT) in congenital hyperinsulinism. Hormone Research. 2006;66(1):40–2.
2. Shield JPH. Fluorine-18 L-3,4-dihydroxyphenylalanine positron emission tomography: Improving surgery and outcome in focal hyperinsulinism. Hormone Research. 2006;66(1):43–4.
3. Cordes J, et al. Preoperative segmentation of neck CT datasets for the planning of neck dissections. Proc SPIE. 2006.
4. Englmeier, et al. Virtuelle Bronchoskopie mit Positronenemissions- und Computertomographie-Bilddaten. Jahresbericht des GSF-Forschungszentrum für Umwelt und Gesundheit in der Helmholtz-Gemeinschaft. 2005; p. 65–70.

Entwicklung und Evaluation einer Kalibrierungsmethode für 3D-Ultraschall

Christoph Bergmeir[1], Mathias Seitel[1], Christian Frank[2], Raffaele De Simone[2], Hans-Peter Meinzer[1], Ivo Wolf[1]

[1]Abteilung für Medizinische und Biologische Informatik, DKFZ Heidelberg
[2]Abteilung für Herzchirurgie, Universitätsklinikum Heidelberg
c.bergmeir@dkfz.de

Kurzfassung. Wir stellen eine Methode zur Kalibrierung einer 3D-Ultraschallsonde vor. Für Anwendungen in der minimalinvasiven Chirurgie wird die Ultraschallsonde mit einem Trackingsystem verbunden, um dem Aufnahmevolumen eine definierte räumliche Lage zu geben. Die Kalibrierung bringt die Koordinatensysteme des Trackingsystems und des Ultraschallbildes zur Deckung. Hierzu wird ein bekanntes Objekt, das Phantom, aufgenommen und im Ultraschallbild lokalisiert. Die Kalibrierungstransformation wird dann durch ein Verfahren der Hand-Auge-Kalibrierung errechnet. Ein oft übliches Anbringen zusätzlicher Trackingssensoren am Phantom ist damit nicht nötig, was die Kalibrierungsprozedur vereinfacht.

1 Einleitung

Bildgebung mittels Ultraschall ist ein wichtiger Bestandteil vieler diagnostischer und therapeutischer Verfahren in der Medizin. Bringt man Positionssensoren eines Trackingsystems an der Ultraschallsonde an, so kann auf die räumliche Lage des aufgenommenen Bildes geschlossen werden. Hierbei ist eine Kalibrierung nötig, um die Trackingkoordinaten in Bildkoordinaten umrechnen zu können. Neben der Standardanwendung für solch ein System, dem Freihand-3D-Ultraschall [1], existieren auch Anwendungsgebiete in der bildgestützten Chirurgie oder der Bestrahlungstherapie [2, 3]. Für die Kalibrierung werden üblicherweise Aufnahmen eines bekannten Objektes, des Phantoms, gemacht. Dessen Lage wird dann im Bild mit Segmentierungs- und Registrierungsverfahren ermittelt, woraus sich anschließend die Kalibrierungstransformation bestimmen lässt. Wird neben der Sonde auch das Phantom getrackt, so reicht eine einzige Aufnahme zur Kalibrierung aus, es müssen jedoch Trackingsensoren mit hoher Genauigkeit am Phantom angebracht werden. Andernfalls sind mindestens drei Aufnahmen aus verschiedenen Richtungen nötig [4], um die Kalibrierungstransformation mit Verfahren der aus der Robotik bekannten Hand-Auge-Kalibrierung [4, 5] zu errechnen. Die Kalibrierung von 2D- und 3D-Sonden ist nur bedingt vergleichbar. Einerseits kann bei 3D-Sonden durch die große Datenmenge besser Redundanz erzeugt werden und ein bei 2D-Bildern manchmal schwieriges Auffinden des Phantoms und Rückrechnen seiner ursprünglichen Geometrie entfällt. Andererseits jedoch sind die einzelnen Schichten bei 3D meist schlechter aufgelöst. Zur Kalibrierung von 2D-Ultraschallsonden finden sich viele Arbeiten in der Literatur [1]. In Bezug auf 3D-Sonden lassen sich nur wenige Arbeiten finden, sowohl im Hinblick auf getrackte Phantome [3, 6], als auch zu Hand-Auge-Kalibrierungsmethoden [7, 8]. Wir verwenden im Unterschied zu diesen den Algorithmus von Daniilidis [5], welcher auf herkömmlichen Einsatzgebieten der Hand-Auge-Kalibrierung oft zum Einsatz kommt [9, 10]. Der Algorithmus weist einige Vorteile in Robustheit und Genauigkeit gegenüber anderen Verfahren auf [5].

2 Material und Methoden

Wir benutzen ein SONOS 7500 Ultraschallgerät zusammen mit der 3D Ultraschallsonde X4 (beides Philips Medical Systems). Die Sonde wird mit einem optischen System (Polaris, Northern Digital) getrackt. Hierzu sind vier passive Marker an ihr befestigt (Abb. 1).

Als Phantom dient eine Anordnung von fünf Nylonfäden, welche in einer aus Plexiglas gefertigten Vorrichtung eingespannt ist (Abb. 2(a)). Drei Nylonfäden spannen dabei ein orthogonales Kreuz auf, die beiden anderen sind so angebracht, dass das Kreuz unter Rotation eindeutig wird. Das Phantom steht in einer mit Leitungswasser gefüllten Kunststoffbox. Für eine Analyse der Rekonstruktionsgenauigkeit sind auch am Phantom Sensoren des Trackingsystems angebracht, deren Positionsdaten als Goldstandard dienen. Die Sonde ist an einem beweglichen Arm montiert (hierzu dient eine handelsübliche Schwanenhalslampe), was sowohl eine einfache Positionierung der Sonde erlaubt als auch gewährleistet, dass die Sonde während der Aufnahmen fixiert ist. Nun können Datensätze aus Ultraschallbildern und zugehörigen Trackingdaten aus verschiedenen Richtungen aufgenommen werden. Während einer Ultraschallaufnahme wird laufend die Position erfasst und anschließend über diese Datensätze gemittelt. Da die

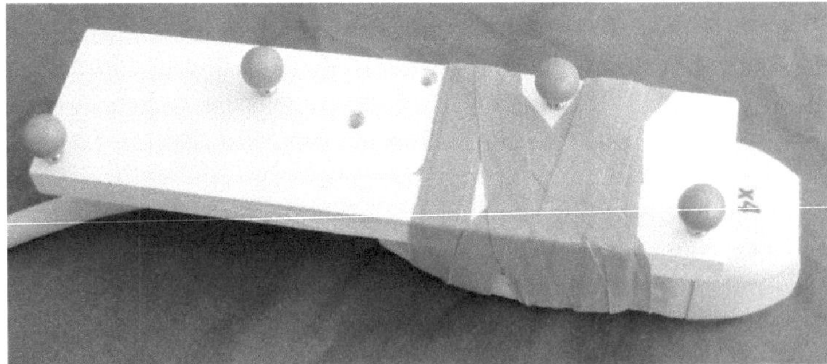

Abb. 1. Eine Ultraschallsonde, welche mit Sensoren eines optischen Trackingsystems kombiniert ist. Somit ist es möglich, die Position und Orientierung der Sonde im Raum zu bestimmen und nach einer Kalibrierung das Bild der Sonde in ein physikalisches Weltkoordinatensystem zu transformieren

Schallgeschwindigkeit in Wasser bei Raumtemperatur von der durchschnittlichen Schallgeschwindigkeit in menschlichem Gewebe abweicht, werden die erhobenen Bilddaten zunächst mit Hilfe eines Skalierungsfaktors von 1.04 vorverarbeitet [1]. Anschließend segmentieren wir das Kreuz mittels eines klassischen Regionenwachstumsverfahrens mit Grauwertintervall und registrieren ein Computermodell der Nylonfäden auf die Segmentierung in einem zweistufigen Verfahren. Im ersten Schritt wird sowohl aus dem Modell als auch aus der Segmentierung durch eine zufällige Abtastung eine Punktwolke erstellt und die quadratischen Abstände der Punktwolken werden minimiert. Da das Ultraschallgerät die Nylonfäden leicht verschwommen darstellt, kann im zweiten Schritt das Originalbild direkt als Distanzkarte dienen, um das Ergebnis des ersten Schrittes weiter zu verbessern (die einzelnen Verarbeitungsschritte illustriert Abb. 2).

Pro Kalibrierung kommen 12 Datensätze zum Einsatz, wobei das Phantom aus vier verschiedenen Raumrichtungen gescannt und die Sonde pro Raumrichtung in drei verschiedene Orientierungen gebracht wird. Die Sonde hat jeweils einen Abstand von ca. 6 cm zum Kreuzmittelpunkt. Zur eigentlichen Hand-Auge-Kalibrierung kommt der geschlossene Lösungsansatz nach Daniilidis [5] zum Einsatz. Dieser beruht darauf, dass gemäß der Screw-Theorie [4] Rotation

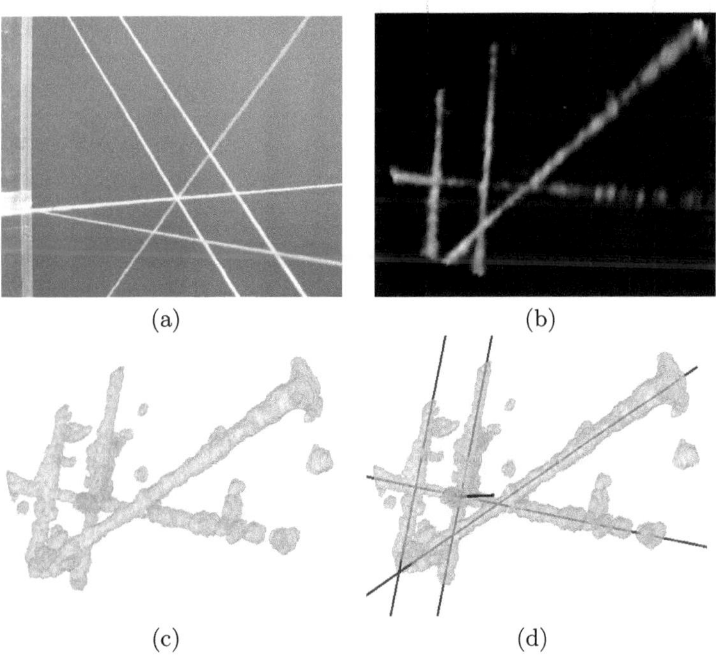

Abb. 2. Die einzelnen Verarbeitungsschritte der Phantomsdetektion. (a) Phantom, bestehend aus Nylonfäden, welche durch eine Plexiglasvorrichtung gespannt werden (am linken Bildrand zu sehen). (b) Ausgewählte Schicht des von der Sonde aufgenommenen Ultraschallvolumens. (c) Dreidimensionale Visualisierung des Ergebnisses des Regionenwachstumsverfahrens. (d) Ergebnis einer Registrierung des Computermodells

und Translation zu einer schraubenförmigen Bewegung zusammengefasst werden können. Algebraisch kann dies durch duale Quaternionen repräsentiert werden. Dadurch lässt sich die Hand-Auge-Kalibrierung in eine Form bringen, welche mit Hilfe einer Singulärwertzerlegung gelöst werden kann.

3 Ergebnisse

Die Kalibrierung wurde 14 mal durchgeführt, wodurch sich insgesamt 168 Datensätze ergaben. Damit bestimmten wir die Kalibrierungswiederholbarkeit. Es ergaben sich Standardabweichungen von 1.26 mm, 1.38 mm und 1.46 mm in den Koordinatenrichtungen und 1.01°, 0.45° und 1.51° in den Eulerwinkeln. Dann berechneten wir die mittlere Kalibrierungstransformation und bestimmten die Rekonstruktionsgenauigkeit, indem wir mit der Kalibrierung die Position und Orientierung des Phantoms in allen Aufnahmen errechneten und diese Daten mit den unabhängig davon erhobenen Daten der am Phantom angebrachten Trackingsensoren verglichen (wodurch dieser Wert auch einen Fehleranteil des als Goldstandard verwendeten Trackingsystems enthält, welcher als klein gegenüber dem Gesamtfehler angenommen wird). Der quadratische Mittelwert des Fehlers ergab sich zu 1.29 mm, 1.84 mm und 1.43 mm in den Koordinatenrichtungen und 1.5°, 1.29° und 1.57° in den Eulerwinkeln. Die Ergebnisse illustriert Abb. 3.

4 Diskussion

Das vorgestellte Verfahren erlaubt eine einfache, schnelle Kalibrierung einer optisch getrackten 3D-Ultraschallsonde. Anders als bei 2D-Sonden entfällt ein aufwändiges Ausrichten der Schnittebene und es reichen bereits wenige Volumenaufnahmen aus, um eine Kalibrierung durchzuführen. Wir konnten zeigen, dass

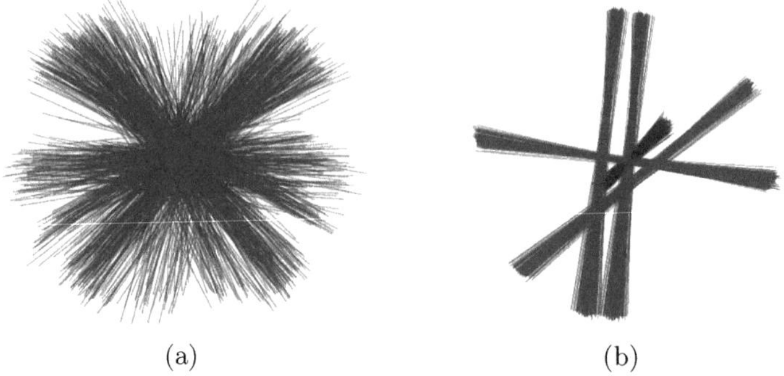

(a) (b)

Abb. 3. Die in den angefertigten Aufnahmen detektierten Kreuze in originaler Lage (a) bzw. mit Hilfe der Kalibrierungstransformation rekonstruiert und auf die als Goldstandard verwendeten Trackingdaten bezogen (b). Die gezeigten Modelle der Nylonfäden haben eine Länge von 26 cm

sich der geschlossene Lösungsansatz von Daniilidis hierfür verwenden lässt, wodurch die Kalibrierung mit wenig Rechenzeit brauchbare Ergebnisse liefert. Die in der Literatur mit getracktem Phantom erreichte Genauigkeit von 1 - 2 mm [3, 6] ist etwas besser als die hier erzielte von ca. 3 - 4 mm. Im Gegenzug ist bei unserer Methode das Tracken des Phantoms überflüssig, was die Prozedur vereinfacht. Für bestimmte Navigationsanwendungen, beispielsweise in der Ausbildung, sollte die von uns erzielte Genauigkeit ausreichen. Im Unterschied zu herkömmlicher Hand-Auge-Kalibrierung einer Kamera besitzt die Ultraschallkalibrierung einige weitere Fehlerquellen, welche die Genauigkeit generell limitieren. So ist die Qualität der Bilder grundsätzlich eher schlecht, was sich negativ auf die Registrierungsgenauigkeit auswirkt. Dadurch, dass die vom Ultraschallgerät angenommene Schallgeschwindigkeit von der im Becken abweicht, können sich zusätzlich systematische Fehler ergeben. Auch wirkt sich die Wahl der Aufnahmerichtungen auf die Genauigkeit aus [9]. Die Ungenauigkeiten resultieren somit weniger aus dem Softwaresystem an sich, als vielmehr aus der Beschaffenheit des Phantoms und dem Versuchsablauf. Einer der nächsten Schritte wird deshalb sein, das Phantom weiter hinsichtlich seiner klaren Sichtbarkeit im Ultraschall zu optimieren und den Versuchsablauf zu standardisieren. Auch liegt es nahe, die ohnehin bereits zur Evaluation erhobenen Trackingdaten des Phantoms zur Kalibrierung zu nutzen, um verschiedene Verfahren vergleichen zu können.

Literaturverzeichnis

1. Mercier L, Lango T, Lindseth F, et al. A review of calibration techniques for freehand 3-D ultrasound systems. Ultrasound Med Biol. 2005;31:449–71.
2. Hassenpflug P, Vetter M, Wolf I, et al. Generation of attributed relational vessel-graphs from three-dimensional freehand ultrasound for intraoperative registration in image-guided liver surgery. Proc SPIE. 2003;5029:222–30.
3. Bouchet LG, Meeks SL, Goodchild G, et al. Calibration of three-dimensional ultrasound images for image-guided radiation therapy. Phys Med Biol. 2001;46:559–77.
4. Chen HH. A screw motion approach to uniqueness analysis of head-eye geometry. Proc IEEE Computer Vision and Pattern Recognition. 1991; p. 145–51.
5. Daniilidis K. Hand-eye calibration using dual quaternions. Int Journ Robotics Res. 1999;18:286–98.
6. Poon TC, Rohling RN. Comparison of calibration methods for spatial tracking of a 3-D ultrasound probe. Ultrasound Med Biol. 2005;31:1095–108.
7. Lange T, Eulenstein S. Calibration of swept-volume 3D ultrasound. Proc Medical Image Understandig and Analysis. 2002.
8. Boctor EM, Iordachita I, Fichtinger G, et al. Ultrasound self-calibration. Proc SPIE. 2006;6141:784–95.
9. Schmidt J, Vogt F, Niemann H. Robust Hand-Eye Calibration of an Endoscopic Surgery Robot Using Dual Quaternions. Proc DAGM. 2003; p. 548–56.
10. Vogt F, Krüger S, Winter M, et al. Erweiterte Realität und 3-D Visualisierung für minimal-invasive Operationen durch Einsatz eines optischen Trackingsystems. Proc BVM. 2005; p. 217–21.

Tracking und Segmentierung baumförmiger, tubulärer Strukturen mit einem hybriden Verfahren

Philipp Wolber[1], Ingmar Wegner[1], Tobias Heimann[1], Michael Puderbach[2], Ivo Wolf[1], Hans-Peter Meinzer[1]

[1]Abt. Medizinische und Biologische Informatik, Deutsches Krebsforschungszentrum
[2]Abt. Radiologie, Deutsches Krebsforschungszentrum
p.wolber@dkfz-heidelberg.de

Kurzfassung. Bereichswachstumsverfahren weisen bei der Segmentierung von tubulären Strukturen geringe Laufzeiten auf, bergen aber die Gefahr von Übersegmentierungen in Form von Auslaufen in benachbarte Strukturen in sich. Modellbasierte Verfahren liefern hier robustere Ergebnisse, sind jedoch deutlich rechenintensiver. Dieser Beitrag beschreibt die Entwicklung eines Verfahrens, welches die Zentralgeometrie eines Gefäßbaumes per erweitertem Bereichswachstum segmentiert und ein modellbasiertes Verfahren für die Peripherie anschließt. Die Ergebnisse zeigen eine Verbesserung der Resultate bei akzeptabler Laufzeiterhöhung gegenüber Bereichswachstumsverfahren.

1 Einleitung

Die Segmentierung baumförmiger tubulärer Strukturen findet in der medizinischen Bildverarbeitung bei der Extraktion von Blutgefäßen, aber auch bei der Kennzeichnung des Tracheobronchialbaums Anwendung. Speziell letztgenannte Anwendung kann für eine Segmentierung mit Bereichswachstumsverfahren problematisch sein. Das Verfahren ist zwar in der Lage, die komplexe Baumstruktur zu erfassen; der sich stetig reduzierende Kontrast zwischen Gefäß und Hintergrund in den unteren Baumebenen bereitet jedoch Schwierigkeiten. Erreicht der Wachstumsprozess die Peripherie, treten durch die Kombination von verminderter Wanddicke und Partialvolumeneffekten im Bild Löcher in der Gefäßwand auf. Dies führt dazu, dass der Wachstumsprozess in umliegende Bereiche ausläuft. Die hieraus resultierende Segmentierung entspricht nicht der gefragten Struktur und muss mit modifizierten Parametern neu erstellt werden, was die Performance des Bereichswachstumsverfahrens stark einschränkt. Das Auffinden des größtmöglichen Intervalls der Grauwerte, in dem kein Auslaufen stattfindet, stellt einen zusätzlichen Aufwand dar.

Modellbasierte Verfahren wie Modell-zu-Bild-Registrierung [1], Pattern Matching [2] oder Aktive Formmodelle [3] sind gegenüber Störungen wie Bildrauschen und Partialvolumeneffekten deutlich robuster. Ihre Performance hängt jedoch stark von der Qualität des zugrundeliegenden Modells ab. In den oberen

Bereichen der Baumstruktur weicht die Form der „Äste“ oft von idealisierten Modellen ab. Krankheitsbedingte Deformationen, beispielsweise durch Tumore, stellen eine zusätzliche Herausforderung dar. Die Erstellung der Modelle (beispielsweise aus Trainingsdatensätzen) ist mit zusätzlichem Aufwand verbunden.

Betrachtet man die Stärken und Schwächen beider Ansätze, liegt folgender Entwurf nahe: Ein hybrides Verfahren, welches mit einem Bereichswachstumsverfahren die Zentralgeometrie mit großer Geschwindigkeit segmentiert, detektiert im Anschluss die peripheren Äste mit einem modellbasierten Tracking. Die Ergebnisse der Verfolgung werden anschließend mit einem lokalen Bereichswachstumsverfahren zu einer Segmentierung erweitert.

2 Material und Methoden

Zur Implementierung des vorgestellten Verfahrens wurden die quelloffenen C++ Klassenbibliotheken Insight Segmentation and Registration Toolkit (ITK) und Medical Imaging Interaction Toolkit (MITK) verwendet.

2.1 Vorsegmentierung

Ein im ITK vorhandener Filter zur Segmentierung per Bereichswachstumsverfahren (Region Growing) wurde dahingehend erweitert, dass in einem Berechnungsdurchgang Segmentierungen für ein ganzes Intervall von Schwellwerten berechnet werden, ohne dabei die Laufzeit gegenüber dem ursprünglichen Verfahren wesentlich zu verlängern. Aus diesen wird derjenige mit maximal möglicher Segmentierung ohne Auslaufen ins Lungenparenchym ausgewählt.Gegebenenfalls kann die automatische Schwellwertbestimmung interaktiv korrigiert werden, wobei eine erneute Durchführung des Verfahrens nicht notwendig ist, was die Bestimmung der optimalen Schwellwerte enorm erleichtert. Ein ähnliches Verfahren, welches auf einer Maximierung des mittleren Gradienten an der Regionengrenze beruht, wurde in [4] präsentiert.

Aus der somit erstellten Segmentierung wird über einen Skelettierungsalgorithmus eine Baumrepräsentation erstellt [5]. Anschließend werden aus dem Baum die Positionen der Blattknoten, sowie deren Orientierung und der Durchmesser der lokal vorliegenden Segmentierung ermittelt. Diese Informationen werden als Startwerte für das anschließende modellbasierte Verfahren verwendet.

2.2 Modellbasiertes Tracking tubulärer Strukturen

Um den weiteren Verlauf der tubulären Struktur auffinden zu können, wird an den identifizierten Endpunkten ein Verfahren gestartet, welches ein Muster (Pattern) mit benachbarten Regionen vergleicht. Das dreidimensionale Pattern kann dabei auf zwei Arten generiert werden:

– Kubusförmige Region; wird an der aktuellen Position aus den Bilddaten erzeugt

– Verwendung eines synthetischen Patterns („idealisierter Zylinder, bzw. Tubus", siehe Abb. 1)

Bei der Erzeugung der synthetischen Patterns wird der enthaltene Zylinder / Tubus stets in die Richtung des aktuellen Translationsvektors ausgerichtet. Hierzu wird initial ein Modell-Pool mit Patterns verschiedener Größe und Orientierung angelegt. So kann zur Laufzeit je nach Bedarf das Modell aufgerufen werden, dass der aktuell verwendeten Patterngröße und der aktuellen Ausrichtung entspricht [6].

Das so erstellte Pattern wird mit benachbarten Regionen gleicher Größe verglichen. Die Summe der quadrierten Differenzen über alle Voxel beider Regionen dient als Kostenfunktion. Die besten Übereinstimmungen werden als Ausgangspunkt für die nächste Iteration verwendet. Periodisch wird überprüft, ob ein Pattern anderer Größe eine bessere Übereinstimmung erzielt. Ist dies der Fall, wird diese Größe bis zur nächsten Überprüfung beibehalten.

Da bei jeder Iteration nicht nur der günstigste Vergleich weiterverfolgt wird, sondern alle, die eine bestimmte Kostenfunktion erfüllen, können sich Pfade über mehrere Iterationen hin durch beispielsweise die Bronchien entwickeln [7]. Hierdurch ist das Verfahren in der Lage, Strukturen auch über Bifurkationen hinweg zu verfolgen.

Nach jeder Iteration wird die Menge der aktiven Pfade auf eine feste Anzahl reduziert. Die Auswahl findet über gleitende Mittelwertbildung der Vergleichskosten statt. Ausgeschlossene Pfade werden als passiv gekennzeichnet und nicht mehr weiter verfolgt. Existieren keine aktiven Pfade mehr oder wurde die Anzahl der maximalen Iterationen erreicht, bricht das Verfahren ab.

2.3 Abschließende Segmentierung

Im vorangegangenen Schritt wurde ein Tracking der tubulären Strukturen durchgeführt, das nun zu einer Segmentierung erweitert werden muss. Für diese wird wiederum ein Bereichswachstumsverfahren angewandt, für welches die aus dem Tracking gewonnenen Koordinaten als Saatpunkte dienen. Ähnlich wie in [8] wird die jeweilige Segmentierung auf eine beschränkte Umgebung des aktuellen Saatpunktes begrenzt. Hierzu dient die Größe des an der jeweiligen Koordinate erfolgreich gematchten Patterns als Region of Interest.

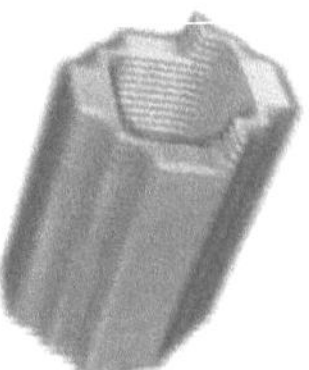

Abb. 1. Volumenvisualisierung eines synthetischen Patterns

3 Ergebnisse

Der Algorithmus wurde erfolgreich auf mehreren CT-Datensätzen getestet, wobei die Verwendung der synthetischen Pattern robustere Ergebnisse lieferte. Der zeitliche Aufwand beträgt hierbei je nach Größe der Bilddaten zwischen 4 und 6 Minuten inklusive Benutzerinteraktion. Der Workflow sieht hierbei vor, zunächst die Segmentierung mit Bereichswachstumsverfahren durchzuführen und ggf. durch einen Schieberegler semiautomatisch anzupassen (ca. 10-30 Sek.) um anschließend das Patternmatching und die abschließende Segmentierung durchzuführen (ca. 3-4 Min.) (P4 2,4 GHz, 2GB RAM). Über die Parameter (max. Matchingkosten, max. aktive Pfade, max. Anzahl Iterationen) kann ihr Ergebnis beeinflusst werden.

Das Gesamtergebnis kann als binäres Segmentierungsbild, als (interaktiver) Baum oder als Oberfläche betrachtet und weiterverarbeitet werden. Bei der Erstellung eines interaktiven Baums können ggf. falsch positiv erkannte Äste markiert und respektiv aus der Segmentierung entfernt werden. Bei der quantitativen Evaluation an CT-Datensätzen war das neue Verfahren in der Lage, im Mittel an 65% der identifizierten Blattknoten den vorliegenden Bronchialast weiter zu verfolgen. Der Anteil falsch positiv erkannter Äste lag bei 3%.

4 Diskussion

Wie Tschirren et al. beschreiben [8], ist eine Evaluation der Segmentierungen von Bronchialbäumen im klassischen Sinne nicht möglich. Dies rührt daher, dass,

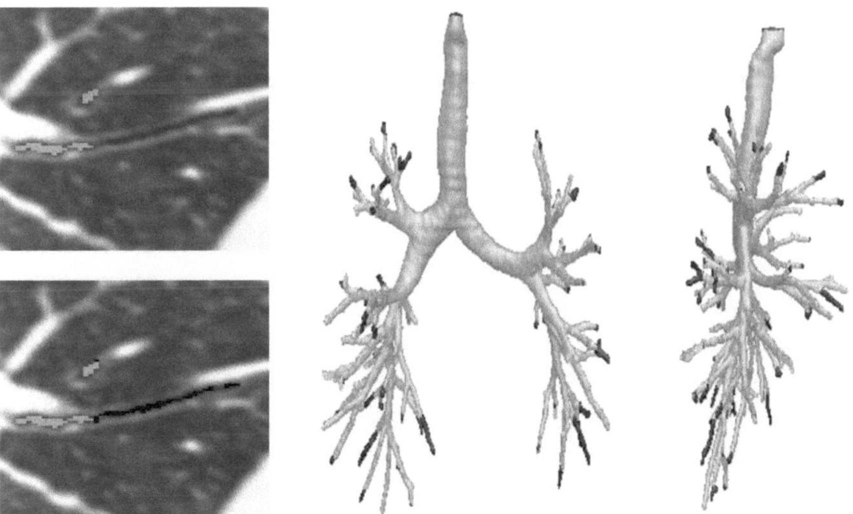

Abb. 2. Vergleich der Ergebnisse des ursprünglichen Verfahrens (hellgrau) mit hybridem Verfahren (schwarz) in 2D und 3D, Bilddaten aus hochaufgelöstem CT des Bronchialbaums

aufgrund des hohen Zeitaufwands und der, durch die hohe Komplexität der anatomischen Struktur bedingte, zu erwartenden Fehlerquote, keine manuellen Segmentierungen als Goldstandard vorhanden sind. Daher werden die Ergebnisse in diesem Bereich häufig mit Resultaten verglichen, die auf Bereichswachstumsverfahren basieren.

Bei der Analyse der Resultate zeigte sich, dass das neue Verfahren an einem Großteil der Blattknoten den Verlauf der vorliegenden Bronchien zuverlässig weiterverfolgen und segmentieren konnte (siehe Abb.2). Die Erweiterung des in Abschnitt 2.1 verwendeten Bereichswachstumsverfahrens auf nachträgliche Adaptierbarkeit der Schwellwerte stellt eine deutliche Beschleunigung und somit Verbesserung des Workflows und eine Erhöhung der Benutzerfreundlichkeit gegenüber dem ursprünglichen Verfahren dar. Durch die Verwendung des Pattern-Pools kann eine deutliche Laufzeitersparnis gegenüber einer Erzeugung der Modelle zur Laufzeit erreicht werden. Die Betrachtung mehrerer Pfade ermöglicht die Verfolgung von tubulären Strukturen über Bifurkationen hinweg. Vereinzelt können falsch positive Ergebnisse auftreten. Diese sind vor allem an Positionen im Bild zu beobachten, an denen die typische Struktur durch Bildartefakte oder ähnliche Störungen deutlich entartet ist.

Zum derzeitigen Stand des Projekts wurde aus Zeitgründen keine Anwendung auf Blutgefäße durchgeführt; hierzu wäre lediglich eine Anpassung des synthetischen Modells notwendig.

Danksagung. Diese Arbeit wurde von der DFG im Rahmen des Projektes „Protektive Beatmungssysteme“ (ME 833/11-1) gefördert.

Literaturverzeichnis

1. Byl N, Wegner I, Wolf I et al . Segmentierung tubulärer Strukturen mittels Modell-zu-Bild-Registrierung. Proc BVM. 2007; p. 126–30.
2. Mayer D, Bartz D, Fischer J et al . Hybrid segmentation and virtual bronchoscopy based on CT images. Academic Radiology. 2004 May;11(5):551–65.
3. de Bruijne M, van Ginneken B, Viergever M et al . Adapting active shape models for 3D segmentation of tubular structures in medical images. Procs IPMI. 2003;2723:136–47.
4. Hojjatoleslami S, Kittler J. Region Growing: A New Approach. Department of Electronic & Electrical Engineering, University of Surrey, Guildford, UK; 1995.
5. Schoebinger M, Thorn M, Vetter M et al . Robuste Analyse von Gefäßstrukturen auf Basis einer 3D-Skelettierung. Proc BVM. 2003; p. 76–80.
6. Heimann T, Baumhauer M, Simpfendörfer T et al . Prostate segmentation from 3D transrectal ultrasoundu using statistical shape models and local histogram matching. In: Proc SPIE; 2008.In print.
7. Schaap M, Schmal I, Metz C et al . Bayesian tracking of elongated structures in 3D images. Procs IPMI. 2007.
8. Tschirren J, Hoffman E A, McLennan G et al . Segmentation and quantitative analysis of intrathoracic airway trees from computed tomography images. In: The Proceedings of the American Thoracic Society. vol. 2; 2005. p. 484–7.

Esophagus Segmentation by Spatially-Constrained Shape Interpolation

Andreas Fieselmann[1,2], Stefan Lautenschläger[2], Frank Deinzer[2], Matthias John[2], Björn Poppe[1]

[1]Medical Radiation Physics, University of Oldenburg, Oldenburg, Germany
[2]Siemens AG Medical Solutions, Forchheim, Germany
andreas.fieselmann.ext@siemens.com

Abstract. The segmentation and visualization of the esophagus is helpful during planing and performing atrial ablation therapy to avoid esophageal injury. Only very few studies have addressed this segmentation problem which is challenging because the esophagus has a low contrast in medical images. In this work we present a technique to segment the esophagus based on the interpolation of Fourier descriptors of manually drawn contours. The interpolation is spatially-constrained using a dedicated correction term to avoid intersections with the convex shaped left atrial posterior wall. Our technique is fast, modality independent and achieves optimal results if at least three input contours are used. We validated our technique successfully with patient data and discuss the use of our technique in the clinical workflow.

1 Introduction

Atrial fibrillation can be treated by catheter ablation of the pulmonary veins inside the left atrium. During this intervention there is a small risk, however, to induce thermal injury to the adjacent esophagus. This can lead to the formation of an atrio-esophageal fistula and air from the esophagus is able to enter into the left atrium [1].

A strategy to avoid this often fatal complication is to decrease the power of the catheter at the contact area of the left atrium and the esophagus. Studies show that the esophagus is always in contact with the left atrium but its route varies widely [2]. Therefore, a segmentation of the esophagus before and during the intervention can help to plan the ablation strategy. The esophagus has a low contrast in cardiac CT, cardiac C-arm CT [3] and cardiac MRI images. This makes segmentation using edge-based techniques difficult.

Research on esophagus segmentation is very rare. Rousson et al. [4] propose a probabilistic shortest path approach to extract the esophagus from CT images. Their method requires a prior segmentation of the left atrium and the aorta. Two points on the centerline of the esophagus are needed as input to the algorithm which is computationally intensive. Ragan et al. [5] use deformable models to segment several organs but fail to accurately contour the esophagus. The work of Huang et al. [6] investigates optical flow to outline the esophagus and other organs. They construct initial 2D contours by Fourier interpolation which is a different concept than the interpolation of Fourier descriptors presented in section 2.1. Jeong and Radke [7] use Fourier descriptors to interpolate contours of the prostate in CT images and present a good overview about alternative shape interpolation techniques like triangulated meshes [8] and implicit functions [9].

In this work we present a technique to segment the esophagus that is independent on the type of modality. Our technique incorporates prior knowledge to avoid intersections with the left atrium. It is robust and faster than existing esophagus segmentation methods because it does not work directly on the image data.

2 Materials and Methods

There are two main assumptions in our segmentation technique. First, the shape of the esophagus contour changes smoothly between axial slices. Second, the esophagus does not intersect with other structures like the left atrium.

We model the esophagus by a sequence of contours along the longitudinal axis (patient axis). As input to our algorithm we expect at least two esophagus contours and a prior segmentation of the left atrium. In the clinical workflow the left atrium is the primary organ of interest and always segmented before the esophagus, so this requirement is not a limitation of our algorithm. The contours between the input contours are determined by a slice-by-slice interpolation in the frequency domain and a correction method is used to ensure that the contours do not intersect with the left atrium. The concept of Fourier descriptors and our interpolation technique are presented below.

2.1 Fourier Descriptors

Fourier descriptors are used to describe the shape of 2D closed curves [10]. They are constructed as follows. A discrete closed curve with coordinates (x_n, y_n) and $n = 0, 1, .., N-1$ can be converted into a complex-valued periodic function a_n by the mapping $\mathbb{R}^2 \mapsto \mathbb{C} : a_n = x_n + j \cdot y_n$ with the imaginary unit j. The discrete Fourier transform $\mathcal{F}$ in (1) is used to transform a_n into the frequency domain. Its inverse transform $\mathcal{F}^{-1}$ is given in (2).

$$A_k = \mathcal{F}\{a_n\} = \frac{1}{N} \sum_{n=0}^{N-1} a_n \cdot \exp\left(-\frac{j2\pi kn}{N}\right) \tag{1}$$

$$a_n = \mathcal{F}^{-1}\{A_k\} = \sum_{k=0}^{N-1} A_k \cdot \exp\left(\frac{j2\pi kn}{N}\right) \tag{2}$$

The coefficients A_k with $k = 0, 1, .., N-1$ are called the Fourier descriptors of the curve. The zeroth descriptor A_0 contains the center of mass of the curve and all other descriptors are invariant to translation. Fourier descriptors are well-suited to describe elliptical shaped curves whose smoothness can be controlled by filtering of the high-frequency coefficients. We keep 6 Fourier descriptors in the following analyses. In order to compute the Fourier descriptors we first resample the curve in the spatial domain by piecewise linear interpolation such that the number of points is the same for all curves.

2.2 Spatially-Constrained Shape Interpolation

The Fourier descriptors $A_{k,z}$ describe the esophagus contour in the axial plane with the longitudinal coordinate z. The shapes of two input contours A_{k,z_1} and A_{k,z_2} with $z_2 > z_1$ are interpolated piecewise-linearly in steps of dz starting from $A_{k,z} = A_{k,z_1}$ according to (3).

$$A_{k,z+dz} = A_{k,z} + dz \cdot \frac{A_{k,z_2} - A_{k,z}}{z_2 - z} \tag{3}$$

After each iteration step the new contour is transformed back into the spatial domain using (2) and checked if it intersects with the left atrium. If the contour intersects it is corrected as follows.

Let $\boldsymbol{r}_i$ $(i = 1, .., M)$ denote the vectors from the center of mass of the contour to the intersecting points. The correction vector $\boldsymbol{t}$ defined in (4) points in the opposite direction of the vectorial sum of all $\boldsymbol{r}_i$ (Fig. 1) and is normalized to one pixel length.

$$\boldsymbol{t} = \begin{pmatrix} t_x \\ t_y \end{pmatrix} = -\frac{1}{M} \sum_{i=1}^{M} \boldsymbol{r}_i \tag{4}$$

In the spatial domain all contour points shifted by $\boldsymbol{t}$. In the frequency domain only $A_{0,z}$ is changed by adding $t_x + j \cdot t_y$. If the contour still intersects then the vectors $\boldsymbol{r}_i$ are updated and the procedure is repeated. All input contours are sorted with respect to their longitudinal coordinate and the interpolation is performed between each neighboring pair.

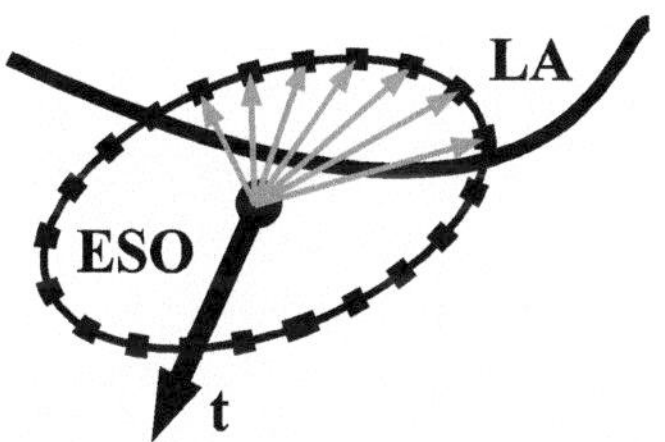

Fig. 1. Intersection of the esophagus (ESO) and the left atrium (LA) generates a correction vector $\boldsymbol{t}$

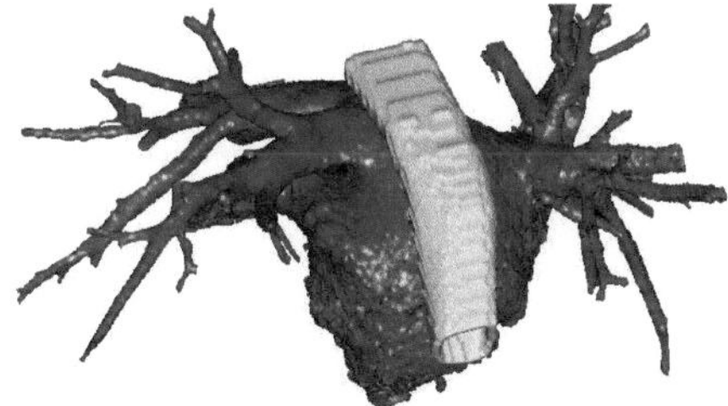

Fig. 2. 3D Volume rendering of the segmented esophagus (light) and the left atrium (dark)

Table 1. Comparison of segmentation results using 2, 3 or 5 input contours. A dice coefficient value $C_D = 1$ indicates complete agreement with the ground truth

patient number	1	2	3	4	5	6	7	8
C_D(2 contours)	0.60	0.61	0.67	0.76	0.49	0.40	0.61	0.65
C_D(3 contours)	0.84	0.70	0.76	0.80	0.79	0.51	0.80	0.81
C_D(5 contours)	0.89	0.81	0.84	0.85	0.86	0.74	0.86	0.88

3 Results

In order to validate our technique we segment the esophagus in 8 CT scans of patients treated with atrial catheter ablation. In each volume the left atrium is segmented using the software *syngo*® InSpace EP (Siemens AG Medical Solutions) and an expert manually draws 9 esophagus contours in equally spaced axial slices. We assume that a segmentation using all 9 contours is a precise segmentation ("ground truth"). We choose 9 contours because it is possible to extract subsets of 2, 3 and 5 equally spaced contours. Then we perform the segmentation using the contours from each subset as input to the algorithm. The dice similarity coefficient C_D [11] defined in (5) is a measure to compare the segmentation results. $|A|$ is the volume of the segmentation with 9 input contours, $|B|$ is the volume of the segmentation with 2, 3 or 5 input contours respectively and $|A \cap B|$ is the intersection of $|A|$ and $|B|$.

$$C_D = \frac{2 \cdot |A \cap B|}{|A| + |B|} \tag{5}$$

The segmentation of the esophagus using all 9 input contours has been assessed by visual inspection and it is very consistent with the true position of the esophagus in all patient data. The results from Table 1 and Fig. 3 show that 3 input contours produce an optimal segmentation with a median dice coefficient of about 0.8 which is similar to the value in [4]. A dice coefficient value greater than 0.7 is usually considered as a good agreement [4]. Two contours may be sufficient for an approximate localization of the esophagus. A volume rendering of the esophagus segmented from 3 input contours is shown in Fig. 2. The time to draw 3 input contours and perform the computations is about 15 seconds.

4 Discussion

Our technique can be used to plan the ablation strategy with cardiac CT scans and is also applicable with cardiac C-arm CT data during the intervention. In order to be modality independent our algorithm does not work directly on the image data. The technique is robust because the input contours profit from human expert knowledge and our correction term avoids intersections with the left atrium. The time needed to segment the esophagus including user interactions is about 15 seconds which is adequate for the clinical workflow and less than other, fully automated techniques usually require. The computational time for the pure

Fig. 3. Shape interpolation of the esophagus contour (thick lines). Two input contours (thin lines) are drawn in (a) and (d). The shown slices are equally space, start at the caudal side of the left atrium (a) and end at the atrial center (d)

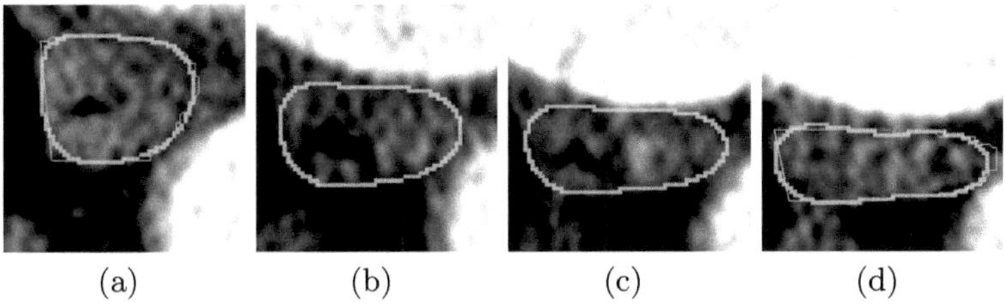

(a) (b) (c) (d)

algorithm is less than a second. The chosen interpolation scheme is well suited for elliptical structures like the esophagus and therefore gives visually pleasing and precise results with only a few input contours. We are currently working on extensions of our technique to find input contours automatically by an algorithm. E.g. air holes inside the esophagus are visible in CT images and can be used to localize the esophagus and detect the esophagus contour.

References

1. Pappone C, Oral H, Santinelli V, et al. Atrio-esophageal fistula as a complication of percutaneous transcatheter ablation of atrial fibrillation. Circulation. 2004;109(22):2724–26.
2. Cury RC, Abbara S, Schmidt S, et al. Relationship of the esophagus and aorta to the left atrium and pulmonary veins: Implications for catheter ablation of atrial fibrillation. Heart Rhythm. 2005;2(12):1317–23.
3. Lauritsch G, Boese J, Wigström L, et al. Towards cardiac C-arm computed tomography. IEEE Trans Med Imaging. 2006;25(7):922–34.
4. Rousson M, Bai Y, Xu C, et al. Probabilistic Minimal Path for Automated Esophagus Segmentation. Proc SPIE. 2006;6144:49–4H.
5. Ragan D, Starkschall G, McNutt T, et al. Semiautomated four-dimensional computed tomography segmentation using deformable models. Med Phys. 2005;32(7):2254–61.
6. Huang TC, Zhang G, Guerrero T, et al. Semi-automated CT segmentation using optic flow and Fourier interpolation techniques. Comput Methods Programs Biomed. 2006;84(2-3):124–34.
7. Jeong Y, Radke RJ. Reslicing axially sampled 3D shapes using elliptic Fourier descriptors. Med Image Anal. 2007;11(2):197–206.
8. Boissonnat JD. Shape reconstruction from planar cross sections. Computer Vis Graph Image Process. 1988;44(1):1–29.
9. Turk G, O'Brien JF. Shape Transformation Using Variational Implicit Functions. Comput Graph (ACM). 1999;33:335–42.
10. Zahn CT, Roskies RZ. Fourier descriptors for plane closed curves. IEEE Trans Comp. 1972;C-21(3):269–81.
11. Heimann T, Thorn M, Kunert T, et al. Empirische Vergleichsmaße für die Evaluation von Segmentierungsergebnissen. Proc BVM. 2004; p. 165–9.

Simultaneous Model-Based Segmentation of Multiple Objects

Astrid Franz[1], Robin Wolz[1], Tobias Klinder[1,2], Cristian Lorenz[1], Hans Barschdorf[1], Thomas Blaffert[1], Sebastian P.M. Dries[1], Steffen Renisch[1]

[1]Philips Research Europe - Hamburg, Sector Medical Imaging Systems
[2]Leibniz University Hannover, Institute of Information Processing
astrid.franz@philips.com

Abstract. Deformable models are used for the segmentation of objects in 3D images by adapting flexible meshes to image structures. The simultaneous segmentation of multiple objects often causes problems like violation of spatial relationships. Here we present two methods for including prior knowledge into the segmentation process: The first deals with objects sliding with respect to each other, and the second considers a pre-defined minimal distance between neighboring objects. Using this prior knowledge improved segmentation results can be reached.

1 Introduction

Segmentation is still one of the main challeging problems in medical image analysis. In order to improve the segmentation, prior knowledge in form of anatomical models is frequently used. For this reason, deformable models of several organs have been earlier developed and used for segmenting the corresponding objects in medical images [1, 2, 3]. In model-based segmentation, flexible meshes, normally triangle meshes, are adapted to the corresponding image structures. Usually this adaptation is carried out for every object separately by optimizing a weighted sum of two competing energies: an external energy E_{ext} driving the mesh triangles towards image features and an internal energy E_{int} preserving the form of the model [4].

The segmentation is often complicated by various factors, like, e.g., no clear boundaries of the object to be segmented, pathologies or intensity similarity of adjacent structures, thus leading to wrong adaptation results. In most cases the segmentation can be improved when not only using prior knowledge of the object's shape but also information about spatial relations to neighboring structures. First attempts to include object relations are described in [5, 6, 7] and references therein. For instance, additional edges connecting neighboring meshes are introduced, or non-overlapping constraints are used.

Here we propose a method for simultaneous segmentation of objects close to each other by introducing additional edges similar to [5]. For these edges, a connection energy is defined in different ways incorporating prior knowledge of the corresponding anatomical region. Hence sliding organs or a required minimal distance of two organs can be represented.

2 Materials and Methods

Let M_i $(i = 1, \ldots, n)$ denote the pre-positioned meshes for n objects which are to be segmented. Then for any two objects being near to each other, a connecting object C_i is defined by a set of additional edges connecting points of the two corresponding meshes $M_{a(i)}$ and $M_{b(i)}$. For each connecting object, a transformation class T_i is chosen which describes the allowed deformations, or a required minimal distance d_i is chosen. Then iteratively the following steps are performed:

1. For each mesh M_i, a feature search is carried out, and the corresponding external energy $E_{\text{ext},i}$ is computed as in [4].
2. For each mesh M_i, a similarity transform, i.e. a rotation matrix r_i and a scaling factor s_i is computed, which best aligns the model mesh with the actual mesh configuration. The remaining deformation results in an internal energy $E_{\text{int},i} = \sum_{(j,k)\in\text{edges}(M_i)} (\hat{x}_j - \hat{x}_k - s_i r_i(x_j - x_k))^2$ [4], where the $\hat{x}_j$ denote the coordinate vectors of the corresponding mesh vertices in the pre-positioned model and the x_j denote the coordinate vectors of the actual mesh configuration.
3. For each connecting object C_i (connecting the meshes $M_{a(i)}$ and $M_{b(i)}$)
   (a) a transformation $t_i \in T_i$ is determined best aligning the pre-positioned model connection object with the actual connection object, and the connection energy $E_{\text{con(a)},i} = \sum_{(j,k)\in\text{edges}(C_i)} (\hat{x}_j - \hat{x}_k - t_i(x_j - x_k))^2$ is computed, or
   (b) two parallel planes are fitted through the vertices, one plane through the vertices belonging to $M_{a(i)}$ and the other plane through the vertices belonging to $M_{b(i)}$. Let ν_i be the normal vector to these planes, going from $M_{a(i)}$ to $M_{b(i)}$. For every edge (j, k) in C_i $(j \in M_{a(i)}, k \in M_{b(i)})$, the scalar product $\langle x_k - x_j, \nu_i \rangle$ is computed, which results in the connection energy $E_{\text{con(b)},i} = \sum_{(j,k)\in\text{edges}(C_i)} (\langle x_k - x_j, \nu_i\rangle - \max(\langle \hat{x}_k - \hat{x}_j, \hat{\nu}_i\rangle, d_i))^2$.
4. The overall energy $E = \sum_{i=1}^{n} \alpha_i E_{\text{ext},i} + \sum_{i=1}^{n} \beta_i E_{\text{int},i} + \sum_{i=1}^{m} \gamma_i E_{\text{con},i}$, with weighting factors α_i, β_i and γ_i, is minimized, resulting in new coordinate vectors for each mesh.

This iteration is repeated for a given number of steps, or it is stopped when the new vertex coordinates do not differ significantly from the ones before.

The transformation class T_i in step 3a can for instance be the class of affine transformations (without reflection). Then shearing is allowed which ensures that the connected meshes can slide with respect to each other. If the distance of the two meshes is to be preserved, the scaling factors of the affine transformation can be restricted. Hence the transformation class can be defined in order to match the requirements of the underlying application.

If two meshes are to have a given minimal distance but this distance can not be reached by pre-positioning, step 3b can be applied. In this step, the connecting edges are projected onto the normal vector of the parallel planes describing the adjacent mesh surfaces. The connection energy penalizes a length of these

Table 1. Mean d_{mean}, maximum d_{max} and standard deviation σ of the distance of the adapted vertebral meshes to the surface of the ground truth meshes for three CT datasets (all numbers are given in mm)

connection energy	dataset 1			dataset 2			dataset 3		
	d_{mean}	d_{max}	σ	d_{mean}	d_{max}	σ	d_{mean}	d_{max}	σ
without	0.90	4.86	0.71	1.35	5.77	1.06	0.72	3.96	0.65
$E_{\text{con(a)}}$	0.83	4.11	0.62	1.24	5.31	0.93	0.57	3.23	0.46
$E_{\text{con(b)}}$	0.81	4.38	0.61	1.23	5.17	0.90	0.61	3.63	0.51

projections smaller than the given minimal distance. Hence an initial mesh overlap (indicated by a negative length of connecting edges) can be corrected during the mesh adaptation process. If, on the other hand, the minimal distance condition is fulfilled, then the projected length of the connecting edge is compared with the projected length in the model, and a deviation is penalized. Hence in this case the distance of the two connected mesh surfaces is to be preserved.

3 Results

A synthetic test example image (size $100 \times 200 \times 100\text{mm}^3$) contains two cubes (size 70^3mm^3) with a light outer region like cortical bone and a dark inner region like cancellous bone (Fig. 1). The two cubes are staggered as for instance vertebrae in the spine may be. The two meshes are pre-positioned in such a way that the upper surface of the lower mesh is closer to the cortex-marrow-transition of the upper cube than to the surface of the lower cube, simluating a typical imperfect pre-positioning (Fig. 1a). Hence an adaptation without a connection energy

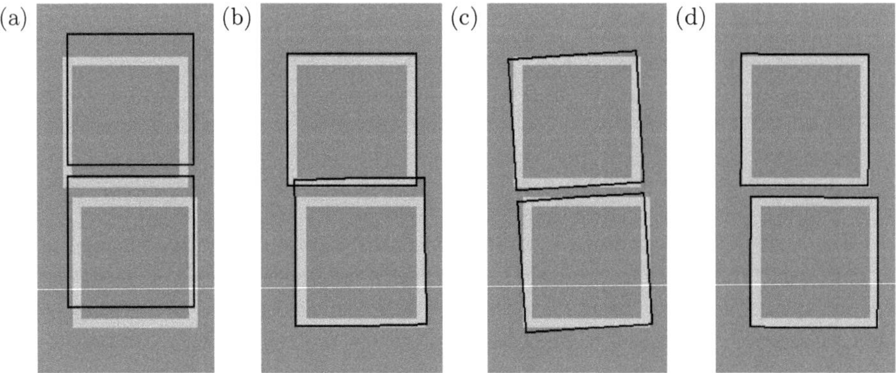

Fig. 1. Synthetic example image of two cubes with two pre-positioned meshes (a), adaptation results without connection energy (b) and with connection energies based on rigid transformation (c) and affine transformation (d). Result (d) is also achieved with the connection energy requiring a minimal distance of 7mm for both starting at configuration (a) or starting at configuration (b)

will fail (Fig. 1b). In contrast, a connection energy $E_{\mathrm{con(a)}}$ based on a rigid or affine transformation can ensure that the upper surface of the lower mesh finds its correct cube surface, since the lower mesh is forced down- wards due to the adaptation of the upper mesh. A rigid transformation keeps the relative positioning of the adjacent mesh surfaces (Fig. 1c), whereas an affine transformation allows for shearing (Fig. 1d). The shearing result in Fig. 1d can also be obtained with the connection energy $E_{\mathrm{con(b)}}$ requiring a minimal distance of 7mm. This connection energy additionally has the potential of correcting initial mesh overlaps: When starting the adaptation process with the mesh configuration shown in Fig. 1b, the result shown in Fig. 1d is achieved as well.

Fig. 3 shows a medical example application. In a computed tomography (CT) image of the spine, the third, fourth and fifth thoracic vertebrae are to be segmented. As the synthetic example illustrated, the transition from cortical to cancellous bone is comparable to the bone boundary, hence a separate adaptation of each vertebra is likely to fail (Fig. 3c). In contrast, the connection energy $E_{\mathrm{con(a)}}$ based on an affine transformation preserves the spatial relationship of the vertebral meshes and hence results in a reasonable segmentation (Fig. 3e). The connection energy $E_{\mathrm{con(a)}}$ requiring a minimal distance of 2mm furthermore corrects for the slight initial mesh overlaps (Fig. 3b). It moves the meshes apart during the adaptation process (Fig. 3f).

We validated our methods for three CT datasets of the 12 thoracic vertebrae with a slice thickness between 2 and 3 mm containing no significant pathologies.

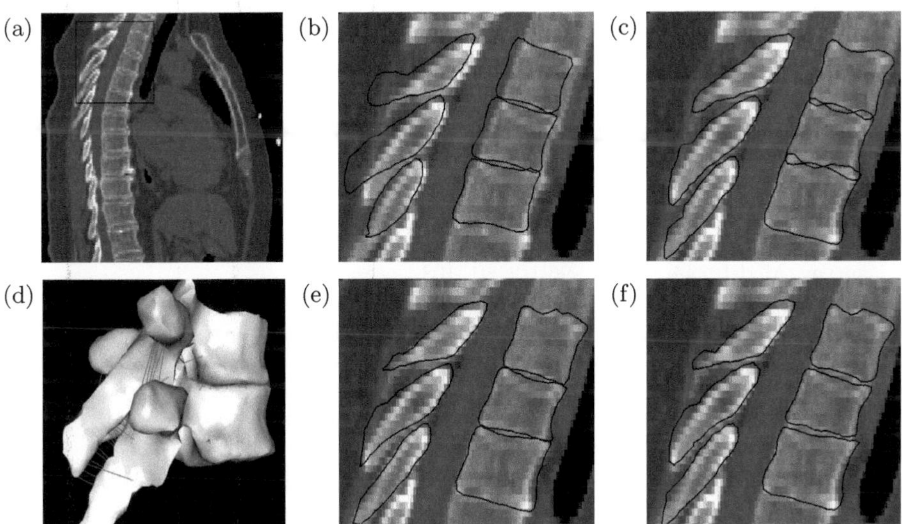

Fig. 2. CT image of the thorax and highlighted region containing the third, fourth and fifth thoracic vertebrae (a), the initial mesh positioning (b) and the adaptation results without connection energy (c) and with a connection energy based on affine transformation (e) and requiring a minimal distance of 2mm (f), based on connecting objects consisting of additional edges connecting two neighboring vertebral meshes (d)

A global manual positioning including rotation and translation of a mean model [8] was used for initialization of the segmentation routines. We compared the segmentation results with manually adapted meshes used as ground truth. The mean, maximum and standard deviation of the distance between the vertices of the adapted meshes to the surface of the ground truth meshes show a decrease of the segmentation error of about 10 % with the introduced methods (Tab. 1).

4 Discussion

As the examples in the previous section illustrate, the introduced connection energies yield an acceptable segmentation of multiple objects close to each other while an independent adaptation of the multiple meshes fails. The kind of connection energy to be applied depends on the requirements of the underlying application. A connection energy based on a rigid transformation keeps the spatial relationship of the pre-positioned meshes and hence avoids mesh overlaps if the mesh initialization is collision-free. A connection energy based on an affine transformation is more flexible allowing for a sliding of adjacent mesh surfaces. This property is important in anatomical regions where organ surfaces may slide with respect to each other. The second variant of a connection energy requiring a minimal distance between two meshes additionally can correct for initial mesh overlaps. Hence a slightly incorrect pre-positioning can be revised during the mesh adaptation process. This strategy absolves the user from a collision-free pre-positioning of the meshes or avoids a computationally expensive collision detection algorithm to be applied prior to mesh adaptation. However, further improvements may be achieded by learning the minimal distance from an ensemble of adapted models. Hence the connection energies bear the potential of correctly segmenting multiple objects with little required user interaction.

References

1. McInerney T, Terzopoulos D. Deformable models in medical image analysis: A survey. Med Image Anal. 1996;1(2):91–108.
2. Kaus MR, McNutt T, Pekar V. Automated 3D and 4D organ delineation for radiation therapy planning in the pelvic area. Procs SPIE. 2004; p. 346–55.
3. von Berg J, Lorenz C. A statistical geometric model of the heart. Procs BVM. 2006; p. 116–20.
4. Weese J, Kaus M, Lorenz C, et al. Shape constrained deformable models for 3D medical image segmentation. Procs IPMI. 2001; p. 380–7.
5. Kaus MR, von Berg J, Niessen W, et al. Automated segmentation of the left ventricle in cardiac MRI. Procs MICCAI. 2003; p. 432–9.
6. Freedman D, Radke RJ, Zhang T, et al. Model-based multi-object segmentation via distribution matching. Procs CVPR. 2004; p. 11.
7. Costa MJ, Delingette H, Novellas S, et al. Automatic segmentation of bladder and prostate using coupled 3D deformable models. Procs MICCAI. 2007; p. 252–60.
8. Klinder T, Lorenz C, von Berg J, et al. Automated model-based rib cage segmentation and labeling in CT images. Procs MICCAI. 2007; p. 195–203.

Edge-Preserving Denoising for Segmentation in CT-images

Eva Eibenberger, Anja Borsdorf, Andreas Wimmer, Joachim Hornegger

Lehrstuhl für Mustererkennung, Friedrich-Alexander-Universität Erlangen-Nürnberg
anja.borsdorf@informatik.uni-erlangen.de

Abstract. In the clinical environment the segmentation of organs is an increasingly important application and used, for example, to restrict the perfusion analysis to a certain organ. In order to automate the time-consuming segmentation process denoising techniques are required, which can simultaneously remove the locally varying and oriented noise in computed tomography (CT) images and preserve edges of relevant structures. We analyze the suitability of different edge-preserving noise reduction methods to be used as a pre-processing step for Geodesic Active Contours (GAC) segmentation. Two popular methods, bilateral filtering and anisotropic diffusion, are compared to a wavelet-based approach, which is adjusted to the CT-specific noise characteristics. We show that robust segmentation results for different organs at varying noise levels can only be achieved using the wavelet-based denoising. Furthermore, the optimal selection of parameters for the bilateral filter and the anisotropic diffusion is highly dependent on the dataset and the segmentation task.

1 Introduction

In computed tomography (CT), the projections acquired at the detector are corrupted by quantum noise. This noise propagates through the reconstruction to the final volume slices. There, noise is non-stationary, its distribution is unknown and directed noise can be present due to high attenuation along certain directions.

In order to improve the reliability of automatic segmentation algorithms, noise has to be removed. The most basic approach is to apply a linear Gaussian filter. The main drawback of low pass filtering is that important image details like edges are smoothed, too. As neighboring structures often show similar intensities, the segmentation may leak into these regions. This effect can be avoided or at least reduced by using edge-preserving noise reduction methods. In this paper the suitability of different denoising approaches as a pre-processing step for edge-based segmentation of organs in CT-images is investigated. Two standard edge-preserving filters are compared to a wavelet-based approach, which adapts itself to the characteristics of noise in CT.

2 Methods

The image data used for the evaluation consists of 2D CT-slices with different amplitudes of noise. The segmentation is performed for the liver, the kidney and the spleen. Certain features, e.g. strong, non-stationary noise, changing contrasts at the boundary, small structures due to contrast agent or diffuse boundaries make the selection of optimal parameters for the denoising and segmentation algorithm difficult. For the clinical practice, methods are useless where too many parameters must be adjusted to the specific problem or dataset.

The edge-based GAC approach [1] is used for segmentation. The parameters for the GAC were optimized once ($[propagation, curvature, advection] \in [(1, 1, 3), (1, 2, 4)]$) and then left unchanged, because here the influence of the pre-processing should be investigated. The considered noise reduction methods are: the bilateral filtering [2], the anisotropic diffusion [3] and a combination of two wavelet approaches based on thresholding [4] and correlation analysis [5]. Several parameters can be adjusted for the examined denoising methods. For the bilateral filtering, σ_D and σ_R, the standard deviations for the image domain and image range, as well as the mask size m have to be specified. The anisotropic diffusion requires the number of iterations N_{iter} and the contrast parameter λ. For the wavelet-based method, the mode of thresholding (hard or soft), a factor k specifying the amount of thresholding and a parameter N defining the amount of noise suppression of the correlation analysis have to be selected.

For each filter the parameter combination resulting in the best segmentation was determined for each organ in the medical data. We used the manual segmentation of a medical expert as reference. Afterwards, the results were analyzed on the basis of simulated water-phantoms with inlaid objects of different contrasts and with varying noise amplitudes. The quality of the segmentation result was quantified through sensitivity and specificity. During the evaluation, especially the robustness with respect to parameter variations, changing organs and varying noise amplitudes were examined.

3 Results

For each organ in both datasets and all filtering methods, it was possible to find segmentation contours almost perfectly fitting the manual segmentation in Fig. 1(a). However, some important differences could be observed with respect to the robustness of the segmentation result regarding the parameter selection of the denoising. These differences are now described on the example of one segmented liver. Similar results were observable for all other investigated organs.

Figure 1(e) shows the best liver segmentation for the bilateral filtering. If the contrast-dependent σ_R was increased, the segmentation contour leaked at the region near the kidney (Fig. 1(f)), as the boundary is slightly diffuse and of low contrast here. It could be observed that for higher noise amplitudes the sensitivity to parameter variations was intensified. The best segmented liver for the anisotropic diffusion is shown in Fig. 1(b). Both Fig. 1(c) and Fig. 1(d) illustrate the segmentation results when the contrast parameter λ was varied slightly.

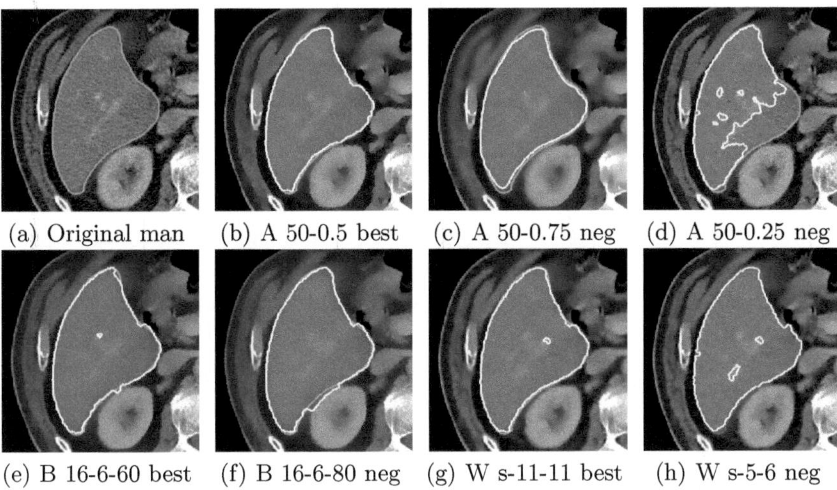

(a) Original man (b) A 50-0.5 best (c) A 50-0.75 neg (d) A 50-0.25 neg

(e) B 16-6-60 best (f) B 16-6-80 neg (g) W s-11-11 best (h) W s-5-6 neg

Fig. 1. GAC segmentation of a liver. Top row: manual segmentation of medical expert and anisotropic diffusion N_{iter}-λ. Bottom row: bilateral filtering m-σ_D-σ_R and wavelet-based filtering $soft$-k-N. The manual segmentation (gray) and the results of the automatic segmentation (white) are plotted in the denoised images in (b)-(h): man = manual segementation; best = best segmentation; neg = negative example

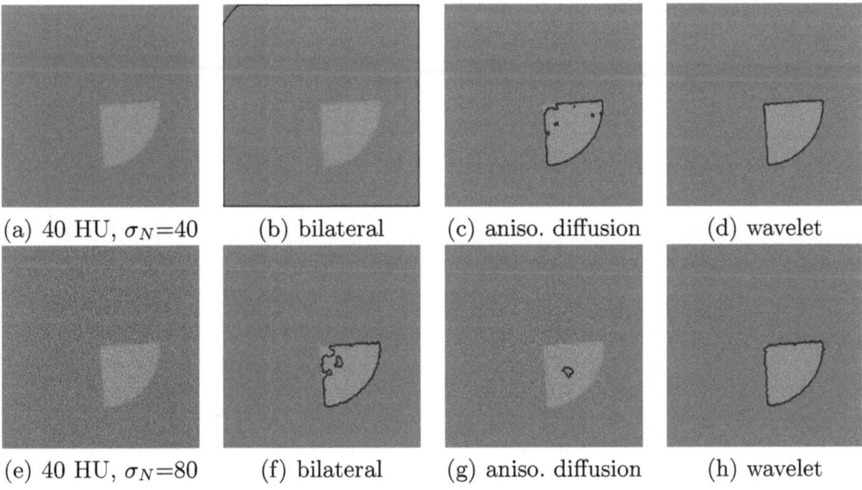

(a) 40 HU, σ_N=40 (b) bilateral (c) aniso. diffusion (d) wavelet

(e) 40 HU, σ_N=80 (f) bilateral (g) aniso. diffusion (h) wavelet

Fig. 2. GAC segmentation results: Filtering performed with the same parameter combination on a phantom image with a contrast of 40 HU but different noise (σ_N). The ideal contour (gray) and segmentation results (black) are plotted in the denoised images

Table 1. Best segmentation results for the example of the liver and the spleen

	without denoising		best linear		best bilateral		best anisotropic		best wavelet	
	iter.	s.×s.	iter.	s.×s.	iter.	s.×s.	iter.	s.×s.	iter.	s.×s.
liver	290	0.08	1449	0.94	794	0.98	911	0.97	847	0.97
spleen	155	0.53	515	0.94	717	0.99	460	0.98	503	0.98

An increasing λ decreased the slope of the edge and the curve evolution process, starting in the interior of the liver, stopped before the ideal contour was reached. If λ was selected too small, the segmentation process stopped after few iterations without covering the whole liver. It can be observed that especially there strong noise could not be removed but was even amplified. The best segmented liver achieved with the wavelet-based filter is shown in Fig. 1(g). It is visible that structures like vessels filled with contrast agent could not be covered during the curve evolution, as during the filtering process even those edges were preserved. If the amount of noise suppression was substantially reduced, (Fig. 1(h)) the outer contour of the liver still matched, however, the holes in the interior increased.

Another observation was that only for the wavelet-based noise reduction method one single parameter combination could be found, leading to good segmentation results for all organs in both datasets. For the anisotropic diffusion and the bilateral filtering even organs of the same dataset could not be segmented without adapting parameters. This is also confirmed by the analysis of simulated phantom images. Figure 2 shows results obtained when for each filter one single parameter set, determined from optimization in real medical data, is applied to images with constant contrast but varying noise level. In contrast to the bilateral filtering and the anisotropic diffusion, the wavelet-based denoising allowed good segmentations for all different noise levels ($\sigma_N \in \{20, 40, 60, 80\}$).

In Table 1 the best achieved results for two examples are listed. The quality of the segmentation is quantified with the product of sensitivity and specificity, leading to values in the range between 0 and 1. The larger the value, the better the result of the segmentation. Furthermore, the numbers of iterations used for the segmentation are included. For better comparison the values for the segmentation without any pre-filtering and the best results achieved with a linear Gaussian filtering are shown. The segmentation contours obtained in the liver without pre-filtering, with optimized Gaussian filtering (σ=2) and too strong Gaussian filtering (σ=4) are shown in Fig. 3 together with the initial segmentation curve. It is obvious that for segmentation a pre-filtering is needed. If too strong linear filtering is performed, the segmentation contour can leak or the precision of the result is reduced. Table 1 shows that with edge-preserving denoising either the number of elapsed iterations could be reduced (example of the liver) or the precision of the segmentation results improved (both examples).

Fig. 3. Comparison of segmentation results (white) without pre-filtering and with linear Gaussian filtering

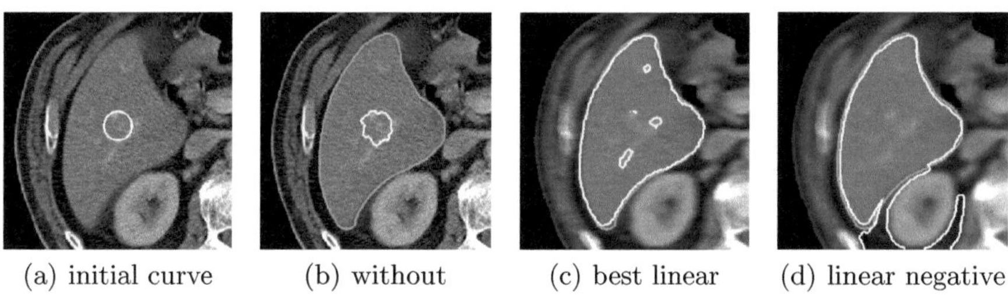

(a) initial curve (b) without (c) best linear (d) linear negative

4 Discussion

The evaluation presented above clearly shows that for the segmentation of organs in medical CT-images a noise-reducing pre-processing step is required. In contrast to linear Gaussian filtering, edge-preserving denoising methods improved the precision of the segmentation contours. Furthermore, the number of elapsed iterations could be decreased for some organs.

By analyzing and comparing different edge-preserving noise reduction methods, it was evident that the parameters of the bilateral filtering and the anisotropic diffusion had to be adapted to each organ in each dataset separately in order to result in precise segmentations. However, for clinical use it is desirable to optimize parameters for the segmentation and its pre-processing once and then used them for all segmentation tasks. In contrast to the bilateral filtering and the anisotropic diffusion, the wavelet-based method allowed the robust and precise segmentation of different organs with varying noise levels with a single parameter combination, as it automatically adapts itself to the CT-specific noise characteristics.

References

1. Caselles V, Kimmel R, Sapiro G. Geodesic active contours. Int J Comp Vis. 1997;22(1):61–79.
2. Tomasi C, Manduchi R. Bilateral filtering for gray and color images. Proc ICCV. 1998; p. 839–46.
3. Perona P, Malik J. Scale space and edge detection using anisotropic diffusion. IEEE Trans Pattern Anal Mach Intell. 1990;12(7):629–39.
4. Borsdorf A, Raupach R, Hornegger J. Separate CT-reconstruction for orientation and position adaptive wavelet denoising. Proc BVM. 2007; p. 232–6.
5. Borsdorf A, Raupach R, Hornegger J. Wavelet-based noise reduction by identification of correlations. Lect Note Comp Sci. 2006;4174:21–30.

Intuitive Mapping of Perfusion Parameters to Glyph Shape

Steffen Oeltze[1], Arvid Malyszczyk[1], Bernhard Preim[1]

[1]Institut für Simulation und Graphik, Otto-von-Guericke Universität Magdeburg
stoeltze@isg.cs.uni-magdeburg.de

Abstract. Perfusion data characterize the regional blood flow in human tissue. For each voxel, a time-intensity curve (TIC) represents the enhancement of a contrast agent (CA). Parameters describing the TIC shape, e.g. the area below the curve (1), maximum (2), and slope (3), characterize the perfusion and have to be derived and integrated for diagnosis. We present the integrated visualization of perfusion parameters based on their intuitive mapping to glyph shape. Glyph attributes such as size, vertical extension and orientation are modified according to (1), (2), and (3) respectively, thereby generating an easy to interpret coding of TIC shape. We further introduce a multi-resolution glyph display and couple our visualizations with a feature specification component.

1 Introduction

In perfusion imaging, the distribution of a contrast agent (CA) is registered to assess blood flow and tissue kinetics. For each voxel, a time-intensity curve (TIC) characterizes the CA enhancement (Fig. 1). How long it takes until the maximum amount of CA is delivered (TTP), which maximum ($Peak$) is achieved, the velocity of CA wash-in ($Slope$), the overall amount of CA ($Integral$), the first momentum of the curve (MTT), as well as other parameters are derived voxel-wise from these curves and stored in parameter volumes. The derived parameters are substitutes for physiological parameters such as tumor perfusion and vessel permeability [1]. The integrated analysis of several parameters is essential. For ischemic stroke diagnosis, e.g., if the blood flow is delayed in a particular region, it is crucial to evaluate if the overall blood flow is also reduced [2].

A straightforward method to analyze several parameters is the side-by-side presentation of color-coded parameter maps (slice in a parameter volume) [2]. However, this requires a mental integration of suspicious regions. Multiparameter visualizations, integrating several perfusion parameters in one image, were introduced in [3] and [4]. Apart from color icons though, none of the presented techniques facilitates the examination of the regional distribution of more than three parameters. However, in perfusion diagnosis, 5-7 relevant parameters may be derived from a TIC (Fig. 1). To accomplish an integrated analysis of the regional distribution of perfusion parameters, we adopt glyphs as a standard technique from the visualization of multi-field data. A glyph is a simple geometric primitive which is positioned with respect to the original data points in space and whose attributes, e.g., color, extension, size, and orientation, are modified according to the represented parameter values. Superquadric tensor glyphs have been applied for tensor field visualization based on data from diffusion tensor imaging [5]. In [6], color-coded ellipsoids are employed for visualizing the myocardial strain based on a model and finite element simulations. The glyph-based integrated visualization of multi-modal cardiac MR-data has been presented in [7]. In [8], a surface-based glyph placement strategy is proposed for the visualization of multi-modal volumetric datasets. Inspired by previous work, we present the integrated glyph-based visualization of perfusion parameters. We focus on an intuitive mapping of parameters to glyph attributes.

2 Materials and Methods

We applied our techniques to cerebral MR perfusion datasets and to Dynamic Contrast Enhanced (DCE) MR mammography datasets. The latter have been motion-corrected according to [9]. Parameter volumes have been pre-computed for all datasets and all relevant parameters (Fig. 1). The presented techniques have been integrated in the MeVisLab platform (www.mevislab.de).

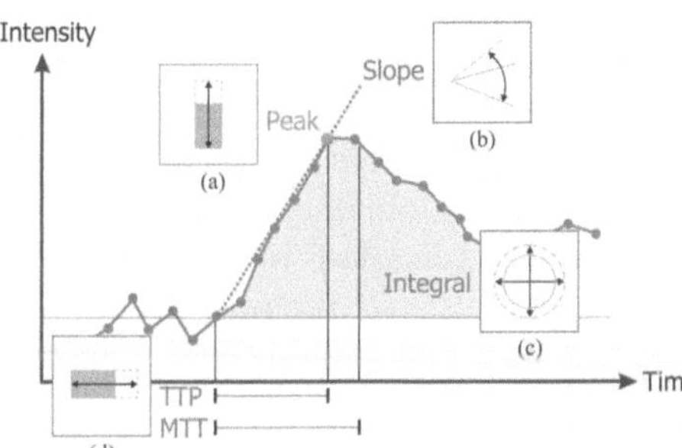

Fig. 1. A typical time-intensity curve in cerebral perfusion annotated with the essential parameters. Glyph attributes which are suitable for an intuitive mapping of parameters are indicated in (a)–(d), e.g., *TTP* should be mapped to the horizontal extension similar to a time axis, *Slope* to orientation and *Integral* to size.

Feature Specification. The diagnostic evaluation of the multi-field parameter data is challenging and time-consuming due to its complexity. Hence, we integrate a feature-based approach to direct the user to suspicious areas. Motivated by the work of Doleisch et al. [10], we apply the concept of linking & brushing. A scatterplot opposing two perfusion parameters is linked to the glyph display. Once an interesting subset of the parameter data is interactively brushed in the plot, the glyph visualization is restricted to this subset. To account for the uncertainty involved in the definition of the subset, smooth brushing is supported. In contrast to a binary decision, this allows a gradual course from uninteresting (context) to definitely interesting (focus). This course is integrated in the glyph display by mapping the so-called *degree of interest (DOI)* to a glyph attribute.

Glyph Design and Placement. We decide in favor of a 2D slice-based glyph placement considering that medical scientists are used to a slice-based exploration. The 2D glyph shapes are presented within the context of an original slice. The slice is rendered as a texture on a 2D plane and scaled such that a single texel (texture element similar to a pixel in an image) covers more than one pixel on the screen. The glyphs are laid out texel-wise and slightly jittered about the texel centers to avoid visual irritations caused by grid patterns. To facilitate an intuitive mapping, we implemented several glyph shapes with different suitable visual attributes besides color (Fig. 1): circular discs (size), rectangles (horizontal and vertical extension), ellipses (size, orientation), toroids (size, roundness, thickness), and oriented toroids (equal to toroids plus orientation).

Multi-resolution Glyph Display. Initial tests showed that a texel-wise glyph placement results in very small glyphs due to the limited space per texel. For example, a screen area S_{xy} of 512×512 pixels reserved for the texture display of a dataset matrix $M_{xy} = 128 \times 128$ leads to an upper glyph size bound B of $S_x/M_x \times S_y/M_y = 4 \times 4$ pixels. This glyph size prevents the readability of subtle changes in glyph shape. A straightforward uniform scaling leads to overlapping artifacts. Hence, we implemented a multi-resolution glyph-display incorporating different resolution layers. The bottommost layer L_0 represents the highest resolution with one glyph per texel. For the above mentioned example, $B_0 = 4 \times 4$ pixels. In each following layer $L_i, i \in [1, n]$, a glyph covers the area of four quadratically arranged neighboring texels in L_{i-1}. A useful maximum number of layers n has been determined empirically so far. For our example, n has been set to three. With $B_i = 2^i \cdot S_x/M_x \times 2^i \cdot S_y/M_y, i \in [1, n]$ pixels, this results in upper glyph size bounds $B_1 = 8 \times 8$, $B_2 = 16 \times 16$, and $B_3 = 32 \times 32$ pixels. For lower resolution layers, the parameter values which determine the glyph attributes have to be computed. Simple averaging of voxel values may suppress pathologies. Instead, we propose to compute the minimum or maximum value dependent on the particular parameter and the application. In tumor perfusion, e.g., high "Slope"values indicate suspicious tissue. Hence, the maximum value is coded in the next lower resolution layer. The user may interactively explore the layers starting with the initially displayed topmost layer.

3 Results

First, a cerebral perfusion dataset from ischemic stroke diagnostics has been analyzed (Fig.2, (a)-(c)). In (a), one circular disc has been placed per texel. The glyph placement is restricted to regions with high TTP and small $Peak$ values (delayed and diminished perfusion). This restriction has been defined via smooth brushing to detect the infarcted tissue. While the glyph color is easily distinguishable, changes in size are hard to evaluate. Zooming in, as illustrated by the inlet, improves the readability but involves a loss of context information and spatial orientation. Therefore, we applied our multi-resolution glyph display (b). The layer with $B_2 = 16 \times 16$ pixels is presented, i.e. a glyph represents 4×4 voxels. Since the glyph size is modified according to $Integral$, whose small values are of special interest in cerebral perfusion, the minimum voxel value is mapped to size. Though the representation of small values by small glyphs is intuitive, interesting regions should immediately grab the viewers attention. Therefore, the mapping is inverted. In (c), the discs are replaced by rectangles since this primitive better fills in the rectangular region it represents. The glyph color is modified based on the respective DOI value.

Furthermore, a DCE mammography has been analyzed (Fig.2, (d)). Ellipses are used to code the two most relevant parameters in tumor perfusion. The

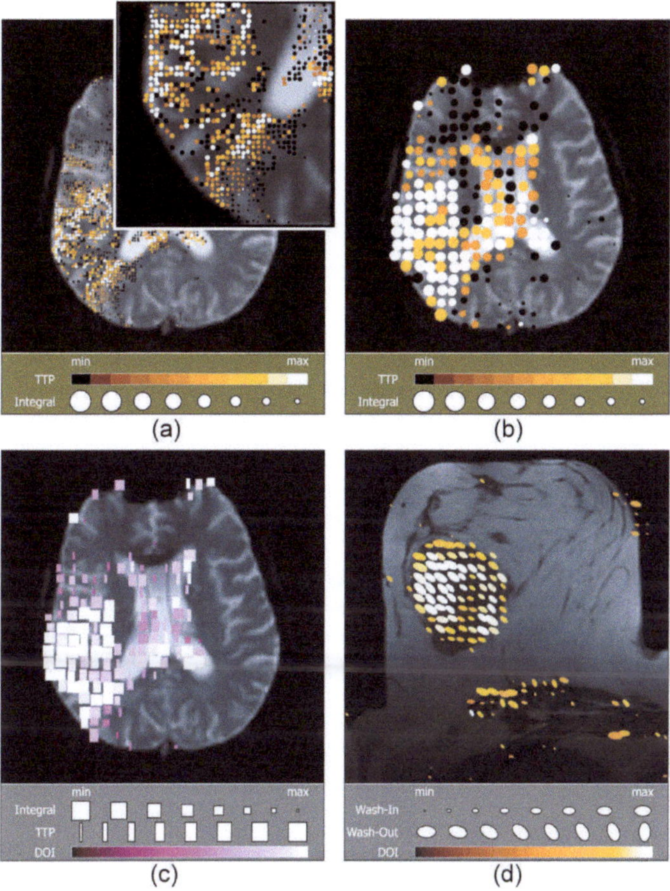

Fig. 2. Visualization examples based on the analysis of a cerebral perfusion ($(a) - (c)$) and a DCE mammography dataset (d). The glyph display in all images has been restricted to suspicious regions by means of smooth brushing. In (a), one circular disc is placed per texel. Changes in glyph size are hard to interpret. A magnification (inlet) improves the readability but involves a loss of context information and spatial orientation. The application of a lower resolution layer (B_2) solves the problem (b). In (c), the discs are replaced by rectangles since this primitive better fills in the rectangular region it represents. The DOI values are integrated by a color mapping. In (d), ellipses are used to code the two most important parameters in tumor perfusion. Probably malignant tissue is indicated by large, vertically oriented ellipses.

Slope (also called *Wash-In* in tumor diagnostics) is mapped to size while the velocity of the CA *Wash-Out* is mapped to orientation. The glyph placement is restricted to regions with large *Wash-In* values (suspicious enhancement). Probably malignant tissue is indicated by large, vertically oriented ellipses which represent strong perfusion and a high vessel permeability. In (d), the resolution layer with $B_3 = 32 \times 32$ pixels is presented, i.e. a glyph represents 8×8 voxels. The glyph size is modified according to the maximum voxel value.

4 Discussion

The developed glyph visualizations have been applied for detecting pathologies in three datasets so far. Initial tests indicated that, in spite of the multi-resolution display, some glyph attributes, such as roundness and thickness of toroids, are hard to interpret. Furthermore, the inverse mapping violates our concept of an intuitive mapping. To examine if our hypothesis of an easy to interpret coding of TIC shape is still supported, a clinical evaluation will be carried out.

Acknowledgement. We thank J.Wiener (Boca Raton Comm. Hosp., Florida) for providing the image data and MeVis Research for providing advanced MeVis-Lab features.

References

1. Choyke PL, Dwyer AJ, Knopp MV. Functional tumor imaging with dynamic contrast-enhanced magnetic resonance imaging. J Magn Reson Imaging. 2003 May;17(5):509–20.
2. König M, Klotz E, Heuser L. Perfusion CT in acute stroke: Characterization of cerebral ischemia using parameter images of cerebral blood flow and their therapeutic relevance. Electromedica. 1998;66(2):61–7.
3. Kohle S, Preim B, Wiener J, et al. Exploration of time-varying data for medical diagnosis. Proc VMV. 2002; p. 31–8.
4. Oeltze S, Grothues F, Hennemuth A, et al. Integrated visualization of morphologic and perfusion data for the analysis of coronary artery disease. Proc EuroVis. 2006; p. 131–8.
5. Kindlmann G. Superquadric tensor glyphs. Proc VisSym. 2004; p. 147–54.
6. Wünsche BC, Lobb R, Young AA. The visualization of myocardial strain for the improved analysis of cardiac mechanics. Proc GRAPHITE. 2004; p. 90–9.
7. Paasche L, Oeltze S, Hennemuth A, et al. Integrierte Visualisierung kardialer MR-Daten zur Beurteilung von Funktion, Perfusion und Vitalität des Myokards. Proc BVM. 2007; p. 212–6.
8. Ropinski T, Specht M, Meyer-Spradow J, et al. Surface glyphs for visualizing multimodal volume data. Proc VMV. 2007; p. to appear.
9. Rueckert D, Sonoda LI, Hayes C, et al. Nonrigid registration using free-form deformations: Application to breast MR images. IEEE Trans Med Imaging. 1999;18(8):712–21.
10. Doleisch H, Gasser M, Hauser H. Interactive feature specification for focus+context visualization of complex simulation data. Proc VisSym. 2003; p. 239–48.

A Scientific Workflow Platform for Generic and Scalable Object Recognition on Medical Images

Manuel Möller, Christopher Tuot, Michael Sintek

German Research Center for Artificial Intelligence (DFKI), Kaiserslautern, Germany
manuel.moeller@dfki.de

Abstract. In the research project THESEUS MEDICO we aim at a system combining medical image information with semantic background knowledge from ontologies to give clinicians fully cross-modal access to biomedical image repositories. Therefore joint efforts have to be made in more than one dimension: Object detection processes have to be specified in which an abstraction is performed starting from low-level image features across landmark detection utilizing abstract domain knowledge up to high-level object recognition. We propose a system based on a client-server extension of the scientific workflow platform Kepler that assists the collaboration of medical experts and computer scientists during development and parameter learning.

1 Introduction

Rapid advances in imaging technology have dramatically increased the amount of medical image data generated every day (e.g., University Hospital of Erlangen, Germany has approx. 150,000 medical examinations producing 13 TB per year). This data is produced in different modalities such as CT, MRI, ultrasound and PET/CT which each have their own characteristics.

In recent years great improvements have been made in object recognition on medical images [1]. However, they have not yet resulted in more flexible or generic image understanding techniques. Instead, the analysis methods are still very object specific and difficult to scale across different applications (e.g. [2]). Consequently, current image search is still dependent on the manual and subjective association of keywords to images. On the other side there are declarative representations of medical knowledge in formal ontologies like the foundational model of anatomy (FMA) [3].

Our approach aims to integrate existing pattern recognition algorithms with formal ontologies. The benefit of this integration is twofold: Firstly, ontologies are used to improve the image analysis through checking the output from the pattern recognition algorithms for their medical consistency. Secondly, the mapping of images to concepts in an ontology allows semantic and cross-modal information retrieval. We propose to use a scientific workflow engine to make the complexity of our approach tractable and aid the collaboration of medical experts and computer scientists.

2 Materials and Methods

As presented in [4] we seek a deep fusion of sub-symbolic pattern recognition algorithms and domain knowledge represented in formal ontologies. We aim to eventually allow a fully automatic image segmentation and semantic annotation.

The adoption of domain knowledge from ontologies like the FMA (we rely on the OWL [5] version by [6]) has great potentials. It allows iterative processes of interaction between purely sub-symbolic pattern recognition algorithms and reasoners like Pellet [7] based on these ontologies.

To give an example: In the first step a couple of pattern matching algorithms is applied to a particular image. They output a list of detected objects. The domain knowledge can be used in conjunction with a reasoner to rule out results like a ventricle and a knee joint next to each other on the same image since this combination is anatomical nonsense.

On the other hand, the adoption of formal ontologies entails a higher complexity of the object recognition processes which makes them harder to develop, adjust and maintain. Fig. 1 shows our proposal for a system that has sub-symbolic feature extractors above the "controller" which operate on bit vector representations of the images. They are complemented by high-level object recognition algorithms and a reasoner interfacing medical ontologies and knowledge bases to provide the system with domain knowledge. The input in form of plain images is fed in from the left. The output is twofold: low-level features are returned to be saved in a database for content based image retrieval (CBIR) based on *visual* similarity like in [8]. Concepts are returned which map image regions to corresponding concepts in the ontology to support retrieval based on *semantic* similarity. This technique allows to answer a query for the "heart" with images from various modalities which can look different from each other but all contain information about the heart.

When a medical expert performs object recognition for an image, e.g. to detect lymph nodes in a CT volume data set, he follows an implicit process

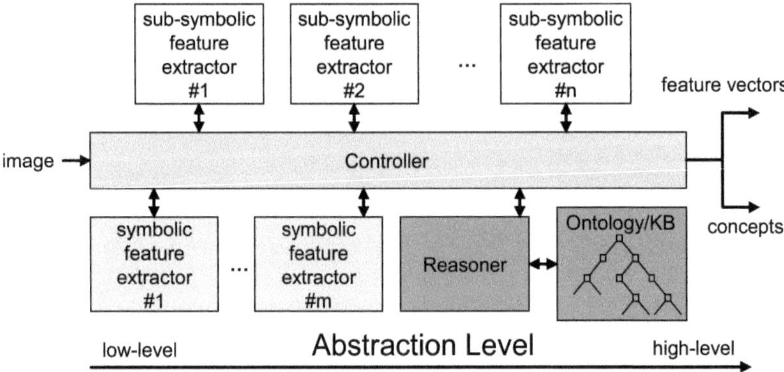

Fig. 1. Integration of feature extraction and background knowledge

consisting of several steps. Throughout this document we will use the term "process" to describe sequences of steps that have to be performed to reach a certain goal while a "workflow" is a formalization of such a process to be processed by a computer. Our architecture aims to make such workflows explicit and implement them (to a reasonable extent) in the controller component. It coordinates the feature extractors, interacts with the domain knowledge base (represented by reasoner and ontology) and directs data streams.

Therefore we base our framework on the open-source scientific workflow platform Kepler [9]. It is based on Ptolemy II, a system for heterogeneous, concurrent modeling and design developed at UC Berkeley. In Kepler, workflows can be designed following a 100% visual programming principle which allows medical experts with non or slight programming skills to design workflows and execute them remotely on a high-performance Grid-computing system.

3 Results

Fig. 2 shows a screenshot of our client/server extension to the Kepler system with a sample workflow for the detection of lymph nodes. Starting from the image reader the Generic Shape Detector performs a first preprocessing of the image. The output of this actor is passed to the Body/Non-Body Border Detection to separate the image into body and non-body regions. In parallel the Anatomical Shape Detector tries to select those shapes which are likely to belong to anatomical structures. Based on these shapes, a vertebrae detection is performed that tries to detect a vertebra as a landmark. Based on this data the reasoner searches the anatomical ontology for possible locations of lymph nodes. A resulting list of image region is subsequently processed by the Lymph Node Detector Grid. The results of this grid are checked for anatomical consistency. Anatomically unlikely or impossible location combinations are passed back to the Lymph Node Detector Grid to be checked again.

4 Discussion

Visual Representation

We believe that a formal and visual representation of the processes has benefits for all involved persons. As discussed above, the knowledge transfer from the medical experts into computers is a complicated problem. Our system addresses this fact by aiding the collaboration of medical experts and computer scientists. The clear visual representation is of substantial help when it comes to modeling complex processes. Misunderstandings between both groups can be detected easier, since the workflow is presented visually right right after it is modeled and even before it is executed for the first time.

Separation of Workflows from Application Logic

To our knowledge, all approaches which integrate symbolic and sub-symbolic techniques fuse them into monolithic applications. These approaches work well for particular tasks (e.g. [10]) but make maintenance and reusability difficult and do not scale for other object recognition tasks. Our proposed workflows have a greater maintainability since they are no longer hard-coded into the application code but are modifiable remotely, via a graphical user interface. Additionally, this architecture supports the distribution and coordination of a complex architecture of remote services independent of hardware platform and physical location. This is a great benefit, since it allows to perform data intensive calculations near to where the data is stored. The Kepler platform has also built-in support for the distribution of multiple tasks over a battery of equal webservices. This feature allows to parallelize long running computing across several machines easily.

Support for Parameter Learning

For medical image analysis often object recognition algorithms are used which incorporate inductive learning. They require a set of labeled samples compiled by medical experts who annotate image regions with particular descriptions. These descriptions can be used to train the inductive algorithm. Usually, the training phase of the classifier includes tweaking various parameters. This parameter adjustment has to be repeated several times, is time consuming and requires

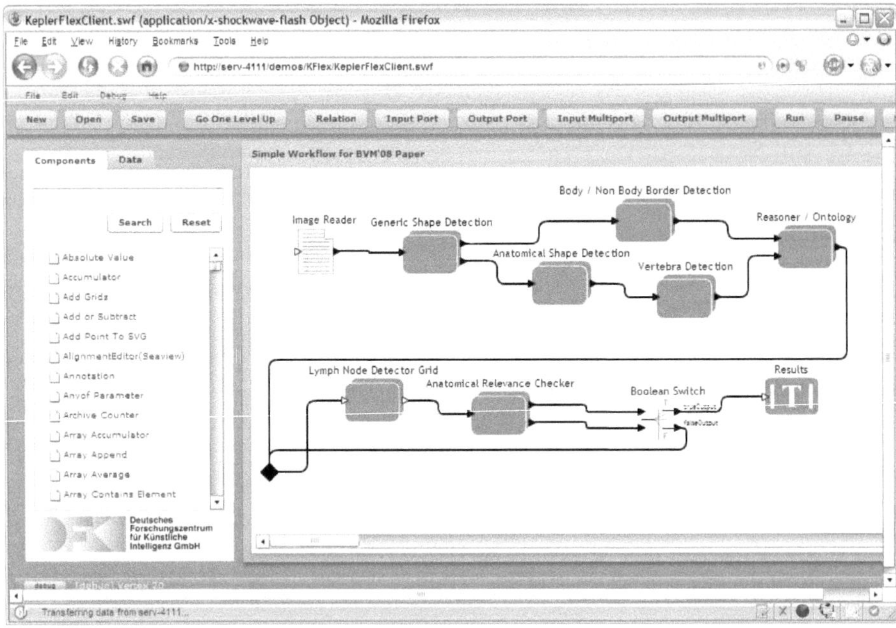

Fig. 2. Screenshot of the interface

human interaction. Apart from the object recognition workflows our system also supports the visual modeling of the processes which train and evaluate the classifiers. It even allows parameter tweaking for workflows containing multiple data preprocessing steps with additional parameters.

Current State and Next Steps

Currently, our implementation of the system architecture is based on an extension of the search engine Lucene[1] and the Lucene Image Retrieval Image Retrieval (LIRE) library.[2] Among our next steps are the integration of a reasonable number of existing object recognition algorithms and the definition of workflows which connect these algorithms to proceed towards a generic image understanding.

Acknowledgement. This research has been supported in part by the THESEUS Program in the MEDICO Project, which is funded by the German Federal Ministry of Economics and Technology under the grant number 01MQ07016.

References

1. Tu Z, Zhou XS, Bogoni L, et al. Probabilistic 3D polyp detection in CT images: The role of sample alignment. Proc IEEE Computer Vision and Pattern Recognition. 2006;2:1544–51.
2. Chan AB, Moreno PJ, Vasconcelos N. Using statistics to search and annotate pictures: An evaluation of semantic image annotation and retrieval on large databases. Proc JSM. 2006.
3. Rosse C, Mejino JLV. A reference ontology for bioinformatics: The foundational model of anatomy. J Biomed Inform. 2003;36:478–500.
4. Möller M, Sintek M, Buitelaar P, et al. Medical image understanding through the integration of cross-modal object recognition with formal domain knowledge. Proc HealthInf. 2008.
5. McGuinness DL, van Harmelen F. OWL Web Ontology Language Overview; 2004.
6. Noy NF, Rubin DL. Translating the foundational model of anatomy into OWL. In: Stanford Medical Informatics Technical Report; 2007.
7. Sirin E, Parsia B. Pellet: An OWL DL reasoner. CEUR Workshop Proceedings. 2004;104.
8. Deselaers T, Weyand T, Keysers D, et al. FIRE in ImageCLEF 2005: Combining content-based image retrieval with textual information retrieval. Working Notes of the CLEF Workshop. 2005.
9. Ludäscher B, Altintas I, Berkley C, et al. Scientific workflow management and the Kepler system. In: Concurrency and Computation: Practice & Experience. vol. 18; 2006. p. 1039–65.
10. Mechouche A, Golbreich C, Gibaud B. Towards an hybrid system using an ontology enriched by rules for the semantic annotation of brain MRI images. Lect Note Comp Sci. 2007;4524:219–28.

[1] http://lucene.apache.org/

[2] http://www.semanticmetadata.net/lire/

A Knowledge-Based System for the Computer Assisted Diagnosis of Endoscopic Images

Andreas Kage, Christian Münzenmayer, Thomas Wittenberg

Fraunhofer Institute for Integrated Circuits (IIS) Erlangen
kage@iis.fraunhofer.de

Abstract. Due to the actual demographic development the use of Computer-Assisted Diagnosis (CAD) systems becomes a more important part of clinical workflows and clinical decision making. Because changes on the mucosa of the esophagus can indicate the first stage of cancerous developments, there is a large interest to detect and correctly diagnose any such lesion. We present a knowledge-based system which is able to support a physician with the interpretation and diagnosis of endoscopic images of the esophagus. Our system is designed to support the physician directly during the examination of the patient, thus prodving diagnostic assistence at the point of care (POC). Based on an interactively marked region in an endoscopic image of interest, the system provides a diagnostic suggestion, based on an annotated reference image database. Furthermore, using relevant feedback mechanisms, the results can be enhanced interactively.

1 Introduction

1.1 Background

Every year more than 4000 people in Germany are diagnosed with esophageal cancer. Although that is only a small number of all cancers (2%) diagnosed, there is a big interest to detect esophagus cancer at an early stage. The prediction for this cancer shows that more than 80% of all men diagnosed with esophagus cancer will not survive the first five years after the first diagnosis [1]. Thus it can be pointed out that this type of cancer has one of the worst prediction rates. Therefore, it is of the highest importance to detect any change of the esophagus tissue surface as early as possible. The standard diagnosis process for the esophageus is based on an visual examination of the esophagus, cardia and corpus tissues, usually by the use of video tip-chip endoscopes. During the examination the physician interprets the acquired images delivered by the endoscope and shown on a high-resolution monitor. The interpretation is not an easy task, since small variations and changes of the tissue are not unusual. But not all changes are related to a dysplastic or a cancerogenous changes of the mucosa. Therefore we have designed and built a system to support the physician with the interpretation of endoscopic images during the examination process by presenting him a second opinion in an easy and intuitive way at the point of care (POC).

1.2 State of the Art

Computer-Assisted-Diagnosis (CAD) systems support the physician with the interpretation of complex image data acquired from modalities such as CT, MRI, Mammography or Endoscopy. Such CAD systems might become a very important part of clinical workflows and clinical decision making processes for several reasons. First, the use of a CAD system provides an objective second opinion without the need for a second physician. This can save costs as well as time. Secondly, in contrast to physicians, CAD systems will always provide a constant quality for the decision support. Finally, CAD systems can use multimodal knowledge databases which can comprise more information than any physician could ever keep in mind.

Due to the fact that CAD systems for digital endoscopy are currently hardly known in clinical routine, not much literature can be found. Tjoa and Krishnan [2] have suggested an image processing system for the automatic detection and classification of lesions in the colon. Illgner et al [3] presented a method to distinguish between normal and dysplastic taypes of tissue on the vocal folds based on color extended GLCM features. Karkanis et al. [4] as well as Maroulis et al. [5] have proposed methods based on combined color and texture analysis for the the classificaion of polyps in the colon. For that purpose Karkanis et al. have applied color wavelet features. Ji et al [6, 7] have suggested a new set of texture primitives to describe the tissue of the cervix acquired by colposcopy.

2 Material and Methods

The proposed system is based on a knowledge database. This reference database currently contains 482 images of the esophagus, cardia and corpus tissue, obtained from over 60 cases. In these images 482 regions of interest have been marked and classified by clinical experts. All findings and classifictions have been confirmed by a histological biopsy. To compute the features for all marked regions, we use statistical geometrical features [8] and second order textual statistics [9] in color extensions suggested by [10]. These algorithms simultaneously extract spatial (textural) and spectral (colour) information of every region of interest to form a combined feature vector. This feature vector is computed for every annotated region in the image data set, and the complete set of feature vectors is stored in the knowledge database.

The CAD system is designed in such way to enable the physician to interactively mark a region of interest (ROI) on a touch screen while he is examining the patient. After a lesion has been marked as a region of interest, the corresponding feature vector for this ROI is computed automatically. Then the feature vector

Table 1. Confusion matrix and classification rates for the diagnosis of lesions in the eosophagous

true	Corpus	Epithelium	Barett's	$\sum$	%
Corpus	145	2	31	178	81
Epithelium	10	172	0	182	95
Barett's	29	0	94	122	76
$\sum$	184	174	124	482	85

is classified based on the knowledge database, using a kNN classifier. The classifier searches for the k nearest neighbours in the complete database to form a result. The images and lesions related to the k closest neighbours in the database are shown in order of their distance on the screen. The physician has now the possibility to influence the presented results interactively using relevance feedback [11]. From several relevance feedback algorithms available, we have chosen a *Query-Point-Movement* and have used the *Rocchio* formula:

$$q_i = \alpha q_i + \beta v_r \tag{1}$$

where q_i denotes the feature vector of the input image and v_r the avarage sum of all *relevant* reference images. After the physician has assessed the relevance of all reference images, the system re-computes the distances to the reference vectors and re-shows a new result.

To support the clinical workflow, the CAD- system consists additionally of a touchscreen and a footbutton to enable the physician to use the system while examining the patient.

3 Results

We have created a knowledge-based system for the Computer-Assisted-Diagnosis of endoscopic images of the oesophagus. Classification results for the 3-class problem (epithelum, corpus and cardia, Barett's mucosa) are presented in Table 1. Using a leaving-one-out analysis (n-fold-cross-validation) [12] a combined classification rate of 85% could be achieved. The individual classification rates for the corpus and cardia class was 81%, for the epithelium 96% and for the Barett's mucosa 76%. Furthermore, using the relevance feedback for that image data set and simulating the input of the physician, the classification rate could be increased up to over 90% after 2 iterations. A screenshot of the graphical user interface (GUI) is presented in Figure 1.

4 Discussion

The use of CAD systems becomes a more important part of clinical workflows today. These systems can provide a second opinion without the need of a second physician and thus might save cost and time.

We have presented a system for the interpretation of endoscopic images of the esophagus which is able support the physician while he is examining the patient using a gastroscopic video tip-chip endoscope. That makes it possible to integrate the system easily into the existing workflows to provide the physician a second opinion at the point of care (POC) immediately. The diagnosis assistance we provide is based on a validated knowledge database. The database we use contains 482 annotated image regions. The database includes cases of all usual changes of the surface tissue. Therefore the system is able to handle all these changes.

The feature extraction algorithms have also a big influence on the performance of the complete system. We use the algorithms which are presented in [10] and which seem to fit the requirements of our task. The use of other feature extraction algorithms can surely increase the accuracy and will be tested in the future.

The statistics for esophageal cancer show that there are several additional factors which can influence the risk. Such known factors include the weight, the age, the consumption of tobacco and alcohol and the existence of similar cancers

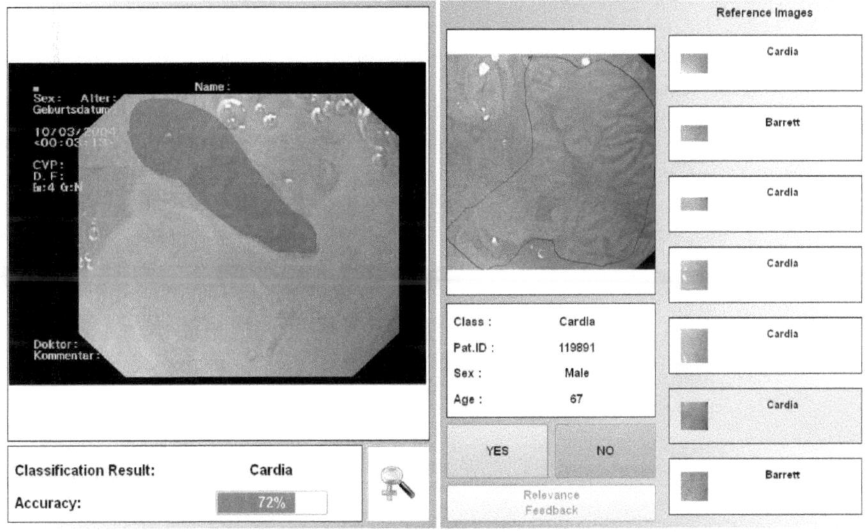

Fig. 1. Screenshot of the GUI of the proposed system. On the left pane the actual endoscopic *live* image is depicted. The user has the possibility to capture and freeze the current live image by pushing a foot-button. Then a region of interest can be interactively marked in the acquired image as shown in the screenshot. Within the next instant, the system computes a classification result and presents it to the user immediately. On the right hand side a list of all database entries which have been used to create the result is presented. All of these reference images can be reviewed by the user and marked as *relevant* or *not relevant*. After doing that the system uses this feedback to compute a new refined result

in the patient's family. The inclusion of these anamnestic parameters as well as the inclusion of the patients demographic data is likely to further increase the accuracy of the diagnosis assistance and will be part of our future work.

References

1. Bertz J, Giersiepen K, Haberland J, et al. Krebs in Deutschland: Häufigkeiten und Trends. Saarbrücken: GEKID & RKI; 2006.
2. Tjoa MP, Krishnan SM. Feature extraction for the analysis of colon status from the endoscopic images. Biomed Eng OnLine. 2003;2(9):1–17.
3. Illgner JH, , Palm C, et al. Colour texture analysis for quantitative laryngoscopy. Acta Otolaryngol. 2003;123:730–4.
4. Karkanis SA, Iakovidis DK, Maroulis DE, et al. Computer-aided tumor detection in endoscopic video using color wavelet features. IEEE Trans Inform Tech Biomed. 2003; p. 141–51.
5. Maroulis DE, Iakovidis DK, Karkanis SA, et al. ColD: A versatile detection system for colorectal lesions in endoscopy video-frames. Comp Meth Prog Biomed. 2003;70:151–66.
6. Ji Q, Engel J, Craine E. Classification cervix tissue patterns with texture analysis. J Pattern Recogn. 2000;33(9):1–13.
7. Ji Q, Engel J, Craine E. Texture analysis for classification of cervix lesions. IEEE Trans Med Imaging. 2000;19(11):1144–9.
8. Chen YQ. Novel techniques for image texture classification [PhD Thesis]. Dept. of Electronics and Computer Science, University of Southampton; 1995.
9. Unser M. Sum and Difference Histograms for Texture Analysis. IEEE Trans Pattern Anal Mach Intell. 1986;8(1):118–25.
10. Münzenmayer C. Color Texture-Analyis in Medical Applications. Tönning: Der andere Verlag; 2006.
11. Münzenmayer C, Hirsch A, Paulus D, et al. Diagnostic reasoning supported by content-based image retrieval. Proc Koblenzer Farbworkshop. 2005;3(3):141–8.
12. Handels H. Medizinische Bildverarbeitung. Teubner, Stuttgart; 2000.

A Global Criterion for the Computation of Statistical Shape Model Parameters Based on Correspondence Probabilities

Heike Hufnagel[1,2], Xavier Pennec[1], Jan Ehrhardt[2], Nicholas Ayache[1], Heinz Handels[2]

[1] INRIA Asclepios Project, 06902 Sophia Antipolis, France
[2] Medizinische Informatik, Universität Hamburg, 20246 Hamburg
h.hufnagel@uke.uni-hamburg.de

Abstract. A fundamental problem when building a statistical shape model (SSM) is the correspondence problem. We present an approach for unstructured point sets where one-to-one correspondences are replaced by correspondence probabilities between shapes which are determined using the Expectation Maximization - Iterative Closest Points registration. We propose a unified MAP framework to compute the model parameters which leads to an optimal adaption of the model to the observations. The optimization of the MAP explanation with respect to the observation and the generative model parameters leads to very efficient and closed-form solutions for (almost) all parameters. Experimental results on synthetic data and brain structures as well as a performance comparison with a statistical shape model built on one-to-one correspondences show the efficiency and advantages of this approach.

1 Introduction

In order to analyze shape variability it is necessary to determine correspondences between the observations of the training set. Several techniques were developed to automatically find exact correspondences [1], some in combination with the search for the SSM [2, 3] or a shape analysis [4]. An interesting approach proposes an entropy based criterion to find shape correspondences [5]. However, these methods are not easily adaptable to point sets as exact correspondences can only be determined between continuous surfaces, not between point cloud representations of surfaces. The SoftAssign algorithm tries to solve this problem with an initial probabilistic formulation [6]. In order to build a SSM for unstructured point sets, we advance the probabilistic concept of [7] using the EM-ICP registration which proved to be robust, precise, and fast [8]. The approach solves for the mean shape and the eigenmodes in a unique criterion *without* the need of one-to-one correspondences as is usually required by the PCA. This article focuses on the validation of the work presented in [9].

2 Methods and Experiments

We first realize a MAP estimation of the model and observation parameters which leads to a unique criterion. We then compute the SSM which best fits the given data set by optimizing the global criterion iteratively with respect to all model and observation parameters. A key part of our method is that we can find a closed-form solution for nearly each of the parameters.

2.1 Statistical Shape Model Built on Correspondence Probabilities

In the process of computing the SSM, we distinguish strictly between model parameters and observation parameters. The generative SSM is explicitly defined by 4 model parameters: The mean shape $\bar{M} \in \mathbb{R}^{3N_m}$ parameterized by N_m points $m_j \in \mathbb{R}^3$, the eigenmodes v_p consisting of N_m 3D vectors v_{pj}, the associated standard deviations λ_p which describe the impact of the eigenmodes, and the number n of eigenmodes. Using the generative model $\Theta = \{\bar{M}, v_p, \lambda_p, n\}$ of a given structure, the shape variations of that structure can be generated by $M_k = \bar{M} + \sum_{p=1}^{n} \omega_{kp} v_p$ with $\omega_{kp} \in \mathbb{R}$ being the deformation coefficients. The shape variations along the modes follow a Gaussian probability with variance λ_p and $\Omega_k = \{\omega_{kp}, p = 0, ..., n-1\}$.

$$p(M_k|\Theta) = p(\Omega_k|\Theta) = \prod_{p=1}^{n} p(\omega_{kp}|\Theta) = \frac{1}{(2\pi)^{n/2} \prod_{p=1}^{n} \lambda_p} \exp\left(-\sum_{p=1}^{n} \frac{\omega_{kp}^2}{2\lambda_p^2}\right) \quad (1)$$

In order to account for the unknown position and orientation of the model in space, we introduce the linear transformation T_k. A model point m_j can then be deformed and placed in space by the linear transformation T_k with $T_k \star m_{kj} = T_k \star (\bar{m}_j + \sum_p \omega_{kp} v_p)$. Finally, we model each observation point s_{ki} as a Gaussian measurement of a (transformed) model point m_j. As we do not know the originating model point for each observation point s_{ki}, the probability of a given s_{ki} is described by a Mixture of Gaussians and the probability for the whole scene S_k becomes:

$$p(S_k|M, T_k) = \prod_{i=1}^{N_k} \frac{1}{N_m} \sum_{j=1}^{N_m} p(s_{ki}|m_j, T_k) \quad (2)$$

with $p(s_{ki}|m_j, T_k) = (2\pi)^{-3/2} \sigma^{-1} \exp(-\frac{1}{2\sigma^2}(s_{ki} - T_k \star m_j)^T.(s_{ki} - T_k \star m_j))$. We summarize the observation parameters as $Q_k = \{\Omega_k, T_k\}$.

2.2 Derivation of the Global Criterion Using a MAP Approach

When building the SSM, we use N observations $S_k \in \mathbb{R}^{3N_k}$, and we are interested in the parameters linked to the observations $Q = \{Q_k\}$ as well as the unknown model parameters Θ. In order to determine all parameters of interest, we optimize a MAP on Q and Θ.

$$\text{MAP} = -\sum_{k=1}^{N} \log(p(Q_k, \Theta|S_k)) = -\sum_{k=1}^{N} \log\left(\frac{p(S_k|Q_k, \Theta)p(Q_k|\Theta)p(\Theta)}{p(S_k)}\right) \quad (3)$$

As $p(S_k)$ does not depend on Θ and $p(\Theta)$ is assumed to be uniform, the global criterion integrating our unified framework is the following:

$$C(Q, \Theta) = -\sum_{k=1}^{N} \left(\log(p(S_k|Q_k, \Theta)) + \log(p(Q_k|\Theta)) \right) \quad (4)$$

The first term describes the ML criterion (eq. (2)) whereas the second term is the prior on the deformation coefficients ω_{kp} as described in eq.(1). Dropping the constants, our criterion simplifies to $C(Q, \Theta) \sim \sum_{k=1}^{N} C_k(Q_k, \Theta)$ with

$$C_k(Q_k, \Theta) = \sum_{p=1}^{n} \left(\log(\lambda_p) + \frac{\omega_{kp}^2}{2\lambda_p^2} \right) - \sum_{i=1}^{N_k} \log\left(\sum_{j=1}^{N_m} \exp\left(-\frac{\|s_{ki} - T_k \star m_{kj}\|^2}{2\sigma^2} \right) \right) (5)$$

This equation is the heart of the unified framework for the model computation and its fitting to observations. By optimizing it alternately with respect to the operands in $\{Q, \Theta\}$, we are able to determine all parameters we are interested in. In a first step, all observations are aligned with the initial mean shape by estimating the T_k using the EM-ICP. In order to robustify, we used a multi-scaling scheme concerning the variance σ^2, for details please refer to [9]. Starting from the initial model parameters Θ, we then fit the model to each of the observations. Next, we fix the observation parameters Q_k and update the model parameters. This is iterated until convergence.

2.3 Experiments

We present two experiments we ran in order to evaluate our approach. A typical correspondence problem: One of our arguments against the concept of enforcing homologies between points representing surfaces is the fact that certain shape structures of one observation might not appear on all observations of the training set. We constructed a synthetic data set containing 20 observations in order to illustrate this problem, see figure 1 a). Half of the ellipsoids are equipped with a bump, and the other half are not. A reliable SSM should be able to represent both classes by including this distinction in its variability model. In order to compare the results, we generated two SSMs, one by using our new method, the other one by using the traditional ICP and PCA.

Our data set consists of $N = 21$ left segmented putamen observations (approximately $20mm \times 20mm \times 40mm$) which are represented by min 994 and max 1673 points (Fig. 1c)). In order to assess the quality of a SSM, we measure two performance measures as proposed in [10]. A good generalization ability is

Table 1. Performance Measures. Shape distances found in generalization experiments (7 leave-one-out tests) and in specificity experiments (500 random shapes) with our SSM approach and with an ICP+PCA approach using 18 eigenmodes

Generalization ability	ICP+PCA model	our SSM
average mean distance + standard deviation in mm	0.610 ± 0.089	0.447 ± 0.101
average max. distance + standard deviation in mm	4.388 ± 0.930	2.426 ± 0.712
Specificity	ICP+PCA model	our SSM
average mean distance + standard deviation in mm	0.515 ± 0.117	0.452 ± 0.020

important for recognition purposes as a SSM must be able to adopt the shape of an unseen observation which comes from the same structure type. We test it in a series of leave-one-out experiments. The SSM is first aligned with the unseen observation, then the matching is optimized by finding the best deformation coefficients ω. Finally, the distance of the deformed SSM to the left-out observation is measured. The specificity of a SSM must be high for shape prediction purposes as the SSM should only adopt shapes similar to the ones in the underlying training set. We generated random shapes x which are uniformly distributed with σ being equal to the standard deviation of the SSM. Next, we computed the distance of the random shapes to the closest observations in the training data set. As we do not have surface representations, we chose a distance measure which computes the average minimum point distance between the deformed model points and the observation points.

3 Results

For our SSM, the following parameters were chosen: $\sigma_{\text{start}} = 4$mm, reduction factor $= 0.85$, 10 iterations (EM-ICP) with 5 SSM iterations. For the ICP+PCA SSM, we iterated the ICP 50 times. The results for the experiments concerning the typical correspondence problem are shown in Figure 1 a),b). For both meth-

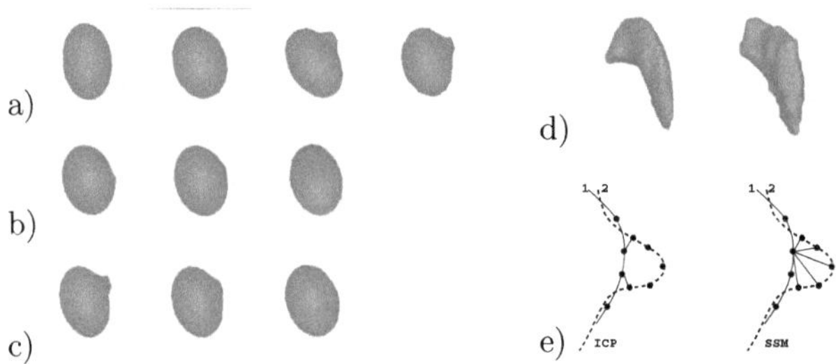

Fig. 1. SSM on synthetic data set: (a) Ellipsoid observation examples; (b) Results SSM/ICP; (c) Results SSM/EM-ICP with final mean shape (middle), and the mean shapes deformed with respect to the first eigenmode ($\bar{M} - 3\lambda_1 \boldsymbol{v}_1$ and $\bar{M} + 3\lambda_1 \boldsymbol{v}_1$); (d) Putamen observation examples; (e) Exact correspondence versus correspondence probabilities. Left: ICP, right: EM-ICP.

ods, we chose the initial model from the ellipsoid class without bump. The first row shows the mean shape and eigenmodes for the SSM built by the ICP+PCA SSM whereas the second row shows those for our SSM.

The results of the testing series for the generalization ability and the specificity for both our SSM and the ICP+PCA SSM on putamen data are depicted in table 1. We performed the leave-one out test for 7 different unknown observations. The specificity was computed for 500 random shapes. We computed the average and maximal distances as well as the variances.

4 Discussion

We proposed a mathematically sound and unified framework for the computation of model parameters and observation parameters and succeeded in determining a closed form solution for optimizing the associated criterion alternately for all parameters. Experiments showed that our algorithm works well and leads to plausible results. It seems to be robust to different initial mean shape choices and is stable even for small numbers of observations. We showed the efficiency of our approach compared with a SSM built by the traditional ICP and PCA for a typical correspondence problem on synthetic data: The SSM based on the EM-ICP models the whole data set, it is able to represent the ellipsoids featuring a bump and those without as that deformation information is included in its variability model. On the other hand, the results show that the SSM based on the ICP is not able to model the bump. This is due to the fact that the ICP only takes into account the closest point when searching for correspondence, thus, the point on top of the bump is not involved in the registration process. The EM-ICP, however, evaluates the correspondence probability of *all* points, therefore, also the point on top of the bump is matched. We illustrated these two concepts in figure 1d). Furthermore, in the test series on putamen data, our SSM achieved superior results in both performance measures. Especially the values of the maximal distance illustrate the benefit of the new approach. From a theoretical point of view, a very powerful feature of our method is that we are optimizing a unique criterion. Thus, the convergence is ensured.

Acknowledgement. This work is supported by a grant from the DFG, HA2355.

References

1. Besl PJ, McKay ND. A method for registration of 3D shapes. IEEE Trans Pattern Anal Mach Intell. 1992;14:239–56.
2. Davies RH, Twining CJ, Cootes TF. A minimum description length approach to statistical shape modeling. IEEE Medical Imaging. 2002;21(5):525–37.
3. Heimann T, Wolf I, Williams T, et al. 3D Active shape models using gradient descent optimization of description length. Proc IPMI. 2005;3565:566–77.
4. Tsai A, Wells WM, Warfield SK, et al. An EM algorithm for shape classification based on level sets. Med Image Anal. 2005;9:491–502.

5. Cates J, Meyer M, Fletcher PT, et al. Entropy-based particle systems for shape correspondences. Proc MICCAI. 2006; p. 90–9.
6. Rangarajan A, Chui H, Bookstein FL. The softassign procrustes matching algorithm. Proc IPMI. 1997;1230:29–42.
7. Hufnagel H, Pennec X, Ehrhardt J, et al. Point-based statistical shape models with probabilistic correspondences and affine EM-ICP. Proc BVM. 2007; p. 434–8.
8. Granger S, Pennec X. Multi-scale EM-ICP: A fast and robust approach for surface registration. Lec Not Comp Sci. 2002;2525:418–32.
9. Hufnagel H, Pennec X, Ehrhardt J, et al. Shape analysis using a point-based statistical shape model built on correspondence probabilities. Proc MICCAI. 2007;1:959–67.
10. Styner M, Rajamani KT, Nolte LP, et al. Evaluation of 3D correspondence methods for model building. Proc IPMI. 2003;2732:63–75.

Verbesserte Visualisierung der Koronararterien in MSCT-Daten mit direkter Vergleichbarkeit zur Angiographie

Christina Lacalli[1], Marion Jähne[2], Stefan Wesarg[2]

[1]Abteilung Cognitive Computing & Medical Imaging, Fraunhofer IGD Darmstadt
[2]Graphisch-Interaktive Systeme, Technische Universität Darmstadt
christina.lacalli@igd.fraunhofer.de

Kurzfassung. In diesem Beitrag stellen wir neue, automatisierte Verfahren zur Visualisierung der Koronararterien einerseits und für eine direkte Vergleichbarkeit mit konventionellen Angiogrammen andererseits vor. Unser Ansatz umfasst Methoden für die automatische Extraktion des Herzens aus kontrastverstärkten CT-Daten, sowie für die Maskierung grosser kontrastmittelgefüllter Kavitäten des Herzens, um die Sichtbarkeit der Koronararterien bei der Darstellung mittels Volumenrendering zu verbessern. Zum direkten Vergleich mit konventionellen Angiographien wurde ein Verfahren zur automatischen Generierung von Projektionsansichten aus den CT-Daten entwickelt.

1 Einleitung

Bis heute stellt die invasive Koronarangiographie den *Goldstandard* in der Analyse der Koronararterien dar. Die neueste Generation der MSCT-Scanner ermöglicht eine schonendere, nicht-invasive Untersuchung, wobei sich die Frage stellt, inwieweit die auf den CT-Daten basierenden Analyseergebnisse mit dem etablierten Verfahren konkurrieren können. Dies verlangt nach einer direkten Vergleichsmöglichkeit der beiden Modalitäten.

Ein allgemeines Problem bei der Visualisierung von kardiologischen CT-Daten mittels Volumenrendering ist die eingeschränkte Sichtbarkeit auf das Herz und die Koronararterien. Eine einfache und in der klinischen Praxis angewandte Lösung ist ein manuelles, aber zeitaufwendiges Beschneiden der CT-Daten. Es existieren bereits Verfahren zur automatischen Extraktion des Herzens [1, 2]. Im Gegensatz zu diesen Ansätzen verwenden wir weniger Annahmen über die Lage des Herzens.

Eine direkte Vergleichsmöglichkeit zwischen CT-Daten und Angiogrammen erfordert jedoch eine Darstellungsform, bei der beide Daten einander entsprechen. Eine Möglichkeit ist die 3D-Rekonstruktion der Koronararterien aus multiplanaren Angiogrammen und der Vergleich derselben mit dem aus den CT-Daten segmentierten Gefäßbaum [3, 4, 5]. Umgekehrt ist es möglich, den aus den CT-Daten extrahierten Gefäßbaum auf eine Bildebene zu projizieren [6]. Wir stellen eine alternative, automatisierte Methode vor, die ohne explizite Segmentierung, aus den CT-Daten sogenannte *Digitally Reconstructed Radiographies* (DRRs) generiert.

2 Material und Methoden

Im Folgenden beschreiben wir unsere beiden Methoden für die verbesserte Visualisierung der Koronararterien in volumengerenderten CT-Daten. Wir zeigen, wie eine dem Angiogramm ähnliche Projektionsansicht aus den CT-Daten generiert werden kann, um eine direkte Vergleichbarkeit zwischen den beiden Modalitäten zu ermöglichen. Abb. 1 gibt eine Übersicht über die einzelnen Verfahren.

2.1 Extraktion des Herzens

Bei der Visualisierung kardiologischer CT-Daten ohne Vorverarbeitung stören anatomische Strukturen (Rippen, Brustbein) die Sicht auf das Herz (Abb. 1 (a)). Wir präsentieren eine Methode mit der diese Strukturen zuvor entfernt werden, um eine störungsfreie Sicht auf das Herz zu erhalten.

Die Grauwerte in den CT-Daten korrelieren mit den anatomischen Strukturen. Mit Otsu's automatischem Schwellwertverfahren [7] teilen wir die Original CT-Daten in drei Grauwertklassen ein. Die dunkelste Grauwertklasse entspricht Luft, die mittlere Fett- und Muskelgewebe und die hellste entspricht Knochen und den kontrastmittelgefüllten Kavitäten. In den axialen Schichten wird der Schwerpunkt über die beiden hellsten Grauwertklassen berechnet.

Vom berechneten Schwerpunkt wird ein radiales Suchstrahlmuster [8] ausgesendet, um die äußere Begrenzung des Herzens zu ermitteln. Klare hell-dunkel Übergänge werden detektiert. An Bereichen an denen das Herz angewachsen ist (Aorta, Brustbein) sind die Suchstrahlen zu lang und werden mittels Strahllängeninterpolation korrigiert. Aus den Endpunkten der Suchstrahlen wird eine binäre Maske erzeugt, die in den Original CT-Daten die störenden äußeren Strukturen entfernt (Abb. 1 (b)).

2.2 Direkter Vergleich zwischen CT-Daten und Angiogrammen

Die Verwendung der Original CT-Daten für die DRR-Generierung führt zu Problemen hinsichtlich der Sichtbarkeit der Koronararterien in den erzeugten Projektionsansichten. Einerseits verdecken auch hier die umliegenden Knochenstrukturen die Sicht auf das Herz. Da das Kontrastmittel systemisch verabreicht wird, werden die Koronararterien zusätzlich durch die grossen Herzkavitäten (Ventrikel, Atria) überdeckt. Durch Anwendung der oben generierten Maske können die umliegenden Strukturen entfernt werden. Wir stellen nun ein Verfahren vor, das zusätzlich die störenden Herzkavitäten automatisch aus den CT-Daten entfernt.

Die kontrastmittelgefüllten Kavitäten wurden in 2.1 dem hellsten Grauwertbereich zugeordnet. Durch ein einfaches Thresholding erzeugen wir aus den gelabelten CT-Daten zunächst eine binäre Maske, die sowohl die grossen Kavitäten als auch die Koronararterien aus den CT-Daten entfernt. Unter Verwendung

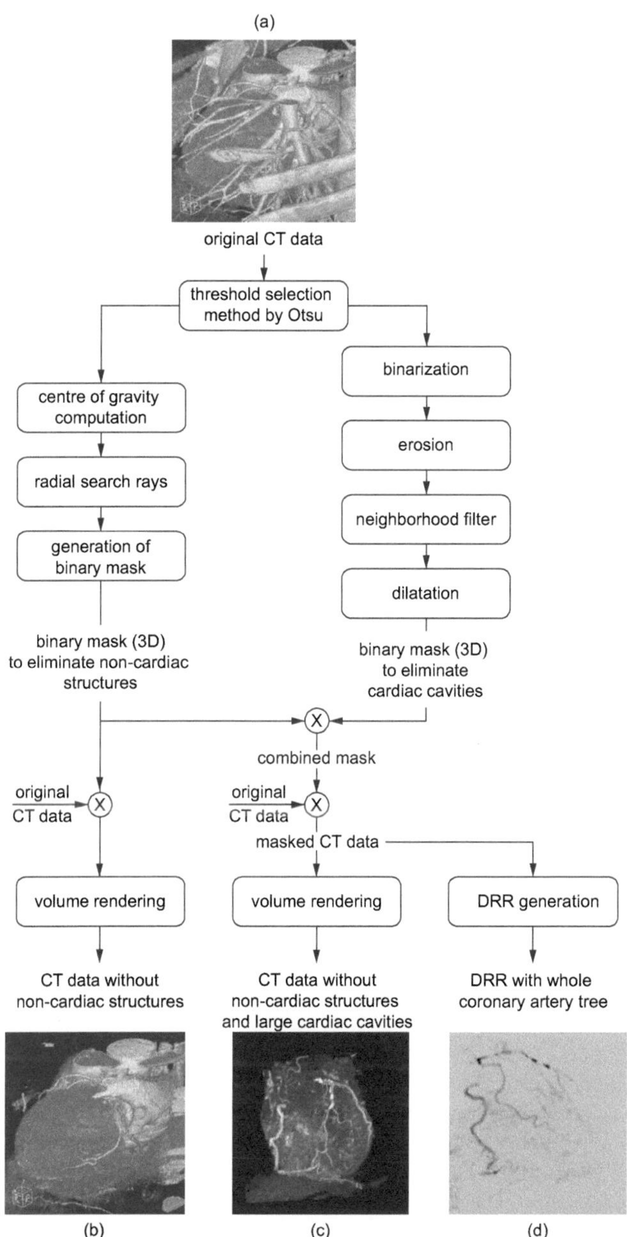

Abb. 1. (a) Original CT-Daten. (b) CT-Daten ohne störende äußere Strukturen. (c) CT-Daten ohne störende äußere Strukturen und ohne störende grosse Kavitäten. (d) Aus den maskierten CT-Daten generiertes DRR. Sowohl störende äußere Strukturen als auch störende grosse Kavitäten werden ausgeblendet

morphologischer Operatoren wird die binäre Maske so verändert, dass sie nur die kontrastmittelgefüllten Kavitäten, nicht aber die Koronararterien in den bereits in den Aussenbereichen des Herzens maskierten CT-Daten entfernt.

Die Erzeugung künstlicher Projektionsansichten aus den maskierten CT-Daten basiert auf einem perspektivischen Projektionsmodell. Die relevanten geometrischen Parameter, um aus den CT-Daten eine dem Angiogramm entsprechende Ansicht zu generieren, werden automatisch aus deren DICOM-Header bestimmt. Die Intensität eines jeden Pixels des zu generierenden DRRs wird durch Summation der Grauwerte aller Voxel entlang des virtuellen Röntgenstrahls berechnet.

3 Ergebnisse

Die Verfahren zur Extraktion des Herzens und der erweiterten Maskierung wurden mit 25 CT-Datensätzen getestet. Dabei konnten jeweils in einem einzigen Verarbeitungsschritt die das Herz umgebenden Strukturen, als auch störende Herzkavitäten erfolgreich ausmaskiert werden (Abb. 1 (b) und (c)). Die Generierung der DRRs wurde für solche 8 Datensätze getestet, für die entsprechende Angiogramme vorlagen, und lieferte in 5 von 8 Fällen morphologisch äquivalente Ansichten der Koronararterien zu denen in konventionellen Angiogrammen (Abb. 2 (b)). Insgesamt lag die Bearbeitungszeit bei durchschnittlich 7 bis 11 Sekunden (2 GHz AMD Athlon).

4 Diskussion

Die Extraktion des Herzens und die Maskierung der grossen, kontrastmittelgefüllten Kavitäten ermöglichen dem Radiologen eine störungsfreie Sicht auf das Herz und die Koronararterien in volumengerenderten CT-Daten. Eine einfache, direkte Vergleichsmöglichkeit, um Korrespondenzen zwischen pathologischen Strukturen zu finden, wird dem Radiologen durch die Erzeugung von DRRs gegeben.

Im Gegensatz zu [1] finden wir die äußere Herzbegrenzung ausgehend von dem automatisch bestimmten Mittelpunkt des Herzens. Wir benötigen daher weniger Vorwissen über die Lage des Herzens in den CT-Daten. Damit ist unser Ansatz flexibler für unterschiedliche Fields-of-View einsetzbar. [2] bestimmen zunächst einige Punkte innerhalb des Herzens und einige Punkte ausserhalb des Herzens. Dabei gehen sie jedoch davon aus, dass die Rippen symmetrisch um das Herz verteilt sind. Da die Bildakquisition in der klinischen Routine nicht standardisiert ist, ist jedoch nicht immer der komplette Brustkorb in kardiologischen CT-Daten enthalten. Dies könnte ein Grund dafür sein, warum die Initialisierung nicht immer gelingt. Der Vorteil der vorgestellten DRR-Generierung ist neben der automatisierten Berechnung, dass wir ohne vorhergehende Segmentierung des Gefäßbaumes, weder in den CT-Daten noch in den Angiogrammen, auskommen.

Abb. 2. (a) Konventionelles Angiogramm der linken Koronararterie (RAO 30.9 / CRAN 0.1). (b) Aus den maskierten CT-Daten generiertes DRR. Der gesamte Gefäßbaum ist sichtbar. (c) Um nur die linke Koronararterie darzustellen, werden die maskierten CT-Daten vor der Projektion geclippt

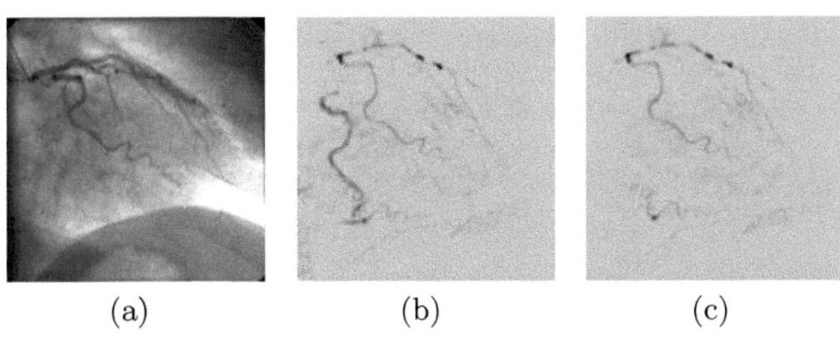

Da die CT-Daten vollständig in die Berechnungen der einzelnen Verfahren einfliessen, hängt die Qualität der Ergebnisse von der Qualität der Original CT-Daten ab. Erfolgte beispielsweise die Rekonstruktion der CT-Daten zu einem Zeitpunkt, zu dem das Kontrastmittel ungleichmäßig verteilt war, ist eine klare Einteilung der kontrastmittelgefüllten Kavitäten in die hellste Grauwertklasse schwierig. Um derartige Probleme zu umgehen, ist es dem Radiologen möglich, Parameter, wie die Anzahl der Schwellwerte, anzupassen.

Derzeit arbeiten wir an einer Registrierung der erzeugten DRRs mit den entsprechenden Angiogrammen. Darauf aufbauend könnten Parameter aus der CT-Analyse direkt in die Angiogramme eingeblendet werden. Dies wäre ein weiterer Schritt, um das Vertrauen des Radiologen in das nicht-invasive Untersuchungsverfahren MSCT zu erhöhen.

Literaturverzeichnis

1. Lorenz C, Lessick J, Lavi G, et al. Fast automatic delineation of cardiac volume of interest in MSCT images. Proc SPIE. 2004 may;5370:456–66.
2. Funka-Lea G, Boykov Y, Florin C, et al. Automatic heart isolation for CT coronary visualization using graph-cuts. Proc ISBI. 2006; p. 614–7.
3. Großkopf S, Hildebrand A. Three-dimensional reconstruction of coronary arteries from X-ray projections. In: Lanzer P, editor. Diagnostics of Vascular Diseases. Principles and Technology. Berlin; Heidelberg: Springer; 1997. p. 307–14.
4. Sang N, Peng W, Li H, et al. 3D reconstruction of the coronary tree from two X-ray angiographic views. Proc SPIE. 2006;6144:1591–8.
5. Blondel C, Malandain G, Vaillant R, et al. Reconstruction of coronary arteries from a single rotational X-ray projection sequence. IEEE Trans Med Imaging. 2006;25:653–63.
6. Schnapauff D, Dübel H, Scholze J, et al. Multislice computed tomography: angiographic emulation versus standard assessment for detection of coronary stenoses. Eur Radiol. 2007;17:1858–64.
7. Otsu N. A threshold selection method from gray level histograms. IEEE Trans Syst Man Cybern. 1979;9:62–6.
8. von Berg L. Fast automated object detection by recursive casting of search rays. Int Congress Series. 2005;1281:230–5.

3D Blood Flow Reconstruction from 2D Angiograms

Esther-S. Platzer[1], Frank Deinzer[2], Dietrich Paulus[3], Joachim Denzler[1]

[1]Institut für Mathematik/Informatik, Friedrich-Schiller-Universität, 07743 Jena
[2]Siemens AG, Medical Solutions, 91301 Forchheim
[3]Institut für Computervisualistik, Universität Koblenz-Landau, 56070 Koblenz
platzer@informatik.uni-jena.de

Abstract. A method for 3-d blood flow reconstruction is presented. Given a 3-d volume of a vessel tree and a 2-d sequence of angiograms, the propagation information can be back-projected into the 3-d vessel volume. In case of overlapping vessel segments in the 2-d projections, ambiguous back-projection results are obtained. We introduce a probabilistic blood flow model for solving these ambiguities. Based on the last estimated state and known system dynamics the next state is predicted, and predictions are judged by the back-projected information. The discrete realization is done with a particle filter. Experiments prove the efficiency of our method.

1 Introduction

In the field of vessel diagnostics, 2-d digital subtraction angiographies (DSA) and 3-d reconstructions of the vessel trees belong to the state of art. Since a 2-d DSA only provides 2-d+t information and a 3-d reconstruction offers non-temporal information about the vessel morphology, a fusion of both is necessary to visualize spatial and temporal coherences.

Establishing a 2-d/3-d mapping allows the look up of the bolus arrival time (BAT) for every voxel from the 2-d angiograms. Unfortunately, the mapping between 2-d pixels and 3-d voxels is usually ambiguous due to the loss of information caused by dimensionality reduction. State of the art work offers several ways to establish the mapping between pixels and voxels. Schmitt et. al [1], for example, cluster the 3-d vessel tree by a region growing algorithm and look up the BAT for every cluster in the 2-d angiograms by projecting the clusters to the detector plane. In case of ambiguities, correction of the cluster BAT with help of a median filter and heuristic assumptions is done. In [2] the mapping is established by artificial projections of the 3-d volume, which allows a 2-d/2-d mapping between angiogram and artificial projection. Ambiguities are solved for by the use of a bi-plane angiography system, associated with an increased exposure dose for patients. A third approach are numerical flow simulations, also called computational fluid dynamics (CFD). They simulate the blood flow through a given 3-d model of the vessel tree based on physics and the navier-stokes equations [3]. This simulation is very time-consuming and has to be done for every

3-d-model individually. Under use of actual hardware, this is not acceptable for clinical course of life.

We present a probabilistic model of blood flow for dissolving ambiguous mappings based on recursive state estimation. The blood flow model evaluates the probability of the back-projection results with simultaneous consideration of the existing knowledge from previous time steps. So uncertainty is decreased by the integration of additional knowledge in every new time step.

2 Materials and Methods

Our goal is to create a probabilistic model of the 3-d blood flow. With the knowledge we get from the 2-d angiograms, modelling was done by a Bayesian filter that estimates the non-measurable state $\boldsymbol{q}_t$ of a system based on the observation $\boldsymbol{o}_t$ and the actual belief of the previous state. $\langle \boldsymbol{o} \rangle_t$ is the observation sequence of all observations made from $t = 0$ until now:

$$p\left(\boldsymbol{q}_t \mid \langle \boldsymbol{o} \rangle_t\right) = \underbrace{p\left(\boldsymbol{o}_t \mid \boldsymbol{q}_t\right)}_{\text{evaluation}} \int \underbrace{p\left(\boldsymbol{q}_t \mid \boldsymbol{q}_{t-1}\right)}_{\text{prediction}} \underbrace{p\left(\boldsymbol{q}_{t-1} \mid \langle \boldsymbol{o} \rangle_{t-1}\right)}_{\text{recursion}} d\boldsymbol{q}_{t-1} \tag{1}$$

For non-linear and non-gaussian, multimodal state estimation problems normally no analytic, closed-form solution exists. Therefore a discrete realization was done using a particle filter [4, 5] in combination with the Condensation algorithm [6].

Given an initial belief of the fill state of the vessel tree and assumptions on the actual velocity and direction of the bolus front, a prediction of the covered vessel distance in the next step is possible. In the discrete case, this motion model is based on a uniform weighted voxel graph [7]. The costs of edge traversal from one voxel to another represent the distances in the vessel tree, which are weighted by a gaussian distribution with a mean corresponding to the actual velocity. For every particle, its new position can be predicted under use of a shortest-path algorithm.

The evaluation step is performed with help of sensor data, called observation $\boldsymbol{o}$, where $\boldsymbol{o}_t$ is represented by the extracted and back-projected flow information from the 2-d angiogram at time t. Particle weighting is done accordingly to the back-projected flow information and results in a corrected belief at time t.

By taking the corrected estimate as initial belief of the next time step, the gathered knowledge is propagated and increased over time. Practically, this knowledge propagation is done by resampling from the previous particle set accordingly to the particle weights.

Because no a priori knowledge is given for the initial state, it is modeled by a uniform distribution. A robust estimation in the first time steps is not possible. This will become clear in Fig. 3. Given Fig. 4(b) and a uniform particle distribution in Fig. 4(c), particles in the left and right vessel ends would gain a good evaluation in the first steps, resulting in a propagation of flow in both vessel arms. Smoothing-filters [8] allow the evaluation of a density on past and future observations. They are motivated by the fact, that the density $p(\boldsymbol{q}_T \mid \langle \boldsymbol{o} \rangle_T)$ contains all information from all angiograms and can be described by the following formula, where $\langle \boldsymbol{o} \rangle_T$ denotes all observations from angiograms 0 till T:

$$p(\boldsymbol{q}_t \mid \langle \boldsymbol{o} \rangle_T) \propto \underbrace{p(\boldsymbol{q}_t \mid \langle \boldsymbol{o} \rangle_{1:t})}_{\text{Forward Filter}} \underbrace{p(\langle \boldsymbol{o} \rangle_{t+1:T} \mid \boldsymbol{q}_t)}_{\text{Backward Filter}} \tag{2}$$

The use of a forward-backward smoother in combination with Condensation is described in [9]. The forward part of the filter is given by a simple Condensation run, resulting in a robust estimate of $\boldsymbol{q}_T$. Using this estimate as initial belief of an analogue backward run eliminates ambiguous estimates and returns a good estimate of the initial state. Usually, in the prediction step of the backward-filter, state changes are restricted to the states predetermined by the forward step:

$$p(\langle \boldsymbol{o} \rangle_{t+1:T} \mid \boldsymbol{q}_t) = \int p(\langle \boldsymbol{o} \rangle_{t+1:T} \mid \boldsymbol{q}_{t+1})\, p(\boldsymbol{q}_{t+1} \mid \boldsymbol{q}_t)\, d\boldsymbol{q}_{t+1} \tag{3}$$

In our work, we changed this restriction and used the same motion model as in the forward step, in order to compensate for the failure of observations in a sequence of 2-d-angiograms, caused by vessel overlaps. (3) changes to:

$$p(\langle \boldsymbol{o} \rangle_{t+1:T} \mid \boldsymbol{q}_t) = \int p(\langle \boldsymbol{o} \rangle_{t+1:T} \mid \boldsymbol{q}_{t+1})\, p(\boldsymbol{q}_t \mid \boldsymbol{q}_{t+1})\, d\boldsymbol{q}_{t+1} \tag{4}$$

In the evaluation step, a correction of the gained particle weights of the forward-step is performed:

$$p(\langle \boldsymbol{o} \rangle_{t:T} \mid \boldsymbol{q}_t) = p(\boldsymbol{o}_t \mid \boldsymbol{q}_t)\, p(\langle \boldsymbol{o} \rangle_{t+1:T} \mid \boldsymbol{q}_t) \tag{5}$$

In case of vessel bifurcations, the underlying densities become multimodal and two bolus fronts have to be propagated. At vessel ends, the underlying densities are unimodal, even if in-between vessel bifurcations enforce multimodal densities. In the forward step, the split-up of blood flow is supported by the motion model, but in the backward step the propagation of particles into the bifurcated vessel segments is restricted due to inverse traversal of the vessel tree. A schematic illustration of this problem is given in Fig. 1, where a particle propagation at

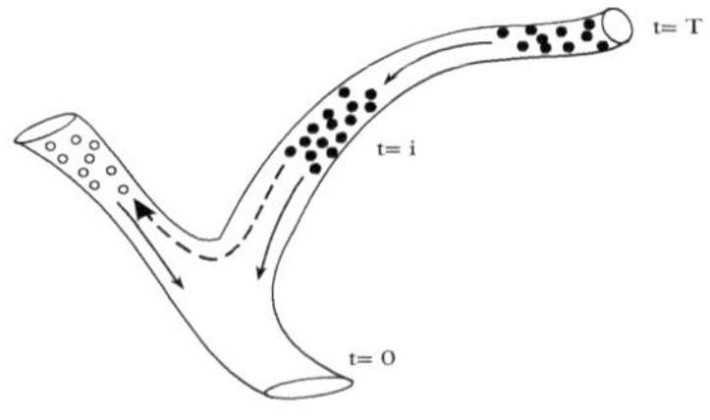

Fig. 1. Restriction of the change from an unimodal (black) to a multimodal (outlined) density. The distance in the graph is marked with the dashed line

$t = i$ into the left vessel segment is prohibited because of too large distances. This problem was solved by an additional, slightly modified forward run, offering the data for a correct visualization. It relies on the robust estimate of the initial state, returned by the forward-backward smoother and uses $\langle \boldsymbol{o} \rangle_t$ instead of $\boldsymbol{o}_t$ for the likelihood estimation in order to compensate for the different velocities in the bifurcated vessel segments.

3 Experiments and Results

Evaluation was done on different angiography sequences of a vessel phantom, including views resulting in many overlaps, especially at beginning and the end of the vessels (Fig. 3 (a)-(b)). Fig. 4(c) shows the 3-d reconstruction of the vessel phantom. All acquisitions were done on a Siemens Artis dFA, and for all computations an AMD Athlon64 X2 3800+ was used. Computation time for one time step with 15000 particles lies at approximately 30-40 seconds were most time is spent on the evaluation process. All experiments were performed with different-sized particle sets ranging from 1000 till 15000 particles. We compared our results to those of pure back-projection. Additionally, for ground-truth evaluation, the ambiguous back-projection information was solved for manually, and the number of correct particles regarding a non-ambiguous flow was determined. In all experiments a particle size of 2000 copes a feasible 3-d blood flow reconstruction. All ambiguities could be dissolved, even in case of overlapping vessel segments at the beginning of the sequence. Furthermore, the failure of observations can be compensated due to the estimation process based on the system dynamics. Observation failures result from artefacts avoiding a correct extraction of flow information, as well as huge vessel overlaps that cause mutual subtraction of the flow information (Fig. 4(b)). Fig. 2 shows the number of correct particles out of all good-evaluated particles reconstructed from Fig. 4(b). In the first forward run (Fig. 2(a)), the number of correct particles (shaded) is less than that of all good-evaluated particles (solid), whereas in the second forward run (Fig. 2(b)) all ambiguities could be resolved. Snapshots of the 3-d reconstruction and its visualization of blood flow are shown in Fig. 3(d)-(f).

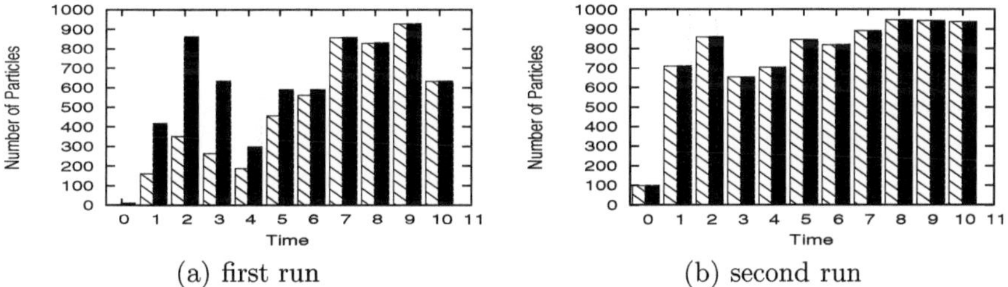

(a) first run (b) second run

Fig. 2. Number of correct particles (shaded) related to the number of all good-evaluated particles (solid) for both forward runs (1000 particles)

Fig. 3. Angiograms from frontal (a) and side view (b), 3-d reconstruction of the vessel phantom (c) and results of the 3-d blood flow visualization (d)-(f)

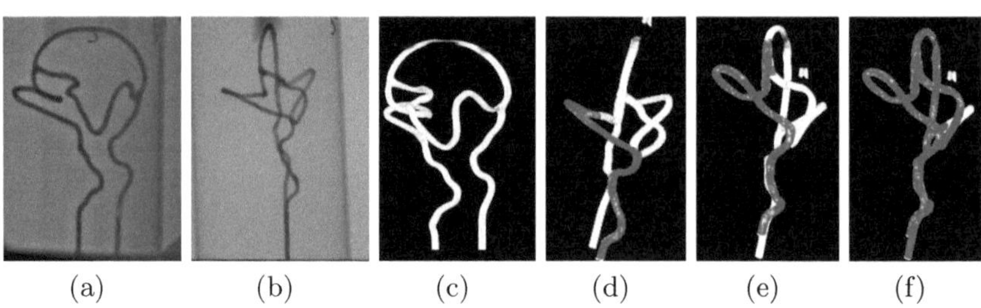

(a) (b) (c) (d) (e) (f)

4 Discussion

A method for 3-d reconstruction of blood flow with help of the propagation information, gathered from a 2-d angiography sequence, was presented. Our probabilistic model relies on the theory of state estimation in a dynamic system, and discrete realization was done with a forward-backward-forward particle filter. Weak point of our model is the motion model. Because system dynamics not being stable, especially in case of vessel bifurcations, the motion model has to be updated during the whole estimation process. The computational overload could be reduced by the use of adaptive particle filters [5], and the motion model could be improved by CFD-methods which allow further modelling of non-observable flow characteristics in aneurysms or the diffusion of blood and contrast agent.

References

1. Schmitt H, Grass M, Rasche V, et al. An X-ray-based method for the determination of the contrast agent propagation in 3-d vessel structures. IEEE Trans Med Imaging. 2002;21(3):251–62.
2. Hüllmandel T. Räumliche und zeitliche Rekonstruktion in der Neuroradiologie [Diplomarbeit]. Universität Würzburg; 2004.
3. Ford MD, Stuhne GR, Nikolov HN, et al. Virtual angiography for visualization and validation of computational models of aneurysm hemodynamics. IEEE Trans Med Imaging. 2005 12;24(12):1586–92.
4. Arulampalam S, Maskell S, Gordon N, et al. A tutorial on particle filters for on-line non-linear/non-Gaussian Bayesian tracking. IEEE Trans Signal Process. 2002;50(2):174–88.
5. Doucet A, de Freitas N, Gordon N. Sequential Monte Carlo Methods in Practice. Springer, Berlin; 2001.
6. Isard M, Blake A. CONDENSATION: Conditional density propagation for visual tracking. Int J Computer Vis. 1998;29(1):5–28.
7. Xu L. Konzipierung und Realisierung eines interaktiven Editors für Gefäßgraphen. DKFZ Heidelberg; 2005.
8. Kitagawa G. Monte Carlo filter and smoother for non-Gaussian nonlinear state space models. J Comput Graph Stat. 1996;5(1):1–25.
9. Isard M, Blake A. A smoothing filter for Condensation. Proc ECCV. 1998;1:767–81.

SinusEndoscopy
Ein skalierbares Visualisierungssystem für die virtuelle Endoskopie

Arno Krüger[1], Christoph Kubisch[1], Ilka Richter[2,3], Gero Strauß[3], Bernhard Preim[1]

[1]Institut für Simulation und Graphik, Otto-von-Guericke-Universität Magdeburg
[2]Innovation Center for Computer Assisted Surgery (ICCAS), Leipzig
[3]Abteilung HNO-Heilkunde, Universitätskrankenhaus Leipzig
krueger@isg.cs.uni-magdeburg.de

Kurzfassung. Für komplizierte endoskopische Operationstechniken im Bereich der Nasennebenhöhlen (NNH) ist eine sorgfältige Planung des Eingriffs notwendig. Aufgrund des eingeschränkten Sichtfeldes stehen dem Operateur während der Operation weniger Informationen über das Umfeld im Arbeitsbereich zur Verfügung. Um sich an diese erschwerten Bedingungen zu gewöhnen bieten Systeme zur virtuellen Endoskopie die Möglichkeit, sich mit der Umgebung vertraut zu machen. In diesem Beitrag wird ein neuartiges System vorgestellt, das, basierend auf direktem Volumenrendering, den gängigen Funktionsumfang virtueller Endoskopie Systeme bietet, mit besonderem Fokus auf eine realistische Darstellung. Die Bildqualität der Endoskopiesicht lässt sich derart skalieren, dass außer einer modernen Grafikkarte keine Spezialhardware zum Einsatz kommen muss, um eine interaktive Darstellung zu erreichen. Gezielt werden dabei Besonderheiten des Einsatzzwecks zur Optimierung des Volumenrenderings verwendet.

1 Einleitung

Zur Planung und Übung minimal-invasiver endoskopischer Operationstechniken wird die virtuelle Endoskopie bereits in verschiedenen Bereichen erfolgreich unterstützend eingesetzt [1, 2]. Beim endoskopischen Eingriff kann der Operateur nur auf einem Bildschirm die Auswirkungen seiner Handlungen beobachten. Die Reduktion auf ein zweidimensionales Abbild ist dabei eine besondere Herausforderung. Virtuelle Endoskopie zur HNO-Operationsplanung ermöglicht es dem Operateur, sich Landmarken einzuprägen, an denen er sich zum Zeitpunkt des Eingriffs orientieren kann. Die ohnehin zur Operationsvorbereitung aufgenommenen CT-Daten können dabei für die virtuelle Endoskopie ohne Mehraufwand genutzt werden. Zum besseren Erkennen der zu erlernenden Landmarken ist es sinnvoll, dass die Darstellung in der virtuellen Endoskopie möglichst realistisch ist. Darüber hinaus sollte es dem Chirurg möglich sein, die Daten effizient zu explorieren, welches der größte Kritikpunkt für den klinischen Einsatz von existierenden Systemen ist. Das hier vorgestellte System widmet sich demzufolge vor allem der Verbesserung der Handhabung und der Darstellung bei der virtuellen Planung von NNH-Operationen.

2 Stand der Forschung und Zielstellung

Es gibt bereits eine Reihe von Systemen, die zur virtuellen Endoskopie eingesetzt werden [1, 3, 4]. Sie unterscheiden sich neben dem Einsatzgebiet meist auch im Renderingverfahren der Volumendaten. Grundsätzlich unterscheidet man zwischen indirektem und direktem Volumenrendering. Bei ersterem werden die Dichtewerte in eine Isooberfläche umgewandelt, d.h der Übergang von einem definierten Grenzwert wird als Fläche definiert. Ein Algorithmus dafür ist die Erstellung von Dreiecksnetzen mit dem Marching Cube Algorithmus [5]. Der Vorteil hierbei ist, dass sich die Dreiecksnetze sehr effizient und einfach mit heutigen Grafikkarten darstellen lassen. Allerdings sind meist aufwändige Vor- und Nachbearbeitungsschritte notwendig, um visuell ansprechende Ergebnisse zu erzielen und mit den großen Datenmengen umzugehen. Ein weiteres Verfahren ist die Isooberfläche mittels Ray-Casting zu generieren. Neubauer et al. [6] stellten hierfür diverse Beschleunigungsmöglichkeiten vor.

Direkte Verfahren benutzen die Dichtewerte des Volumens und bestimmen den finalen Farbwert als Funktion über alle Dichtepartikel entlang des Sichtstrahls. Heutige Grafikkarten lassen sich auch geeignet für diese Art der Darstellung einsetzen, da sie die 3D Volumendaten direkt laden und über parallele Schnitte das Volumen sichtbar machen können [7]. Der besondere Vorteil hierbei ist, dass den Dichtwerten über eine Transferfunktion verschiedene Farb- und Transparenzwerte zugeordnet werden können und die verlustbehaftete Reduktion auf eine Oberfläche entfällt. Doch war lange Zeit die gängige Hardware für diese Verfahren zu langsam und Beleuchtungseffekte, die für die Formwahrnehmung wichtig sind, waren nicht effizient realisierbar. Die Fortschritte bei der Entwicklung von Grafikkarten erlauben moderne Techniken, wie von Scharsach et al. [4] vorgestellt, welche die Vorteile verschiedener Verfahren vereinen.

Eine weitere Anforderung an die Darstellung ist, neben der Qualität und Leistung, auch die Integration von anderen 3D Modellen. Die virtuelle Endoskopie bietet den Vorteil, dass bereits vorher segmentierte Strukturen, wie Organe und Tumore, hinter der Gewebeoberfläche sichtbar gemacht werden können. Dabei werden entweder die Volumendaten transparenter dargestellt [4] oder die Segmentierten Daten überlagert [3]. Für das hier vorgestellte System wurden deshalb gerade diese neuen Techniken evaluiert und für den Anwendungsfall, der egozentrischen Sicht innerhalb des Volumens, hin optimiert. Sie bieten die größtmögliche Flexibilität, was den dargestellten Wertebereich angeht, bei einem Minimum an Vorverarbeitung. Ein weiterer Bestandteil, neben der Darstellung der Daten, ist die Kamerainteraktion, wofür mindestens ein einfaches Kollisionserkennungssystem notwendig ist.

Ziel ist es, ein skalierbares System zu entwickeln, welches auf herkömmlicher Hardware, im Idealfall auch Laptops, zum Einsatz kommen kann. Für die Entwicklung musste das System deshalb Vergleichsmöglichkeiten der Bildqualität in

Abhängigkeit von der Leistung bieten, denn sowohl verschiedene Datensätze als auch Techniken müssen getestet werden. Realitätsnahe Oberflächendetails, wie Nässe und Textur, sollten sichtbar sein.

3 Umsetzung

Das SinusEndoscopy-System enthält ein Hauptmodul, welches die Benutzeroberfläche erstellt und das Laden von Volumen- und segmentierten Daten sowie den Darstellungstechniken verwaltet. Es bietet auch einige grundlegende Kontrollmechanismen, die vor allem die 3D Darstellung beeinflussen. So können Werte wie Sichtweite, die Transparenz der segmentierten Modelle oder die Eigenschaften der Transferfunktion interaktiv verändert werden. Als Transferfunktion wurde eine 1D-Rampenfunktion gewählt, da diese performant evaluiert werden kann und ausreichende Freiheiten für die Anwendung aufweist. Die Techniken können auf diese Werteanfragen individuell reagieren, so dass es möglich ist, das Framework zum Testen verschiedener Techniken zu benutzen. Jede Technik kann darüber hinaus eigene Kontrollmechanismen bereitstellen, mit der für die Technik relevante Werte verändert werden können. Das Hauptmodul kann darüber hinaus ein erneutes Laden aller Techniken oder Daten auslösen, so dass zur Laufzeit Änderungen vorgenommen werden können. Diese Möglichkeiten des Neuladens sowie dem interaktiven Anpassen von Werten haben die Entwicklungseffizenz steigern können und erleichtern zudem die Vergleiche zwischen den Techniken.

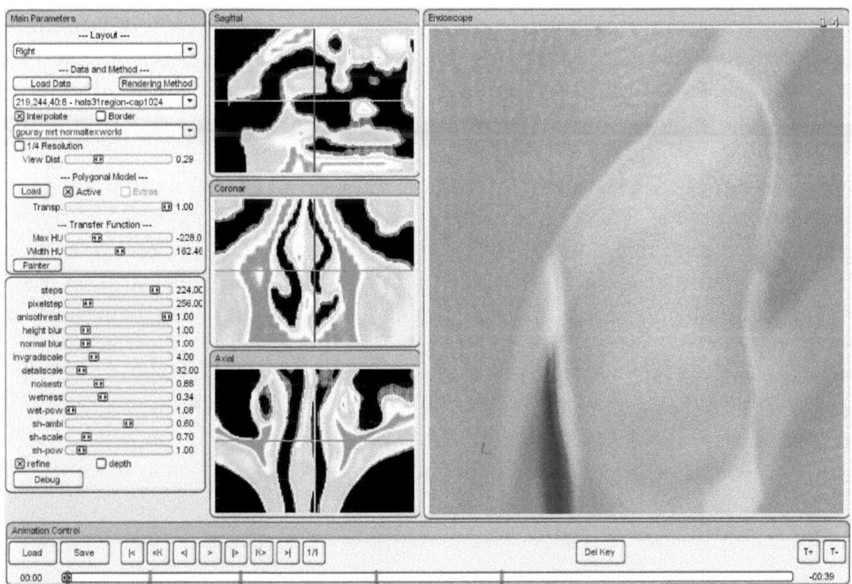

Abb. 1. Übersichtsdarstellung der Benutzeroberfläche. Links: Parameterwerte für die aktuelle Renderingtechnik; Mitte: Orthogonale Schnittansichten; Rechts: Ansicht des virtuellen Endoskops; Unten: Kontrollelemente für die Pfadanimation

Um die Navigation und Übersicht zu verbessern, gibt es in der vorgestellten Anwendung neben der perspektivischen Endoskopsicht auch drei orthogonale Schnittansichten entlang der Hauptachsen, die an die Lage der Kamera im Raum gekoppelt sind (Abb. 1). Die Bewegung der Kamera erfolgt entweder durch Ziehen der Maus innerhalb der Endoskopsicht oder per Klick in den Schnittansichten. In jedem Fall wird zuvor die Transferfunktion für die neue Position evaluiert und so verhindert, dass sich der Benutzer innerhalb solider Regionen bewegt. Ein Animationsmodul ermöglicht es dem Benutzer Schlüsselpositionen und -rotationen zu verschiedenen Zeitpunkten zu erstellen. Die Abspielfunktion interpoliert zwischen diesen und hebt dabei die Kollisionsüberprüfung auf, so dass in wenigen Schritten Animationen erstellt werden können.

Die größte Aufmerksamkeit der Entwicklung galt der Evaluierung verschiedener GPU-basierter Volumenrenderingtechniken. Das heißt, die CPU Nutzung sollte auf ein Minimum begrenzt sein und dafür die Grafikkarte die Hauptlast tragen, um die CPU für andere Aufgaben parallel nutzen zu können. Als Basis unseres Ansatzes diente die von Neubauer et al. [3] vorgestellte Technik zum Rendern von Isooberflächen. Aus dem berechneten Tiefenbild lassen sich die Gradienten für Oberflächennormalen gewinnen und aus der Kombination schließlich für jeden Pixel diverse Schattierungseffekte erzielen. Die Methode, im Bildraum die Oberflächeneffekte zu berechnen, ist auch als Deferred Shading bekannt und wird derzeit vor allem bei modernen Computerspielen eingesetzt. Für das Anwendungsgebiet war, neben den Tiefenwerten der festen Flächen, auch die Darstellung weniger dichter Materie (eine Art Schleim) wichtig. Daher wurde die Oberfläche mit einer organisch wirkenden Textur überzogen und um einen zusätzlichen Effekt für nasse Oberflächen ergänzt, um den Grad des Realismus zu erhöhen und die Tiefenwahrnehmung zu verbessern. Da beim Deferred Shading am Ende ein Kompositionsschritt steht, kann hier auch auf die Interaktion mit vorher gerenderten (segmentierten) anatomischen Landmarken eingegangen werden. In einer Variante werden diese mit einer Art Stipplingeffekt dargestellt, wie aus technischen Zeichnungen bekannt, um verdeckte Elemente besonders zu kennzeichnen.

Der entwickelte Renderer besteht aus verschiedenen Bausteinen, die nicht alle benutzt werden müssen und in erster Linie der Bildartefaktbeseitigung dienen. Die Berechnungspräzision sowie die Genauigkeit der Ein- und Ausgangsdaten lassen sich verändern, so dass durch die Permutation der Bausteine mehrere Techniken entstehen, die sich in Qualität und Leistung vergleichen lassen. So kann je nach Leistungsstärke der Hardware oder dem Grad der benötigten Interaktivität eine passende Technik ausgewählt werden.

4 Ergebnisse

Das System konnte erfolgreich auf verschiedenen Hardwarekonfigurationen getestet werden. Für den Einsatz der moderneren Techniken ist ein Grafikprozessor erforderlich, der auf Pixelebene bedingte Sprünge und Schleifen unterstützt. Diese Hardware ist seit 2004 in diversen Leistungsvarianten auf dem Massenmarkt verfügbar. Aktuelle Standardmodelle bieten genug Speicher an, um CT Daten von 512×512×256 Auflösung bei 16-Bit Präzision darzustellen. Für den endoskopischen Eingriff ist ohnehin nur ein Teilausschnitt der Daten relevant. Wegen des modularen Aufbaus des Renderers ließen sich auf aktuellen, drei Jahre alten und mobilen Rechnern interaktive Bildraten ($\geq$ 15 fps) erzielen. Auch in der Minimalvariante blieben dabei wichtige Eigenschaften, wie die interaktive Transferfunktion und Schattierungshinweise zur Tiefenwahrnehmung, erhalten.

5 Evaluierung und Diskussion

Zukünftig sind einige Erweiterungen des Systems geplant. Derzeit gibt es beispielsweise noch keinen übergeordneten Regelmechanismus, der je nach Hardwareleistung eine passende Technik wählt. Auch gibt es eine Vielzahl an Parametern, die entscheidend die Bildqualität beeinflussen, allen voran die Sichtweite. Da der Renderer für die Endoskopie optimiert ist, kommt es zum Leistungsabfall, wenn die Kamera sich außerhalb des Volumens befindet oder wenn dieser große Leerräume aufweist. Es gibt weiterführende Techniken die hier Verbesserungen bringen [4]. Ein wichtiger Schritt wäre auch die Verbesserung der Kamerasteuerung. Diese ließe sich in einer geführten Variante anbieten, zum Beispiel durch die Gewinnung von Distanzfeldern, wie in [8] beschrieben. Durch das Deferred Shading ergibt sich aber auch die Möglichkeit nicht-realistische Visualiserungstechniken zu verwenden. Gerade im medizinischen Anwendungsgebiet sind derartige Darstellungen oft besser geeignet, was sich auch positiv auf die Operationsplanung auswirken kann, wie in [9] erläutert.

Literaturverzeichnis

1. Bartz D. Virtual endoscopy in research and clinical practice. Comp Graph Forum. 2005;24:111–26.
2. Wolfsberger S, Forster MT, Donat M, et al. Virtual endoscopy is a useful device for training and preoperative planning of transsphenoidal endoscopic pituitary surgery. Minim Invasive Neurosurg. 2002;47:214–20.
3. Neubauer A, Wolfsberger S, Forster MT, et al. STEPS: An application for simulation of transsphenoidal endonasal pituitary surgery. In: Proc IEEE Vis; 2004. p. 513–20.
4. Scharsach H, Hadwiger M, Neubauer A, et al. Perspective isosurface and direct volume rendering for virtual endoscopy applications. In: Proc Eurovis; 2006. p. 315–22.
5. Lorensen WE, Cline HE. Marching cubes: A high resolution 3D surface construction algorithm. Proc SIGGRAPH. 1987; p. 163–9.
6. Neubauer A, Mroz L, Hauser H, et al. Fast and flexible ISO-surfacing for virtual endoscopy. In: Proc CESCG; 2002.
7. Cullip TJ, Neumann U. Accelerating Volume Reconstruction With 3D Texture Hardware. University of North Carolina at Chapel Hill; 1994.
8. Bartz D, Straßer W, Skalej M, et al. Interactive exploration of extra- and intracranial blood vessels (case study). Proc IEEE Vis. 1999; p. 389–92.
9. Preim B, Tietjen C, Doerge C. NPR: Focussing and emphasis in medical visualizations. In: Simulation und Visualisierung. SCS; 2005. p. 139–52.

Creating a Vision Channel for Observing Deep-Seated Anatomy in Medical Augmented Reality

A Cut-Away Technique for In-Situ Visualization

Felix Wimmer[1], Christoph Bichlmeier[1], Sandro M. Heining[2], Nassir Navab[1]

[1]Chair for Computer Aided Medical Procedures (CAMP), TU München, Germany
[2]Trauma Surgery Department, Klinikum Innenstadt, LMU München, Germany
felix.wimmer@gmail.com

Abstract. The intent of medical Augmented Reality (AR) is to augment the surgeon's real view on the patient with the patient's interior anatomy resulting from a suitable visualization of medical imaging data. This paper presents a fast and user-defined clipping technique for medical AR allowing for cutting away any parts of the virtual anatomy and images of the real part of the AR scene hindering the surgeon's view onto the deep-seated region of interest. Modeled on cut-away techniques from scientific illustrations and computer graphics, the method creates a fixed vision channel to the inside of the patient. It enables a clear view on the focussed virtual anatomy and moreover improves the perception of spatial depth.

1 Introduction

Using Augmented Reality (AR) for in-situ visualization of medical data has been a subject of intensive research during the last two decades [1, 2]. The objective of this research is the use of AR technology for preoperative diagnoses and surgical planning as well as intraoperative navigation. The purpose of medical AR is to augment the surgeon's real view on the patient with the patient's interior anatomy. A stereo video see-through head mounted display and an external optical tracking system allow for precise registration of visualized medical imaging data such as computed tomography (CT), magnetic resonance imaging (MRI) and ultrasound with the patient [3].

Improving data presentation for correct perception of depth, relative distances and layout of "hidden and occluded objects", for instance the position of anatomy inside the human body from the surgeons point of view, is a major issue in AR [4, 5]. In one of the first publications [6] about medical AR, Bajura et al. already identified the problem of misleading depth perception when virtual anatomy occludes the patient. To handle the problem, they render a "synthetic hole [...] around ultrasound images in an attempt to avoid conflicting visual cues".

Following this model of creating a virtual hole inside the body of the patient, we developed a fast and user-defined clipping technique, which enables the user to cut away parts of the virtual anatomy and the camera image. The method allows for a clear visibility of the focussed virtual anatomy and furthermore improves the perception of spatial depth. In a preparative step the medical imaging data is segmented into a region of the anatomy the user is interested in (the focus) and an unimportant region. The user defines and positions a volume cutting away all parts of the pre-segmented unimportant region lying inside of it. The pre-defined focus region is not clipped and remains inside the volume. Shape and size of the clipping volume can be defined individually by the user. The remaining part of the unimportant region outside the volume and the borders of the volume provide context information and thus positional and depth cues.

Medical imaging data usually includes a barrage of information. The present cut-away technique is capable of reducing this information to an important fraction of the data set and to reveal the view onto the focussed anatomy. We combine cut-away views known from technical and medical illustrations and various approaches in the field of computer graphics [7, 8, 9] with the beneficial potentials of medical AR technology.

2 Materials and Methods

Medical imaging data taken from a CT or MRI scan is presented using a stereoscopic video see-through HMD. The entire tracking system allowing for tracking the HMD, the patient and several surgical instruments is described in detail at [10]. We use pre-segmented surface models to visualize the anatomy.

The application of the present cut-away technique is illustrated in Figures 1. Different shapes can be used for the clipping volume. Figures 1 (a) and (b) show a box and Figure 1 (c) a sphere used as clipping volume. The clipping technique is intended to be applied in conjunction with a technique described at [10] used to modify the transparency of the camera image. Figure 1 (a) shows a clipping box without integrating the transparency modulation technique (ghosting), whereas Figures 1 (b) and (c) illustrate the combination of clipping volumes and the transparency modulation technique.

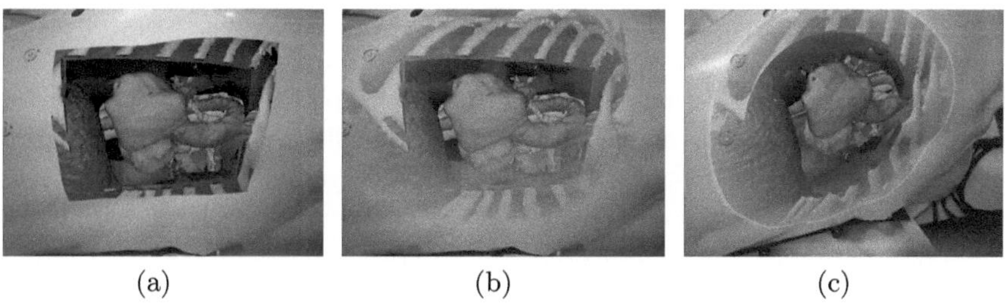

(a) (b) (c)

Fig. 1. Cut-away with Volume Clipping: (a) using a box as the clipping volume, (b) the clipping box in conjunction with ghosting of the skin [10] and (c) the usage of a clipping sphere in conjunction with ghosting of the skin [10]

The present technique generates a depth map by grabbing the depth buffer after off-screen rendering of the skin and the chosen clipping volume. This depth map is used to clip objects in the scene by performing a depth test in a shader program.

2.1 Setting up Size and Position of the Clipping Volume

When using a box for clipping, the user is able to interactively define the coordinates of each vertex of the box by key-pressing, mouse movement or movement of his head (see Figure 2 (a)). If a sphere or a cylinder has been chosen, the user can define the position and the radius of the volume. When the user found the right location and size of the volume, it can be fixed permanently to this position.

2.2 Generation of the Clipping Depth Map

In order to generate the depth map, first all buffers are cleared and the skin is rendered to the depth buffer. Afterwards the depth test is flipped, which means that fragments pass the depth test, that have a higher depth value than those, which are already in the depth buffer. Consequentially the clipping volume is rendered to the depth buffer. The depth values of the clipping volume are stored in the depth buffer at the corresponding pixel positions, if they are greater than those of the previously rendered skin. Additionally the stencil bit[1] is set at the corresponding pixel positions. The resulting stencil mask is used to clip the camera image and to display the volume. The depth values of the skin remain in the buffer at all pixel positions where they are bigger than the depth values of the clipping volume. The resulting depth buffer is stored to a designated buffer called depth map.

2.3 Clipping of Virtual Anatomy and the Camera Image

A render mode chosen by the user determines, if a segmented virtual object should be clipped or not and thus if it should be a focussed object or not. When rendering an object that should be clipped, a fragment shader program is performing a second depth test in addition to the standard depth test, using the previously created depth map as an input parameter. This shader performs a lookup into the depth map at the screen coordinates of the fragment and compares the received depth value with the depth value of the fragment. If the depth value is smaller (closer to the eye), the fragment is discarded. For this reason every fragment, which has a smaller depth value than the corresponding fragment of the clipping volume is discarded and thus the part of the dataset lying inside the clipping volume is clipped.

[1] The stencil buffer is an additional buffer beside the color buffer and depth buffer, and available on usual modern computer graphics hardware.

Fig. 2. (a) Setting up the clipping volume and (b) texturing the clipping volume

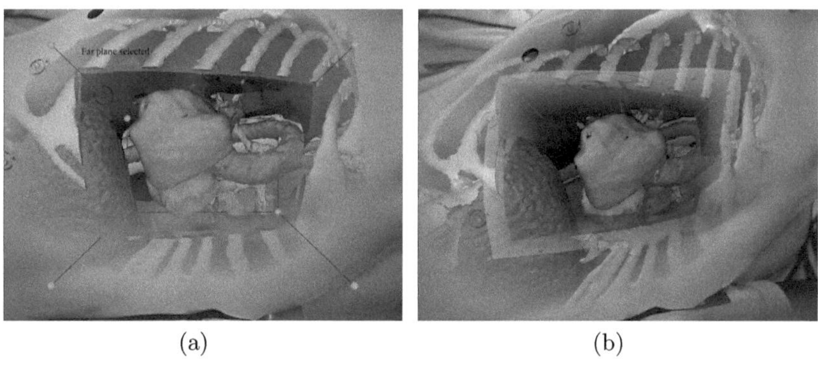

(a) (b)

The camera image gets only clipped, if the clipping volume is not used in conjunction with ghosting of the skin. If applied without ghosting of the skin, the generated stencil mask can be utilized to display the camera image only at those screen positions where the stencil bit is not set. In this way, every part of the skin lying inside the clipping volume is clipped and a window on the skin is generated offering the depth cue occlusion for improved perception of virtual anatomy (see Figure 1 (a)).

2.4 Displaying and Texturing the Clipping Volume

In order to provide further depth cues, the borders and planes of the clipping volume can also be displayed. Therefore, fragments of the clipping volume lying in front of the skin are removed using the generated stencil mask. The borders of the clipping volume can be displayed in a semi-transparent or opaque way. Shading and texturing the clipping volume provides further context information for perceiving the focussed anatomy. Figure 2 (b) illustrates these effects. Here a semi-transparent texture showing a linear gradient from white (close to the observer) to dark (distant to observer) was chosen to improve depth estimation.

3 Results

We used a thorax phantom to evaluate qualitatively the present visualization technique. Originally, the phantom only consisted of a spinal column installed inside the phantom. However, we extended the virtual anatomy by surface models segmented from the Visible Korean Human (VKH)[2] data set. Virtual models are registered manually with the thorax phantom, which is in our case sufficient for evaluating the visualization method.

2 The Visible Korean Human project provides different full body data sets: CT, MRI and anatomical images http://vkh3.kisti.re.kr/new

4 Discussion

The present method uses polygonal surface models to allow for real time visualization. Surface models have to be segmented and triangulated before the visualization can be performed. Future work will include the integration of this approach into a ray cast based volume renderer to be able to render volumetric CT or MRI data directly without time wasting, preparative steps. However, such a rendering technique requires powerful hardware to obtain real-time rendering.

Acknowledgement. We want to express our gratitude to the radiologists and surgeons of Klinikum Innenstadt München, Frank Sauer, Christopher Stapleton, Mohammad Rustaee and the NARVIS group for their support. This work was granted by the BFS within the NARVIS project (www.narvis.org).

References

1. Cleary K, Chung HY, Mun SK. OR 2020: The operating room of the future. Laparoendosc Adv Surg Tech. 2005;15(5):495–500.
2. Peters TM. Image-guidance for surgical procedures. Phys Med Biol. 2006;51(14):R505–R540.
3. Sauer F, Khamene A, Bascle B, et al. Augmented reality visualization in iMRI operating room: System description and pre-clinical testing. Proc SPIE. 2002;4681:446–54.
4. Furmanski C, Azuma R, Daily M. Augmented-reality visualizations guided by cognition: Perceptual heuristics for combining visible and obscured information. In: Proc. IEEE and ACM Int'l Symp. on Mixed and Augmented Reality (ISMAR). Washington, DC, USA: IEEE Computer Society; 2002. p. 215.
5. Sielhorst T, Bichlmeier C, Heining S, et al. Depth perception a major issue in medical AR: Evaluation study by twenty surgeons. Lect Notes Computer Sci. 2006; p. 364–72.
6. Bajura M, Fuchs H, Ohbuchi R. Merging virtual objects with the real world: Seeing ultrasound imagery within the patient. Proc SIGGRAPH. 1992; p. 203–10.
7. Feiner S, Seligmann DD. Cutaways and ghosting: Satisfying visibility constraints in dynamic 3D illustrations. Vis Comp. 1992;8(5&6):292–02.
8. Diepstraten J, Weiskopf D, Ertl T. Interactive cutaway illustrations. Comp Graph Forum. 2003;22(3):523–32.
9. Weiskopf D, Engel K, Ertl T. Volume clipping via per-fragment operations in texture-based volume visualization. In: Proc IEEE Vis. Washington, DC, USA: IEEE Computer Society; 2002. p. 93–100.
10. Bichlmeier C, Wimmer FJ, Heining SM, et al. Contextual anatomic mimesis: Hybrid in-situ visualization method for improving multi-sensory depth perception in medical augmented reality. In: Proc. IEEE and ACM Int'l Symp. on Mixed and Augmented Reality (ISMAR); 2007. p. 129–38.

A Novel Two-Step Method for CT Reconstruction

Michael Felsberg

Computer Vision Laboratory, Dept. EE, Linköping University, Sweden
mfe@isy.liu.se

Abstract. In this paper we address the parallel beam 2D computer tomography reconstruction. The proposed method belongs to the field of analytic reconstruction methods and is compared to several methods known in the field, among other the two-step Hilbert-transform method. In contrast to the latter, the derivative data is multiplied with an orientation vector and the Hilbert transform is replaced with the Riesz transform. Experimental results show that the new method is superior to established ones concerning aliasing, noise, and DC errors.

1 Introduction

Given a number of line projections of an object, we want to reconstruct its density. This type of problem typically occurs in context of parallel beam computer tomography (CT) reconstruction. For this paper, we consider a simplified 2D setting neglecting a number of physical phenomena (Fig. 1a). The measuring unit consists of a source emitting parallel rays and a detector measuring the intensity of each incoming ray for each position s. The object between source and detector attenuates the rays depending on its density. The problem to solve for CT reconstruction is to compute the 2D density distribution of the object from the set of its line projections at different rotation angles θ.

The object is located at the origin of the 2D coordinate system $(x, y)^T$. The coordinate system of the measuring unit $(s, t)^T$ and is rotated by θ around the

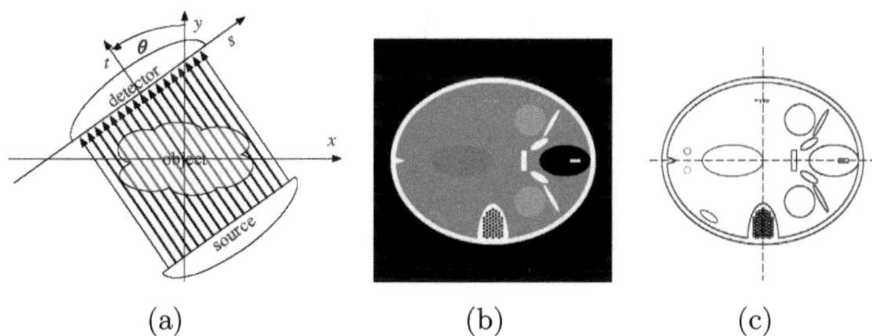

Fig. 1. (a) 2D geometry for the projections. Note that the s-axis was moved to the detector in order to visualize that s is at the same time the position on the detector. (b) Phantom used for experiments. (c) Edge map of phantom in (b)

Fig. 2. Different options for analytic linear reconstruction. (a) ramp-filtered back-projection. (b) two-step reconstruction using the Hilbert transform [2]. (c) post-filtered back-projection [3]. (d) three-step Hilbert method [4]. Proposed method

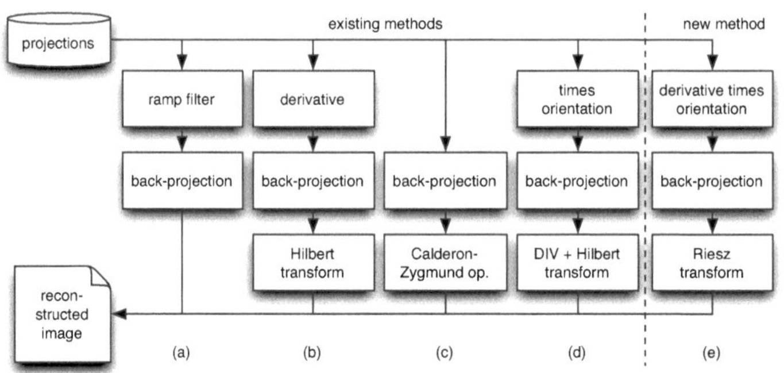

origin. The Radon transform [1] is obtained by integrating the object density $f(x, y)$ along t: $p_\theta(s) = \int_{-\infty}^{\infty} f(x, y)\, dt = \int_{-\infty}^{\infty} f(s\cos\theta - t\sin\theta, s\sin\theta + t\cos\theta)\, dt$.

Various analytic methods for reconstruction have been suggested in the literature. We have summarized the relevant methods in Fig. 2. Starting point for all considered approaches is the projection slice theorem [5] resulting in $f(x, y) = \int_{-\infty}^{\infty} \int_0^{\pi} P_\theta(m) \exp(i2\pi m(\cos\theta x + \sin\theta y))|m|\, d\theta\, dm$, where $P_\theta(m)$ is the 1D Fourier transform[1] of $p_\theta(s)$. For what follows, we define the back-projection operator as $\mathcal{B}\{g_\theta\} = \int_0^{\pi} g_\theta(\cos\theta x + \sin\theta y)\, d\theta$, where g_θ is a family of 1D functions parametrized by θ.

For the ramp-filtered back-projection, p_θ is filtered with the 1D ramp filter, corresponding to $|m|$, and then back-projected, cf. Fig. 2 (a). Denoting the ramp-filtered projection as p_θ^r, we obtain $f(x, y) = \mathcal{B}\{p_\theta^r\}$. For the post-filtered back-projection, the back-projected image is filtered with the 2D ramp filter $\sqrt{u^2 + v^2}$, the Calderon-Zygmund operator [3], cf. Fig. 2 (c): $f(x, y) = \left[\int_{-\infty}^{\infty} \int_{-\infty}^{\infty} \sqrt{u^2 + v^2} \exp(i2\pi(ux + vy))\, du\, dv\right] * \mathcal{B}\{p_\theta\}$.

For the two-step reconstruction using the Hilbert transform, which goes back to the original work of Radon [1], the term $|m|$ is split into two factors $|m| = (im)(-i\text{sign}(m))$, where the first factor corresponds to the derivative in the spatial domain (up to a factor 2π) and the second factor is the Hilbert transform. The latter is computed after the back-projection [2], cf. Fig. 2 (b): $f(x, y) = 2\pi\mathcal{H}\{\mathcal{B}\{p_\theta'\}\}$, where $\mathcal{H}$ is the Hilbert transform operator acting in an arbitrary direction[2] and p_θ' denotes the derivative of the projection. For the three-step Hilbert method, the projection data is multiplied with the orientation vector before back-projection and the Hilbert transform is computed on the divergence of back-projected vector field [4], cf. Fig. 2 (d): $f(x, y) = 2\pi\mathcal{H}_y\left\{\langle\nabla; \mathcal{B}\{(\cos\theta, \sin\theta)^T p_\theta\}\rangle\right\}$, where $\langle\cdot;\cdot\rangle$ denotes the scalar product and $\nabla = (\partial_x, \partial_y)^T$ is the gradient operator.

[1] 1D Fourier kernel: $\exp(-i2\pi ms)$; 2D Fourier kernel: $\exp(-i2\pi(ux + vy))$

[2] For the sake of simplicity we apply the vertical transform in what follows.

2 Materials and Methods

For the novel reconstruction method, we split the Calderon-Zygmund operator into two parts:

$$\sqrt{u^2+v^2} = \langle i(u,v)^T; -i\frac{(u,v)^T}{\sqrt{u^2+v^2}}\rangle = \langle i(u,v)^T; R^T(u,v)\rangle \tag{1}$$

where the left factor corresponds to the 2D gradient (up to a factor of 2π) and the right factor corresponds to the Riesz transform, a rotation-invariant generalization of the Hilbert transform [6]. The method of rotation [6] results in a relation between the 1D Hilbert transform and the 2D Riesz transform [7], which can be applied in this case for expressing the 2D gradient in the projection domain as $(\cos\theta, \sin\theta)^T p'_\theta(s)$, leading to the final reconstruction formula

$$f(x,y) = 2\pi\mathcal{R}\left\{\mathcal{B}\{(\cos\theta, \sin\theta)^T p'_\theta\}\right\} \ , \tag{2}$$

where $\mathcal{R}$ is the Riesz transform operator. The latter is defined by $\sqrt{-\Delta} = \langle\nabla|\mathcal{R}\rangle$, where $\Delta = \langle\nabla|\nabla\rangle = \partial_x\partial_x + \partial_y\partial_y$ is the Laplace operator. The Riesz operator in the reconstruction (2) should be interpreted as a scalar product, i.e., the respectively first and second component of $\mathcal{R}$ is applied to the first and second component of the integral.

For periodic boundary conditions, $\mathcal{R}$ corresponds to the frequency response $R(u,v)$. For Neumann boundary conditions, the solution has been given in [8]. For the here considered problem, the ideal setting would be to restrict the computation to a circular domain, but practical considerations require a rectangular domain. The reasons are twofold: a) images are typically rectangular shaped and b) the rectangular domain solution can be computed by FFT algorithms.

Hence, we require the reconstruction to be zero outside a rectangular domain, i.e., the reconstruction has compact support. Consequently, all projections have a finite support and so do the derivatives. Applying the back projection to the projection derivatives, however, results in a 2D function with infinite support. This can easily be verified by either considering the projection geometry or the non-locality of the Riesz kernel. If we back-project onto a finite image, we cut of the tails of the filtered gradient image. Hence, our task is to compute the finite Riesz transform of an infinite gradient signal which is truncated, knowing that the result is zero outside the considered domain.

Assume that $b(x,y) = \mathcal{B}\{(\cos\theta, \sin\theta)^T p'_\theta\}$ is the back-projected oriented derivative on the domain $(x,y) \in (0; x_{\max}) \times (0; y_{\max})$. Define the modified signal $b_m(x,y)$ on the domain $(x,y) \in (-x_{\max}; x_{\max}) \times (-y_{\max}; y_{\max})$ by

$$b_m(x,y) = \begin{pmatrix} \text{sign}(y) & 0 \\ 0 & \text{sign}(x) \end{pmatrix} b(|x|,|y|) \tag{3}$$

i.e., the components of b are mirrored at the coordinate axes, with anti-symmetry with respect to the y- and x-axis, respectively. As a result, the signal tails which should exist in the back-projected image b compensate each other and a good approximation of the Riesz transform with finite data becomes possible.

The Riesz transform of the signal $b(x, y)$ under the side condition of zero continuation outside of $(0; x_{\max}) \times (0; y_{\max})$ is computed using the DFT and the frequency response of the Riesz transform:

$$\mathcal{R}\{b\} = \mathrm{iDFT}\langle -i\frac{(u, v)^T}{\sqrt{u^2 + v^2}}|\mathrm{DFT}\{b_m\}\rangle \tag{4}$$

The new method described in the previous paragraphs has slightly higher computational complexity than ramp-filtered back-projection, post-filtered back-projection, and the two-step Hilbert method. Similar to the three-step Hilbert method, two images need to be back-projected and back-projection is the computationally most demanding step in all cases. The higher complexity can be justified by three significant advantages, some of which are shared with some of the methods from the literature, but not with a single one:

- *Aliasing.* The two-step Hilbert method and the Riesz-method use DC-free projection data, which suppresses DC aliasing altogether without any particular efforts for the design of the interpolation filter.
- *SNR.* The Riesz-method shows (together with the three-step Hilbert method) significant lower noise levels since both methods reconstruct orientation dependent and noise is typically unoriented.
- *DC estimation.* In contrast to the two Hilbert-methods, the Riesz-method only needs to be complemented by a single DC estimate, whereas the Hilbert-methods need an additional DC estimate for each column of the reconstructed image.

The experiment that we use to verify these properties is based on noisy projections from the phantom in Fig. 1 (b). For verifying the alias components visually, we apply a Prewitt edge detector to the resulting images. The SNR is measured along the dashed lines in Fig. 1 (c). The DC estimation problematic is verified by visually inspecting reconstructed images without edge detection.

3 Results

The reconstruction results can be found in Fig. 3.

4 Discussion

Comparing the results in Fig. 3 with respect to aliasing, SNR, and DC estimation, we draw the following conclusions:

- *Aliasing.* As claimed before, the methods which are back-projecting a derivative do not show the aliasing artefacts that are visible in the other methods, cf. (b) and (d) vs. (a) and (c).
- *SNR.* The noise level in the methods without orientation vector is more than 10% higher than for the other methods, cf. (a) and (d) vs. (b) and (c).

Fig. 3. Reconstructed densities. Note that the intensity range in (e) is amplified compared to (f) in order to show the presence of the weaker structures

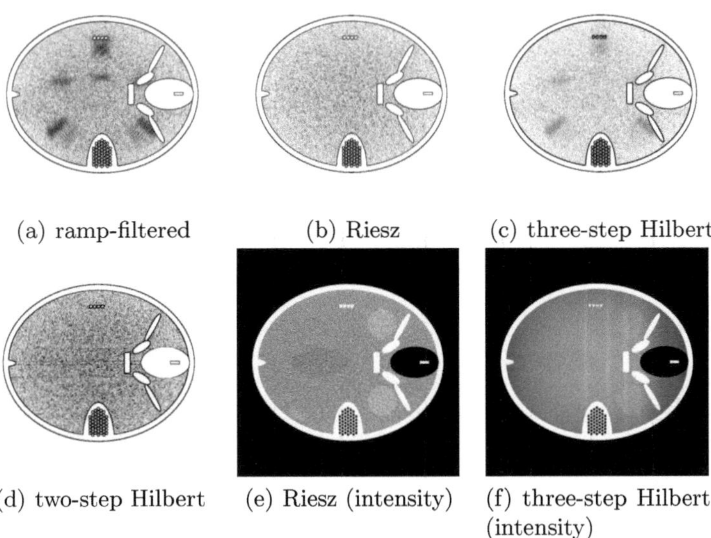

(a) ramp-filtered (b) Riesz (c) three-step Hilbert

(d) two-step Hilbert (e) Riesz (intensity) (f) three-step Hilbert (intensity)

- *DC estimation.* The DC estimation for the Hilbert-based methods is fairly tricky without prior knowledge about the object, cf. (f) vs. (e).

Summarising the experimental results, we conclude that the Riesz method combines all positive properties of the compared methods in a single method.

References

1. Radon J. On the determination of functions from their integral values along certain manifolds. IEEE Trans Med Imaging. 1986;5:170–6.
2. Noo F, Clackdoyle R, Pack JD. A two-step Hilbert transform method for 2D image reconstruction. Phys Med Biol. 2004;49:3903–23.
3. Solmon DC. Asymptotic formulas for the dual Radon transform and applications. Math Z. 1987;195:321–43.
4. Zeng GL. Image reconstruction via the finite Hilbert transform of the derivative of the backprojection. Med Phys. 2007;34:2837–43.
5. Bracewell RN. Two-Dimensional Imaging. Prentice Hall Signal Processing Series. Prentice Hall, Englewood Cliffs; 1995.
6. Stein EM, Weiss G. Introduction to Fourier Analysis on Euclidean Spaces. Princeton University Press, New Jersey; 1971.
7. Felsberg M, Sommer G. The monogenic signal. IEEE Trans Signal Process. 2001;49:3136–44.
8. Felsberg M, Duits R, Florack L. The monogenic scale space on a rectangular domain and its features. Int J Comput Vis. 2005;64.

Automatische Detektion von Lymphknoten in CT-Datensätzen des Halses

Lars Dornheim, Jana Dornheim

Institut für Simulation und Graphik, Otto-von-Guericke-Universität Magdeburg
lars@isg.cs.uni-magdeburg.de

Kurzfassung. Zur computergestützten, präoperativen Planung von HalsLymphknoten-Ausräumungen (Neck Dissections) ist eine Detektion aller vergrößerten Lymphknoten wünschenswert. Diese erfolgt zur Zeit ausschließlich manuell durch einen Radiologen und ist ein zeitaufwändiger und fehleranfälliger Prozess. Wir präsentieren ein Verfahren zur automatischen Detektion von Lymphknoten in CT-Datensätzen des Halses mit Hilfe dreidimensionaler Stabiler Feder-Masse-Modelle (SMSMs). Die Detektion erfolgt durch Abgleich aller in Frage kommenden Datensatzbereiche mit einem deformierbaren 3D-Modell des Lymphknotens, welches Form, Grauwerte und Kanteninformation gleichermaßen modelliert. Das Verfahren wurde an 29 vergrößerten (> 8 mm) Lymphknoten eines klinischen CT-Datensatzes evaluiert und zeigte daran eine Detektionsrate von 100 % bei 9 falsch-positiven Kandidaten.

1 Einleitung

Die Neck Dissection (Hals-Lymphknoten-Ausräumung) wird häufig im Rahmen von Tumorerkrankungen des Kopf- und Halsbereiches durchgeführt, um metastatische (vergrößerte) Lymphknoten zu entfernen. Für die präoperative Planung dieses Eingriffs ist es entscheidend, Lage und Ausdehnung der relevanten Lymphknoten zu kennen, sowie ihren Bezug zu Risikostrukturen (Blutgefäße, Muskeln, etc.). Die dreidimensionale Visualisierung und Vermessung der einzelnen Strukturen und Abstände zur Planungsunterstützung erfordert eine Detektion und anschließende Segmentierung der Lymphknoten.

Zur Segmentierung von Lymphknoten existieren bereits automatische Verfahren [1, 2, 3], die jedoch alle an der Position der zu segmentierenden Lymphknoten initialisiert werden müssen. Dies setzt eine Lymphknotendetektion voraus, die zur Zeit nur manuell erfolgt und sowohl langwierig als auch fehleranfällig ist (z. B. Übersehen einzelner Lymphknoten). In [4] wird die manuelle Detektionsrate von Halslymphknoten in CT experimentell mit weniger als 55% Trefferquote (bei einer Betrachtungszeit von maximal 180 Sekunden) bestimmt.

Die hier vorliegende Arbeit baut auf der Arbeit von Dornheim und Seim [3] zur Lymphknotensegmentierung in CT-Datensätzen auf. Darin wird ein dreidimensionales Stabiles Feder-Masse-Modell [5] in Form einer doppelwandigen, formflexiblen Kugel nach erfolgter Initialplatzierung erfolgreich zur automatischen Segmentierung von Lymphknoten eingesetzt. Es ist robust gegenüber der

Initialplatzierung, so daß es bei nahezu beliebiger Platzierung des Modells im Lymphknoten (auch am Rand) zu einer erfolgreichen Segmentierung führt [6].

Automatische Verfahren zur Lymphknotendetektion existieren derzeit nicht. Rigide Objekt-Detektionsverfahren wie Template Matching, erweiterte Hough-Transformation, etc., können auf Grund ihrer Unflexibilität bzgl. der zu suchenden Objekte nicht mit Erfolg auf die Detektion variabler Strukturen wie Lymphknoten (verschiedene Größen, Ausrichtungen, Detailformen und benachbarte Strukturen) in schwierigen medizinischen Daten (unklare Abgrenzungen und Anzahl, viele ähnliche Formen) angewendet werden.

2 Material und Methoden

2.1 Methode

Die Detektion der Lymphknoten wird durch Abgleich eines deformierbaren Form- und Grauwertmodells des Lymphknotens mit allen in Frage kommenden Lymphknotenpositionen im Datensatz durchgeführt. Dabei handelt es sich um ein dreidimensionales Stabiles Feder-Masse-Modell mit 100 Massen und 338 Federn und einer Ausgangsgröße von 3 mm, wie in [3] beschrieben.

Das hier vorgestellte Prinzip der Lymphknotendetektion basiert auf einer Populationssuche mit Hilfe dieser Modelle. Hierzu werden entlang eines Gitters mit dem Abstand d Modelle dicht verteilt über den Datensatz platziert und synchron gestartet. Jedes dieser Modelle strebt nun, wie beim Segmentierungsprozess, in seiner lokalen Umgebung zu Strukturen, welche die charakteristischen Lymphknoteneigenschaften hinsichtlich Form, Grauwert und Kanteninformation aufweisen, soweit das möglich ist. Damit führt es im Prinzip eine lokale Suche nach der Struktur, die es modelliert, durch.

Mittels der in [7] beschriebenen Methode kann für ein beliebiges SMSM zur Laufzeit effizient die Anpassungsgüte in jedem Simulationsschritt beurteilt werden. Diese wird durch einen Wert zwischen 0 (keine Anpassung) und 1 (ideale Anpassung) ausgedrückt und beschreibt, wie gut die vom Modell erwarteten Form- und Grauwertspezifika im Datensatz wiedergefunden werden. So kann für jedes Lymphknotenmodell der Population verfolgt werden, ob es sich an eine Struktur anpasst, die die Lymphknoteneigenschaften aufweist.

Um den Rechenaufwand von Anfang an möglichst gering zu halten, wird jedes Modell des Gitters nur dann initialisiert, wenn es innerhalb einer *binären Erwartungskarte* liegt, die beschreibt, an welchen Stellen im Datensatz nach Lymphknoten gesucht werden soll. Diese Karte spiegelt in vereinfachter Form die anatomische Lage verschiedener Lymphknotengruppen wieder. Sie hat den Wert 1 an allen Voxeln, die maximal 25 mm von V. jugularis, A. carotis, M. sternocleidomastoideus oder Unterkiefer entfernt sind, den Wert 0 in allen anderen Voxeln und den genannten Strukturen selbst.

Zusätzlich werden Modelle während der Suche aus der Population entfernt, wenn sie sich nicht mehr an Lymphknoten in der Nähe ihrer Startposition anpassen können. Das ist in folgenden Situationen definitiv der Fall:

1. Ein Modell hat sich zu weit von seiner Startposition entfernt und befindet sich nun im Aktionsbereich eines anderen Modells.
2. Ein Modell ist in einem lokalen Minimum zum Stillstand gekommen und hat keine ausreichende Anpassungsgüte erreicht.
3. Ein Modell hat sich so stark verformt, daß es sich an keine Lymphknoten mehr anpassen wird.
4. Ein Modell stimmt nicht mehr mit dem charakteristischen Grauwertbereich eines Lymphknotens (1000–1130 in einem Bereich von 0–4095 HU) überein.

Alle vier Punkte treten nicht auf, wenn ein Modell sehr nahe an oder in einem Lymphknoten gestartet wird, da es dann eine ordnungsgemäße Segmentierung ohne Verformung, Abdriften oder Stillstand an falscher Stelle durchführt.

Das Verfahren endet, wenn alle Modelle der Population zum Stillstand gekommen oder verworfen worden sind, bzw. nach einer maximalen Simulationsdauer, in der im Schnitt alle erfolgreichen Segmentierungen von Lymphknoten abgeschlossen sind (250 Schritte im Fall unseres Modells). Als Lymphknoten-Kandidaten kommen die Modelle mit der besten Anpassungsgüte in Frage. Sie werden mittels eines Schwellenwertes von 0.8 für die Anpassungsgüte ausgewählt, der sich in Experimenten als geeignet herausgestellt hat. Aus den so erhaltenen Lymphknotenkandidaten können direkt die Positionen der auf diese Weise detektierten Lymphknoten abgelesen werden. Oft liegt auch bereits eine gute Segmentierung des Lymphknotens vor.

2.2 Material

Das vorgestellte Verfahren wurde an 29 vergrößerten Lymphknoten im CT-Datensatz eines Patienten mit glottischem Larynxkarzinom und beidseitigem Lymphknotenbefall untersucht. Die originale Auflösung des Datensatzes betrug 0.41 mm in X/Y-Richtung und 1,5 mm in Z-Richtung.

Aus dem vorhandenen Datensatz wurden vier Teilregionen ausgewählt, die in der Summe alle klinisch relevanten Lymphknoten des Datensatzes enthielten. Die Teilregionen lagen jeweils um die V. jugularis, sowie am Unterrand des Unterkiefers links und rechts. Zur korrekten Berechnung der Gradienteninformation musste ein lineares Resampling aller ausgewählten Teilregionen auf isotrope Voxelgröße (0.41 mm) durchgeführt werden. Tabelle 1 zeigt die Größe und Auflösung der ausgewählten Regionen sowie die Anzahl enthaltener Lymphknoten.

Als Gitterabstand für die Initialplatzierung der Modellpopulation wurden 3.5 mm gewählt, da dies knapp unter der doppelten Abtastdichte für Lymphknoten von 8 mm Größe liegt, unterhalb derer sie klinisch nicht als auffällig gelten.

3 Ergebnisse

Aufgrund der Erwartungs- und Grauwertkarten wurden 958 Modelle gestartet. Nach Ende des Verfahrens blieben davon 38 Modelle übrig, deren Anpassungsgüte mehr als 0.8 betrug. Die gesamte Laufzeit für alle 4 Teilregionen lag bei ca. 17 Minuten auf einem modernen PC (Pentium 4, 3.1 GHz, 1 GB RAM).

Tabelle 1. Übersicht der gewählten Teilregionen aus dem untersuchten CT-Datensatz

Teilregion	Lagebeschreibung	Lymphknoten (> 8 mm)	Größe nach Resampling (in Voxeln)		
			X	Y	Z
Region 1	V. jugularis rechts	7	80	113	233
Region 2	V. jugularis links	12	110	137	222
Region 3	Unterkiefer rechts	4	142	110	76
Region 4	Unterkiefer links	6	106	110	80

Die verbliebenen Modelle arrangierten sich in Clustern, da oftmals mehrere Modelle denselben Lymphknoten detektiert hatten (Abb. 3). Für die Bezifferung der richtig-positiven und falsch-positiven Detektionsergebnisse (Tab. 2) wurde deshalb die Anzahl der Cluster betrachtet. Ein Lymphknoten galt dabei als detektiert, wenn er durch mindestens ein Modell gefunden wurde.

Alle 29 Lymphknoten über 8 mm Größe wurden durch das vorgestellte Verfahren detektiert. Neben den gefundenen Lymphknoten wurden 9 falsch-positive Kandidaten gefunden. Unter diesen waren 6 Detektionen von Blutgefäßen und 2 Detektionen des Platysma. Modelle unter 8 mm Durchmesser wurden automatisch herausgefiltert und flossen somit nicht in die Betrachtung mit ein.

4 Diskussion

In der vorliegenden Arbeit wurde erstmalig ein vollautomatisches Verfahren zur Detektion vergrößerter Lymphknoten in CT-Datensätzen des Halses entwickelt und an 29 realen Lymphknoten eines CT-Datensatzes evaluiert. Die Detektionsrate von 100% liegt deutlich über der in [4] angegebenen manuellen Erkennungsrate von 55 % und muss als sehr zufriedenstellend bewertet werden. Sehr positiv ist auch die geringe Anzahl falsch-positiver Lymphknotenkandidaten zu bewerten, die leicht von Hand durch den Benutzer eliminiert werden können.

Die Laufzeit des Suchverfahrens ist derzeit für einen routinemäßigen klinischen Einsatz noch etwas zu lang, erfordert jedoch keine Interaktion des Benutzers und kann daher auch im Hintergrund während anderer Tätigkeiten ablau-

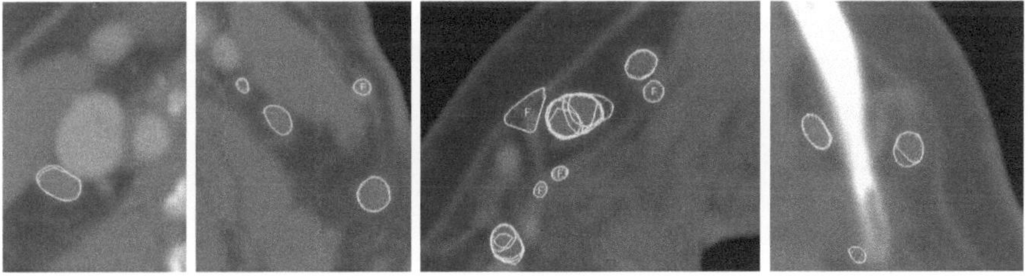

Abb. 1. beispielhafte Ergebnisse der Lymphknotendetektion in den Teilregionen 1 bis 4 (falsch-positive Kandidaten mit einem „F“ markiert)

Tabelle 2. Ergebnisse der Detektion vergrößerter Lymphknoten

Teilregion	gestartete Modelle	erfolgreiche Modelle	richtig-positiv (Detektionsrate)	falsch-positiv	Blutgefäß detektiert
Region 1	294	7	7 (100%)	0	0
Region 2	346	18	12 (100%)	6	4
Region 3	184	7	4 (100%)	3	2
Region 4	134	6	6 (100%)	0	0
Summe	958	38	29 (100%)	9	6

fen. Möglichkeiten zur deutlichen Reduzierung der Laufzeit liegen in der frühzeitigen Elimination nicht erfolgreicher Modelle aus der Population, gezielterer Einschränkung der Erwartungskarten, sowie in der hervorragenden Parallelisierbarkeit des Verfahrens (z. B. auf mehrkernigen Prozessoren in modernen PCs).

Eine weitere Reduktion der Laufzeit, aber auch der falsch-positiv gefundenen Kandidaten, lässt sich durch die Vermeidung der ungewollten Blutgefäßdetektion erzielen, da diese den größten Anteil unter den falsch-positiven Ergebnissen ausmacht. Hierzu würde es bereits genügen, die betreffenden Blutgefäße des Halses im Vorfeld der Lymphknotendetektion zu segmentieren und ebenfalls aus der Erwartungskarte zu entfernen. Gleiches gilt für das fälschlicherweise detektierte Platysma.

Literaturverzeichnis

1. Honea D, et al. Three-dimensional active surface approach to lymph node segmentation. Proc SPIE. 1999;3361:1003–11.
2. Yan J, et al. Lymph node segmentation from CT images using fast marching method. Comput Med Imaging Graph. 2004;28:33–8.
3. Dornheim J, et al. Segmentation of neck lymph nodes in CT datasets with stable 3D mass-spring models. Proc MICCAI. 2006.
4. Schreyer AG, et al. Vergleich der Genauigkeit und Effizienz koronarer und axialer Rekonstruktionen zur Lymphknotendetektion bei einem 16-Zeilen-Spiral-CT am Beispiel von Halslymphknoten. Rofo. 2005;177(10):1430–5.
5. Dornheim L, et al. Stable dynamic 3D shape models. Proc ICIP. 2005.
6. Dornheim J, et al. Segmentation of neck lymph nodes in CT datasets with stable 3D mass-spring models. Academic Radiol. 2007.
7. Dornheim L, et al. Quality of fit of stable mass spring models. In: Proc 7th Open German/Russian Workshop on Pattern Recognition and Image Understanding; 2007.

Haptic Landmark Positioning and Automatic Landmark Transfer in 4D Lung CT Data

Matthias Färber[1], Björn Gawenda[1,2], Christian-Arved Bohn[2], Heinz Handels[1]

[1]Department of Medical Informatics, University Medical Center Hamburg-Eppendorf
[2]Computergraphics & Virtual Reality, University of Applied Sciences Wedel
m.faerber@uke.uni-hamburg.de

Abstract. Manual landmark positioning in volumetric image data is a complex task and often results in erroneous landmark positions. The landmark positioning tool presented uses image curvature features to precompute suitable candidates for landmark positions on surface data of anatomical structures. A force-feedback I/O device is then used to haptically guide the user during the definition of the correct landmarks in the 3D data volume. Furthermore, existing landmarks in a time-point of a sequence of 3D volumes (4D data set) can iteratively be transferred to other time-points using a surface based registration technique. First results show significant time savings and small interobserver variability (IROV) compared to the IROV of manually defined landmark positions using orthogonal slices of the image data.

1 Introduction

Medical landmarks are definite points in human anatomy that can be described using medical terminology (e.g. bifurcatio tracheae) or unique location definitions (e.g. "apex of the left lung"). They are required to determine quantitative measures like distances or angles, they represent significant points for navigation purposes and can be used for further image processing (e.g. landmark based registration). In this work landmarks are determined in 4D CT lung data to quantify motion of lung structures due to breathing motion. Usually the landmark positions are defined manually using orthogonal (sagittal, coronal, axial) slices of the image data. As orientation and navigation in 3D image data volumes is a complex task even for experienced medical experts, the correct manual positioning of landmarks is a time-consuming process and it often results in misplaced landmarks. For these reasons a tool has been developed to support and guide the user during the positioning and to transfer landmarks between 3D volumes of a 4D data set.

Previous work in the direction of automatic detection of landmarks has been presented in [1, 2]. The detection of landmark candidates in our work is based on the work of Hartkens et al. [3], and some ideas of Ehrhardt et al. [4] are used for landmark transfer between time-points. A technique for haptic guidance during the interactive positioning of landmarks has not yet been proposed.

2 Materials and Methods

The assistance during the positioning of landmarks on surface models is split up into three parts: The automatic detection of landmark candidates (2.1), the haptic guidance to these candidates (2.2) and the transfer of landmarks between time-points of a 4D data set (2.3).

2.1 Detection of Landmark Candidates

This work is focussed on the detection of landmarks that lie at bifurcations of the bronchus tree. We restrict the landmark positions to the surface of this organ. Therefore these landmarks are located at saddle points of hyperbolic shaped surfaces and can further be characterized by a strong image curvature. In a first step different measures for surface curvature (Gaussian curvature, mean curvature, and moment based curvature [4]) have been evaluated to detect the saddle points. It turned out, that Gaussian and mean curvature strongly depend on the quality and smoothness of the surface meshes and therefore are inappropriate to detect the landmarks. The moment based curvature approach is more stable to quality issues but has some disadvantages in discriminating saddle points and points on flat surfaces. A combination of moment based and Gaussian curvature where candidates have been defined at positions with minimal Gaussian and small moment based curvature showed better results but was still depending on surface smoothing.

To be independent of surface quality and smoothness it was decided to use an image curvature measure instead. According to the results presented in Hartkens et al. [3] the Rohr operator k_{Rohr} is used to calculate the image curvature. It is defined by the determinant $\det \underline{C}$ of the structure tensor $\underline{C}$ which is built of the mean image gradients $\nabla g = (g_x, g_y, g_z)^T$ of a local neighborhood in a three-dimensional image $g(x, y, z)$:

$$\underline{C} = \overline{\nabla g (\nabla g)^T} \tag{1}$$

Fig. 1(a) shows the results of the Rohr operator transferred to the bronchus surface. The maxima of this measure are located at the bifurcations of the bronchus tree. The resulting landmark candidates (Fig. 1(b)) are computed in a local distance around the surface and therefore incorporate points with a high k_{Rohr} that do not exactly lie on the surface. Each candidate features a k_{Rohr} of at least 30% of the maximum k_{Rohr} of the entire bronchus area. Furthermore, only the points with highest k_{Rohr} in a local neighborhood ($3 \times 3 \times 3$) are chosen.

2.2 Force Calculation for Haptic Guidance

A haptic I/O-device (Sensable Phantom Omni) is used to place the landmarks on the organ surface. The visualization toolkit (VTK) and Sensable´s OpenHaptics library have been combined, to enable haptic feedback from surface objects that are graphically rendered through the VTK-pipeline [5]. Thus the user is able to touch the surface with the haptic device to place landmarks on it.

Furthermore, magnetic forces $\boldsymbol{f}_{mi}$ between the landmark candidates $\boldsymbol{p}_{li}$ and the device tip $\boldsymbol{p_t}$ are rendered around the landmark candidates within local areas with radius r and center points $\boldsymbol{p}_{li}$:

$$\boldsymbol{f}_{mi} = \begin{cases} k \cdot \boldsymbol{v}_n \cdot \frac{|\boldsymbol{v}|^2}{r^2} & \text{, if } |\boldsymbol{v}| < r \\ k \cdot \boldsymbol{v}_n \cdot \frac{r^2}{|\boldsymbol{v}|^2} & \text{, if } |\boldsymbol{v}| >= r \end{cases} \quad \text{where } \boldsymbol{v} = \boldsymbol{p}_t - \boldsymbol{p}_{li} \text{ and } \boldsymbol{v}_n = \frac{\boldsymbol{v}}{|\boldsymbol{v}|}. \qquad (2)$$

These forces guide the user to the exact positions of landmark candidates when the device enters the area around a candidate $\boldsymbol{p}_{li}$. The first case in eq. 2 ($|\boldsymbol{v}| < r$) is used to avoid vibration artifacts when the device reaches a landmark candidate. The magnetic forces $\boldsymbol{f}_{mi}$ of all candidates are summed up to build a resulting force $\boldsymbol{F} = \sum_i \boldsymbol{f}_{mi}$. $\boldsymbol{F}$ is then added to the surface rendering force.

2.3 Automatic Landmark Transfer

Landmarks in a 4D data set are traced by iteratively transferring the existing landmarks in the image volume of one time-point to the following image volumes. A non-linear surface based registration approach [4] is used to transfer the landmarks by matching the area around a given landmark (surface patch) to a corresponding area on the destination surface of the next time-point. Supposed a landmark $\boldsymbol{p}_l$ is placed on a triangulated surface patch consisting of n vertices $\boldsymbol{p}_{s,i}$. This surface patch is then deformed to match a set of vertices $\boldsymbol{p}_{d,i}$ that build up the corresponding surface patch at the next time-point. Surface constrained diffusion [6] which is based on Gaussian smoothed displacement fields is used to iteratively deform the surface patch. Corresponding vertices are found using a distance measure d that is a weighted sum of the Euclidean distance $d_e = |\boldsymbol{p}_d - \boldsymbol{p}_d|$, the distance of the normals $d_n = -\frac{\boldsymbol{n}_s \cdot \boldsymbol{n}_d}{2} + 0.5$, and the distances

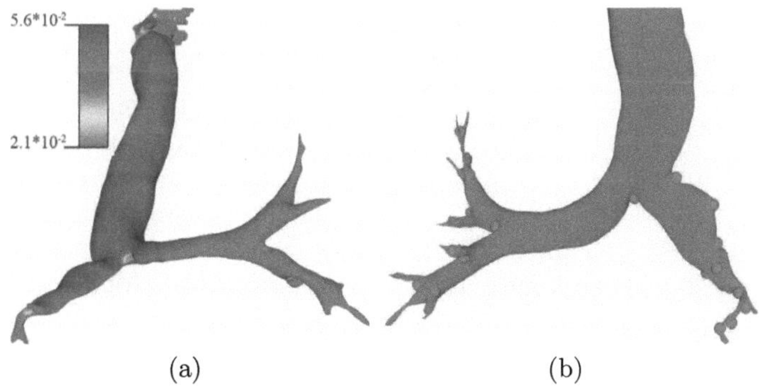

(a) (b)

Fig. 1. (a) Rohr operator results on the bronchus surface. (b) Back of the bronchus showing the resulting landmark candidates

Table 1. Standard deviations (σ) and mean distance $\overline{d}$ between landmarks of different users (IROV). $\overline{d}_{hm}$: Mean distance between manually and "haptically" placed landmarks (IAOV)

	haptically (in mm)				manually (in mm)				
ID	σ_x	σ_y	σ_z	$\overline{d}$	σ_x	σ_y	σ_z	$\overline{d}$	$\overline{d}_{hm}$
0	0.561	1.159	0.623	1.106	0.977	0.488	3.326	2.687	0.47
1	0.957	1.106	1.384	1.627	3.937	3.686	13.500	11.188	4.39
2	0.206	0.803	0.521	0.686	1.229	0.977	2.839	2.401	1.53
3	0.675	0.688	0.526	0.854	4.980	13.351	5.612	13.026	10.39
4	1.099	1.005	0.567	1.158	6.398	4.809	6.364	8.728	8.85
5	1.266	0.680	1.119	1.485	6.404	13.493	10.247	15.633	12.14

of the image curvature k_{Rohr} at the vertex positions $d_c = |k_{\text{Rohr}}(\boldsymbol{p}_d) - k_{\text{Rohr}}(\boldsymbol{p}_s)|$:

$$d = \omega_e \cdot d_e + \omega_n \cdot d_n + \omega_c \cdot d_c \tag{3}$$

The resulting displacement of the landmark $\boldsymbol{p}_l$ is then derived by interpolating the displacement vectors of the corners of the underlying triangle of $\boldsymbol{p}_l$.

2.4 Evaluation

A first evaluation has been done by placing landmarks of the bronchus tree in three time-points of a 4D lung CT data set. Four users with different medical experience manually positioned 6 landmarks using orthogonal slice-views of the volumetric image data at three time-points. Then each user placed the landmarks of the first time-point on the surface of the bronchus guided by the haptic device. These landmarks have been iteratively transferred to the next time-points allowing the user to correct misplaced landmarks using the haptic device.

3 Results

The time used to manually position all required landmarks took 30 to 35 min. compared to 7 to 10 min. consumed for haptically guided positioning and landmark transfer. The time to segment the bronchus and to generate the required surface models took about 10 min. Tab. 1 shows the interobserver variability (IROV) for haptically and manually placed landmarks (σ_y and $\overline{d}$) and the mean intraobserver variability (IAOV) as mean distance between the corresponding landmarks of each user $\overline{d}_{hm}$. The results of Tabelle 1 are supported by user opinions that conclude a higher intuitiveness during the guided positioning.

4 Discussion

The results show that it is hard to find the correct positions for some landmarks (especially no. 1, 3, and 5, which are located deep in the bronchus tree), when no

Fig. 2. GUI of the landmark positioning tool showing orthogonal slices of the image data (right) and a 3D visualization overlaid with an image of the haptic device

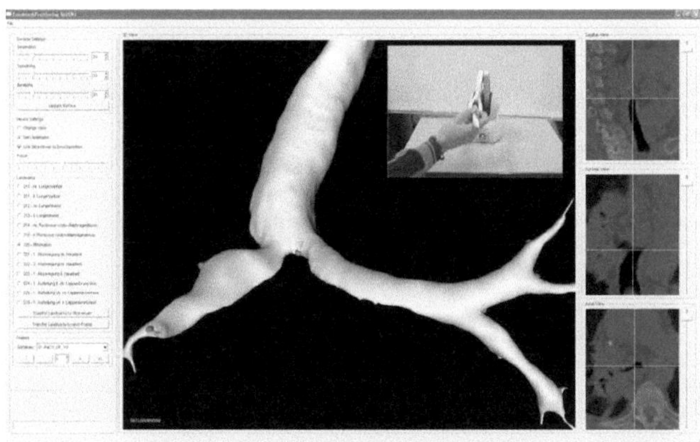

haptic guidance can be used. Therefore the landmark positioning tool presented forms an intuitive and reproducible way of placing landmarks of lung structures in 4D data. It offers significant time-savings and smaller inter- and intraobserver variability than the manual alternative. The guided navigation with the haptic device makes it easy to find the correct landmark positions and the transfer to the next time-point reduces further interaction time.

A restriction of our method is the need for surface models of the lung structures which require a segmentation. In case of the bronchus this can be done nearly automatically using volume growing. But as segmentation is not always such an easy task, our plans for the future include to make the tool independent from surface models using volume rendering techniques.

References

1. Wörz S, Rohr K. Localization of anatomical point landmarks in 3D medical images by fitting 3D parametric intensity models. Med Image Anal. 2006;10(1):41–58.
2. Berlinger K, Roth M, Sauer O, et al. Fully automatic detection of corresponding anatomical landmarks in volume scans of different respiratory state. Med Phys. 2006;33(6):1569–72.
3. Hartkens T, Rohr K, Stiehl HS. Evaluation of 3D operators for the detection of anatomical point landmarks in MR and CT images. Comput Vis Image Underst. 2002;86(2):118–36.
4. Ehrhardt J, Handels H, Plötz W, et al. Atlas-based recognition of anatomical structures and landmarks and the automatic computation of orthopedic parameters. Methods Inf Med. 2004;43(4):391–7.
5. Färber M, Drescher F, Ehrhardt J, et al. Integration von haptischen Ein-/Ausgabegeräten zur intuitiven Interaktion mit virtuellen Körpern in OP-Planungssysteme. Proc GMDS. 2006; p. 71–2.
6. Andresen PR, Nielsen M. Non-rigid registration by geometry-constrained diffusion. Med Image Anal. 2001;5(2):81–8.

Iterative Reconstruction of SPECT Images Using Adaptive Multi-level Refinement

Hanno Schumacher[1,3], Stefan Heldmann[1], Eldad Haber[2], Bernd Fischer[1]

[1]University of Lübeck, Institute of Mathematics, Wallstr. 40, 23560 Lübeck, Germany
[2]Emory University, Mathematics and Computer Science, Atlanta, GA 30322, USA
[3]MiE GmbH, Hauptstr. 112, 23845 Seth, Germany
schumaha@math.uni-luebeck.de

Abstract. We present a novel method for iterative reconstruction of high resolution images. Our method is based on the observation that constant regions in an image can be represented at much lower resolution than region with fine details. Therefore, we combine adaptive refinement based on quadtrees with iterative reconstruction to reduce the computational costs. In our experiments we found a speed up factor of approximately two compared to a standard multi-level method.

1 Introduction

Imaging systems are important tools in today's clinical routine. Tomographic images as, e.g., MRI, CT, PET, or SPECT images, have become standard for diagnosis and clinical testing. However, due to existing techniques, image reconstruction from tomographic data is still an open and active research field.

Here, we focus on iterative reconstruction methods particularly for SPECT. Such algorithms are able to compute high resolution high quality images and they are particularly useful when dealing with noisy data. Nevertheless, computing high quality images comes not for free. The complexity of such algorithms depends on the desired (high) target resolution. Typical dimensions are 128^3, 256^3, or 512^3 involving huge amount of data and thus lead to a non-neglectable computational effort.

Our new approach reduces the computational complexity without reducing the desired resolution. The basic idea is that regions of (almost) constant intensities can be represented at a very low resolution. To this end, we combine iterative reconstruction with adaptive multi-level refinement. Starting from a very low resolution, we locally refine regions where we expect details in the image while other regions with, e.g., only background information, stay coarse. Due to their simplicity and the rectangular pixel-structure of image, we propose quad- (2D) and octrees (3D) for the local refinement [1].

The ideas of representing images with local low and high resolutions as well as adaptive refinement are not new. These techniques are well known and have already been used in many other fields, too. Recent examples particularly incorporating quad-/octrees include image registration [2, 3, 4], computer graphics

[5], or inverse problems [6]. A similar approach for image reconstruction using a fixed non-uniform mesh generated from external knowledge is presented in [7]. However, to our best knowledge adaptive multi-level refinement has not been used for image reconstruction, yet.

The paper is organized as follows. In section 2 we state the image reconstruction problem and describe our new method. Subsequently, we present a real SPECT data and an academic example in section 3. Finally we discuss the results in section 4.

2 Materials and Methods

Here we focus on reconstruction of SPECT images [8]. Therefore, emitted radiation of an injected radioactive contrast agent is measured at different position around the object. Then, the measured projection data d is used to reconstructed an image f such that the image f represents the distribution of the contrast agent. Formally, this leads to the problem

$$\mathcal{A}f = d \quad s.t. \quad f \geq 0 \tag{1}$$

with a linear projection operator $\mathcal{A}$ describing the SPECT measurement. The constraint $f \geq 0$ is required to guarantee a positive distribution since negative concentrations are not physical. It is well known that (1) is an ill-posed problem [9, 10]. Therefore, additional constraints and/or regularization is needed. Furthermore, real measured data d comes with non-neglectable noise such that solving $\mathcal{A}f = d$ for f exactly will not produce wanted results. Therefore, instead of trying to solve (1) directly, we consider the optimization problem

$$\text{minimize} \quad \mathcal{J}(f) = \frac{1}{2}\|\mathcal{A}f - d\|_{L_2}^2 + \alpha\mathcal{R}(f) \quad s.t. \quad f \geq 0 \tag{2}$$

Here, $\frac{1}{2}\|\mathcal{A}f - d\|_{L_2}^2$ forces fitting the data d and $\mathcal{R}$ is a regularizer addressing the ill-posedness and the noise in the data. Typically, $\mathcal{R}$ forces smoothness of the image f such that the parameter $\alpha > 0$ weights the influence of the regularizer versus the (noisy) data fit. In particular, here we choose

$$\mathcal{R}(f) = \frac{1}{2}\sum_{i=1}^{n} \|\partial_i f\|_{L_2}^2 \tag{3}$$

where n is the dimension of the image f ($n = 2$ or $n = 3$).
To compute a numerical solution we first discretize (2) on a given quad- or octree. We proceed analog to [1, 2, 3, 6]. Quad- and octrees are an efficient way to compress structured data. To make the idea clear, let us consider a regular discretization of a image composed of pixels/voxels with uniform size. For the quad-/octree we combine square blocks of pixels and represent each of theses blocks by a single large pixel, i.e., lower resolution. See Figures 1,2 for

2D quadtree examples. Thus, we discretize the image on cell-centers of the given quad-/octree such that the discretized problem reads

$$\text{minimize} \quad \mathbf{J}(\mathbf{f}) = \frac{1}{2}\|\mathbf{A}\mathbf{f} - \mathbf{d}\|_2^2 + \frac{\alpha}{2}\mathbf{f}^\top \mathbf{B}^\top \mathbf{B}\,\mathbf{f} \quad s.t. \quad \mathbf{f} \geq 0 \tag{4}$$

where the matrix $\mathbf{A}$ is a discretization of the $\mathcal{A}$ and the $\mathbf{f}^\top \mathbf{B}^\top \mathbf{B}\,\mathbf{f}$ is a finite difference approximations to the regularizer $\mathcal{R}(f)$ [5].

Our overall method is an adaptive multi-level scheme. We start with discretizing the problem on a coarse regular grid say 8 by 8 and compute a minimizer of (4). Subsequently, we locally refine our discretization due to some criteria explained below and compute a minimizer of (4) discretized on the new grid. Then, we locally refine again, solve the problem on the new grid and so on. We proceed until the finest cells in our discretization have reached the target resolution.

To compute a minimizer of (4) on a fixed level we use Newton's method with projecting each iterate to the constraints $\mathbf{f} \geq 0$. The method is similar to the gradient-projection algorithm described in [11] except that for fast convergence we take a Newton search direction instead of the negative gradient. Therefore, in each step we have to solve a large linear system. Here we spend the main computational efforts and this is also the point where we get the major benefit from our method by reducing the number of unknowns. Our experiments show that we gain a speedup of a factor 2 compared to a standard method.

Our local refinement strategy is based on the general idea that constant regions of an image can be represented with low resolution than regions with rapidly changing gray values, i.e., edges. To this end, we consider the gradient of the image and do a refinement where it is large. Since we do not have an analytic gradient, we compute a finite difference approximation [5, 6]. Let $\mathbf{g}_j$ be an approximation to the image gradient on the j-th cell of our current grid such that $\mathbf{g}_j \approx \nabla f(\text{cell}_j)$. Then we subdivide the j-th cell into four sub-cells if $\|\mathbf{g}_j\|_\infty > \gamma$ where $\gamma > 0$ is a chosen parameter.

3 Results

We present two 2D examples where we compare our adaptive method with a standard uniform refinement. In the first academic example, we reconstruct a Shepp-Logan-Phantom (256^2 pixels, max. gray value 255) where the artificial projection data was generated from an ideal noise-free image. The aim of this experiment is to demonstrate that we are able to reconstruct high quality images on quite sparse quadtrees. For the second example we reconstruct images (128^2 pixels, max. gray value 800) from real SPECT data. Here, we demonstrate the use of our method for real data with noise. In both experiments we started our multi-level method from a coarse 8 by 8 grid and the regularization parameter α was set to 10^{-3}.

For the Shepp-Logan-Phantom we simulated 120 SPECT projections with 256 pixels each. We evaluated several choices for the refinement parameter γ. The resulting images and quadtrees are presented in Figure 1. As expected, the

Fig. 1. Results for the Shepp-Logan-Phantom

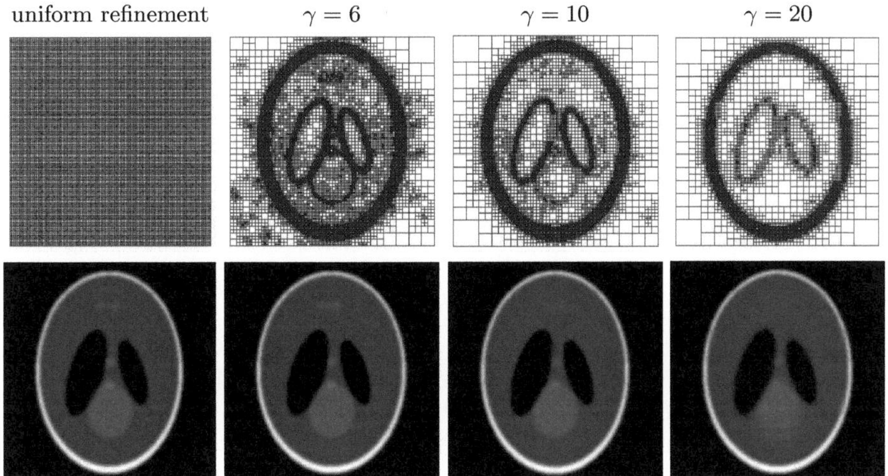

results show that with increasing γ the resulting quadtrees become more sparse and the number of pixels is drastically reduced. Nevertheless, the visual quality of the images remains reasonable even for very large values of γ.

In our real data example, 120 projections of the Benchmark-Jaszczak-Phantom were measured with a SPECT system from the MiE company in Seth, Germany. In contrast to the academic example, here we have to deal with noise that is included in the data. However, we are able to compute images on sparse quadtrees that are visually indistinguishable from the result when using a standard uniform refinement (Fig. 2).

In both experiments we successfully apply our adaptive refinement strategy that drastically reduces computational efforts. Basically, we found that we only need 30–50% of the pixels resulting an overall speedup factor of approximately 2. The computational results for both experiments are presented in Table 1.

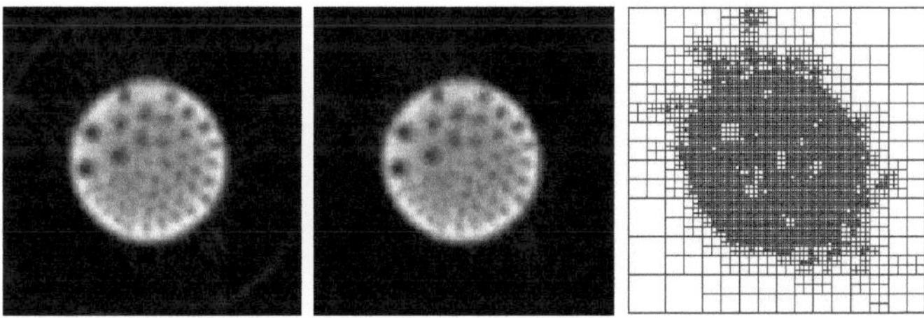

Fig. 2. Results for the Benchmark-Jaszczak-Phantom. Left result for uniform refinement, middle + right result after adaptive refinement ($\gamma = 40$)

Table 1. Computational results for the finest level computed in Matlab

Data	refinement	#iter	average time per iter	#pixels	resolution
Shepp-Logan	uniform	6	5.39 sec	65,536	256^2
Shepp-Logan	$\gamma = 6$	3	2.96 sec	22,198	256^2
Shepp-Logan	$\gamma = 10$	4	2.22 sec	16,732	256^2
Shepp-Logan	$\gamma = 20$	4	1.52 sec	11,749	256^2
Real-data	uniform	4	1.25 sec	16,384	128^2
Real-data	$\gamma = 40$	4	0.60 sec	5,782	128^2

4 Discussion

We have presented a novel multi-level reconstruction scheme using an adaptive refinement strategy based on quadtrees. The method is able to produce high quality images at the same level of detail as standard methods while significantly reducing the computational costs. Moreover, no external knowledge about the image content is used. In our experiments we found a speedup factor of roughly 2. Our examples demonstrate the potential of the new method and its successful use with real data having noise.

The presented results are basically 2D and can be used for slice-wise reconstruction of 3D data. However, in future work the approach shall be extended to fully 3D, i.e., by using 3D octrees instead of 2D quadtrees. Furthermore, we aim for an automatic estimate of the refinement parameter γ.

References

1. Samet H. The Design and Analysis of Spatial Data Structures. Boston, MA, USA: Addison-Wesley Longman Publishing Co., Inc.; 1990.
2. Haber E, Heldmann S, Modersitzki J. An OcTree method for parametric image registration. SIAM J Sci Comp. 2006;Accepted.
3. Haber E, Heldmann S, Modersitzki J. Adaptive mesh refinement for non-parametric image registration. SIAM J Sci Comp. 2007;Submitted.
4. Szeliski R, Lavallée S. Matching 3-D anatomical surfaces with non-rigid deformation using Octree-splines. Proc SPIE. 1993;2031.
5. Losasso F, Gibou F, Fedkiw R. Simulating water and smoke with an octree data structure. ACM Trans Graph. 2004;23(4):457–62.
6. Haber E, Heldmann S, Ascher U. Adaptive finite volume methods for distributed non-smooth parameter identification. Inverse Problems. 2007;23:1659–76.
7. Brankov JG, Yang Y, Wernick MN. Tomographic image reconstruction based on a content-adaptive mesh model. IEEE Trans Med Imaging. 2004;23(2):202–12.
8. Groch MW, Erwin WD. SPECT in the Year 2000: Basic principles. J Nucl Med Technol. 2000;28(4):233–44.
9. Natterer F, Wübbeling F. Mathematical Methods in Image Reconstruction. Philadelphia: Society for Industrial and Applied Mathematics; 2001.
10. Bruyant P. Analytic and iterative reconstruction algorithms in SPECT. J Nucl Med. 2002;43(10):1343–58.
11. Nocedal J, Wright SJ. Numerical Optimization. Springer; 1999.

Automatic Ascending Aorta Detection in CTA Datasets

Stefan C. Saur[1], Caroline Kühnel[2], Tobias Boskamp[2], Gábor Székely[1], Philippe Cattin[1,3]

[1]Computer Vision Laboratory, ETH Zurich, 8092 Zurich, Switzerland
[2]MeVis Research GmbH, 28359 Bremen, Germany
[3]CMBE, University Basel, 4003 Basel, Switzerland
saur@vision.ee.ethz.ch

Abstract. The assessment of coronary arteries is an essential step when diagnosing coronary heart diseases. There exists a wide range of specialized algorithms for the segmentation of the coronary arteries in Computed Tomography Angiography datasets. In general, these algorithms have to be initialized by manually placing a seed point at the origins of the coronary arteries or within the ascending aorta. In this paper we present a fast and robust algorithm for the automatic detection of the ascending aorta in Computed Tomography Angiography datasets using a two-level threshold ray propagation approach. We further combine this method with an aorta segmentation and coronary artery tree detection algorithm to achieve a fully automatic coronary artery segmentation.

1 Introduction

The assessment of coronary arteries is an essential diagnostic tool as coronary heart diseases account for approximately 40% of deaths in both the male and female population in the European Union [1]. Computed Tomography Coronary Angiography is a frequently used modality for the detection of coronary artery diseases as it visualizes the 3D course of the coronary arteries and shows a good correlation with the gold standard, the conventional coronary angiography [2].

Automatic segmentation of the coronary arteries is desired for the diagnosis of plaques, aneurysms, or stenoses. Nowadays, a variety of specialized methods like fast marching [3], region growing [4], or model-based segmentation [5] exists for the segmentation of the coronary arteries. A detailed overview of existing segmentation algorithms for tubular structures can be found in [6]. While available algorithms perform the segmentation automatically, they still need a manual initialization in form of seed points in the origins of the coronary arteries. With the proposed ascending aorta detection, we can close this gap towards a fully automatic segmentation. The shape of the ascending aorta can be described as circular or elliptical in the slices along the z-direction. Thus, approaches like the Hough Transform used in [7] or the search ray approach described in [8] are suitable methods for an automatic localization of the ascending aorta. The disadvantage of the Hough Transform, however, is its limited computational efficiency. Furthermore, it is sensitive to noise and deviations of the model shape.

2 Methods

The proposed procedure is based on the method described by Lorenz *et al.* [8] for the detection of the descending aorta. Within a fixed volume of interest (VOI) in a dataset, a search ray passes the voxels in x-direction (left to right), line by line (top-down), for each axial slice (Fig. 1(a)). For voxels above a predefined intensity threshold, several geometric criteria are evaluated that a candidate point for the ascending aorta must fulfill. In contrast to the descending aorta, our VOI contains more elliptical structures (e.g. right atrium, right ventricle) that fulfill the criteria used by Lorenz *et al.* [8]. Therefore, additional constraints were introduced to validate circularity. The detection algorithm looks as follows:

1. Trace search ray in x-direction while gray values stay below a given primary threshold th_p (Fig. 1a).
2. If primary threshold is met, continue with search ray and look for an intensity transition that falls below a secondary threshold th_s (Fig. 1b).
3. If transition is reached, search backwards to above th_p (Fig. 1b).
4. If the diameter d_x of the found structure is within $d_{\min}$ and $d_{\max}$, compute center p_x between both transition points and search from this center with the procedure as described above for the extension d_y in y-direction. Compute center point p_y in y-direction and search for extension $d_{+\pi/4}$ and $d_{-\pi/4}$ in direction of the two angle bisectors in the xy-plane (Fig. 1c).
5. Compute ratio $a = |d_y/d_x - 1|$.
6. If $d_{\min} < d_i < d_{\max} \forall d_i, d_i \in \{d_x, d_y, d_{+\pi/4}, d_{-\pi/4}\}$ and ratio a is below threshold th_a, add p_y to the candidate list $\mathcal{L}$.
7. Set search ray to the next line or slice, respectively, and continue with step 1 until whole VOI is processed.

Neighborhood clusters are computed out of the list $\mathcal{L}$ of candidate points. An initial cluster is defined with the first candidate point of $\mathcal{L}$. For each remaining point p_l of $\mathcal{L}$, it is checked if a cluster already contains an element that is less than a given euclidian distance d_{clust} away from p_l. If yes, the candidate point p_l is added to this cluster. Otherwise, a new cluster is initiated. The cluster containing the most elements is taken as the representant of the ascending aorta.

In addition to Lorenz *et al.* we introduced the ratio a and the diameters $d_{+\pi/4}$ and $d_{-\pi/4}$ along the direction of the two angle bisectors as extra constraints for the candidates. To speed up the detection process, the search ray is not propagated voxel by voxel, but is incremented by Δ_x, Δ_y, and Δ_z, in x-, y-, and z-direction, respectively. A priori anatomical knowledge about the expected position of the ascending aorta is used to define the VOI.

We used 100 computed tomography angiography (CTA) datasets (standard cardiac protocol, Siemens Definition) to fix a set of parameters that minimizes the number of false detections: $\Delta_x = 1$mm, $\Delta_y = 5$mm, $\Delta_z = 1$mm, $th_p = 180$HU, $th_s = 100$HU, $d_{\min} = 20$mm, $d_{\max} = 70$mm, $d_{\text{clust}} = 5$mm (isotropic), $th_a = 0.25$, $\text{VOI}_x = 0 - 0.75$, $\text{VOI}_y = 0.25 - 0.70$, $\text{VOI}_z = 0.50 - 1.00$. The VOI is given as a percentage of the total dataset extension in the corresponding direction whereby the z-direction is defined in cranial direction.

As a benchmark for the proposed algorithm, we used the method developed by Hennemuth *et al.* [9] to segment the ascending aorta and to detect voxel clusters at the coronary artery origins. Initialized with the detected seed point in the ascending aorta, the algorithm relies on a statistical analysis of areas segmented by a 2D region growing algorithm to segment the ascending aorta in caudal direction. The method automatically stops at the aortic valve and detects the origins of the coronary arteries. As the focus of this work was on the automatic detection of the ascending aorta, we did not evaluate the performance of different coronary artery segmentation approaches, although it is possible to combine the presented method with any algorithm that needs a point within the ascending aorta or the origins of the coronary arteries for its initialization.

For the initialization of the ascending aorta segmentation, a cluster point has to be selected that is sufficiently above the aortic valve and below the aortic arch. We sort the points of the largest cluster by their z-coordinate such that the first point in the list is closest to the aortic valve. The cluster point at the 90% quantile of the sorted list is finally selected as the seed point for the following segmentation process. The ground truth was defined by three experienced readers who manually placed a seed point within the ascending aorta for all datasets. Each reader - blinded to the seed points of the others - was instructed to mark a point within the ascending aorta well above the aortic valve and below the aortic arch. The seed point was then used as an initialization for the ascending aorta segmentation method as described above.

3 Results

We evaluated the presented method on 297 CTA datasets from different Siemens CT scanners (Definition, Sensation 64, Sensation Cardiac 64, Sensation 16) whereby the datasets for the parameter optimization were not included in this

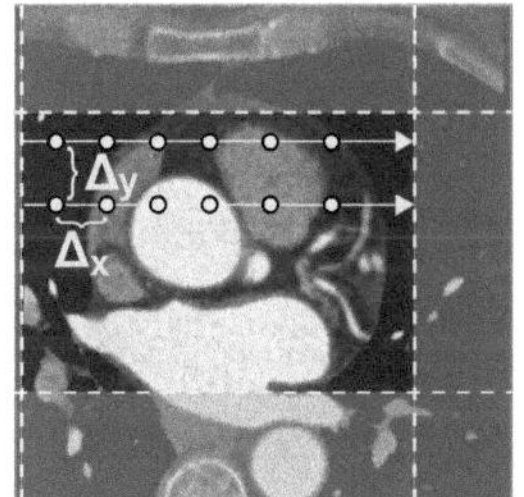

(a) VOI and ray propagation

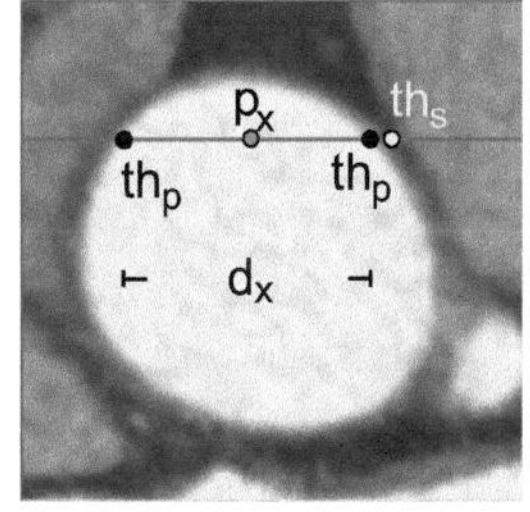

(b) Extension in x-direction

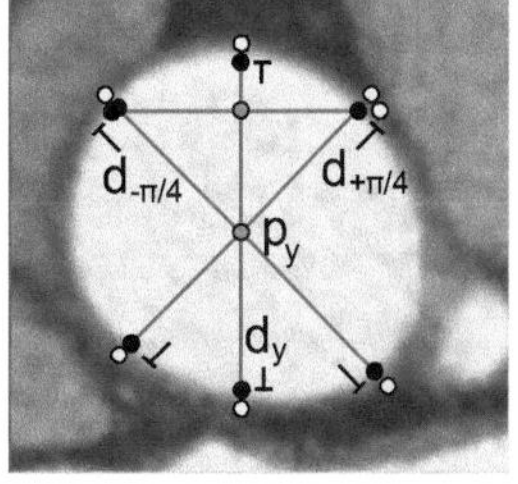

(c) Candidate point p_y

Fig. 1. Detection of the ascending aorta. Within a predefined volume of interest (VOI), search rays are propagated (a) following a two-level threshold approach to compute the extension in x-direction (b) and afterwards in y-direction as well as in direction of the two angle bisectors (c). If geometric constraints are fulfilled, the point p_y is added to the list of ascending aorta candidates.

Table 1. As a benchmark, we initialized an ascending aorta segmentation and coronary artery detection algorithm for both automatically detected and manually placed seed points. We evaluated the successful segmentation of the ascending aorta down-to the aortic valve as well as the detection of the left and right coronary artery tree (CAT) origin, respectively. Values are given as successful number/total number (percentage)

	Detection of ascending aorta	Segmentation of ascending aorta	Detection of left CAT origin	Detection of right CAT origin
Our method	288/297 (97.0%)	284/288 (98.6%)	261/284 (91.9%)	263/284 (92.6%)
Reader 1	297/297 (100.0%)	292/297 (98.3%)	270/292 (92.5%)	271/292 (92.8%)
Reader 2	297/297 (100.0%)	296/297 (99.7%)	275/296 (92.9%)	279/296 (94.3%)
Reader 3	297/297 (100.0%)	295/297 (99.3%)	274/295 (92.9%)	273/295 (92.5%)

evaluation. The in-plane resolution ranged from 0.236-0.512 mm and the slice thickness varied between 0.3-0.8 mm. Each slice contained 512x512 voxels and the number of slices varied between 150 and 591.

A seed point was correctly placed in the ascending aorta in 288 (97.0%) datasets. For 9 datasets, the aorta could not be detected and a point within the right ventricle (8 times) or descending aorta (once) was chosen by the algorithm. In these cases, the second largest cluster represented the ascending aorta. The mean detection time for the ascending aorta was 0.30 s and ranged from 0.13-0.77 s on a Pentium 4 with 3 GHz and 2 GB RAM.

In 98.6% of the cases where our automatic detection succeeded, the aorta could be segmented down to the aortic valve. With this correct ascending aorta segmentation, a detection rate of 91.9% for the left coronary artery tree (CAT) origin and 92.6% for the right CAT origin could be achieved.

Based on different placed seed points by the readers, the aorta segmentation rate varied between 98.3% and 99.7% which led to a detection rate of 92.5%-92.9% for the left and 92.5%-94.3% for the right CAT origin, respectively. A detailed comparison of the results for the segmentation of the ascending aorta and the detection of the origins for the left and right CAT is listed in Table 1.

4 Discussion and Conclusion

We presented a fast and robust algorithm for the automatic detection of the ascending aorta in CTA datasets using a two-level threshold ray propagation approach. The method has been tuned on 100 CTA datasets and has been successfully evaluated on 297 scans from different CT devices. A detection rate of 97.0% confirms the robustness of the presented method. Figure 2 exemplarily shows four detected aortas. In all 9 cases where the largest candidate cluster did not represent the ascending aorta, it was identified by the second largest cluster. Thus, our future work will focus on the definition of additional features for the two largest clusters to further improve the detection rate.

With a successfully detected ascending aorta, the performance of the aorta segmentation and coronary artery tree origin detection was within the variability

Fig. 2. Screenshots of four different datasets with varying contrast agent distribution and anatomical shape: In 97.0% of all cases, our presented algorithm automatically found a point within the ascending aorta (black circle)

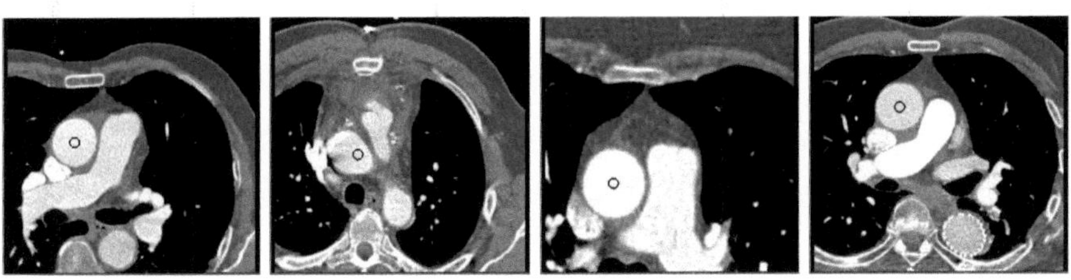

range given by the results of manually placed seed points. Hence, the developed method is suitable to speed up the diagnostic process by automatically presegmenting the coronary arteries.

Therefore, our method can close the gap to a fully automatic vessel segmentation by combining the developed ascending aorta detection with an aorta and coronary artery tree segmentation algorithm.

Acknowledgement. The authors thank the radiology departments from the Universitätsspital Zürich, Universitätsklinikum Erlangen, Radiological University Hospital Tübingen, University Hospital of Munich, PUMC Hospital and PLA Hospital in Beijing for providing the CTA datasets. This work has been supported by the CO-ME/NCCR research network of the Swiss National Science Foundation (`http://co-me.ch`).

References

1. Jougla E. Health Statistics - Atlas on mortality in the European Union. European Communities; 2003.
2. Leschka S, Alkadhi H, Plass A, et al. Accuracy of MSCT coronary angiography with 64-slice technology: First experience. Eur Heart J. 2005;26(15):1482–7.
3. Lorenz C, Renisch S, Schlathölter T, et al. Simultaneous segmentation and tree reconstruction of the coronary arteries in MSCT images. Proc SPIE. 2003;5031(1):167–77.
4. Boskamp T, Rinck D, Link F, et al. New vessel analysis tool for morphometric quantification and visualization of vessels in CT and MR imaging sata sets. Radiographics. 2004;24(1):287–97.
5. Wörz S, Rohr K. Segmentation and quantification of human vessels using a 3-D cylindrical intensity model. IEEE Trans Image Process. 2007;16(8):1994–2004.
6. Kirbas C, Quek F. A review of vessel extraction techniques and algorithms. ACM Computing Surveys. 2004;36(2):81–121.
7. Kovacs T, Cattin P, Alkadhi H, et al. Automatic segmentation of the vessel lumen from 3D CTA images of aortic dissection. Proc BVM. 2006; p. 161–5.
8. Lorenz C, Lessick J, Lavi G, et al. Fast automatic delineation of cardiac volume of interest in MSCT images. Proc SPIE. 2004;5370(1):456–66.
9. Hennemuth A, Boskamp T, Fritz D, et al. One-click coronary tree segmentation in CT angiographic images. Proc CARS. 2005;1281:317–321.

Aufnahme, Analyse und Visualisierung von Bewegungen nativer Herzklappen in-vitro

Oliver Weiß[1], Sven Friedl[1,2], Markus Kondruweit[2], Thomas Wittenberg[1]

[1]Fraunhofer Institut für Integrierte Schaltungen IIS, Erlangen
[2]Universitätsklinikum Erlangen
weissor@iis.fraunhofer.de

Kurzfassung. Die hohe Zahl an Transplantationen von Herzklappen und viele nötige Re-Operationen machen eine detaillierte Analyse der Strömungen und Klappenbewegungen klinisch interessant. Ein neuer Ansatz ist hierbei der Einsatz von Hochgeschwindigkeitskameras um Bewegungsabläufe der Herzklappen beobachten und auswerten zu können. Die hohen Datenraten erfordern allerdings eine möglichst automatisierte Analyse und möglichst komprimierte Darstellung des Schwingungsverhaltens. In dieser Arbeit wird ein Ansatz vorgestellt, bei dem Bewegungen nativer Herzklappen in-vitro aufgenommen, analysiert und kompakt visualisiert werden.

1 Einleitung

Bei den zurzeit etablierten und eingesetzten Herzklappenprothesen bzw. Rekonstruktionsmethoden zeigen sich im klinischen Verlauf mehrere Probleme. Implantierte Bioprothesen verkalken im Verlauf zunehmend und entwickeln dadurch eine Dysfunktion, die bis zur Re-Operation führen kann [1]. Bei mechanischen Herzklappenprothesen, insbesondere in Aortenposition, zeigen sich häufig hohe Bewegungsgradienten über der Klappe, die einer Erholung eines bereits vorgeschädigten Herzens entgegenstehen und somit die Lebenserwartung des Patienten limitieren [2].

Um die Ursachen und Einflussparameter von Kalzifikationen an Herzklappen qualitativ und quantitativ zu untersuchen, werden seit einiger Zeit in verschiedenen Einrichtungen Aufnahmen von Herzklappenbewegungen mit Hilfe von Hochgeschwindigkeitskameras durchgeführt [3, 4]. Da derartige Kamerasysteme Bewegungen mit einer Datenrate von bis zu 4000 Bildern pro Sekunde aufnehmen können, ist für die Auswertung und Aufbereitung des derart erfassten Datenmaterials eine automatische und quantitative Methode wünschenswert und sinnvoll.

Die direkte Beobachtung und bildbasierte Analyse von Herzklappenbewegungen mittels Hochgeschwindigkeitskameras ist eine relativ junge Disziplin. Daher existieren kaum Arbeiten auf dem Gebiet. [3, 5] haben sowohl flächen- als auch kantenbasierte Ansätze zur Segmentierung der Herzklappen vorgestellt. Der flächen-basierte Ansatz besteht aus einer Pixelklassifikation über globale und lokale Schwellwerte über ein Zwei-. Mehr bzw. einem Finite Mixture-Model sowie einer Nachbearbeitung der Fläche. Als kantenbasierte Ansätze, auch in [4] vorgeschlagen, werden Aktive Konturen zur Segmentierung eingesetzt. Ansätze zur Visualisierung von Bewegungsfunktionen von Organen aus Bildsequenzen mit einem einzigen Bild wurden für die Analyse von Stimmlippen vorgestellt [6]. Dieser Ansatz wird im Rahmen dieser Arbeit für die Visualisierung von Herzklappen weiterentwickelt.

2 Methoden

2.1 Aufnahme

Zur Analyse des Schwingungsverhaltens der nativen Herzklappen werden diese mit einem Hochgeschwindigkeitskamerasystem in-vitro aufgenommen. Dazu wird ein explantiertes Schweineherz über eine Herz-Lungen-Maschine reanimiert. Die Koronararterien werden darüber mit sauerstoffreichem Blut versorgt und mit der Zugabe von Nährstoffen und Medikamenten wird die Kollabierung des Organs verzögert. Um die Bewegungen der Klappen beobachten zu können, wird Wasser in den linken Vorhof geleitet und passiert über die linke Herzkammer die Aortenklappen. Durch Reduktion des Aortendurchmessers werden physiologische Druckverhältnisse hergestellt. Die Hochgeschwindigkeitskamera blickt über ein 0°-Endoskop durch die erste Abzweigung der Aorta auf die nun sichtbare Herzklappe. Durch die Aufnahmengeschwindigkeit von 2000 Bildern pro Sekunde bei einer Ortsauflösung von 256×256 Bildpunkten können die biomechanischen Bewegungsabläufe der Herzklappen detailliert aufgezeichnet und ausgewertet werden. Das Aufnahmeverfahren besitzt den einmaligen Vorteil, dass die Aufnahmen unter physiologischen Bedingungen im schlagenden Herzen stattfinden. Dadurch kann das Schwingungsverhalten naturgetreu analysiert werden.

2.2 Segmentierung

Die von der Hochgeschwindigkeitskamera gelieferten, Datenmengen mit 2000–6000 Bildern pro Aufnahme erfordern eine automatisierte Analyse der Klappenbewegungen. Dabei sind für medizinische Aussagen nur Zeitintervalle relevant,

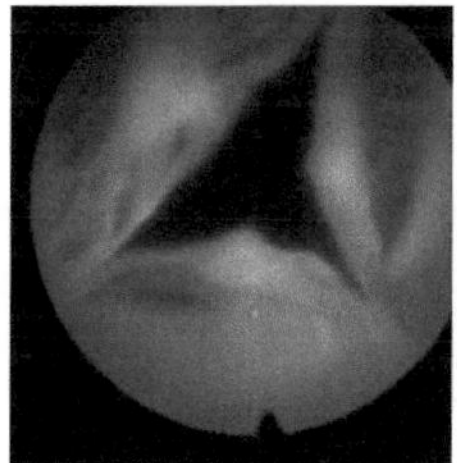
(a) Orginalbild $f(i,j)$

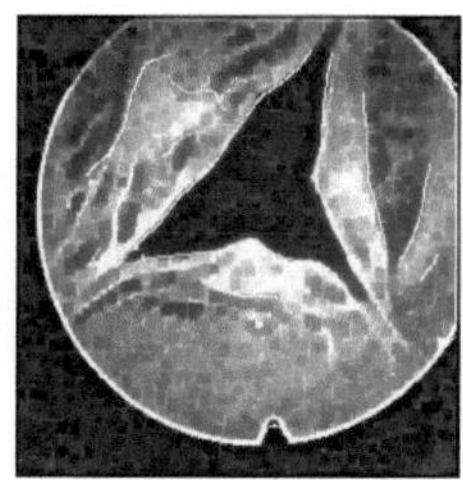
(b) Kantenbild $g(i,j)$

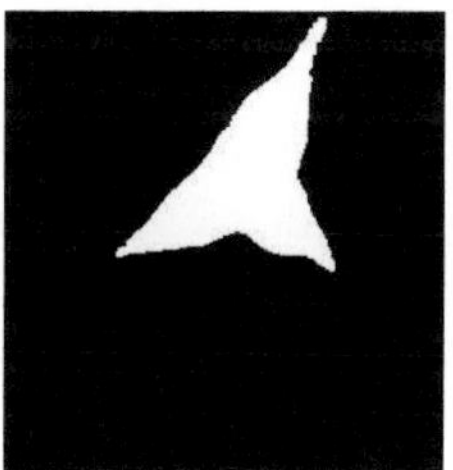
(c) Binärbild $b(i,j)$

Abb. 1. Barrieren durch Betonung von Kanten und resultierendes Binärbild

in denen ausgeprägte Bewegungen stattfinden. Maximale und minimale Öffnung der Herzklappen werden mittels einer Abschätzung des Öffnungsgrades durch die mittlere Bildenergie $E(t)$ für jedes Einzelbild zum Zeitpunkt t und der Berechnung von lokalen Extrema bestimmt. Die Bildindizes $t_{\text{Max},l}$, t_{Min} und $t_{\text{Max},r}$ beschreiben den kompletten Öffnungs- und Verschlussvorgang einer Öffnungsperiode und werden automatisch aus den Energiekurven ermittelt.

Mit einem Regionenwachstumsverfahren erfolgt die Segmentierung der Öffnungsfläche zwischen $t_{\text{Max},l}$ und $t_{\text{Max},r}$. Als Ausgangspunkt der Segmentierung wird die Lage eines Saatpunktes innerhalb der zu segmentierenden Fläche automatisch bestimmt. Der Saatpunkt wird als dunkelster Grauwert innerhalb eines Quadrates angenommen, das um einen initialen Punkt gebildet wird. Als erstes, zu verarbeitendes Bild wird das Einzelbild zum Zeitpunkt t_{Min} der jeweiligen Sequenz mit maximal geöffneten Klappen gewählt, da der Schwerpunkt der ROI bereits innerhalb dessen Öffnungsfläche liegt. Jeder weitere initiale Punkt ist als Schwerpunkt der vorangegangenen Segmentierung gegeben. Ausgehend vom Zeitpunkt t_{Min} erfolgt die Verarbeitung chronologisch in beide Richtungen, bis die Bilder erreicht sind, die den benachbarten Maxima $t_{\text{Max},l}$ und $t_{\text{Max},r}$ entsprechen.

Um ein Überlaufen zu verhindern, werden Objektkanten betont und Barrieren für den Wachstumsprozess geschaffen. Die Anwendung einer 5×5-Laplace-Filtermaske, ergänzt um eine Liniendetektion mittels Canny-Operator, erzeugt die erforderlichen geschlossenen Kanten. Eingangsbilder $g(i,j)$ des Wachstumsalgorithmus' werden durch eine gewichtete Summe aus Kantenbildern und Orginalbild $f(i,j)$ gemäß $g(i,j) = \lceil a \cdot f_{\text{Laplace}}(i,j) + b \cdot f_{\text{Canny}}(i,j) + c \cdot f(i,j) \rceil$ berechnet, wobei $a, b, c \in [0,1]$ heuristisch zu bestimmende Gewichtungsfaktoren sind.

Das verwendete Homogenitätskriterium basiert auf einem Schwellwertverfahren. Der Schwellwert θ berechnet sich aus dem normalisierten Grauwerthistogramm. Unter der Annahme, dass dieses in zwei Klassen unterteilt werden kann, läßt sich der Schwellwert durch Maximierung von verschiedenen Kennzahlen berechnen. Die beiden verwendeten Größen sind die Summe der Entropien der Klassen [7] und die Varianz zwischen den Klassen [8]. Wurde eine ausreichende Menge von Bildpunkten segmentiert, kann auf den adaptiven Schwellwert $\theta = \mu + 3\sigma$ zurückgegriffen werden. Hierbei bezeichnet μ den linearen Mittelwert und σ die Standardabweichung der bereits segmentierten Grauwerte.

Gegebenenfalls weist die segmentierte Fläche Einschlüsse von Pixeln auf. Zur Korrektur wird ein morphologisches Closing verwendet, mit dem auch Fehlerstellen in den Randbereichen zwischen den Segmenten entfernt werden. Große Störungen in den Flächensegmenten lassen sich mit einer Anwendung von Regionenwachstum beseitigen, bei dem der Saatpunkt in den Bereich außerhalb der Öffnungsfläche gesetzt wird. Teilschritte der Segmentierung sind in Abb. 1 dargestellt.

2.3 Visualisierung

Für eine kompakte Visualisierung der Herzklappenbewegungen, werden sogenannte Kardiovibrogramme nach dem Vorbild der Phonovibrogramme [6] eingeführt. Sie repräsentieren einen interessanten Aspekt der Herzklappendynamik: Die Bewegung der Klappenränder in Relation zur Klappenmitte. Die Grundidee zu dieser Visualisierungstechnik ist eine Abstandsmessung zwischen einem zentralen Punkt S und ausgewählten Randpunkten R. S wird durch eine lineare Interpolation zwischen den Schwerpunkten der segmentierten Flächen bestimmt, die den Bildern mit maximal und minimal geöffneten Klappen entsprechen. Zur Berechnung der Punkte R werden ausgehend vom Startpunkt S Strahlen traversiert, die abhängig von einem Winkel α in unterschiedliche Richtungen verlaufen. Schnittpunkte mit dem Rand der Öffnungsfläche liefern die gesuchten Randpunkte R. Die grauwertcodierten Euklidischen Abstände zwischen dem Punkt S und den Punkten R werden in einen Spaltenvektor eingetragen. Erfolgen die Messungen für alle Bilder einer Teilsequenz und werden die Spaltenvektoren entsprechend der Bildnummer entlang der Abszisse platziert, entsteht ein Kardiovibrogramm.

3 Ergebnisse

Die Anzahl der zur Verfügung stehenden Aufnahmen nativer Herzklappen invitro ist mit etwa 25 Sequenzen noch sehr gering. Der vorgestellte Ansatz zur Segmentierung und Visualisierung der Herzklappenbewegungen wurde an allen Aufnahmen evaluiert. Eine automatisierte Auswertung ist dabei nur bei den jüngeren Aufnahmen mit besserer Bildqualität möglich. Ein großer Teil der älteren Aufnahmen lässt sich nicht oder nur mit manueller Hilfe auswerten, da der Segmentierungsansatz hier nicht immer vollständig stabil ist.

Bei den erfolgreich ausgewerteten Sequenzen ermöglicht die Visualisierung der Herzklappenbewegungen durch Kardiovibrogramme eine kompakte Darstellung des Schwingungsverhaltens in einem einzigen Bild. Somit müssen zur Bewertung nicht mehrere tausend Einzelbilder betrachtet und bewertet werden. Die Helligkeitsänderungen in Abb. 2 zwischen den Kommissurlinien entlang der Zeitachse zeigen deutlich das Öffnungs- und Verschlussverhalten der Herzklappen. Symmetrien und Auffälligkeiten im Bewegungsablauf lassen sich somit einfach erkennen.

4 Diskussion

Wie zu erwarten, hängen die Ergebnisse stark von der Aufnahmequalität ab. Der kritische Teil des Verfahrens ist hierbei insbesondere die Segmentierung der Öffnungsfläche, die direkten Einfluss auf die nachgestellte Visualisierung hat. Die schwierige Aufnahmesituation und geringer Kontrast zwischen Gewebe und Öffnungsfläche machen eine vollautomatische Segmentierung zur Herausforderung. Durch die Hervorhebung der Kanten als Grenzen des Regionenwachstums

Abb. 2. Kardiovibrogramm einer Herzklappenschwingung und Auswirkungen der Segmentierung. (1) Kommissurlinien, (2) Übersegmentierung, (3) Untersegmentierung

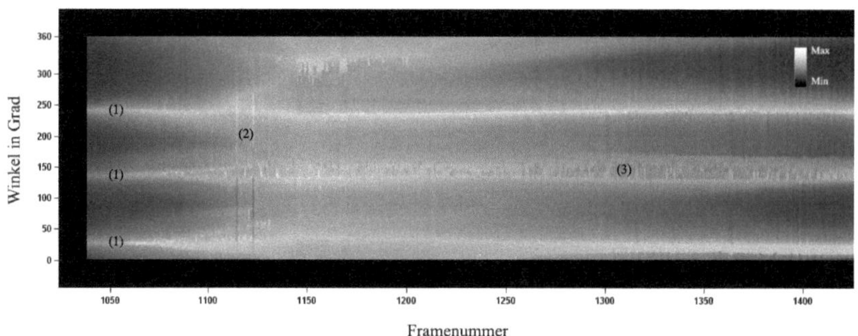

können Übersegmentierungen weitgehend vermieden werden. Bei weit geöffneten Klappen werden zum Teil tieferliegende Strukturen, wie etwa die Innenwand der Herzkammer sichtbar. Dies kann zu einer Untersegmentierung der Öffnungsfläche führen. Dies zeigt sich auch in den daraus resultierenden Kardiovibrogrammen wie Abb. 2 zeigt. Für qualitativ hochwertige Aufnahmen sind aber weitgehend automatisierte Segmentierungen und entsprechende Visualisierungen möglich und auch trotz kleinerer Fehler im Segmentierungsverlauf lässt sich das Schwingungsverhalten abbilden. Die neuartige und bisher wenig erforschte Operations- und Aufnahmemodalität erfordert noch Erfahrung um hochwertige Aufnahmen in größerer Anzahl zu erzeugen. Im Vergleich der ersten Aufnahmen zeigt sich jedoch, dass mit steigender Erfahrung die Aufnahmequalität steigt und somit auch die Auswertungen stabiler werden.

Literaturverzeichnis

1. Jamieson W, et al. Re-operation for bioprosthetic aortic valve structural failure-risk assessment. Eur J Cardiothorac Surg. 2003;24:873–8.
2. Tarantini G, et al. Aortic valve replacement in severe aortic stenosis with left ventricular dysfunction: Determinants of cardiac mortality and ventricular function recovery. Eur J Cardiothorac Surg. 2003;24:879–85.
3. Hahn T, et al. Automatic in-vitro orifice area determination and fluttering analysis for tricuspid heart valves. Proc BVM. 2006; p. 21–5.
4. Wittenberg T, et al. High-Speed-Camera recordings and image sequence analysis of moving heart-valves: Experiments and first results. In: Adv Med Engineer. vol. 114; 2007. p. 169–74.
5. Condurache P, et al. Automatic measuring of quality criteria for heart valves. Proc SPIE. 2007;6512:2Q1–2Q11.
6. Doellinger M, et al. Phonovibrography: The fingerprint of vocal fold vibrations. Proc IEEE ICASSP. 2007; p. I381–4.
7. Paulus D, Hornegger J. Applied Pattern Recognition. Viehweg & Sohn; 2003.
8. Otsu N. A threshold selection method from gray-level histograms. IEEE Trans Syst Man Cybern. 1979;9(1):62–6.

Kontinuierliche Wanddickenbestimmung und Visualisierung des linken Herzventrikels

Lars Dornheim, Peter Hahn, Steffen Oeltze, Bernhard Preim, Klaus D. Tönnies

Institut für Simulation und Graphik, Otto-von-Guericke-Universität Magdeburg
lars@isg.cs.uni-magdeburg.de

Kurzfassung. Zur Bestimmung von Defekten in der Herztätigkeit kann die Veränderung der Wanddicke des linken Ventrikels in zeitlichen MRT-Aufnahmesequenzen gemessen werden. Derzeit werden für diese Bestimmung im allgemeinen nur die aufwändig manuell erstellte Segmentierungen der Endsystole und Enddiastole benutzt. Wir stellen ein bis auf die Startpunktinitialisierung automatisches Verfahren zur Bestimmung der Wanddicke des linken Ventrikels und ihrer Veränderung vor, das auf einer vollständigen Segmentierung der Herzwand in allen Zeitschritten durch ein dynamisches dreidimensionales Formmodell (Stabiles Feder-Masse-Modell) basiert. Dieses Modell nutzt bei der Segmentierung neben der Grauwertinformation eines Zeitschrittes auch die Segmentierungen der anderen Zeitschritte und ist so aufgebaut, dass die Wanddicken direkt gemessen und visualisiert werden können. Auf diese Weise werden die lokalen Wanddickenextrema über den gesamten Aufnahmezeitraum detektiert, auch wenn sie nicht in die Endsystole bzw. -diastole fallen. Das Verfahren wurde auf sechs 4D-Kardio-MRT-Datensätzen evaluiert und stellte sich als sehr robust bzgl. der einzig nötigen Interaktion heraus.

1 Einleitung

Lokale Defekte des Herzmuskels (Myokard) in Folge koronarer Herzerkrankung verursachen Einschränkungen der Leistungsfähigkeit des Herzens. Durch Perfusionsanalyse von Kardio-MRT-Aufnahmen kann das geschädigte Gewebe sichtbar gemacht werden. Für die Beurteilung der Auswirkungen auf die verbliebene Kontraktionsfähigkeit des Myokards ist jedoch eine funktionelle Analyse notwendig. Neben der Bestimmung globaler Funktionsparameter (Schlagvolumen, Auswurffraktion) konzentriert sich ein wesentlicher Teil aktueller Forschung auf die Analyse von Bewegungs- und Deformationsparametern wie Wanddickenveränderung und Wandbewegung des Myokards.

Derzeit findet die überwiegende Zahl klinischer Untersuchungen auf der Basis manuell erzeugter Segmentierungen statt. Bedingt durch den dadurch entstehenden hohen Arbeitsaufwand, werden zur Bestimmung der Wanddickenveränderungen daher oft nur die Endsystole und -diastole betrachtet, obwohl in den zeitlichen MRT-Daten ein vollständiger Herzzyklus vorhanden ist. Das hierfür am häufigsten [1] eingesetzte Verfahren ist die Centerline-Methode [2].

Eine Reihe existierender Arbeiten setzt sich mit der funktionellen Analyse und Modellierung des Myokards auseinander. Dabei liegt der Schwerpunkt der Arbeiten auf der Modellierung und Visualisierung. Viele Arbeiten benötigen als Eingabe weiterhin eine auf manueller Abgrenzung oder einfachen bildbasierten Verfahren beruhende Segmentierung (z. B. Schwellenwertverfahren). So stellen Euseman et al. [3] die Analyse funktionaler Parameter mittels eines deformierbaren Modells vor, welches eine manuelle Segmentierung des gesamten Herzzyklus vorraussetzt. Bardinet et al. [4] nutzen Superquadriken, um durch Schwellenwertverfahren aus einer CT-Sequenz gewonnene Segmentierungen des Myokards zu modellieren. Montagnat et al. [5] setzen Simplex-Meshes zur 4D-Segmentierung des linken Ventrikels in MRT-Daten ein. Interessant ist, dass hier neben Raum- auch Zeitbedingungen einfließen. Die Initialisierung ist jedoch sehr aufwändig und die resultierenden Segmentierungen scheinen zu grob für eine Wanddickenbestimmung. Wesarg et al. [6] stellen ein automatisches Verfahren zur Bestimmung von Wanddickenveränderung und Wandbewegung vor, welches auf einer Kette bildbasierter Verfahren und Radialstrahlen basiert und bis auf eine Glattheitsbedingung kein weiteres Modellwissen nutzt. Kuehnel et al. [7] verwenden ein modifiziertes Region-Growing zur Segmentierung des linken Ventrikelvolumens sowie ein Active-Shape-Model zur Segmentierung des Myokards.

2 Material und Methoden

In dieser Arbeit wird ein Stabiles Feder-Masse-Modell (SMSM) [8] des linken Herzventrikels, nach erfolgter manueller Initialisierung im ersten Zeitpunkt in jedem weiteren Zeitpunkt dynamisch und automatisch an die Bilddaten angepasst, um so die Wanddicke des linken Ventrikels zu jedem Zeitpunkt berechnen zu können.

Dieses Modell ist ein allgemeines, nicht patienten-spezifisches Modell. Es wurde aus einem durchschnittlichen, patienten-spezifischen Modell erstellt, dessen individuelle Merkmale durch deutliche Glättungen entfernt wurden. Es besteht

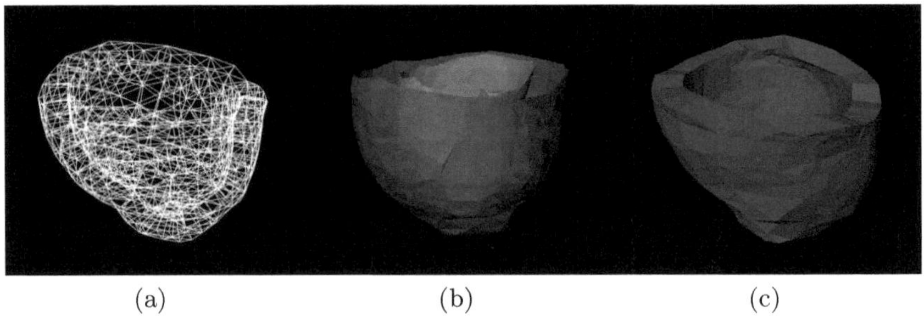

(a) (b) (c)

Abb. 1. (a): verwendetes stabiles Feder-Masse-Modell. (b), (c): Farbkodierung der Wanddickenveränderung auf der äußeren bzw. der gesamten Modelloberfläche (rot: hohe / blau: geringe Wanddickenvariabilität)

Tabelle 1. Segmentierungsgüte der modellbasierten Segmentierungen im Vegleich zum Goldstandard

Datensatz	1	2	3	4	5	6
mittlere Oberflächendistanz in mm (Systole)	2.80	2.00	2.40	1.90	4.10	2.20
Tanimoto-Koeffizient (Systole)	0.46	0.61	0.53	0.66	0.39	0.63
mittlere Oberflächendistanz in mm (Diastole)	1.60	1.80	2.30	1.90	2.00	1.80
Tanimoto-Koeffizient (Diastole)	0.60	0.54	0.44	0.58	0.44	0.57

aus zwei miteinander vernetzten Masse-Schichten, welche die innere und die äußere Grenze der Herzwand modellieren (Abb. 1). Diese Massen sind mit Datensensoren assoziiert, die die Masse-Schichten zu Kanten im Bilddatensatz ziehen. Dabei werden nur Kanten im Datensatz betrachtet, deren Normalenrichtung denen im Modell ähnlich sind. Weitere Massen liegen innerhalb der modellierten Herzwand und im Inneren des modellierten Ventrikels, deren assozierte Sensoren sie zu den entsprechenden, an ihren Positionen im Modell erwarteten Intensitäten (niedrige Intensitäten innerhalb der Herzwand und hohe im Ventrikelinneren) streben lassen.

Beide Masse-Schichten bestehen aus feinen, topologisch äquivalenten Dreiecksnetzen, deren jeweils korrespondierenden Massen durch Federn direkt verbunden sind. Dadurch kann die Wanddicke für jeden Zeitpunkt direkt aus dem angepaßten Modell abgelesen werden.

Die Segmentierung erfolgt durch sukzessive Modellsimulation auf den 3D-Datensätzen aller Zeitschritte. Im ersten Zeitpunkt muss das Ventrikelmodell durch einen Mausklick grob auf dem linken Ventrikel im Datensatz platziert werden. Danach wird das Modell vollautomatisch angepasst, bis es konvergiert. Auf Grund der zeitlichen Kohärenz der Bilder kann das Modell im nächsten Zeitschritt von der Position und mit der Form starten, die es bei der Konvergenz im vorigen Zeitschritt hatte, was erneute Initialisierungen unnötig macht.

Nach der vollständigen Segmentierungen aller Zeitschritte kann aus den Längen der die beiden Masse-Schichten verbindenden Federn direkt die Dicke verschiedener Wandstellen zu jedem Zeitpunkt abgelesen werden. Die Segmentierung kann schichtweise, dreidimensional oder über die Zeit visualisiert werden. Zudem wird die Variabilität der Wanddicke w (siehe Gleichung (1)) farbkodiert auf der Ventrikelmodelloberfläche oder im Bulls-Eye-Plot der American Heart Association dargestellt (Abb. 1(b),(c)). Des Weiteren ist die dynamische Darstellung der Ventrikelbewegung möglich.

$$v = \frac{w_{max} - w_{min}}{w_{min}} \tag{1}$$

3 Ergebnisse

Das Verfahren wurde auf sechs uns zur Verfügung stehenden 4D-Kardio-MRT-Datensätzen evaluiert, die jeweils einen kompletten Herzzyklus beinhalten. Die Datensätze haben ein Auflösung von $208 \times 256 \times 10 \times 30$ Voxel bei einer Voxelgröße

Tabelle 2. minimale, durchschnittliche und maximale Wanddickenvariabilität v der modellbasierten und manuellen Segmentierungen

Datensatz	1	2	3	4	5	6
minimal (modell-basiert)	0.04	0.02	0.03	0.03	0.10	0.07
durchschnittlich (modell-basiert)	0.26	0.43	0.57	0.41	0.67	0.50
maximal (modell-basiert)	0.40	0.80	1.06	1.00	1.33	1.03
minimal (manuell)	0.00	0.00	0.00	0.00	0.00	0.00
durchschnittlich (manuell)	0.46	0.62	0.69	0.78	0.54	0.92
maximal (manuell)	1.30	3.30	2.63	2.94	1.89	2.91

von 1,4 mm×1,4 mm×6,0 mm in Zeitschritten von ca. 0.045 sec gemessen. Für die Modellanpassung wurden die Datensätze auf isotrope Voxel (Kantenlänge 1,4 mm) reformatiert und durch anisotrope Diffusion geglättet.

Die Modelle wurden jeweils durch einen Mausklick ungefähr in der Mitte des linken Ventrikels initialisiert. Die automatische Segmentierung erfolgte dann jeweils in ca. 6,5 Minuten auf einem Standard-PC (P4, 3.2 GHz, 1 GB RAM).

Als Goldstandard lagen manuelle Segmentierungen der Endsystole bzw. Enddiastole des linken Ventrikels vor, die von einem Experten angefertigt wurden. Für diese Zeitpunkte wurde die Segmentierungsgüte ermittelt. Tab. 1 zeigt die Tanimoto-Koeffizienten [9] und mittleren Oberflächendistanzen für die 6 vorhandenen Datensätze. Tab. 2 gibt einen Überblick über die gemessenen Wanddickenvariabilitäten v in den modellbasierten bzw. manuellen Segmentierungen.

Die Segmentierung des linken Ventrikels mit dem vorgestellten Stabilen Feder-Masse-Modell war sehr robust gegenüber seiner Startplatzierung. Verschiedenste Startpunkte des Modells innerhalb des Ventrikelinneren führten stets zu einer immer ähnlichen und guten Segmentierung (siehe Abb. 2). Grund für dieses Verhalten sind die über das gesamte Volumen verteilten Intensitätssensoren des Modells, die schon bei einer geringen Startüberlappung das Modell zielstrebig an die richtige Position steuern, bevor die Kantenanpassung an die Zielstruktur durch die Kantensensoren erfolgt. Lediglich die Abgrenzung der äußeren Ventrikelwandbegrenzung war in einigen Fällen auf Grund der unklaren Kanteninformation einiger Bereiche problematisch.

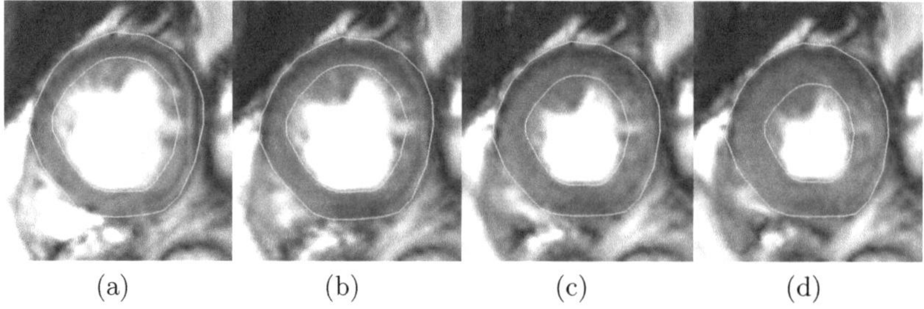

(a) (b) (c) (d)

Abb. 2. erfolgreiche Segmentierung des linken Ventrikels mit einem Stabilen Feder-Masse-Modell (Ausschnitte einer Zeitsequenz von der Diastole (a) zur Systole (d))

4 Diskussion

Die Ergebnisse aus Abschnitt 3 zeigen, dass sowohl die Segmentierungen, aber auch die Wanddickenvariabilitäten im Bereich der Goldstandards liegen. Weiterhin ist in der zeitlichen Visualisierung des angepassten Ventrikelmodells deutlich die sich drehend zusammenziehende Bewegung des linken Ventrikels zu sehen. Zukünftig gilt es zu untersuchen, in wie weit die Bildwertkorrespondenz unseres Modells mit den einzelnen Organregionen auch über die Zeit erhalten bleibt (z. B. durch Nutzung getagter MRT-Aufnahmen) und somit auch eine Analyse der Drehbewegung des Myokards zulässt.

Mit Hilfe unserer Ergebnisse können pathologische Veränderungen in der Herzbewegung deutlicher als bisher (z. B. in Volume-Rendering-Sequenzen) aufgespürt werden. Zudem vermitteln die farbkodierten dreidimensionalen Modelldarstellungen einen klaren Eindruck über die geschädigten Ventrikelwandregionen, die zum Teil deutlich über die eigentliche, in der Perfusionsaufnahme zu sehende Infarktnarbe hinausgehen und so gezielter therapiert werden können.

Zusammenfassend ermöglicht die vorgestellte halbautomatische Ventrikel-Segmentierung mit einem SMSM eine sehr robuste und hinreichend genaue Möglichkeit zur Messung und Visualisierung der Wanddickenvariabilität und Ventrikelbewegung in Funktions-MRT-Bildern, die damit für den klinischen Alltag sehr geeignet ist. Zusammen mit dem Wissen über die Infarktnarbe aus Perfusionsaufnahmen, können hier nicht zuletzt geschädigte, aber therapierbare Regionen des linken Herzventrikels sehr effizient und deutlich ausgemacht werden.

Literaturverzeichnis

1. Frangi AF, Niessen WJ, Viergever MA. Three-dimensional modeling for functional analysis of cardiac images, a review. IEEE Trans Med Imaging. 2001;20(1):2–5.
2. Sheehan FH, Bolson EL, Dodge HT, et al. Advantages and applications of the centerline method for characterizing regional ventricular function. Circulation. 1986;74:293–305.
3. Eusemann CD, Ritman EL, Bellemann ME, et al. Parametric display of myocardial function. Comput Med Imaging Graph. 2001;25(6):483–93.
4. Bardinet E, Cohen LD, Ayache N. Tracking and motion analysis of the left ventricle with deformable superquadrics. Med Image Anal. 1996;1(12):129–49.
5. Montagnat J, Delingette H. Space and time shape constrained deformable surfaces for 4D medical image segmentation. Proc MICCAI. 2000.
6. Wesarg S, Nowak S. An automated 4D approach for left ventricular assessment in clinical cine MR images. In: Hochberger C, editor. Informatik 2006. Informatik für Menschen. vol. 1. Gesellschaft für Informatik; 2006. p. 483–90.
7. Kuehnel C, Hennemuth A, Boskamp T, et al. New software assistants for cardiovascular diagnosis. Proc GI Annual Conference. 2006; p. 491–8.
8. Dornheim L, Tönnies KD, Dornheim J. Stable dynamic 3D shape models. In: Proc ICIP; 2005.
9. Heimann T, Thorn M, Kunert T, et al. Empirische Vergleichsmaße für die Evaluation von Segmentierungsergebnissen. Proc BVM. 2004; p. 165–9.

Approximation dreidimensionaler Oberflächenmodelle der Lippen-Kiefer-Gaumen-Region durch aktive Polygonnetze

Frank Weichert[1], Christoph Ewerlin[1], Christian Büttner[1], Ali Shamaa[2], Constantin Landes[3], Roland Linder[4], Mathias Wagner[5]

[1]Lehrstuhl für graphische Systeme, Technische Universität Dortmund
[2]Department of Oral Biology, Al Minia University, Ägypten
[3]Kiefer- und Plastische Gesichtschirurgie, Universitätsklinikum Frankfurt
[4]Institut für Medizinische Informatik, Universität zu Lübeck
[5]Institut für Allgemeine und Spezielle Pathologie, Universität des Saarlandes
`frank.weichert@udo.edu`

Kurzfassung. In dieser Arbeit wird ein Verfahren zur Rekonstruktion eines dreidimensionalen Oberflächenmodells aus Serienschnitten vorgestellt, die sich von Lippen-Kiefer-Gaumenspalten (kurz LKG) ableiten und insbesondere die in der chirurgischen Behandlung relevanten medizinischen Strukturen berücksichtigen. Die Intention ist, ein aktives Polygonnetz (deformierbares Oberflächennetz) zur Rekonstruktion der Struktur zu verwenden. Initial wird ein Netzprototyp als grobe Approximation der Struktur erstellt und dann mithilfe eines Gradient Vector Flow (GVF)-Kraftfeldes deformiert. Inhärenter Aspekt der Deformation ist die Beachtung eines resultierenden überschneidungsfreien Oberflächennetzes. Die rekonstruierte Oberfläche eignet sich aufgrund ausgezeichneter Eigenschaften als Eingabe für eine Kräftesimulation mittels Finite-Elemente-Methoden.

1 Einleitung

Lippen-Kiefer-Gaumenspalten sind eine Fehlbildung bei Neugeborenen, die durch unvollständige oder fehlerhafte Verschmelzungen von Gesichtswülsten während der Embryonalentwicklung entstehen. Neben funktionellen Einschränkungen fühlen sich die Betroffenen auch durch das Stigma der Fehlbildung im Gesicht beeinträchtigt. Daher ist eine operative Intervention unumgänglich, wobei aber das genaue Behandlungskonzept noch nicht abschließend geklärt ist [1]. Daher ist es das Ziel dieser Arbeit, die Auswirkungen unterschiedlicher Operationsansätze über eine virtuelle Operationsplanung mittels Kräftesimulation durch Finite-Elemente-Methoden miteinander zu vergleichen. Der Grundtenor der Umsetzung ist die Erstellung eines Volumenmodells (z.B. aus Tetraedern) der an der LKG-Problematik beteiligten Strukturen [2]. Aufgrund unterschiedlicher Artefakte in den Datensätzen, beispielsweise inhärenter Fehler bei der Gewebeaufbereitung oder Segmentierungsfehler, muss der Ansatz robust genug sein, diese Probleme zu handhaben. Daher wird dieses mit einem aktiven Oberflächennetz realisiert, welches nachfolgend in ein FE-konformes Volumennetz überführt wird. Alternative Rekonstruktionsansätze wie Alpha Shapes oder MPUs (Multi-Level Partition of Unity Implicits) wären prinzipiell auch möglich, sie genügen aber nicht den gestellten Anforderungen (vgl. Kapitel 4). Bei fast allen Strukturen treten Selbstüberschneidungen vor allem dadurch auf, dass Verzweigungen in der Segmentierung nicht berücksichtigt werden. Dieses Problem wird in dieser Arbeit mithilfe eines neuen Rekonstruktionsansatzes gelöst.

2 Material und Methoden

Der vorgestellte Rekonstruktionsansatz gliedert sich in verschiedene Teilaspekte auf, die im Folgenden beschrieben werden. Initial wird aus den von Medizinern segmentierten Daten ein Kraftfeld generiert, damit sich ein aktives Polygonnetz während der Deformation an die segmentierten Strukturen anpassen kann. Ausgangspunkt der Deformation ist ein Netzprototyp, welcher dieselbe Topologie wie die zu approximierende Struktur aufweist. Dieser kann nachfolgend mithilfe eines aktiven Oberflächenmodells deformiert werden, bis er sich an die segmentierte Struktur anpasst.

2.1 Feldgenerierung

Initialer Aspekt der Generierung des approximierenden Netzes ist die Erzeugung einer äußeren Kraft für die Deformation aus den Segmentierungsinformationen. Erstellt wird ein Kraftfeld $\mathbf{v}_F : \mathbb{R}^3 \rightarrow \mathbb{R}^3$, welches jedem Punkt $\mathbf{x} = (x, y, z)$ einen Kraftvektor $\mathbf{v}_F(\mathbf{x})$ zuordnet. Die besondere Herausforderung der Feldgenerierung besteht darin, auch zwischen den Schichten ein sinnvolles Feld zu interpolieren. Erreicht wird diese Anforderung durch die Verwendung eines GVF-Feldes $\mathbf{v}_F : \mathbb{R}^3 \rightarrow \mathbb{R}^3$, $\mathbf{v}_F(\mathbf{x}) = (u(\mathbf{x}), v(\mathbf{x}), w(\mathbf{x}))$, definiert als das Minimum des Funktionals

$$\mathcal{E}(\mathbf{v}_F) = \int \mu(|\nabla u|^2 + |\nabla v|^2 + |\nabla w|^2) + |\nabla P|^2 |\mathbf{v}_F - \nabla P|^2 d\mathbf{x} \qquad (1)$$

wobei P eine berechnete Potentialfunktion ist [3].

2.2 Prototypgenerierung

Für die Approximation einer segmentierten Struktur durch Deformation ist ein Netzprototyp notwendig, der bereits möglichst viele der aus der Segmentierung bekannten Informationen (Topologie eines Segments) berücksichtigt. Gewährleistet wird dieses durch den so genannten k-DOP-Prototyp (Discrete Oriented Polytopes) [4]. Dazu ist zunächst ein Verbindungsgraph aus der Segmentierung zu erstellen, der die Verbindungsinformationen (Muskeltopologie) des Segments verwertet. Die Polygone eines Segments werden durch einfache, konvexe Geometrien ersetzt und die DOPs mithilfe fester Regeln miteinander verbunden, wie es sich aus dem Verbindungsgraphen ergibt.

2.3 Deformation

Die Deformation eines erzeugten Netzprototypen beruht auf dem Prinzip eines deformierbaren Modells gemäß Park et al. [5], aber u.a. zusätzlich verbessert um die Behandlung von Selbstüberschneidungen und der Verwendung eines GVF-Feldes als äußere Kraft (Abb. 1). Zuerst wird der Deformationsschritt durchgeführt, in dem die Positionen der Knoten im Dreiecksnetz angepasst werden. Die eigentliche Dynamik der Knoten ist durch eine diskretisierte Formulierung des Kräftegleichgewichts für deformierbare Modelle gegeben. Jedem Knoten $i \in V$ im Dreiecksnetz ist eine Position $\mathbf{x}_i \in \mathbb{R}^3$, ein Geschwindigkeitsvektor $\mathbf{v}_i = d\mathbf{x}_i/dt \in \mathbb{R}^3$ und ein Beschleunigungsvektor $\mathbf{a}_i = d^2\mathbf{x}_i/dt^2 \in \mathbb{R}^3$ zugeordnet. Alle Knoten besitzen die gleiche Masse $m \in \mathbb{R}$ und den gleichen Dämpfungskoeffizienten $\gamma \in [0,1]$, woraus sich folgende diskretisierte Form der Gleichgewichtsbedingung ergibt:

$$m\mathbf{a}_i + \gamma\mathbf{v}_i = \mathbf{F}_{\text{int},i} + \mathbf{F}_{\text{ext},i} \tag{2}$$

$\mathbf{F}_{\text{int},i} \in \mathbb{R}^3$ und $\mathbf{F}_{\text{ext},i} \in \mathbb{R}^3$ sind die inneren bzw. äußeren Kräfte, die auf den Knoten i wirken. Zu einem Zeitpunkt t werden die momentan auf den Knoten i wirkenden Kräfte $\mathbf{F}_{\text{int},i}(t)$ und $\mathbf{F}_{\text{ext},i}(t)$ berechnet - daraus ergibt sich die momentane Beschleunigung $\mathbf{a}_i(t)$. Folglich können die Geschwindigkeit $\mathbf{v}_i(t+step_t)$ und die Position $\mathbf{x}_i(t+step_t)$ zum Zeitpunkt $t+step_t$ berechnet werden. Die auf einen Knoten i wirkende innere Kraft $\mathbf{F}_{\text{int},i}$ setzt sich aus einer Spannungskraft $\mathbf{F}_{\text{stretch,i}}$ und einer Krümmungskraft $\mathbf{F}_{\text{bend},i}$ zusammen, die durch zwei Parameter w_{stretch} und w_{bend} gewichtet werden:

$$\mathbf{F}_{\text{int},i} = w_{\text{stretch}}\mathbf{F}_{\text{stretch},i} + w_{\text{bend}}\mathbf{F}_{\text{bend},i} \tag{3}$$

Hierbei kontrolliert die Spannungskraft $\mathbf{F}_{\text{stretch},i}$ die Abstände des Knotens i zu seinen Nachbarknoten $\mathbf{N}(i)$, wobei alle Verbindungskanten als elastische Federn modelliert werden. Zusätzlich verhindert die Krümmungskraft $\mathbf{F}_{\text{bend},i}$ eine zu starke Krümmung der Netzoberfläche. Die bei der Deformation auf einen Knoten i wirkende äußere Kraft $\mathbf{F}_{\text{ext},i}$ wird durch das GVF-Feld generiert. Da

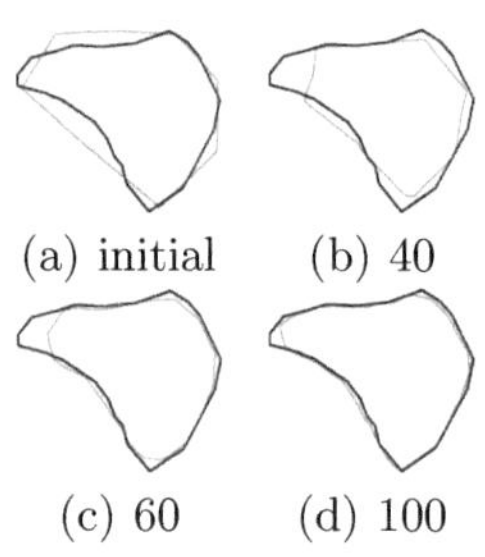

(a) initial (b) 40 (c) 60 (d) 100

Abb. 1. Schnittpolygon bei unterschiedlichen Deformationsschritten

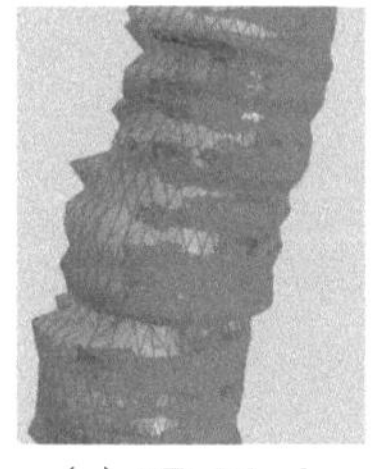

(a) 3D-Mesh

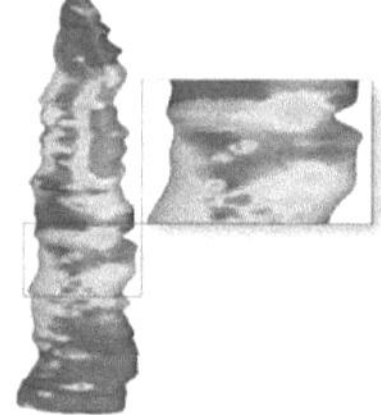

(b) FE-Simulation

Abb. 2. Dreidimensionale Approximation der anatomischen Strukturen, hier *muskulus masseter* und farbliche Darstellung der von-Mises Spannungen

nach jedem Deformationsschritt Selbstüberschneidungen im Dreiecksnetz auftreten können, müssen diese im Hinblick auf ein überschneidungsfreies Dreiecksnetz behoben werden. Die Identifizierung möglicher Kollisionspaare geschieht hierbei mehrstufig. Zunächst werden räumlich nah beieinander liegende Dreieckspaare durch das sehr effiziente Spatial Hashing - Verfahren identifiziert und über einen Schnitttest die Axis Aligned Bounding Boxes (AABBs) überprüft. Weitere Teilaspekte der Deformation sind die globale Verfeinerung, die lokale Neuvernetzung und die Verschmelzung kurzer Kanten in der ersten Phase der Neuvernetzung.

3 Ergebnisse

Resultierend steht eine Approximation der gewünschten anatomischen Struktur zur Verfügung (Abb. 2), die sowohl den medizinischen Anforderungen gerecht wird, aber auch robust gegenüber Segmentierungsfehlern. Abbildung 1 zeigt hierzu den Verlauf der Deformation anhand eines ausgewählten Polygons (in 2D). Das segmentierte Polygon ist schwarz visualisiert, das jeweilige Schnittpolygon nach einer bestimmten Anzahl von Iterationen rot. Dargestellt ist, dass die Abweichung von der ursprünglichen Segmentierung im Verlauf der Deformation immer geringer wird — dieses wird im Folgenden quantitativ näher untersucht. Ein entscheidender Qualitätsfaktor ist die Flächendifferenz über den Verlauf der Deformation (Abb. 3). Erkennbar ist, dass sich die Flächendifferenz der Schnittpolygone zu den segmentierten Polygonen im Verlauf der Deformation deutlich verkleinert und zum Ende der Deformation nach 100 Iterationen nur noch 2.4 Prozent beträgt. Neben der Approximationsqualität ist auch die Performanz relevant (Abb. 4). Für die 50 Iterationen der ersten Phase werden 8.45 Sekunden benötigt, nach der ersten globalen Neuvernetzung für die 35 Iterationen der zweiten Phase der Deformation 65.23 Sekunden und für die letzten 15 Iterationen nach der zweiten globalen Neuvernetzung 91.84 Sekunden, bzw. 55.48 Prozent der gesamten Zeit. Im Durchschnitt entspricht dies 6.12 Sekunden je Iteration. Die für die Kräfteberechnung benötigte Zeit ist mit einem Anteil von 0.33 Prozent an der Gesamtzeit vernachlässigbar klein, ebenso die Neuvernetzung (1.81 Prozent). Ein Zeitanteil von über 95 Prozent entfällt hingegen auf die Kollisionserkennung und die Kollisionsbehandlung. Auf einem AMD Athlon 3700+ Prozessor mit 2GB RAM benötigt die Approximation eines durchschnittlichen Muskels ca. 160 Sekunden.

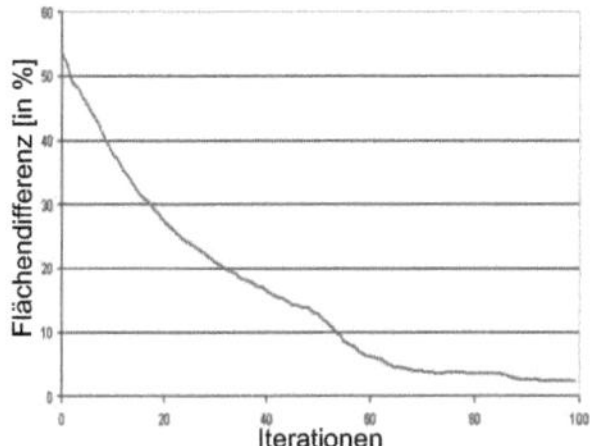

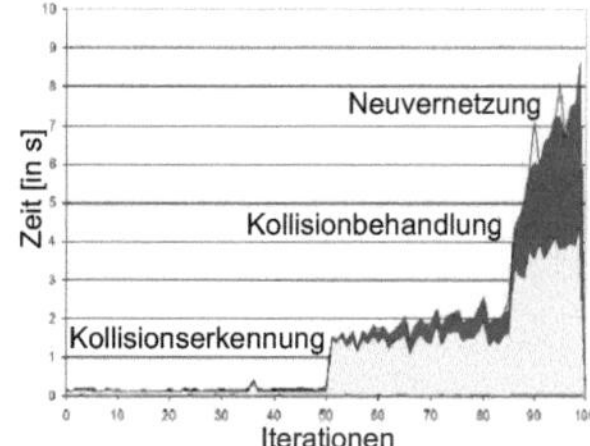

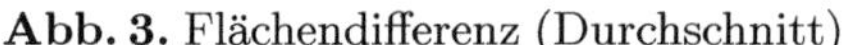

Abb. 3. Flächendifferenz (Durchschnitt)

Abb. 4. Benötigte Zeit pro Iteration

Abb. 5. Rekonstruktionsansätze im direkten Vergleich

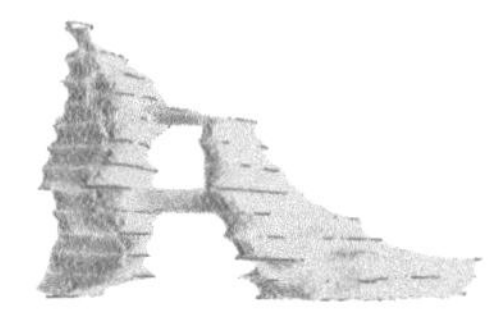
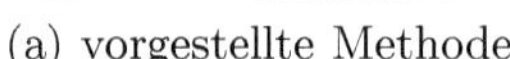
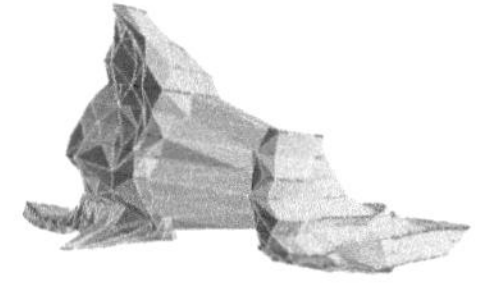
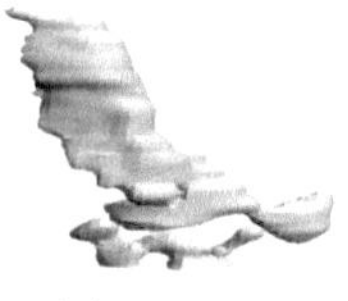

(a) vorgestellte Methode (b) *AlphaShapes* (c) *MPUs*

4 Diskussion

Die rekonstruierte Oberfläche zeigt insgesamt nur eine geringe Abweichung zu der realen Oberfläche des Segments. Zum Vergleich wird die Rekonstruktion des *musculus veli palatini* in Abbildung 5 den Ergebnissen der Rekonstruktion mit *AlphaShapes* und *MPUs* gegenüber gestellt. Beide Verfahren basieren ausschließlich auf der Rekonstruktion von Punktwolken und beziehen die Verbindungen zwischen den Polygonen nicht in ihre Berechnung ein. Aus diesem Grund können die beiden Verzweigungen nicht akkurat rekonstruiert werden und die Verfahren eignen sich nicht für die notwendige Rekonstruktion. Im Gegensatz zu anderen Prototypen wird bei der Generierung des DOP-Prototypen die Verbindungsinformationen (Topologie) des Segments mit einbezogen. Kollisionen werden zudem nach jedem Deformationsschritt mithilfe von Spatial Hashing effizient erkannt und durch eine rekursive Kollisionsbehandlung aufgelöst. Das rekonstruierte Oberflächennetz ist dadurch garantiert überschneidungsfrei. Insgesamt lässt sich festhalten, dass das vorgestellte Verfahren zur Oberflächenrekonstruktion das Verarbeitungsschema für LKG-Daten auf dem Weg zu einer virtuellen OP-Simulation um eine wichtige Stufe erweitert. Durch die überschneidungsfreie Oberflächenrekonstruktion fast aller Segmente und der Bereitstellung eines FE-konformen Netzes ist es möglich, verschiedene Simulationsmodelle vergleichend anzuwenden. Abbildung 2(b) zeigt hierzu das Ergebnis einer Berechnung über eine farbliche Repräsentierung der von-Mises Spannungen.

Literaturverzeichnis

1. Bitter K. Chirurgische Erstbehandlung der Lippen-Kiefer-Gaumen-Spalten im Jahr 2000. Mund-, Kiefer- und Gesichtschirurgie. 2000;4(7):49–60.
2. Landes C, Weichert F, Geis P, et al. Evaluation of two 3D virtual computer reconstructions for comparison of cleft lip and palate to normal fetal microanatomy. Anat Rec A Discov Mol Cell Evol Biol. 2006;288(3):248–62.
3. Xu C. Deformable models with application to human cerebral cortex reconstruction from magnetic resonance images. John Hopkins University; 1999.
4. Klosowski JT, Held M, Mitchell JSB, et al. Efficient collision detection using bounding volume hierarchies of k-DOPs. IEEE Trans Vis Comp Graph. 1998;4(1):21–36.
5. Park JY, McInerney T, Terzopoulos D, et al. A non-self-intersecting adaptive deformable surface for complex boundary extraction from volumetric images. Comp Graph. 2001;25:421–40.

Schnelles Voxel-Resampling für DRR-Raycasting-Verfahren in der 2D/3D-Registrierung

Axel Newe[1], Richard Rascher-Friesenhausen[1,2], Heinz-Otto Peitgen[2]

[1]Hochschule Bremerhaven
[2]Mevis Research gGmbH, Bremen
axl@axelnewe.de

Kurzfassung. Das Raycasting ist ein etabliertes Verfahren zur Berechnung von Digital Rekonstruierten Röntgenbildern (DRRs), auf Basis von CT-Daten approximierten Radiographien, die vorwiegend für die 2D/3D-Registrierung und die Strahlentherapieplanung eingesetzt werden. Das Strahlresampling ist der mit Abstand langwierigste Schritt des Raycastings. Es wird ein Algorithmus vorgestellt, der diesen Vorgang auf das absolute Minimum reduziert, aber trotzdem die Berechnung von DRRs ermöglicht, die qualitativ für die meisten Anwendungen in der 2D/3D-Registrierung ausreichen.

1 Einleitung

Digital Rekonstruierte Röntgenbilder (DRRs) sind auf Basis von CT-Daten approximierte Projektionen eines dreidimensionalen CT-Volumens auf eine zweidimensionale Bildebene. Sie werden vorwiegend für die 2D/3D-Registrierung und die Strahlentherapieplanung eingesetzt. Das ursprüngliche und naivste Verfahren zur Berechnung von DRRs ist das Raycasting: die Verfolgung einer Anzahl von virtuellen Röntgenstrahlen durch einen virtuellen Patienten hindurch. Für die Ermittlung der Voxel eines CT-Datensatzes, die ein solcher Strahl durchquert (Resampling) sind verschiedene Verfahren beschrieben; besonders der Algorithmus von Siddon [1], der sich durch eine hohe Genauigkeit auszeichnet und jener von Amanatides und Woo [2], der einen Kompromiss zwischen Geschwindigkeit und Qualität darstellt, werden häufig zitiert. Mit dieser Arbeit wird ein Algorithmus vorgestellt, der die Berechnungen auf das absolute Minimum reduziert und daher sehr schnell ist. Weiterhin wird gezeigt, dass die daraus erzielte DRR-Qualität für die Anwendung in der 2D/3D-Registrierung ausreichend ist.

2 Material und Methoden

Als Plattform für die Entwicklung und den Test des im Folgenden vorgestellten Algorithmus' diente ein IBM-kompatibler PC mit 3.4-GHz-Prozessor und 2 GB Hauptspeicher. Die Implementierung erfolgte in Form eines Moduls für die von der MeVis Research GmbH (Bremen) entwickelte Rapid-Prototyping-Bildverarbeitungssoftware MeVisLab (http://www.mevislab.de).

Der entwickelte Algorithmus tastet ein Voxelvolumen schichtweise ab und sampelt nur das dem Strahl naheliegendste Voxel jeder Schicht. Dieses „Nearest Neighbour"-Prinzip ist dem Algorithmus von Bresenham [3] ähnlich, berücksichtigt jedoch alle drei Dimensionen und wird (auf zwei Dimensionen reduziert) in Abb. 1 veranschaulicht.

Gegeben sei ein zu sampelnder Strahl mit dem Startpunkt S und dem Endpunkt E in einem kartesischen Koordinatensystem. Der erste Schritt des Algorithmus' besteht in der Berechnung eines Vektors $\overrightarrow{V}$ mit den Komponenten V_x, V_y und V_z, anhand dessen im späteren Schleifendurchlauf einer Anwendung von einem Voxel zum nächsten gesprungen wird („Nachbar-Vektor"). Dieser Vektor verläuft entlang des zu sampelnden Strahls und ist dahingehend normiert, dass der Betrag der größten Komponente zu 1 wird und sich für jene Komponente ergibt, die zur Achse α mit der größten Steigung gehört.

Im abgebildeten Beispiel ist die y-Achse die maßgebende Achse, da der Strahl in y-Richtung die größte Steigung aufweist. Der Normierungsquotient n berechnet sich mit E_α als α-Komponente des Endpunkts und S_α als α-Komponente des Startpunkts wie folgt:

$$n = |E_\alpha - S_\alpha| \tag{1}$$

Dieser Normierungsquotient n entspricht gleichzeitig der Anzahl der später zu absolvierenden Schleifendurchläufe.

Die einzelnen Komponenten des Vektors $\overrightarrow{V}$ berechnen sich demnach aus

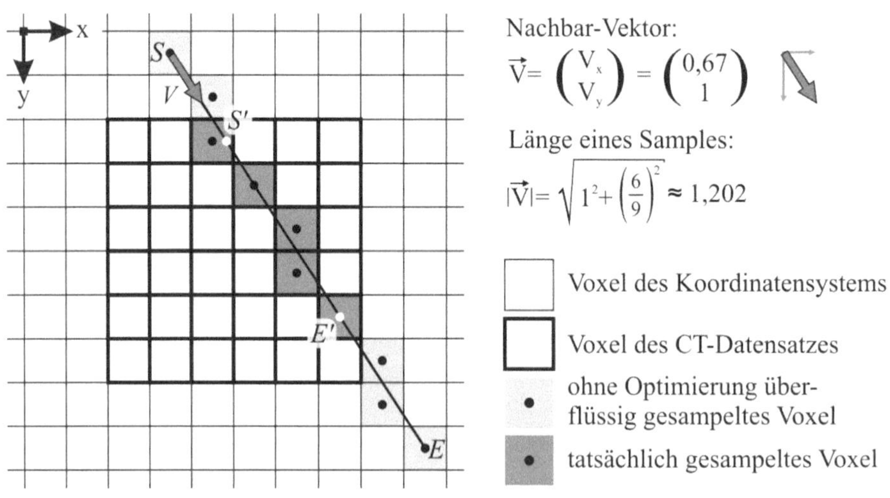

Abb. 1. 2D-Skizze zum „Nearest Neighbour"-Resampling-Algorithmus

Tabelle 1. Durchschnittliche Berechnungszeiten aus zehn Messungen für das Resampling eines Strahls nach „Nearest Neighbour"- und Siddon-Algorithmus in Abhängigkeit von Eingangsdatensatz und Projektionswinkel (Rotation um die z-Achse)

Volumendatensatz	Projektionswinkel	„Nearest Neighbour"	Siddon
Thorax-CT, 82×82×78 Voxel	0°	0,04 ms	1,93 ms
Thorax-CT, 82×82×78 Voxel	30°	0,04 ms	2,29 ms
Femur-CT, 512×512×130 Voxel	0°	0,24 ms	6,20 ms
Femur-CT, 512×512×130 Voxel	30°	0,27 ms	7,30 ms

$$V_x = \frac{E_x - S_x}{n}, V_y = \frac{E_y - S_y}{n}, V_z = \frac{E_z - S_z}{n} \in [-1, 1] \quad (2)$$

Sind alle Einzelkomponenten V_x, V_y und V_z des Nachbar-Vektors ermittelt, so wird im zweiten Schritt die Länge eines einzelnen Strahlabschnittes pro Voxelschicht aus der euklidische Länge $|\vec{V}| = \sqrt{V_x^2 + V_y^2 + V_z^2}$ des Nachbar-Vektors berechnet. Hier wird deutlich, dass bei diesem Algorithmus - im Gegensatz zum Verfahren nach Siddon - alle Strahlabschnitte (Samples) die gleiche Länge und damit die gleiche Wichtung für die Ergebnisberechnung aufweisen.

Im letzten Schritt schließlich erfolgt das eigentliche Resampling, in dem ausgehend vom Startpunkt S und mit dem Nachbar-Vektor als Zeiger auf das jeweils nächste Voxel alle Grauwerte der betroffenen Voxel des Eingangsbilds ermittelt und zusammen mit der zuvor berechneten Länge $|\vec{V}|$ gespeichert werden.

Der Algorithmus wurde in der Implementierung dahingehend optimiert, dass das Sampling nicht beim tatsächlichen Startpunkt S beginnt und beim Endpunkt E endet, sondern vom ersten im CT-Datensatz enthaltenen Voxel S' bis zum letzten enthaltenen Voxel E' läuft (mit entsprechender Anpassung von (1)).

In Pseudocode lässt sich das Resampling dann wie folgt beschreiben:

```
voxelPosition = S'
loop n times:
    sample.greyValue = getVoxelGreyValueAt(voxelPosition)
    sample.length = |V|
    store(sample)
    voxelPosition = voxelPosition + V
```

3 Ergebnisse

Der beschriebene Algorithmus wurde gemeinsam mit dem Siddon-Algorithmus in ein Bildverarbeitungsmodul für MeVisLab implementiert und sowohl hinsichtlich der Berechnungsgeschwindigkeit als auch der praktischen Qualität getestet.

Es wurde die Zeit ermittelt, die für das Resampling eines Strahls nötig ist. Hierfür wurden zwei Eingangsdatensätze (ein Thorax-CT mit 82×82×78 Voxeln und ein Femur-CT mit 512×512×130 Voxeln) mit den beiden Resampling-Methoden für zwei verschiedene Projektionswinkel (0° und 30° Rotation um die

z-Achse) getestet. Die Ergebnisse sind in Tabelle 1 aufgeführt. Es ist deutlich zu erkennen, dass das Strahlresampling nach Siddon bei diesen Tests um etwa den Faktor 25 bis 60 langsamer ist als der vorgestellte Algorithmus.

Zur Beurteilung der Qualität wurden nach beiden Verfahren berechnete DRRs in einer Applikation zur 2D/3D-Registrierung getestet; dort konnte kein bedeutender Unterschied in der Qualität des Registrierungsergebnisses festgestellt werden. In Abb. 2 sind zwei Ähnlichkeitskurven dargestellt.

4 Diskussion

Der vorgestellte „Nearest Neighbour"-Algorithmus ist sehr schnell und für die Anwendung in der 2D/3D-Registrierung ausreichend genau. Es werden alle Schichten des Voxelvolumens einer Hauptrichtung durchlaufen und durch Abtastung äquidistanter Punkte entlang eines virtuellen Strahls nur diejenigen Voxel gesampelt, deren Mittelpunkte diesem Strahl in der jeweiligen Schicht am nächsten sind. Dadurch kann die Anzahl der in einem Programm nötigen Schleifendurchläufe auf das absolute Minimum (die Anzahl der betroffenen Voxelschichten) beschränkt werden.

Es gehen jedoch - im Gegensatz zu den Verfahren nach Siddon oder Amanatides und Woo, die jedes durchquerte Voxel berücksichtigen - Informationen verloren. Im ungünstigsten Fall (d.h. bei isotropen Voxeln und einem Projektionswinkel von 45°) kann diese Ungenauigkeit bei annähernd 50% liegen. Dieses auf den ersten Blick erhebliche Problem relativiert sich aber, wenn man berücksichtigt, dass die benachbarten Voxel eines CT-Datensatzes nur selten sehr große Unterschiede in den Grauwerten aufweisen. Selbst starke Kontraste in der Röntgendichte (beispielsweise am Übergang von Weichteil- zu Knochengewebe) ergeben sich technisch bedingt kaum von einem Voxel zum nächsten, sondern sind in der Regel über einige Voxelnachbarn verteilt. Dadurch wird der nachteilige Effekt des ungenauen Grauwert-Resamplings deutlich abgeschwächt. Weiterhin

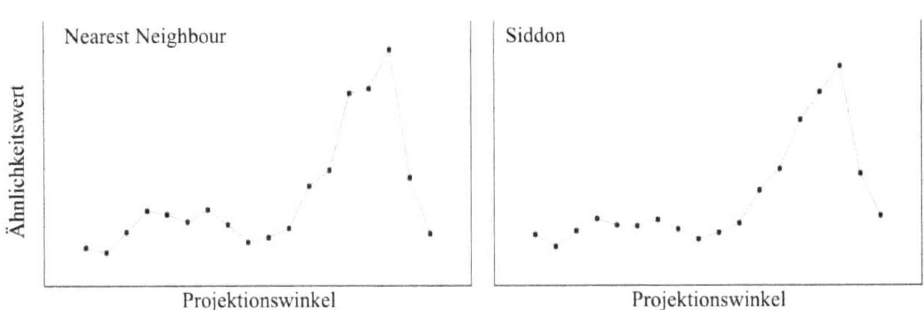

Abb. 2. Kurven der Ähnlichkeitswerte (Mutual Information) aus einer Applikation zur 2D/3D-Registrierung. Links für DRRs, die mittels „Nearest Neighbour" berechnet wurden, rechts für DRRs, die auf dem Siddon-Algorithmus basieren. Das Registrierungsergebnis (höchster Wert) ist für beide Verfahren das gleiche; auch die Verläufe der Kurven sind sehr ähnlich

Abb. 3. Vergleich eines mit dem beschriebenen „Nearest Neighbour"-Algorithmus erzeugten DRRs mit einem auf dem Siddon-Algorithmus basierenden DRR bei dem für den „Nearest Neighbour"-Algorithmus ungünstigsten Fall eines Projektionswinkel von 45° Rotation um die z-Achse des Eingangsbilds. Das Siddon-Bild zeichnet sich durch feinere Strukturierung und stärkeren Kontrast kleiner Details aus (Pfeilmarkierungen). Auch beim „Nearest Neighbour"-Bild sind aber alle Strukturen deutlich zu erkennen und für die Anwendung in der 2D/3D-Registrierung ausreichend

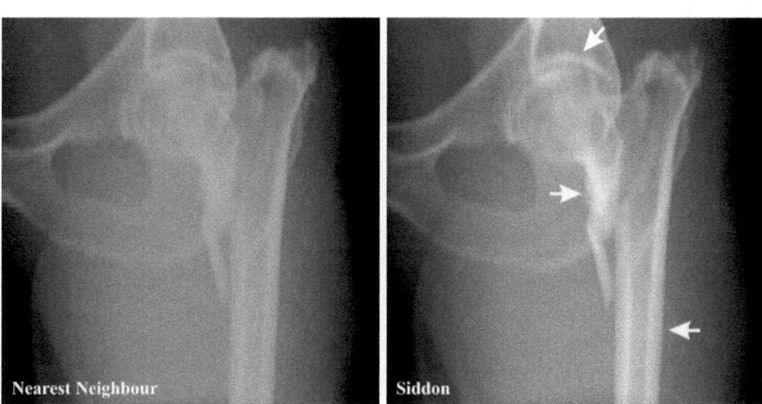

ist zu bedenken, dass die Auswirkung der Ungenauigkeit auf das Ausgangsbild direkt von der Voxelgröße des Eingangsbilds abhängt. Für ein DRR mit einer Pixelgröße von $2 \times 2\,\mathrm{mm}^2$ wäre das „Nearest Neighbour"-Resampling aus einem Eingangsbilddatensatz mit einer Voxelgröße von $2 \times 2 \times 2\,\mathrm{mm}^3$ akzeptabel, da der absolute Fehler auf maximal eine halbe Voxelgröße limitiert ist. Zur Veranschaulichung der Bildqualität des „Nearest Neighbour"-Algorithmus' sind in Abb. 3 zwei DRRs (Pixelgröße $1{,}79 \times 1{,}79\,\mathrm{mm}^2$) gegenübergestellt, die auf Basis von CT-Daten mit einer Voxelgröße von etwa $0{,}43 \times 0{,}43 \times 2\,\mathrm{mm}^3$ erstellt wurden.

Wie oben und in Abb. 2 dargestellt, stellt es für das Registrierungsergebnis keinen nennenswerten Unterschied dar, ob das Strahlresampling mittels „Nearest Neighbour"- oder mittels Siddon-Methode erfolgt. Davon ausgehend kann das Strahlresampling für den Registrierungsvorgang ohne Probleme grundsätzlich mittels „Nearest Neighbour" erfolgen, da der Zugewinn an Qualität durch die Siddon-Methode in keinem Verhältnis zum dafür erforderlichen Rechenaufwand steht und für die Registrierung letztlich nur geeignete und nicht unbedingt perfekte Bilder erstellt werden müssen. Der Zeitfaktor steht hier im Vordergrund.

Literaturverzeichnis

1. Siddon RL. Fast calculation of the exact radiological path for a three-dimensional CT array. Med Phys. 1985;12(3):252–5.
2. Amanatides J, Woo A. Fast voxel traversal algorithm for ray casting. Procs Eurographics. 1987; p. 3–10.
3. Bresenham JE. Algorithm for computer control of a digital plotter. IBM Syst J. 1965;4(1):25–30.

Adaptive Visualization Using the Annealing M-estimator

Ruxandra Lasowski[1], 2, Selim Benhimane[1], Jakob Vogel[1], Tobias F. Jakobs[3], Christoph J. Zech[3], Christoph Trumm[3], Martin Brokate[4], Nassir Navab[1]

[1]Chair for Computer Aided Medical Procedures (CAMP), TU Munich, Germany
[2]Siemens Medical Solutions, Computed Tomography, Forchheim,
[3]Institute for Clinical Radiology, Grosshadern Hospital, University of Munich,
[4]Technical University Munich, Center of Mathematics, TU Munich, Germany
micu@cs.tum.edu

Abstract. This paper presents an adaptive visualization for helping the needle insertion task for RF liver ablation under CT-fluoroscopy (CT-fluoro) guidance. It shows slices of the 3D CT-volume that are resulting from the out-of-plane motion parameters along weighted isosurfaces in the convergence basin of the employed cost function. The visualization is coupled to the uncertainty in estimating the deformation of the liver and brings much more information than a single registered slice. We evaluated the proposed visualization with three experienced interventional radiologists and they pointed out that such visualization revealing the neighborhood with the belonging structures, like vessels and lesion spread, will help the needle guidance.

1 Introduction

Radiofrequency Ablation (RFA) is an interventional procedure applied to patients with unresectable primary liver tumors and metastases. The needle is percutaneously inserted into the lesion and can be performed eg. under CT-fluoro guidance. We would like to help this procedure by displaying high resolution contrasted data corresponding to the actual CT-fluoro slice in the intervention room when further needle insertion becomes difficult. In such cases we would like to enable an interface of triggering an automatic registration process and presenting e.g. the target lesion, neighborhood, vessel structures in the intervention room with the high quality of the contrasted pre-interventional CT-volume. However the deformation due to the breathing, the non-contrasted low resolution CT-fluoro makes it very hard to guarantee the validity of any deformable slice-to-volume registration. Attempts for a non-rigid 2D/3D registration employing the DEMONS algorithm [1] did not succeed even for very small deformations. Rigid slice-to-volume registration for similar applications has been reported in [2, 3]. In [4] a visualization of a subvolume is proposed based on piecewise registration. In contrast to that approach, this paper aims to first obtain a solution to the global registration and then visualize a specific volume that encompasses its neighborhood. In this neighborhood, out-of-plane motion parameters samples on the isosurfaces of the minimized cost function are found using a line search strategy. The defined volume takes into account in which projection parameters the registration is most sensitive, and is obtained from the definition of slices defined by motion parameters on weighted isosurfaces. The visualization of a subvolume in the pre-interventional volume brings much more intuitive information to the interventional radiologist than one single slice. Therefore, the needle guidance toward the lesion is improved. In addition, this could result in less radiation dose for the patient and examiner.

2 Materials and Methods

Due to the noisy nature of the CT-fluoro slice, the needle presence and contrast differences, we are using a robust similarity measure to outliers and adaptive to discontinuities: the annealing M-estimator in conjunction with a GNC (graduated non-convexity) optimization [5] in order to compute the update parameters for the incremental pose $\mathbf{T}(\mathbf{x})$ in the volume that is composed with the current estimate $\widehat{\mathbf{T}}$ such that a cost function is minimized. The cost function $f_\gamma(\mathbf{x})$ is then defined as:

$$f_\gamma(\mathbf{x}) = \frac{\sum_{\mathcal{X}_i}(h_\gamma(d_i)|d_i|)}{\sum_{\mathcal{X}_i} h_\gamma(d_i)} \tag{1}$$

with $h_\gamma(d_i) = 1/(1 + d_i^2/\gamma)$ and $d_i = \mathcal{I}^*(\mathcal{X}_i) - \mathcal{I}(\widehat{\mathbf{T}}\mathbf{T}(\mathbf{x})\mathcal{X}_\mathbf{i})$. Here $\mathcal{I}^*(\mathcal{X}_i)$ is the intensity of the CT-fluoro slice at the pixel $\mathcal{X}_i$ and $\mathcal{I}(\widehat{\mathbf{T}}\mathbf{T}(\mathbf{x})\mathcal{X}_\mathbf{i})$ is the intensity in the CT-volume at the pixel $\mathcal{X}_i$ after being projected at the pose $\widehat{\mathbf{T}}\mathbf{T}(\mathbf{x})$. Since h is continuous it is stable to changes of the difference conditions and $h_\gamma(d_i)/\sum_{\mathcal{X}_i} h_\gamma(d_i)$ is acting as a weight for d_i penalizing outliers. The parameter γ is set initially to a high value such that h is strictly convex and is lowered according to a defined schedule.

For better spatial orientation, and to increase the confidence in the registration result, not only the minimizer of the registration function f is visualized as a 2D view, but also other views "close" to the minimizer. The visualization of the 3D volume gives the intuition of slowly exploring the volume in the neighborhood (in real space) of the minimizer. For a given $\alpha \in \mathbb{R}^+$, an isosurface of the cost function f defined in the equation (1) is a set $\mathcal{C}(\alpha) \subset \mathbb{R}^6$ given by $\mathcal{C}(\alpha) = \{\mathbf{x} \in \mathbb{R}^6 : f_\gamma(\mathbf{x}) = \alpha\}$. Now, let $\widetilde{\mathbf{x}} \in \mathbb{R}^6$ be the estimated minimizer. To find a certain number of parameters $\mathbf{x}_i$ around the minimizer, we use a line search in different directions for points on the isosurface $\mathcal{C}(f_\gamma(\widetilde{\mathbf{x}}) + \varepsilon)$, where ε defines the size of the neighborhood in parameter space. In section 3 we explain how we choose the directions of the line search and the ε defining the size of the neighborhood. Each of these points correspond to a certain pose and therefore to a certain projection of the volume. We call these views *cost-equivalent projections* (CEPs). Once the minimizer of the function $f_\gamma(\mathbf{x})$ is identified and a number of samples on a given isosurface are determined, it is possible to define a trajectory interpolating these points. In order to visualize the volume smoothly, we first need to find an optimal trajectory from the minimizer through all of the isosurface sample points $\mathbf{x}_i$. Ideally, this trajectory follows the shortest path from the minimizer toward the isosurface, stays on the latter exactly, and aims for the minimizer again. As the isosurface itself is not analytically known, we use the sample points computed previously as waypoints, and rearrange them in a way that we visit each point once while following a trajectory of minimal length. We currently use the Euclidean norm as distance metric between parameters in $\mathbb{R}^6$. A smooth path is passing by the ordered points $\mathbf{x}_i$ defined above. We interpolate these points and the transformation matrices denote now the position and orientation of the virtual camera.

3 Results

The registration is performed with a coarse-to-fine strategy, starting at 64×64 and increasing to 128×128 and 256×256. Each time the estimated values are taken as initialization for the next resolution. The optimization procedure is started from the pose obtained by the DICOM Image Position Patient since the

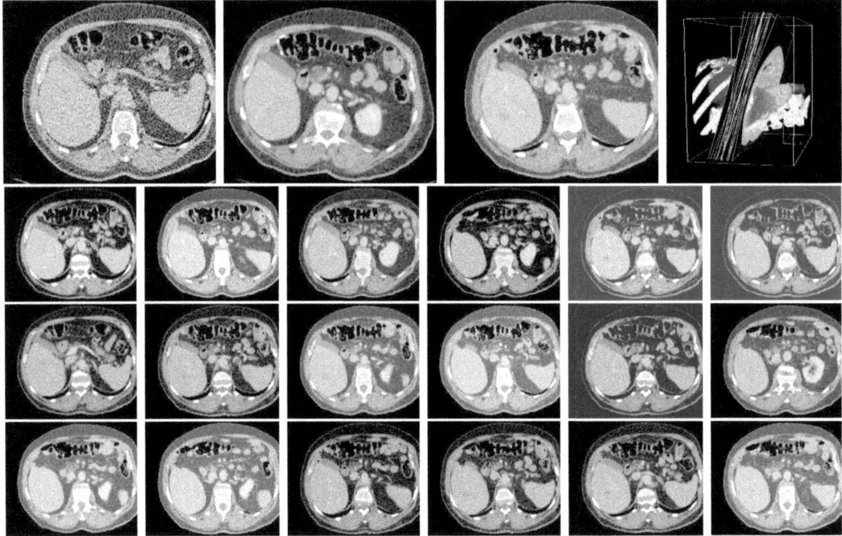

Fig. 1. First top row: the first image represents the CT-fluoro slice, the second one represents the initial pose in the volume and the third one represents the estimated minimum. Note that the lesion is not visible in the CT-fluoro slice. The forth image is showing a 3D view of the generated CEP's. The next rows are 2D views and represent CEPs at motions from out-of-plane parameters: 6 result from the 3 out-of-plane parameters in positive and negative direction, and 12 result from the combination of each of two parameters in positive and negative direction. The subvolume defined by the CEP's and the minimum slice is showed in a smooth animation. This example shows the possible convergence problems: the kidney is present in the initial pose and also in different CEP's whereas the liver shape does not significantly change

patient is not moved from the table. The following experiments were run on a PC with 1.80GHz Intel Pentium processor and 1GB of memory. The average time for the registration for the clinical images was $4s$. The computation of the set of solutions on the isosurface took in average $15s$. A solution set of 18 sampling points on the isosurface is used resulting from search directions obtained by combinations of out-of-plane parameters, i.e. translation along the z axis, rotations about the x and y axis. Here, 6 CEPs result from the 3 out-of-plane parameters in + and - direction, and 12 result from the combination of each of two parameters in + and - direction.

3.1 Linking ε with the Volume

Based on results of the literature, e.g. [6], the deformation in the liver can reach up to 20 mm from the predicted rigid position, while the average across tissue yields about 6 mm. Therefore, we would like the CEPs to represent an average movement between 6–7 mm. We start with an initial guess of $\varepsilon = 0.25$ and adapt it until the average motion of all 3D points $\mathcal{X}_i$ considered in the volume between the minimum view and the views at the CEPs will be in this interval.

3.2 Simulations Without Deformation

To test the registration algorithm, we created a set of Ground-Truth (GT) slices simulating a CT-fluoro slice. We used from one patient a noisy reconstructed volume where we extracted at different poses including rotations and translations four slices. These slices were registered to the same pre-interventional volume but reconstructed without noise. An average RMS between the starting positions and the GT pose is about 35.75 mm for translation and 7.22° for rotation. The results of the RMS calculations between registered noisy slices and the GT give an average RMS for translation of 0.65 mm and for rotation 0.03°.

3.3 Simulations Including Deformation

For deriving synthetic 2D slices that also include deformations, we are using two CT-volumes of one patient, the pre- and the post-interventional datasets. The pre-interventional CT-volume (the template volume) is elastically [7] registered to the post-interventional CT-volume (the reference volume). Since after the intervention, the patient is not any more able to achieve the full inspiration breath-hold as before the intervention, the registration of the pre-interventional toward the post-interventional scan is mimicking a possible expiration movement. The displacement field for the achieved deformation will map the voxels of the deformed volume into the pre-interventional scan. In this way by extracting axial slices of this deformed volume, adding noise, each of these slices represent hypothetical CT-fluoro slices. We are using six axial slices extracted every $1cm$. Visual inspection on 3D views show that the deformation of the liver voxels is included by the estimated CEPs.

3.4 Experiments with Real CT-fluoro Slices

Six routinely acquired datasets (Siemens Somatom Sensation 16) are used together with 3 CT-fluoro slices, which results in 18 examples. Figure 1 shows one example of the 2D views and a 3D view of all 18 estimated CEPs.

3.5 Evaluation of Adaptive Visualization

Evaluation of the CEP visualization versus the visualization of a single slice has been performed by three experienced interventional radiologists. In that setup we used though the results of the M-estimator, but the principles are the same. Two of the radiologists considered in all 18 times (100%) the CEP visualization more valuable than one slice. One of them voted 11 times (61%) for the CEP visualization. A single slice in the CT-volume will confirm or not the right position, but it misses further guidance and neighborhood assessment. On the other hand, this visualization ties up to the familiar view in the radiology.

4 Conclusion

We proposed an adaptive visualization that includes views of the CT-volume determined along flat directions of the out-of-plane motion parameters next to the minimizer where the optimization encounters uncertainty. The views are generated at poses that represent an average movement reported in the literature. In this way the deformation caused by the breathing should be included into the volume defined by the views. The result of the registration and the adaptive visualization were assessed by three experienced interventional radiologists on real CT-fluoro data. The evaluation outcome supports that such visualization in the intervention room enables the examiner to better orientate during the needle insertion.

References

1. Yaniv Z, Stenzel R, Cleary K, et al. A realistic simulation framework for assessing deformable slice-to-volume (CT-fluoroscopy/CT) registration. Proc SPIE. 2006;6141:116–23.
2. Birkfellner W, Figl M, Kettenbach J, et al. Rigid 2D/3D slice-to-volume registration and its application on fluoroscopic CT images. Med Phys. 2007;34(1):246–55.
3. Fei B, Duerk JL, Boll DT, et al. Slice-to-Volume Registration and its Potential Application to Interventional MRI-Guided Radio-Frequency Thermal Ablation of Prostate Cancer. IEEE Trans Med Imaging. 2003;22(4):515–25.
4. Micu R, Jakobs T, Zech C, et al. Evaluation of different subvolume visualizations in CT-Fluoroscopy guided RF Liver Ablation. Proc SPIE. 2007;6509:51–7.
5. Li SZ, Wang H, Soh WYC. Robust estimation of rotation angles from image sequences using the annealing M-Estimator. J Math Imaging Vis. 1998;8(2):181–192.
6. Clifford MA, Banovac F, Levy E, et al. Assessment of hepatic motion secondary to respiration for computer assisted interventions. Comp Aid Surg. 2002;7:291–9.
7. Modersitzki J. Numerical Methods for Image Registration. Oxford University Press; 2004.

Analysis of Cerebral Blood Flow from Small Rodents

Phase Contrast Angiography of Vascular Geometry

Monika Lehmpfuhl[1,2], Andre Gaudnek[3,4], Andreas Hess[3,5], Michael Sibila[3,4]

[1]Dep. of Electronics and Information, Northwestern Polytechnical, Xi'An, China
[2]IGSS, Munich University of Technology , Germany
[3]Bernstein Centre for Computational Neuroscience Berlin, Germany
[4]Neural Information Processing Group, Berlin University of Technology, Germany
[5]Institute for Experimental and Clinical Pharmacology and Toxicology, Friedrich-Alexander University Erlangen-Nuremberg, Germany
idefix@xs.tu-berlin.de

Abstract. The exact knowledge of the blood vessel geometry plays an important role, not only in clinical applications (stroke diagnosis, detection of stenosis), but also for detailed analysis of functional data, such as fMRI or optical imaging data. Here we focus on validating not only the geometry of the extracted vascular pattern, but also its function, namely the fluid dynamics. For validating angiographic data, phase contrast angiography (PC-MRA) sequences are used, as these data contain additionally to the morphological data rheological information. This rheological information can be used to validate the reconstructed geometric model of the vascular system, especially for the detection of missing vessels due to velocity changes in front of bifurcations.

1 Introduction

Phase contrast angiography (PC-MRA) plays an important role in modern diagnosis techniques for the detection of blood vessel diseases such as stenosis or aneurisms. Moreover, exact geometric reconstructions of the blood vessel pattern can also be used for registration of multimodal functional data, such as fMRI and optical image data.

To validate the quality of our automatic reconstruction method we compare different scans from the same animal with each other and with μCT data of the same rat, being the gold standard for vascular geometry [1].

Here, we focus on some functional aspects of the reconstructed vessel pattern, namely its fluid dynamics. Therefore, we use quantitative flow data, gathered with PC-MRA of small rodent brains to i) optimize the calculation and visualization of the measured flow fields and ii) validate the reconstruction of the brain vessel pattern from angiograms. Reconstructed vector fields offer the information of direction and speed of the blood within the vessel. This information can be used i) to validate the reconstructed blood vessel model by analyzing flow, especially in areas of disturbed flow, such as bifurcations, sharp bends and abrupt diameter changes ii) to indicate missing vessels in the reconstruction because the PC-MRA shows flow changes (speed and velocity) and iii) to indicate faulty reconstructed diameters because the PC-MRA shows constant velocities.

2 Materials and Methods

2.1 Data Aquisition

Scanning was performed at a 4.7 T BRUKER Biospec 47/40 scanner, equipped with an actively RF-decoupled coil system. For the rat scan the RF-signal was transmitted with a whole birdcage coil and received with a 3 cm quadrature surface coil, located directly above the head of the rat. A standard PC-MRA with TE = 7.3 ms, TR = 15.6 ms, flip angle = 30°, field of view = 3.5 cm x 3.5 cm x 3.5 cm, matrix size = 256 x 256 x 256, venc = 40cm/s was used. Animals were anesthetized by Isofluorane, the level of which was adjusted to achieve a stable and physiological respiration rate (60 bpm). For keeping the body temperature of the rat at a constant level, heating was achieved via a water bath.

2.2 Data Visualization

Visualization was carried out using the AMIRA (Mercury inc.) software, where our customized image processing modules were implemented. From PC-MRA modulus images, geometric reconstructions of the blood vessels were automatically generated by a self developed software (patent pending) [1], resulting in a surface description of the vascular system providing diameters and directions (Fig. 1,3).

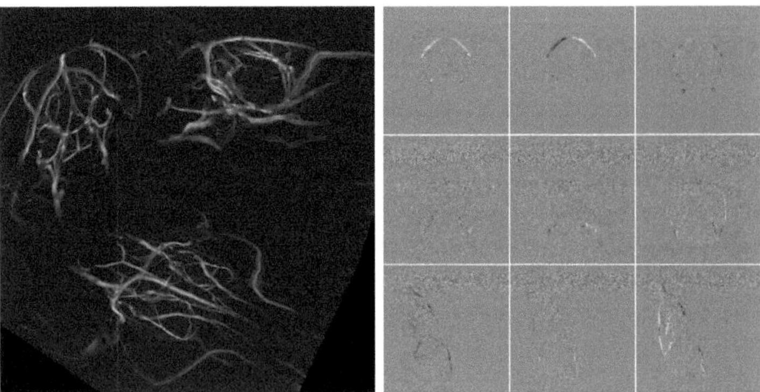

Fig. 1. Maximum intensity projection of a rat brain angiogram, measured with MR-PCA (left); single xy-slice of the measured phases, encoding flow velocity (right top from left: a-p, l-r, h-f direction); same for xz and yz slices (middle bottom)

2.3 Simulation (Pressure Drop in the Blood Vessel System)

For reference data, fluid mechanical approaches were applied. From the reconstructed blood vessel system a line set (skeleton) was constructed. This line set was used to generate a simplified model, in which the velocity in each branch of the vessel system could be estimated. Here we make use of the Krämer [2] model, a model to calculate the pressure drop in the vascular system, but as a simplification of the otherwise unsolvable second order partial differential equations that describe the flow formally.

Under the assumption of laminar flow, Newtonian liquid and a rigid tube, the velocity magnitude within the reconstructed vessel system is calculated. Although, in the vessel system there are periodic variations of blood pressure and velocity, the vessels are elastic and blood is a non Newtonian fluid, a stationary Poiseuille- flow allows an estimation of pressure distribution in the vessel system.

Starting point for the calculation were the two arteries entering the brain (carotids). The starting velocity was set to 40cm/s (maximum from our MR-protocol). The calculation of volume flow and mean velocity after each branching point was calculated with the formulas mentioned in (Fig. 2). The following assumptions were done; i) Starting velocity is the mean velocity in the inflow area of the carotids, ii) In case of interrupted, but ongoing flow, the velocity of the preceding segment is used, iii) In case of non ongoing flow, a new start point velocity was used, namely the MR-measured velocity in the new start point, iv) For circle structures, as they exist often in rat brains, the volume flow in front of and behind the ring structure must be the same (no friction losses).

The line set of the vessel structure was used to determine the direction. Having calculated the velocity in the different branches of the vessel system this mean velocity in each branch was mapped on the reconstructed vessel system (Fig. 4).

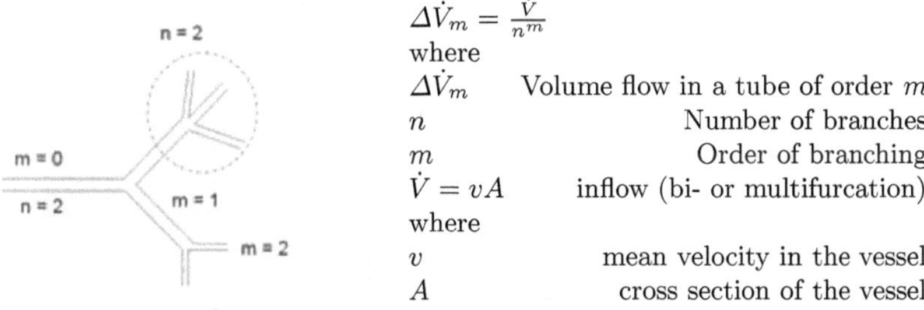

$\Delta \dot{V}_m = \frac{\dot{V}}{n^m}$

where

$\Delta \dot{V}_m$	Volume flow in a tube of order m
n	Number of branches
m	Order of branching
$\dot{V} = vA$	inflow (bi- or multifurcation)

where

v	mean velocity in the vessel
A	cross section of the vessel

Fig. 2. Krämer model of pressure drop for estimation of the mean velocity in each branch of the reconstructed vessel system

3 Results

3.1 Flow Visualization

For visualization of the rheological data (flow velocity and direction) phase images of the PC-MRA are used. As these phase images are noisy and flow quantification does only work correctly in areas where flow is existing, the phase images need to be segmented, using the above mentioned reconstruction method ([1], patent pending) as a mask image. After segmentation the phase images were combined into a three dimensional vector field and streamlines (Fig. 3,4) were generated using a standard streamline algorithm [3]. Due to turbulent flow, small vessel diameters and measurement errors, the calculated vectors are erroneous. This is clearly visible, both in the direct vector visualization and in the streamlines (Fig. 3,4). Due to the curved vessel structure and many bifurcations, streamlines do not follow the vessel structure anymore and when they reach background tissue, the streamlines stop, as background tissue is set to zero. To have streamlines in most parts of the brain vessel system, it is necessary to start the streamlines in different parts of the brain.

3.2 Flow Simulation

As the streamline algorithm is erroneous, and the number of pixels within a vessel is too small to obtain reliable results the mean velocity is mapped on the reconstructed vessel system. This results in a presentation of the velocity in the blood vessel system, but the direction information is lost (Fig. 4).) Based on these observations and the variance of the measured vectors within small test volumes, we derive a confidence measure accessing the quality of a given MR-PCA measurement (noise/diameter, directional variance/diameter etc.).

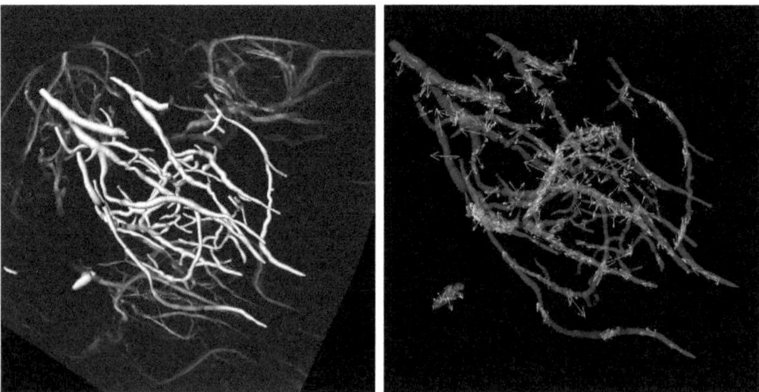

Fig. 3. Blood vessel reconstruction from MR-PCA angiogram (left); direct visualization of vectors, reconstructed from individual phase measurements (right). As reference, the vessel reconstruction is also shown (shaded)

Fig. 4. Flow field visualization using illuminated streamlines (left); visualization of simulated flow as result of an inflow from the right carotid (right). Higher flow is shown using larger diameters and brighter color

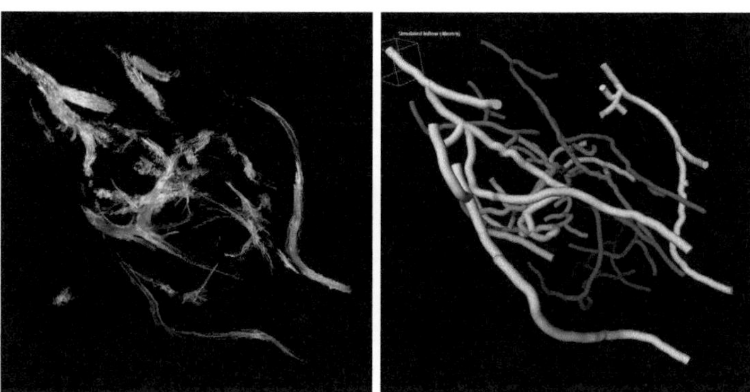

4 Discussion

Numerical errors and image quality remain the main problems for streamline visualization of PC-MRA images. To get meaningful and accurate streamline images the method and the used parameters need to be adapted. However, the proposed method offers an additional tool for accurate registration of small vessels, as both morphological and rheological data are used. The Krämer model, being optimized for low branching orders and relatively large vessels, shows problems due to oversimplified assumptions. The quality of PC-MRA measurements is best in vessels with laminar flow whereas in vessels with turbulent flow signal blackout due to partial volume effects can occur. However, if enough vectors exist in a given vessel and flow is mostly laminar, main flow direction and velocity can be obtained. Based on this information, missing vessel branches can be reconstructed. Moreover, the simulation can be used to correct the measured flow vectors, such that signal voids and other errors can be corrected.

Acknowledgement. This work was supported by Doerenkamp-Lehrstuhl for Innovations in animal and consumer protection, BMBF Verbundprojekt Migräne, BMBF Bernstein centre Berlin, DFG FG 661 small animal imaging.

References

1. Gaudnek MA, Sibila M, Obermayer K, et al. Geometric reconstruction of brain vasculature from small rodents: A comparison of different imaging methods. ISMRM Berlin. 2007.
2. Krämer K. Der Druckabfall in einem laminar durchströmten, regelmäßig verzweigten Rohrleitungssystem mit Anwendung auf den Blutkreislauf des Menschen. Kreislaufforschung. 1967;52:79–95.
3. Buonocore MH. Vizualizing blood flow patterns using streamlines, arrows and particle paths. MRM. 1998;40:210–26.

Quantify Prostate Cancer by Automated Histomorphometry

Ulf-Dietrich Braumann[1], Jens-Peer Kuska[2], Markus Löffler[3], Nicolas Wernert[4]

[1]Translational Centre for Regenerative Medicine, University Leipzig, 04103 Leipzig
[2]Interdisciplinary Centre for Bioinformatics, University Leipzig, 04107 Leipzig
[3]Inst. for Medical Informatics, Statistics & Epidemiology, Univ. Leipzig, 04107 Leipzig
[4]Institute of Pathology, University Bonn, 53105 Bonn
ubraumann@trm.uni-leipzig.de

Abstract. A new method is presented to quantify malignant changes in histological sections of prostate tissue immunohistochemically stained for prostate-specific antigen (PSA) by means of image processing. The morphological analysis of the prostate tissue uses the solidity of PSA-positive prostate tissue segments to compute a quantitative measure that turns out highly correlated with scores obtained from routine diagnosis (Gleason, Dhom).

1 Introduction

Prostate cancer is one of the most frequent cancers in western countries. Routine diagnosis of prostate cancer operates on several levels of resolution. With low microscopic magnification, the shape of the tissues is examined, while on large magnifications on the level of single cells the shape of the cell nucleus and the size of the individual cells is of interest. In the present paper we restrict ourselves to the low magnification scale and look for shape descriptors of the cancer tissue. While a healthy glandular tissue has a regular shape that reflects its function, the cancer tissue has lost this regular structure. We are interested in the quantification of this structural change in prostate cancer. Further, we wish to obtain a quantitative estimate of the cancer shape that compares well to the diagnostic grading obtained by a pathologist. The grading determines the future treatment of the patient, and a more objective measure than the opinion of the pathologist seems to be preferable. The Gleason grading [1] uses the degree of the differentiation of the glandular tissue and the pattern of the glands. The Dhom grading [2] uses additional cytological parameters. We here report on a new algorithm designed to quantify prostate glandular structures and applied this to 26 specimens of 23 patients.

2 Materials and Methods

2.1 Segmentation

All images where preprocessed by a channel-wise total variation filter [3] in RGB space to reduce the spatial noise and obtain more compact regions in the segmentation.

It is typical for immunohistochemical stains that the color distribution may exhibit quite a wide variation in color saturation across different slides or even on the same slide. Our goal was to segment all images with the same set of parameters for the segmentation. For this, a c-means segmentation in the CIE Lu*v* color space was chosen [4, 5]. The result of an individual c-means segmentation are the segmented image and a set of colors that are used as centers in the clustering process. It is always difficult to select initial centers for the c-means segmentation, so we take four centers (rough estimates) and make a first loop over all images that yield new centers for every image. These new centers are averaged over all processed images and taken as starting values for a second c-means segmentation over all images. The resulting segmentations were then used to select the class that corresponds to the prostate tissue in order to later on characterize the shape of the binarized segments. Fig. 1 depicts the result for three samples from the set with an overall of 96 regions of interest (ROIs) out of 26 specimens.

For every connected component (segment, i.e. glandular structure of interest, GOI) referring to a binary mask corresponding to the immunohistochemically stained prostate tissue we compute the solidity of each GOI [6]. The solidity of a single shape i is defined as

$$s_i = \frac{H_i}{A_i} \tag{1}$$

where H_i is the area of the convex hull of the component and A_i is its real area (see Fig. 2).

For convex shapes like disks or rectangles the solidity is always equal to one. For non-convex objects one gets always values larger than one. The solidity is invariant under translation, rotation and scaling. To get a single number for every image we compute a weighted solidity

$$S = \frac{\sum_i A_i \, s_i}{\sum_i A_i} = \frac{\sum_i H_i}{\sum_i A_i}. \tag{2}$$

The summation runs over all i components in the image. The weighting is used, since otherwise small objects should not contribute to the averaged solidity the same way as large objects do. By this averaging process we introduce the important quantity of the size into the calculation that otherwise would be lost by averaging the pure scale invariant solidity.

3 Results

To relate the computed averaged solidities with the gradings obtained from the diagnostic findings box-whisker plots are made from the mean solidity in every

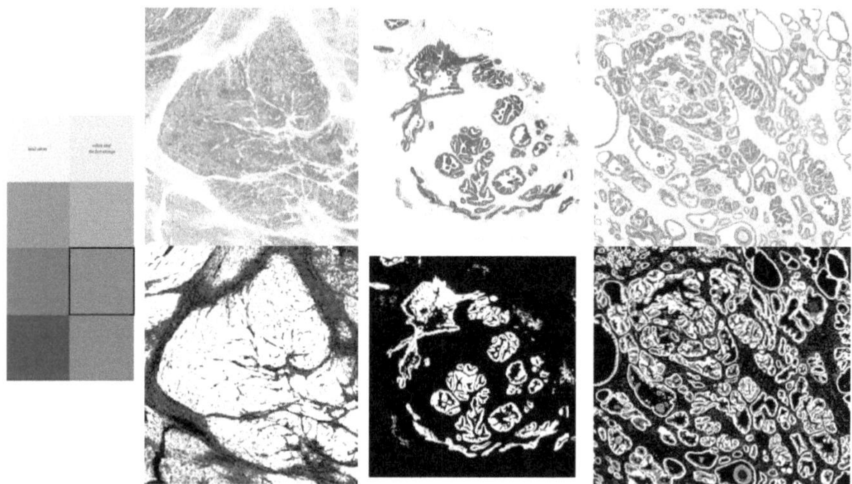

Fig. 1. Left: Colors used as initial centers for the c-means segmentation. That color corresponding to the prostate tissue color is marked by a black frame. Right: Three sample ROIs (upper row) and their segmentation (lower row)

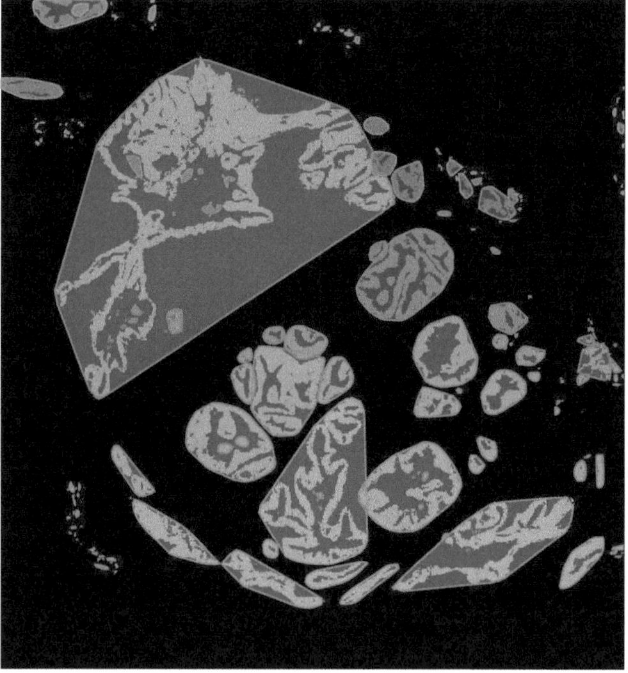

Fig. 2. Solidity for the components (GOIs) determined as ratio of the area of the component's convex hull to the real component's area. For every segmented component (GOI) within this sample ROI, its corresponding convex hull is overlayed in the same label color (shades of green, brown and red) but with 50% transparency

Fig. 3. Box-whisker plots for the mean solidity of the 96 ROIs for Gleason scoring and Dhom grading. The value 0 in both grading systems was assigned cases without malign changes

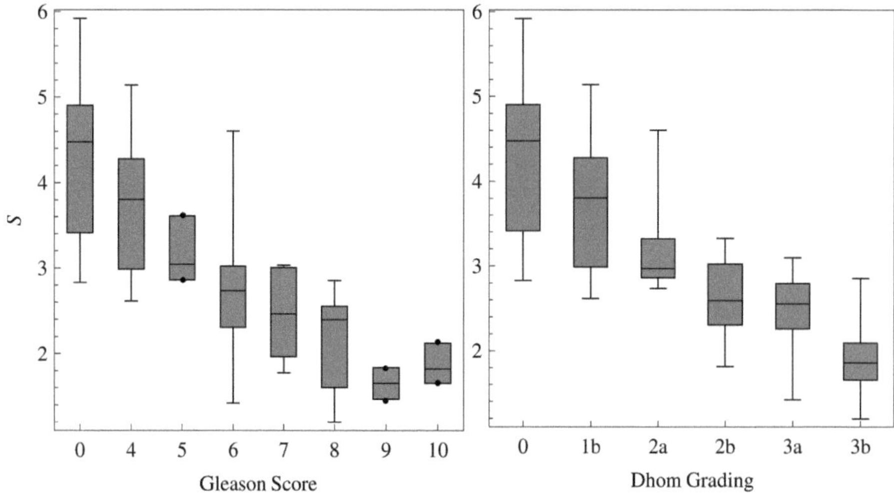

pathological grade class (Fig. 3). For both grading system we obtain a clear correlation of the computed solidities with the grading. Lower mean solidities correspond to higher scores in both grading systems.

4 Discussion

The developed segmentation procedure works well for a wide range of PSA stained samples and allows a robust detection of the PSA-positive prostatic tissue. The mean solidity seems to be a good objective measure for the degree of malignancy of the cancer. It should be noted that the above-mentioned established grading systems as typically are applied in routine pathology – although in good correspondence with our solidity-based histomorphometric assessments – are not considered as gold standards here. Rather, our work is driven by the need of a reliable, reproducible objective quantification and characterization of the malignancy of prostatic changes in order to provide a better basis for prognosis and therapy decisions. With our solidity-based automated histomorphometric approach we have introduced a simple but promising objective method ready for further assessments concerning its appropriateness to support diagnostic findings.

Acknowledgement. The project is supported by the Federal Ministry of Education and Research (BMBF), grant PTJ-BIO/31P4282 (MS CartPro) and grant PTJ-BIO/031390 (TRM Leipzig).

References

1. Gleason DF. Classification of prostatic carcinomas. Cancer Chemotherapy Reports. 1966;50(3):125–8.
2. Helpap B, Böcking A, Dhom G, et al. Klassifikation, histologisches und zytologisches Grading sowie Regressionsgrading des Prostatakarzinoms. Eine Empfehlung des pathologisch-urologischen Arbeitskreises „Prostatakarzinom“. Pathologe. 1985;6:3–7.
3. Chan TF, Osher S, Shen J. The digital TV filter and nonlinear denoising. IEEE Trans Image Process. 2001;10(2):231–41.
4. Linde Y, Buzo A, Gray RM. An algorithm for vector quantizer design. IEEE Trans Commun. 1980;28(1):84–95.
5. Lloyd SP. Least squares quantization in PCM. IEEE Trans Inform Theory. 1982;28(2):129–37.
6. Gonzalez RC, Woods RE. Digital Image Processing. 2nd ed. Prentice Hall; 2002.

Quantifizierung neurodegenerativer Veränderungen bei der Alzheimer Krankheit
Evaluierung eines automatischen Verfahrens

Klaus H. Fritzsche[1], Frederik L. Giesel[2], Philipp A. Thomann[3], Horst K. Hahn[4], Marco Essig[2], Hans-Peter Meinzer[1]

[1]Abteilung für Medizinische und Biologische Informatik, DKFZ Heidelberg
[2]Abteilung Radiologie, DKFZ Heidelberg
[3]Sektion Gerontopsychiatrische Forschung, Universitätsklinikum Heidelberg
[4]MeVis Research, Center for Medical Image Computing, Bremen
k.fritzsche@dkfz-heidelberg.de

Kurzfassung. Die objektive Bewertung neurodegenerativer Prozesse stellt für die Diagnose und Therapiebegutachtung neuropsychiatrischer Krankheiten eine wichtige Grundlage dar. Computerbasierte radiodiagnostische Verfahren können pathologische Veränderungen in verschiedenen Hirnarealen quantifizieren und hierbei die rein visuelle Beurteilung der Bilddaten ergänzen. Inhalt dieser Studie ist die Evaluation einer voll automatischen Methode zur voxelbasierten Messung atrophischer Veränderungen im Gehirn, wie sie bei der Alzheimer-Demenz (AD) oder der leichten kognitiven Störung (LKS) auftreten. Es wurde eine signifikante Korrelation mit den semiautomatisch extrahierten Volumina der Temporalhörner festgestellt. Die Präzision, Benutzerfreundlichkeit, Beobachterunabhängigkeit sowie die kurze Rechenzeit des automatischen Verfahrens sind wichtige Voraussetzungen für den routinemäßigen klinischen Einsatz.

1 Einleitung

Die hohe Inzidenz der Alzheimer-Demenz (AD) im Alter sowie das steigende durchschnittliche Lebensalter in der heutigen Gesellschaft machen die AD zu einer wachsenden Herausforderung für das Gesundheitssystem. Eine frühe und zuverlässige Diagnose der Krankheit ist äußerst wichtig, da der Verlauf der Krankheit - wenn überhaupt - nur im anfänglichen Stadium beeinflusst werden kann. Der Erfolg neuer Behandlungs- und Therapiemöglichkeiten ist somit eng an die Entwicklung von zuverlässigen Markern gebunden. Zusätzlich sind objektive Kennzahlen in der Entwicklungsphase neuer Therapien äußerst wichtig für die Überwachung des Therapieverlaufes.

Bestehende Verfahren zur Quantifizierung zerebraler Atrophie erfordern oft ein gewisses Maß an Interaktion durch einen Spezialisten [1, 2]. Im routinemäßigen klinischen Einsatz können manuelle Ansätze jedoch den Anforderungen in punkto Reproduzierbarkeit, Zeitaufwand oder auch der Benutzerfreundlichkeit oft nicht entsprechen [3].

Neben den *region of interest* (ROI) basierten Methoden haben deshalb vollautomatische morphometrische Methoden viel Aufmerksamkeit auf sich gezogen [4]. Diese erlauben eine ganzheitliche Analyse des Gehirns und sind unabhängig von der die Untersuchung durchführenden Person. In dieser Arbeit wird ein Vergleich durchgeführt zwischen einer vollautomatischen Methode zur Abschätzung der zerebralen Atrophie (Beschreibung in Fritzsche *et al.* [5]) und einer semi-automatischen, ROI-basierten Segmentierungsmethode [6] auf identischen Datensätzen. Laut einer früheren Studie korreliert das semi-automatisch extrahierte Volumen der unteren Ventrikelhörner signifikant mit manuell gemessenen Volumina des Hippokampus und stellt somit eine verlässliche Referenz dar [7].

2 Material und Methoden

2.1 Auswahl der Probanden

Für die Studie wurden 21 Patienten mit leichter kognitiver Störung (LKS) (Durchschnittsalter 65.2 ± 0.9) sowie 21 gesunde Kontrollpersonen (65.3 ± 0.8) aus der Heidelberger Interdisziplinären Längsschnittstudie des Erwachsenenalters (ILSE) ausgewählt. Als zusätzliche Referenzgruppe standen 10 Patienten mit AD (63.8 ± 7.4) aus der Sektion Gerontopsychiatrische Forschung des Universitätsklinikums Heidelberg zur Verfügung. Es bestanden keine signifikanten Unterschiede zwischen den Probanden in Bezug auf Alter, Geschlecht und Bildungsgrad. Alle Probanden wurden ausführlichen neuropsychologischen Tests unterzogen, und es wurden MR Aufnahmen mit einem klinischen 1,5 Tesla Scanner gemacht (Magnetom Vision, Siemens Medical Solutions, 128 T1-gewichtete koronale Schichtbilder, TR=4ms, Flip=13°, FOV=250mm, Matrix=256×256, Schichtabstand 1.8 mm). Ausführlichere Informationen zu Gruppenauswahl und Diagnosemethoden finden sich in Giesel *et al.* [7].

2.2 Semi-automatische Volumenmessung der Ventrikelhörner

Als Referenz wurde eine aktuelle semi-automatische Methode zur Segmentierung der Hirnventrikel herangezogen. Der Segmentierungsalgorithmus basiert hierbei auf mehreren manuell gesetzten Landmarken, welche vom Benutzer an markanten Stellen im Ventrikulärsystem platziert werden. Giesel et al. belegten die Korrelation des so vermessenen Volumens der unteren Ventrikelhörner mit dem manuell gemessenen hippokampalen Volumen in einer früheren Studie [7].

2.3 Vollautomatische Atrophieschätzung

Die vollautomatische Kette von Bildverarbeitungsschritten zur Schätzung des Atrophiefortschritts beinhaltet eine Registrierung der Bilddaten in ein gemeinsames Koordinatensystem [5]. Es folgen Verarbeitungsschritte zum Ausgleich von Abweichungen der Histogramme sowie die Entfernung niedrigfrequenter Artefakte in den Bildern. Die statistische Auswertung der individuellen Volumina anhand eines Modells für Bilddaten gesunder Personen liefert einen Index als Maß

Tabelle 1. Mann-Whitney U-Signifikanztests: ns = nicht signifikant; s = signifikant

	AD/Gesund	AD/LKS	LKS/Gesund
Semi-automatisches Verfahren:			
Volumen untere Ventrikelhörner	$p < 10^{-4}$ (s)	$p < 10^{-4}$ (s)	$p = 0.92$ (ns)
Automatisches Verfahren:			
Atrophie linker Hirnlappen	$p < 10^{-4}$ (s)	$p < 10^{-4}$ (s)	$p = 0.13$ (ns)
Atrophie Hippokampus	$p < 10^{-4}$ (s)	$p < 10^{-4}$ (s)	$p = 0.26$ (ns)

für die Atrophie in dem gewünschten Bereich. Es wurden lokale Messungen in der Hippokampusregion in beiden Hemisphären vorgenommen. Außerdem wurden die zusammengenommenen Bereiche des Frontal-, Parietal-, Temporal- und Insellappens der linken Hemisphäre auf atrophische Veränderungen hin untersucht. Statistisches Wissen über die Morphologie eines gesunden Gehirns wurde hierbei apriori aus 37 gesunden, von der Studie unabhängigen Kontrollpatienten gewonnen.

2.4 Statistik

Der Mann-Whitney U-Test wurde als Signifikanztest herangezogen, um die Qualität der Gruppenauftrennung unter Anwendung der verschiedenen Methoden zu überprüfen. Außerdem wurde die Korrelation der Methoden untereinander mit Hilfe des Pearson-Korrelationskoeffizienten ermittelt.

3 Ergebnisse

Die automatischen sowie die semi-automatischen Auswertungen konnten erfolgreich an allen 52 Probanden vorgenommen werden. Die Messergebnisse in der Gruppe der Kontrollpatienten unterschieden sich hoch signifikant von den Ergebnissen in der Gruppe der AD Patienten (s. Tabelle 1). Die unteren Ventrikelhörner wiesen bei AD Patienten ein größeres Volumen auf als bei Kontrollpatienten (semi-automatisches Verfahren). Die mit dem automatischen Verfahren berechneten Schätzwerte für den Atrophiefortschritt in den Hirnlappen sowie im Hippokampusbereich erreichten ein mit dem semi-automatischen Verfahren vergleichbares Signifikanzniveau. Auch die Gruppe der LKS-Patienten ließ sich anhand beider Verfahren hoch signifikant von der AD-Gruppe trennen. Signifikante Unterschiede zwischen der LKS-Gruppe und der Kontrollgruppe konnten anhand keines der Verfahren festgestellt werden (Abb. 1).

Es zeigte sich eine sehr deutliche Korrelation der automatisch extrahierten Messwerte mit den semiautomatischen Referenzwerten (Tab. 2). Die Messungen des Atrophiefortschrittes im Hippokampusbereich korrelierten außerdem sehr stark mit den Messungen des Atrophiefortschrittes in den Hirnlappen (Tab. 2).

Der Zeitaufwand für die Platzierung der Landmarken während der Ventrikelsegmentierung beträgt zwei bis drei Minuten [7]. Der automatische Ansatz benötigt keine Interaktion und eine Rechenzeit von zirka einer Minute.

Tabelle 2. Pearson-Korrelation der automatisierten Atrophiemessungen untereinander sowie mit den semiautomatisch gemessenen Volumina der Temporalhörner für die Hypothese der Unkorreliertheit: VUV = Volumen untere Ventrikelhörner; LH = Linke Hirnlappen; HIPP = Hippokampusregion

	r	p
VUV / Atrophie LH	0.78	$< 10^{-10}$
VUV / Atrophie HIPP	0.83	$< 10^{-13}$
Atrophie LH / Atrophie HIPP	0.83	$< 10^{-13}$

4 Diskussion

Die hohe Korrelation der Messwerte der beiden Verfahren sowie die vergleichbaren Ergebnisse der Signifikanztests zeigen, dass die automatische Auswertung im Vergleich zu der interaktiven Methode mindestens gleichwertige Ergebnisse liefert.

Mit keinem der Verfahren ist eine signifikante Trennung der Patienten mit LKS von den gesunden Probanden gelungen. Diese Tatsache ist auf den ersten Blick nicht vereinbar mit früheren Ergebnissen (Fritzsche *et al.* [5]). Nach Meinung der Autoren ist die Auswahl der Stichprobe für diesen Effekt verantwortlich. In der vorliegenden Studie wurde die Probandenauswahl rein zufällig und populationsbasiert vorgenommen. In anderen Studien wird oft mit Patienten gearbeitet, die schon mit Problemen zum Arzt kommen und sich somit mit größerer Wahrscheinlichkeit bereits in einem fortgeschrittenen Stadium der LKS befinden.

Die lokale Einschränkung der automatischen Auswertung auf den Bereich des Hippokampus konnte die Aussagekraft der Ergebnisse nicht entscheidend verbessern. Die lokalen Messungen korrelieren stark mit den weit gefassteren Messungen im Bereich der Hirnlappen, auch die erreichten Signifikanzniveaus sind identisch.

Abschließend lässt sich feststellen, dass der hier zu evaluierende, vollautomatische Ansatz zuverlässige und qualitativ hochwertige Ergebnisse liefert. Die

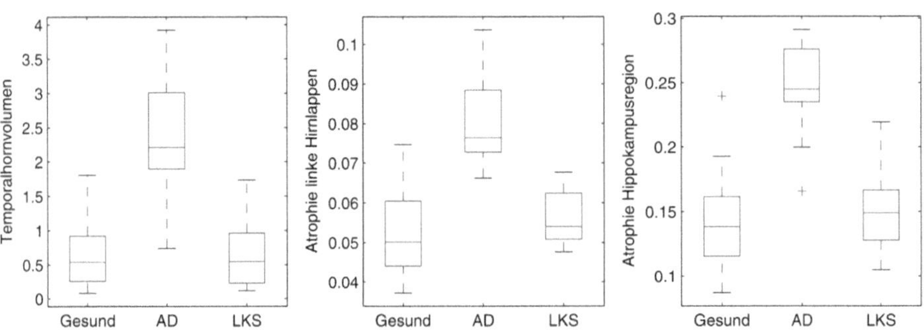

Abb. 1. Gruppenweise Ergebnisse des semi-automatischen Messverfahrens (links) und des automatischen Verfahrens (mitte, rechts)

Methode bringt den Vorteil der Benutzerunabhängigkeit und Reproduzierbarkeit mit sich. Außerdem ist der Zeitaufwand für die Auswertung äußerst gering. Die grundsätzlichen Voraussetzungen für den routinemäßigen Einsatz im Bereich der computergestützten Diagnose sowie bei der Therapiebegleitung sind somit gegeben.

Literaturverzeichnis

1. de Leon MJ, Golomb J, et al. The radiologic prediction of Alzheimer disease: The atrophic hippocampal formation. Am J Neuroradiol. 1993.
2. Bottino CM, Castro CC, Gomes RL, et al. Volumetric MRI measurements can differentiate Alzheimer's disease, mild cognitive impairment, and normal aging. Int Psychogeriatr. 2002;14(1):59–72.
3. Albert M, DeCarli C, DeKosky S, et al. The Use of MRI and PET for Clinical Diagnosis of Dementia and Investigation of Cognitive Impairment: A Consensus Report. Alzheimer's Association Neuroimaging Workgroup; 2004.
4. Lehéricy S, Marjanska M, Mesrob L, et al. Magnetic resonance imaging of Alzheimer's disease. Eur Radiol. 2007;17(2):347–62.
5. Fritzsche K, Wangenheim A, Dillmann R, et al. Automated MRI-based quantification of the cerebral atrophy providing Ddiagnostic information on mild cognitive impairment and Alzheimer's Disease. In: The 19th IEEE International Symposium on Computer-Based Medical Systems; 2006.
6. Hahn K, Rexilius J, Schlüter M, et al. Fast and robust quantification of parahippocampal atrophy via temporal horn index. Proc BVM. 2004; p. 371.
7. Giesel FL, Thomann PA, Hahn HK, et al. Comparison of manual direct and automated indirect measurement of hippocampus using magnetic resonance imaging. Eur J Radiol. 2007.

Measuring the Reliability of Geometries in Magnet Resonance Angiography

A Reference for Multimodal Image Registration?

M. André Gaudnek[1,2], Andreas Hess[2,3], Klaus Obermayer[1,2], Michael Sibila[1,2]

[1]University of Technology, Neural Information Processing Group, Berlin, Germany
[2]Bernstein Centre for Computational Neuroscience, Berlin, Germany
[3]Institute for Experimental and Clinical Pharmacology,
University Erlangen-Nuremburg, Erlangen, Germany
grenjen@cs.tu-berlin.de

Abstract. Magnet Resonance Angiography (MRA) can be used to register MR images of other types (e.g. functional MRI) acquired in the same imaging session as the angiogram since blood vessels are spatially closely confined features. This is only possible if MRA delivers reliable, reproducible images and does not show major random distortions. Therefore, we examine the reliability of MRA over subsequent scanning sessions using an appropriate distance measure on geometric vasculature models obtained from MR angiograms. Additionally we examine the variance between different specimens in order to value the possibility of inter-specimen registration.

1 Introduction

Several applications of MR small animal brain image analysis like the generation of generic functional atlases or the combination of functional data from different modalities [1] rely on the comparison and combination of numerous images of the same or distinct specimens. In this context cerebral vascular MR angiograms play an important role as blood vessels can be used as excellent landmarks for image registration. On the one hand from this application arises the need for reliable, spatially correct angiograms, on the other hand MR images are known to be prone to local distortions. When it comes to the comparison of images from different specimens, additional variability is expected due to the natural variance between each individual's anatomic characteristic.

In order to inspect the spatial reliability of MR angiograms for different MR sequences as well as the cerebral vascular variability between different animals, we use a distance measure that is defined on a geometric model representation of vasculatures.

2 Materials and Methods

All MR angiograms are converted into geometrical representations of the vascular system using an automatic reconstruction algorithm [2]. In these models vessels are represented as chains of connected frustums. The distance measure we use to evaluate the similarity of two distinct vascular models mainly calculates the mean distance between nearest frustum center line segments.

If A, B are two vascular models, then for each frustum a of A the distance $d_{fr}(a)$ is defined as the smallest centerline-to-centerline distance $d_{\text{cen}}(a,b)$ between any point of the center line segment of a and any point of any center line segment in B, i.e.

$$d_{fr}(a) = \min_{b \in B} d_{\text{cen}}(a,b) \tag{1}$$

The distance $d_{\text{mod}}(A,B)$ between both models is then calculated as the mean of the distances of all segments of A to B:

$$d_{\text{mod}}(A,B) = \langle d_{fr}(a) \rangle_{a \in A} \tag{2}$$

This measure is not commutative, i.e. usually $d_{\text{mod}}(A,B) \neq d_{\text{mod}}(B,A)$, but in practice only slight differences should occur.

The calculation of $d_{\text{cen}}(a,b)$ needs only basic mathematics and a couple of case differentiations. The center line segments c_a and c_b of a and b can be expressed using line equations with restricted independent variables t_a and t_b:

$$c_a = \{\boldsymbol{s}_a + t_a \boldsymbol{m}_a | 0 \leq t_a \leq 1, \boldsymbol{m}_a = \boldsymbol{e}_a - \boldsymbol{s}_a\} \tag{3}$$

$$c_b = \{\boldsymbol{s}_b + t_b \boldsymbol{m}_b | 0 \leq t_b \leq 1, \boldsymbol{m}_b = \boldsymbol{e}_b - \boldsymbol{s}_b\} \tag{4}$$

where $\boldsymbol{s}_a$, $\boldsymbol{s}_b$ are the segment starting points and $\boldsymbol{e}_a$, $\boldsymbol{e}_b$ are the segment ending points. There are five distance calculation cases that have to be distinguished, 2 for parallel segments and 3 for non-parallel segments (Fig. 2).

If the segments are parallel, we build two perpendiculars from $\boldsymbol{s}_b$ and $\boldsymbol{e}_b$ onto c_a. This results in two base points $\boldsymbol{p}_s$ and $\boldsymbol{p}_e$ which can also be expressed by specific values for t_a. As the line through $\boldsymbol{s}_b$ and $\boldsymbol{p}_s$ is orthogonal to $\boldsymbol{m}_b$, following equation holds:

$$0 = (\boldsymbol{p}_s - \boldsymbol{s}_b) \cdot \boldsymbol{m}_b \tag{5}$$

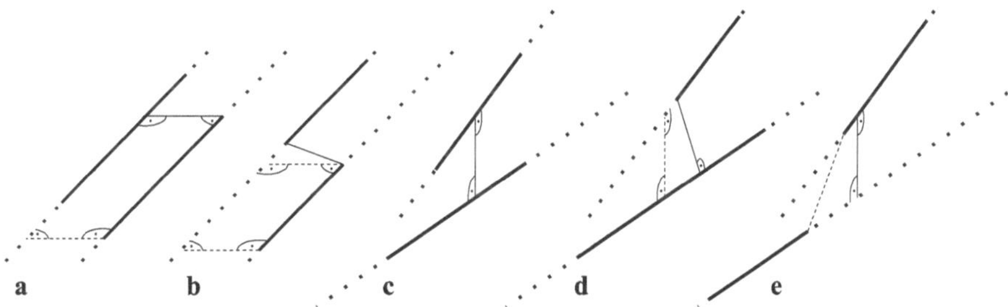

Fig. 1. All segment-to-segment distance calculation cases. Thick solid lines are center line segments, thin solid lines the smallest distance vectors: Segemnts are parallel overlapping (a); parallel non-overlapping (b), non-parallel overlapping (c), non-parallel non-overlapping with smallest distance between endpoint and line segment (d) and with smallest distance between endpoints (e)

$\boldsymbol{p}_s$ is on the line defined in (3), so

$$0 = (\boldsymbol{s}_a + t_{a,ps}\boldsymbol{m}_a - \boldsymbol{s}_b) \cdot \boldsymbol{m}_b \Longleftrightarrow t_{a,ps} = \frac{(\boldsymbol{s}_b - \boldsymbol{s}_a) \cdot \boldsymbol{m}_b}{\boldsymbol{m}_a \cdot \boldsymbol{m}_b} \tag{6}$$

$t_{a,pe}$ is calculated analogically. If $t_{a,pe}, t_{a,ps} < 0$, segment b is completely left of segment a, if $t_{a,pe}, t_{a,ps} > 1$, segment b is completely right of segment a. In both cases the smallest distance $d_{\text{cen}}(a, b)$ between both segments is found between a pair of their end points (Fig. 2b), i.e.

$$d_{\text{cen}}(a, b) = \min\{\|\boldsymbol{s}_b - \boldsymbol{s}_a\|, \|\boldsymbol{s}_b - \boldsymbol{e}_a\|, \|\boldsymbol{e}_b - \boldsymbol{s}_a\|, \|\boldsymbol{e}_b - \boldsymbol{e}_a\|\} \tag{7}$$

In all other cases, there are actually overlapping parts of c_a and c_b, and $d_{\text{cen}}(a, b)$ can be calculated as the distance between $\boldsymbol{s}_b$ and $\boldsymbol{p}_s$ (Fig. 2a):

$$d_{\text{cen}}(a, b) = \|\boldsymbol{s}_a + t_{a,ps}\boldsymbol{m}_a - \boldsymbol{s}_b\| \tag{8}$$

3 Results

If the segments are not parallel, first a normalized vector orthogonal to both lines is constructed as

$$\boldsymbol{n} = \frac{\boldsymbol{m}_a \times \boldsymbol{m}_b}{\|\boldsymbol{m}_a \times \boldsymbol{m}_b\|} \tag{9}$$

$\boldsymbol{n}$ is directed along the shortest perpendicular between both lines, the line-to-line distance $\tilde{d}$ as well as the base point parameters $t_{a,p}$ and $t_{b,p}$ are calculated by solving the linear equation

$$\boldsymbol{s}_a + t_{a,p}\boldsymbol{m}_a + \tilde{d}\boldsymbol{n} = \boldsymbol{s}_b + t_{b,p}\boldsymbol{m}_b \tag{10}$$

If $0 \leq t_{a,p}, t_{b,p} \leq 1$, both base points are actually located on the line segments and the distance is

$$d_{\text{cen}}(a, b) = |\tilde{d}| \tag{11}$$

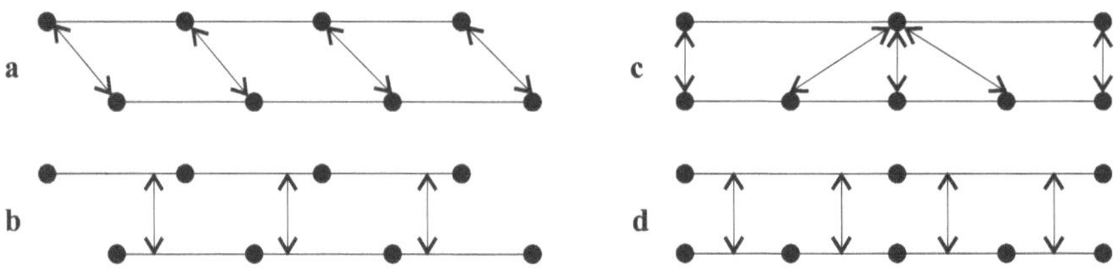

Fig. 2. Shifted segment end points lead to an overestimation when using point-to-point distance (a), whereas the distance is measured correctly using segment-to-segment distance (b). Different point density also leads to distance overestimation with point-to-point distance (c), segment-to-segment distance leads to correct results (d)

If one of the t-values is outside the range [0..1], the shortest distance could be found along a perpendicular from one of the four segment end points onto the corresponding counter-line (Fig. 2d). The t-values for the four perpendiculars are calculated

$$\begin{aligned} t_{a,sb} &= \frac{(\boldsymbol{s}_b - \boldsymbol{s}_a)\cdot \boldsymbol{m}_a}{\|\boldsymbol{m}_a\|^2}, t_{a,eb} = \frac{(\boldsymbol{e}_b - \boldsymbol{s}_a)\cdot \boldsymbol{m}_a}{\|\boldsymbol{m}_a\|^2} \\ t_{b,sa} &= \frac{(\boldsymbol{s}_a - \boldsymbol{s}_b)\cdot \boldsymbol{m}_b}{\|\boldsymbol{m}_b\|^2}, t_{b,ea} = \frac{(\boldsymbol{e}_a - \boldsymbol{s}_b)\cdot \boldsymbol{m}_b}{\|\boldsymbol{m}_b\|^2} \end{aligned} \tag{12}$$

For every t-value in the range [0..1] the corresponding distance can be calculated

$$\begin{aligned} \tilde{d}_{a,sb} &= \|\boldsymbol{s}_a + t_{a,sb}\boldsymbol{m}_a - \boldsymbol{s}_b\|, \tilde{d}_{a,eb} = \|\boldsymbol{s}_a + t_{a,eb}\boldsymbol{m}_a - \boldsymbol{e}_b\| \\ \tilde{d}_{b,sa} &= \|\boldsymbol{s}_b + t_{b,sa}\boldsymbol{m}_b - \boldsymbol{s}_a\|, \tilde{d}_{b,ea} = \|\boldsymbol{s}_b + t_{b,ea}\boldsymbol{m}_b - \boldsymbol{e}_a\| \end{aligned} \tag{13}$$

If none of the t-values is in the valid range, the case shown in fig. 2e applies and the distance is again determined by the smallest distance between an endpoint pair and calculated as in (7). Vessels present in model A but not in model B lead to an overestimation of the mean distance, as their nearest counterpart in B belongs to a different, distant part of the vasculature. Therefore, distances are pruned above an adjustable threshold.

Although more complex and time consuming to calculate, this measure has two major advantages over one that is based on the calculation of minimal distances between centerline segment end points only (Fig. 2):

- It is independent of the end point densities in both models, they may differ considerably.
- Calculation based on end points is prone to bias with specific shifts, which cannot occur using line-to-line distances.

However, the effects are not as drastic as the theoretical reasoning for using the new distance measure induces since the high number of points in our models smoothes the expected strong discontinuities (Fig. 3).

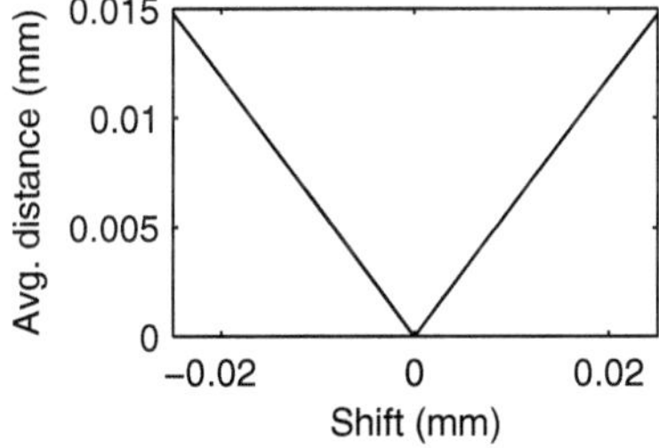

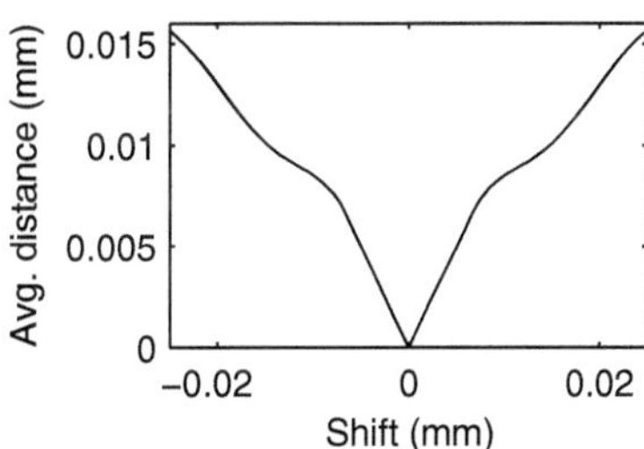

Fig. 3. Measured distance of a vascular system model with 1466 points shifted against a copy of it along one spatial axis. Left: The measure as described in this paper reveals a linear correlation between shift and distance. Right: A simple measure solely based on point-to-point distances results a comparably distorted correlation between shift and measured distance

Table 1. Mean distance and variance in μm between vascular system reconstructions from the same rat but different days (FU1-FU4) and different rats (H156-H341)

	FU1	**FU2**	**FU3**	**FU4**	**H156**	**H209**	**H316**	**H341**
FU1		10.12 ± 0.18	11.46 ± 0.19	10.41 ± 0.14	27.55 ± 0.28	27.73 ± 0.29	28.74 ± 0.32	27.42 ± 0.24
FU2	7.49 ± 0.10		9.04 ± 0.09	8.24 ± 0.07	25.90 ± 0.27	27.17 ± 0.26	26.02 ± 0.26	26.67 ± 0.22
FU3	8.51 ± 0.10	10.65 ± 0.15		9.67 ± 0.14	28.06 ± 0.28	27.85 ± 0.28	25.79 ± 0.29	26.99 ± 0.24
FU4	10.19 ± 0.14	10.87 ± 0.17	9.91 ± 0.16		27.62 ± 0.30	27.82 ± 0.27	26.36 ± 0.28	28.10 ± 0.24
H156	28.62 ± 0.31	28.93 ± 0.35	30.36 ± 0.32	28.13 ± 0.30		28.90 ± 0.30	29.90 ± 0.35	28.21 ± 0.26
H209	26.30 ± 0.28	26.93 ± 0.27	28.07 ± 0.30	27.04 ± 0.27	26.32 ± 0.26		26.53 ± 0.27	25.72 ± 0.24
H316	28.93 ± 0.35	29.58 ± 0.33	29.28 ± 0.36	27.98 ± 0.32	29.47 ± 0.32	28.42 ± 0.31		27.47 ± 0.26
H341	28.17 ± 0.25	28.69 ± 0.24	29.09 ± 0.28	28.90 ± 0.25	28.22 ± 0.24	28.08 ± 0.29	27.10 ± 0.28	

The inspection of 3D TOF scans of the same specimens on subsequent days reveals variances which reside in the range of the scan resolution, no significant distortions are found. 3D TOF scans of distinct specimens reveal considerably higher distances, so it is easy to discriminate using the distance value whether two scans of the same or of different animals are compared (table 1). In general the variance between different animals is smaller for the central brain areas. Although PCA and especially 2D TOF image a different subset of the whole vasculature, common parts are still well aligned.

4 Discussion

Our present results indicate that local MR distortions are of no concern for the vasculature-based registration of MR images. The registration of images from different scan sessions of the same specimen in order to compensate deviating head positions should be possible with high precision in the range of the resolution while the alignment transform for an angiogram obtained in the same session can be used to align functional images.

As the variance of the cerebral vasculature between different animals seems to be acceptable small, it could be possible to generate a digital atlas that encodes mean position and variance of at least the major brain blood vessels, thus subsequently allowing automatic vessel labeling.

The combination of MR angiograms with optical imaging is subject of our current experiments. Assuming OI to deliver as stable imaging as MRA, it should be possible to use 2D projections of vascular models to register MR images with optical images.

References

1. Hess A, Stiller D, Kaulisch T, et al. New insights into the hemodynamic blood oxygenation level-dependent response through combination of functional MRI and optical recording in gerbil barrel cortex. J Neurosci. 2000;20(9):3328–38.
2. Gaudnek M, Hess A, Obermayer K, et al. Geometric reconstruction of the rat vascular system imaged by MRA. Proc IEEE ICIP. 2005; p. 1278–81.

Adaptive Threshold Masking

An Extended Bias Correction Algorithm for Heavily Biased MR Images

M. André Gaudnek[1,2], Andreas Hess[2,3], Klaus Obermayer[1,2], Michael Sibila[1,2]

[1]Neural Information Processing Group, University of Technology, Berlin, Germany
[2]Bernstein Centre for Computational Neuroscience Berlin, Germany
[3]Institute for Experimental and Clinical Pharmacology,
Friedrich-Alexander-University Erlangen-Nuremburg, Germany
grenjen@cs.tu-berlin.de

Abstract. Image bias is a usual phenomenon in MR imaging when using surface coils. It complicates the interpretation as well as the algorithmic postprocessing of such data. We introduce a bias correction algorithm based on homomorphic unsharp masking (HUM) that is applicable on a broad range of image types (as long as fore- and background is separable), simple, fast and requires only minimal user interaction. The results of this new algorithm are superior to HUM, especially with regards to feature separability.

1 Introduction

MR images often suffer from inherent bias throughout the imaged intensity values. The development of specialized coils is an expensive method often not feasible for small animal research imaging, whereas the independent measurement of the bias field using phantoms is laborious and does not guarantee satisfying results. Therefore, we have to circumvent bias artifacts by means of image postprocessing. Our algorithm for bias correction is based on the homomorphic unsharp masking (HUM) [1] which needs very little user interaction – in contrast to e.g. interpolation methods [2] – and needs no specialized a priori knowledge and has less strict requirements on the imaged tissue than statistical bias correction methods [3]. HUM relies on low contrast background tissue and foreground features separable by threshold segmentation. It estimates the bias field by low-pass filtering the background tissue. In the case of rat brain MR angiograms the first requirement is fulfilled, but the separation of vessels from background tissue using only one threshold value is impossible due to the heavy bias. Therefore, we change HUM into an iterative algorithm that estimates the bias field and locally adapts the separation threshold to it alternately.

2 Methods

Our adaptive threshold masking (ATM) algorithm initially works almost identical to HUM. The user has to provide a threshold value indicating an intensity value above which a voxel is considered as foreground feature – in the case of angiograms: vessel – and will not be used for bias field estimation. Additionally a second threshold is provided that masks image background, i.e. out-of-body areas, which are not used for bias field estimation, either. Both threshold values are converted into threshold fields of the same size as the image data field, each threshold field voxel initially set to the corresponding threshold value. Then the algorithm performs following three steps iteratively:

1. Mask foreground and out-of-body background, i.e. every voxel with an intensity above the corresponding value in the foreground threshold field or an intensity below the corresponding value in the out-of-body background threshold field.
2. Create a bias field estimation by low-pass filtering the unmasked tissue. Effectively we use a cube-shaped kernel with uniform voxel weighting as low-pass filter. This can be efficiently implemented using floating average calculation along scan lines in each spatial direction subsequently, leading to a complexity of O(n) regardless of the kernel size.
3. Divide the threshold fields (not the image data!) by the bias field estimation.

Initially the ATM algorithm stopped the iteration when the distance of two subsequent threshold fields fell under a defined value. However, this makes it necessary to keep two copies of the threshold fields in memory. In conjunction with the image resolutions we use, this does not fit into the 3 GB process space of a usual 32 bit PC process, so we use a predefined fixed number of iterations instead. Usually 5 iterations are sufficient. The third iteration step is the crucial extension to the HUM algorithm. Initially in dark image areas the foreground is not masked correctly and thus the bias overestimated. However, by locally adapting the threshold to the bias field estimation it is lowered in these areas and leads to a better segmentation in the next iteration. The image data itself is corrected in a last post iteration loop step by dividing it by the last estimated bias field. If only one iteration is used, the threshold field adaption is never applied: effectively only iteration steps 1 and 2 are performed once, followed by the terminal image data correction, thus leading to the original HUM algorithm as special case of the ATM algorithm.

3 Results

Both HUM and ATM are profound bias correction algorithms that strongly improve the quality of biased images (Fig. 1). However, ATM has some advantages over HUM. Maximum intensity projections emphasize more vessels for ATM, in HUM the bias is still slightly visible and image features are clearly identifiable in the HUM bias field while the ATM bias field is much more independent of the features. Inspection of the histograms show a slightly more uniform intensity distribution after ATM correction compared to HUM. The run time of the ATM algorithm is less than a minute on a usual PC for a 512 voxels^3 data volume and allows several runs in order to achieve the best image quality.

4 Discussion

Adaptive Threshold Masking represents a simply, efficient and fast bias correction algorithm for any type of image that consists of foreground features, a

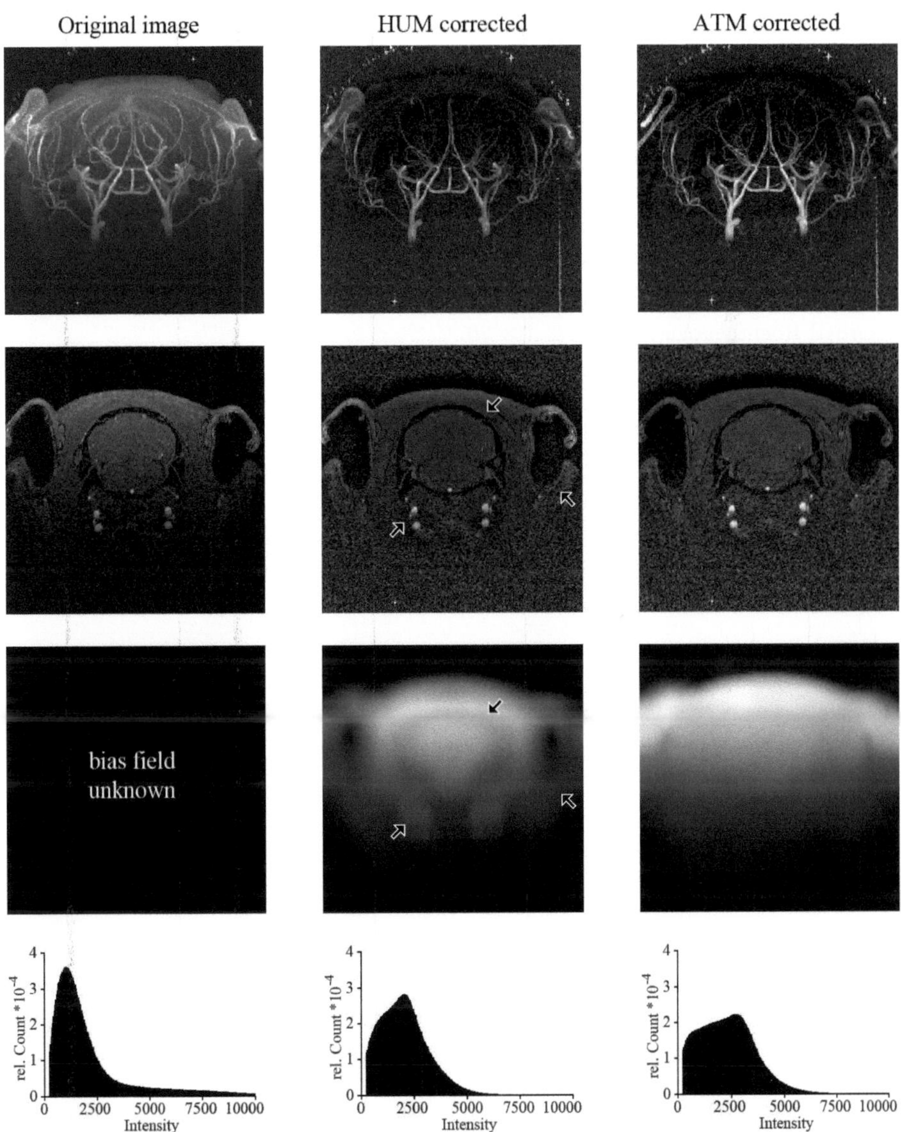

Fig. 1. From top to bottom: maximum intensity projection, exemplary image slice, bias field slice and histogram of the same image without bias correction, after Homomorphic Unsharp Masking and after Adaptive Threshold Masking. Arrows in HUM slices indicate features than are present in the bias field and indicate a faulty separation

low contrast background usable for bias field estimation by means of low-pass filtering and optionally an out-of-body background. It performs a robust and accurate bias field estimation, especially when the bias is so strong that image segmentation is impossible using only one global threshold value. We use ATM on a daily basis as a mandatory preprocessing step for automatic vascular system segmentation and reconstruction [4, 5]. This method strongly depends on possibly unbiased source angiograms and benefits much from the advantages of ATM over HUM, namely the better separability of background and foreground. Although ATM should be adequate for any type of image with the mentioned properties, so far we use it mainly for the bias correction of small animal cerebral vascular MR angiograms.

References

1. Axel L, Costantini J, Listerud J. Intensity correction in surface coil MR imaging. Am J Roentgenology. 1987;148:418–20.
2. Zijdenbos AP, Margolin RA. Correction of intensity variations in MR images for computer-aided tissue classification. IEEE Trans Med Imaging. 1993;12(4):770–81.
3. III WMW, Grimson WEL, Kikinis R, et al. Adaptive segmentation of MRI data. IEEE Trans Med Imaging. 1996;15(4):429–42.
4. Gaudnek M, Hess A, Obermayer K, et al. Geometric reconstruction of the rat vascular system imaged by MRA. Proc ICIP. 2005; p. 1278–81.
5. Gaudnek MA, Sibila M, Obermayer K, et al. Geometric reconstruction of brain vasculature from small rodents: A comparison of different imaging methods. ISMRM Berlin. 2007.

Flow Quantification from 2D Phase Contrast MRI in Renal Arteries Using Clustering

Frank G. Zöllner[1,2], Jan Ankar Monnsen[1], Arvid Lundervold[2], Jarle Rørvik[1]

[1]Department for Radiology, University of Bergen, 5021 Bergen, Norway,
[2]Department for Physiology, University of Bergen, 5009 Bergen, Norway
frank.zoellner@biomed.uib.no

Abstract. We present an approach based on clustering to segment renal arteries from 2D PC Cine MR images to measure blood velocity and flow. Such information are important in grading renal artery stenosis and support the decision on surgical interventions like percutan transluminal angioplasty. Results show that the renal arteries could be extracted automatically and the corresponding velocity profiles could be calculated. Furthermore, the clustering could detect possible phase wrap effects automatically as well as differences in the blood flow patterns within the vessel.

1 Introduction

Renal diseases, caused by e.g. diabetes mellitus or hypertension, can lead to kidney failure that requires renal replacement therapy, where early detection and treatment can delay or prevent this progression towards end-stage renal disease (ESRD). ESDR has an annual mortality of nearly 25%, and in the US the incidence rate of ESRD is 10 new cases per hour. World-wide an accelerating number of people will in the near future suffer from ESRD, with dialysis or kidney transplantation as the costly therapeutic alternatives. Renal artery stenosis (RAS) is

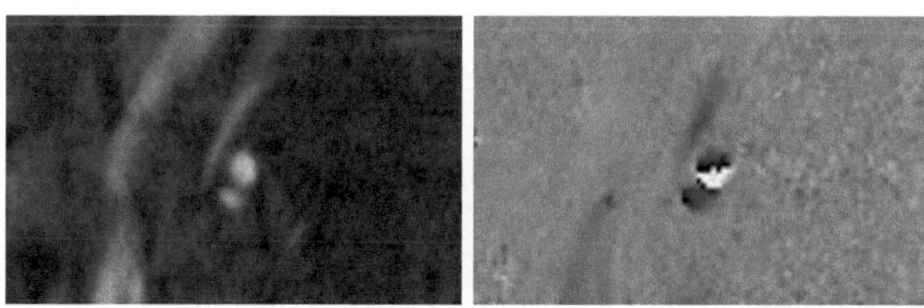

Fig. 1. Images from 2D Cine PC-MRI examination of right renal artery. Left: magnitude image with bright disc shaped region depicting the renal artery, right: corresponding phase image depicting blood flow by grayscale level (midgray level = zero velocity). Dark pixels represent higher blood flow towards the right kidney. The white region next to the dark one depicts a phase wrap effect

the leading cause of secondary hypertension caused by the reduced flow triggering the auto-regulation (renin-angiotesin) of the systemic circulation including the contralateral kidney. By time this may lead to loss of renal parenchyma in the stenosed kidney and microangiopathy in the glomeruli of the non-stenosed contralateral kidney. To be successful, a percutan transluminal angioplasty (PTA) should be performed before these changes have developed past certain limits in flow-reduction, flow velocity, kidney-size and the overall- and split-renal function. Ignoring these measures may lead to a wrong selection of patients treated with PTA and might be a reason why improvement after PTA has shown to be rather low [1]. Thereby, MRI provides a good tool for measuring these processes [2]. Cine Phase-Contrast MR (PC-MRI) blood flow measurements can be used for non-invasive quantification of renal artery blood flow [3]. During acquisition two images are generated, a magnitude image and a phase image (Fig. 1), encoding blood velocity and direction. From these images the blood flow within the vessel can be quantified and abnormalities in the flow or velocity profiles over the cardiac cycle can be assessed and RAS can be graded.

2 State of the Art and New Contribution

Blood flow quantification from PC-MRI acquisition is usually performed by manual or semi-automated delineations of the vessel area [3, 4, 5, 6]. This is time consuming and subject to operator dependent variability. Kozerke et al. [7] proposed an active contour approach for vessel segmentation from PC-MRI. A segmentation approach taking the waveform of the velocities into account and applying correlation and thresholding has been proposed in [8]. In this work we present an approach utilising clustering of time series rather than sequential processing of the images finding the vessel lumen frame-by-frame. By this, a segmentation is obtained by grouping flow patterns that are similar during the cardiac cycle. Furthermore, clustering may detect phase wraps caused by too low velocity encoding (VENC), which might mislead an active contour based segmentation. Also, possible differences in the flow pattern within the lumen, e.g. due to partial stenosis, might be detected. In contrast to the segmentation approaches reported in [7, 8], the complete flow pattern over the cardiac cycle is taken into account. In addition, manual interactions and observer variability are substantially reduced.

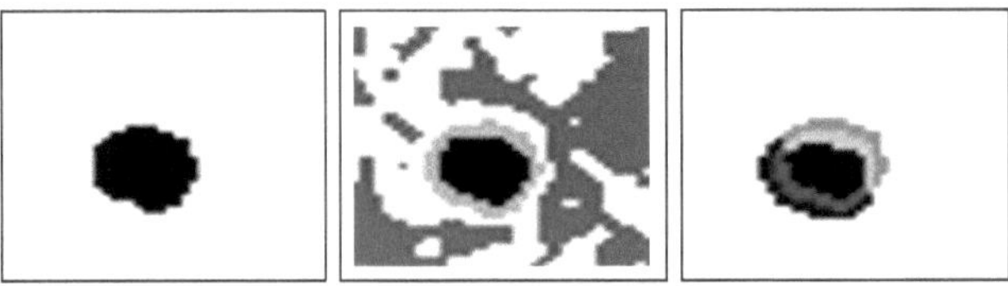

Fig. 2. Clustering results for different K. Left to right K=2,K=4, and K=12 (irrelevant background classes removed for clarity)

3 Methods

Five subjects (3 healthy volunteers, 2 patients) underwent renal blood flow measurements on a 1.5 T scanner. For the acquisition we followed the procedure described by Schönberg et al. [3]. A trans-sectional slice through the renal vessel is set ca. 1-2cm distal of the stenosis for measuring the velocities. We used a ECG gated 2D cine PC-MR sequence with TE=37ms, TR=4ms, flip angle=30°, VENC=100 cm/s. Within the cardiac cycle between 20 and 25 images with matrix 256x192 and spatial resolution 0.9x0.9 mm^2 and slice thickness 6 mm were acquired. The blood velocity is measured by (two) so called flow encoding gradients. Their phase difference($\Delta\phi$) is then proportional to the velocity (ν):

$$\nu = (\frac{\Delta\phi}{\pi})\mathrm{VENC} \qquad -\mathrm{VENC} < \nu < \mathrm{VENC} \tag{1}$$

VENC is an operator defined parameter for each examination and describes the maximum velocity that can be measured. For the flow analysis, the sequence of phase images were transformed into a 2D matrix of size # pixels × time points and then clustered using the K-Means algorithm [9]. We tested three different distance measures (standard euclidean, cosine, and correlation distance) to see which describes the feature space best. Furthermore, we selected several possible numbers of clusters ($K = 2, \ldots, 15$) and evaluated the clustering results by using the DB index [10]. Initialisation of the clustering was by random choice of initial cluster centroids and the clustering was repeated ten times. To increase processing speed the original images were cropped to a small rectangular ROI enclosing the vessel.

4 Results

In all our five subjects clustering could discriminate the renal artery from the surrounding tissue and the corresponding velocity and flow profiles could be assessed. A separation of the renal artery from the background could be realised with choosing only K=2 clusters. The analysis of the optimal number of clusters

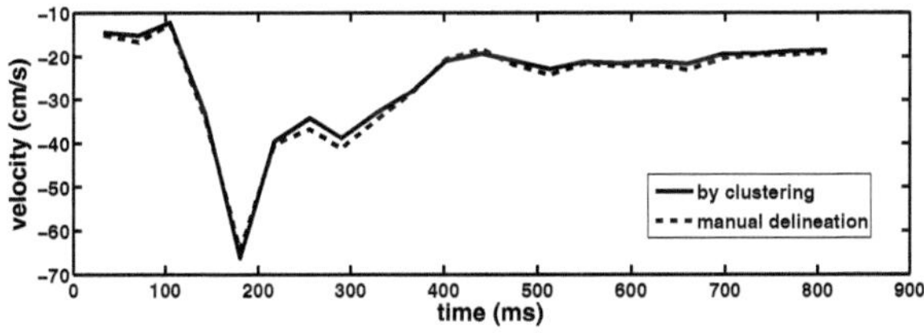

Fig. 3. Calculated mean velocity profiles from manual delineations and from clustering. Data taken from feeding renal artery of the right kidney in a healthy volunteer. Negative velocity values are due to blood flow direction opposite to the read direction in the 2D PC-MR sequence

[10] revealed that usually two local minima (apart from K=2) in the plot of the DB indexes could be observed. This occurred for a small number of clusters (3-5) and a higher one (8-10) depending on the subject and kidney. By selecting such number of clusters, the cluster representing the renal artery was divided in two or more sub-clusters (Fig. 2). Results using the cosine distance and the euclidean metric differed only slightly whereas for the correlation distance, larger regions were segmented.

In one of the data sets, phase wraps occurred (Fig. 1). This could be detected by the clustering approach independently of the number of clusters and distance metric being used (Fig. 4).

Superimposing the resulting clusters onto the original image visually confirms the segmentation results. Also, the calculated velocity profiles in both healthy volunteers and patients have a time course which are typical for those reported in the literature [2]. To better assess our method, we also outlined the vessel lumen manually and calculated the velocity profiles from our datasets. Figure 3 depicts one profile calculated from a manual delineation and results from the clustering. As seen, the two curves show high degree of similarity.

5 Discussion

We have presented an approach to semi-automated extraction of velocity and blood flow information from 2D Cine PC-MR images. This was achieved by using K-means clustering to segment the time series of phase images. Our results show that the images are segmented such that the calculated velocity profiles are similar to those obtained after manual delineation – frame-by-frame – of the vessel.

A segmentation of the images into vessel and background could be obtained simply by selecting K=2 classes. Selecting a larger number of clusters could discriminate between intra-arterial regions with different flow patterns (Fig. 2 & 5). By this approach we could also detect aliasing (phase wrap) automatically as well as blood flow patterns in the renal artery which might not be easily detected when applying whole vessel segmentation only. In addition, manual interaction

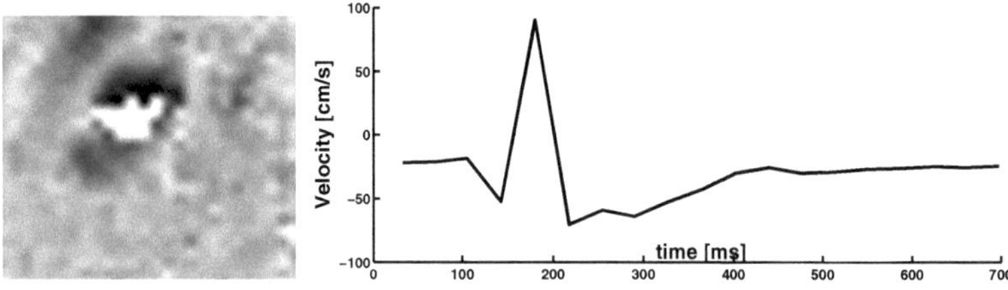

Fig. 4. Clustering result depicting phase wrap in the data. Left: white region represents the phase wrap cluster that is overlayed onto the phase image. Right: calculated velocity profile. At t=190 ms phase wrap occurs. Data is recorded in a healthy volunteer

Fig. 5. Clusters and corresponding velocity profiles. Left and right: cluster regions (white) overlayed on phase images. Middle: corresponding calculated velocity profiles. The solid line corresponds to the left cluster, the dotted line to the right cluster

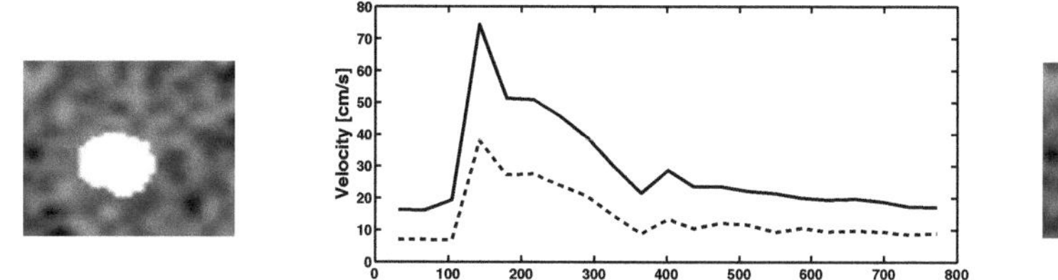

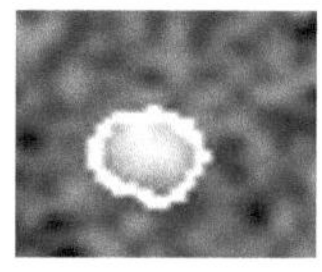

like delineation of the vessel lumen which are mainly performed in clinical practice, are reduced to a simple outlining of a rectangular area containing the vessel in a single frame. In addition, an appropriate number of the clusters has to be selected. We conclude that this approach could be a very helpful tool for clinical assessment and grading of RAS in patients with renal impairment.

References

1. Krijnen P, van Jaarsveld BC, Deinum J, et al. Which patients with hypertension and atherosclerotic renal artery stenosis benefit from immediate intervention? J Hum Hypertens. 2004;18(2):91–6.
2. Michaely HJ, Schoenberg SO, Oesingmann N, et al. Renal artery stenosis: Functional assessment with dynamic MR perfusion measurements–feasibility study. Radiology. 2006;238(2):586–96.
3. Schoenberg SO, Knopp MV, Bock M, et al. Renal artery stenosis: grading of hemodynamic changes with cine phase-contrast MR blood flow measurements. Radiology. 1997;203(1):45–53.
4. Graves MJ, Brewin MP, Priest AN, et al. Automated analysis of cine phase contrast velocity images using scored guided erosion. Proc ISMRM. 2001;9:835.
5. Bax L, Bakker CJG, Klein WM, et al. Renal blood flow measurements with use of phase-contrast magnetic resonance imaging: normal values and reproducibility. J Vasc Interv Radiol. 2005;16.
6. Florez YN, Moratal D, Forner J, et al. Semiautomatic analysis of phase contrast magnetic resonance imaging of cerebrospinal fluid flow through the aqueduct of Sylvius. Magma. 2006;19(2):78–87.
7. Kozerke S, Botnar R, Oyre S, et al. Automatic vessel segmentation using active contours in cine phase contrast flow measurements. J Magn Reson Imaging. 1999;10(1):41–51.
8. Alperin N, Lee SH. PUBS: pulsatility-based segmentation of lumens conducting non-steady flow. Magn Reson Med. 2003;49(5):934–44.
9. MacQueen JB. Some methods for classification and analysis of multivariate observations. Proc Berkeley Symposium on Mathematical Statistics and Probability. 1967;1:281–97.
10. Davies DL, Bouldin DW. A cluster separation measure. IEEE Trans Pattern Anal Mach Intell. 1979;1(2):224–7.

Automatische Rekonstruktion des Verlaufs aneurysmatischer Aorten in postoperativen CTA-Bildern

Frank Schmitt[1], Matthias Raspe[1], Ralph Wickenhöfer[2]

[1]Institut für Computervisualistik, Universität Koblenz-Landau
[2]Abteilung für Radiologie, Bundeswehrzentralkrankenhaus Koblenz
mraspe@uni-koblenz.de

Kurzfassung. Zur Behandlung abdominaler Aortenaneurysmen stellt die minimal-invasive endovaskuläre Stent-Graft-Methode eine wichtige Alternative zur offenen Operation dar. Nach erfolgter Stent-Graft-Implantation sind regelmäßige Nachkontrollen und Analysen der eventuellen Veränderung von Stent und Aneurysmasack nötig, um Undichtigkeiten des Implantats frühzeitig feststellen zu können. Während zur präoperativen Aneurysmasegmentierung bereits erste automatisierte Verfahren zur Verfügung stehen, geschieht die Nachuntersuchung heute meist durch manuelle, nicht-computerunterstützte Analyse der CTA-Aufnahmen. Das in diesem Artikel vorgestellte Verfahren vereinfacht die Nachuntersuchung, indem das Aortenlumen automatisch und robust gegenüber Metallartefakten, wie sie z.B. durch die Prothese erzeugt werden können, segmentiert wird. Ausgehend von der Lumensegmentierung wird mit Hilfe eines Shortest-Path-Verfahrens die Mittellinie durch das Lumen bestimmt. Diese dient als Grundlage für eine kurvenbasierte Reformation, durch die die Länge und der Durchmesser des Aneurysmas leicht bestimmt werden kann.

1 Einleitung

Die Behandlung abdominaler Aortenaneurysmen erfolgt alternativ zur offenen Operation minimal-invasiv durch Implantation eines Stent-Grafts. Da es trotz des verhältnismäßig schonenden Eingriffs zu Folgekomplikationen kommen kann, sind bei diesem Verfahren regelmäßige Nachkontrollen nötig, um Undichtigkeiten des Implantats (Endoleckagen) frühzeitig zu diagnostizieren. Diese Kontrollen geschehen – ebenso wie die Voruntersuchungen – in der Regel auf der Basis von CTA-Aufnahmen. Die Indikatoren für Endoleckagen sind hierbei neben dem offensichtlichen Auftreten von Kontrastmittel im Aneurysmasack ungünstige Veränderungen in der Größe und Form des Aneurysmas. Hierbei muss berücksichtigt werden, dass sich der Aneurysmasack bei erfolgreicher Isolation vom Blutfluss zurückbildet. Dieses „Shrinking" muss somit bei vergleichenden Messungen berücksichtigt werden.

Während für die automatische präoperative Aneurysmasegmentierung bereits einige Methoden publiziert wurden (z.B. [1, 2]) geschieht die Nachkontrolle heute meist noch manuell. Neben der Suche nach Kontrastmittelzuflüssen in den Aneurysmasack wird hierbei in der Regel der maximale Aneurysmadurchmesser bestimmt. Für eine genaue Bestimmung des Durchmessers ist es jedoch notwendig, eine exakt zum Aortaverlauf orthogonale Messung durchzuführen. Weiterhin ist es schwierig, in den klassischen Ansichten die Region der größten Aneurysmaausdehnung zu bestimmen. Wir stellen im folgenden ein Verfahren vor, das ausgehend von einem benutzerdefinierten Start- und Endpunkt das Aortenlumen mit Hilfe des 3-D-CSC-Verfahrens segmentiert und über einen Shortest-Path-Algorithmus die Centerline durch das Lumen errechnet. Diese dient als Grundlage für eine kurvenbasierte Reformation. In dieser Darstellung kann der Nutzer Länge und Durchmesser des Aneurysmas leichter bestimmen. Außerdem lassen sich mit Hilfe des begradigten Aortalängsschnitts neben dem maximalen Durchmesser auch Veränderungen in der generellen Form des Aneurysmas feststellen.

2 Material und Methoden

Ausgangspunkt des Verfahrens sind der zu untersuchende CTA-Datensatz sowie die 3-D-Koordinaten des Start- und Endpunkts des zu untersuchenden Bereichs der Aorta. Der Startpunkt wird im Falle abdominaler Aortenaneurysmen oberhalb der Aortenbifurkation und der Endpunkt unterhalb der Nierenarterienabgänge gesetzt.

Der Datensatz wird zunächst auf die relevanten Schichten beschnitten und mittels einer 3-D-Generalisierung des Kuwahara-Nagao-Filters [3] geglättet. Wir verwenden bewusst keine aufwendigeren Filter wie beispielsweise anisotrope Diffusion, da der folgende Segmentierungsalgorithmus wenig empfindlich gegen leichtes Rauschen ist und somit eine schnellere, parameterlose Methode zu bevorzugen ist.

Im nächsten Schritt wird eine Segmentierung mittels des 3-D-CSC-Verfahrens ([4, 5]) durchgeführt. Der 3-D-CSC ist ein allgemeines 3-D-Segmentierungsverfahren, welches basierend auf einer hierarchischen Zellstruktur beliebige Volumendatensätze in grauwerthomogene, zusammenhängende Regionen (Segmente) einteilt. Er eignet sich sehr gut für das Problem der Lumensegmentierung, da das Aortenlumen bei Auswahl eines passenden Ähnlichkeitsschwellwerts (bei dem typischen Wertebereich von -1024 bis 3071 HU hat sich 75 als geeigneter Schwellwert herausgestellt) bereits fast vollständig zu einem Segment zusammengefasst wird.

Um die durch den 3-D-CSC erzeugten Segmente Gewebeklassen zuordnen zu können, wird das Histogramm des Datensatzes mit Hilfe des K-Harmonic-Means-Algorithmus [6] in fünf Cluster (Luft, Fettgewebe, kontrastmittelfreie Blutgefäße, Kontrastmittel, Knochen/Metallimplantate) eingeteilt. Die Initialisierung der Clustermittelpunkte entspricht dabei den üblichen Werten auf der Hounsfieldskala. Die so gewonnenen Grauwertschwellen erlauben eine Klassifikation der 3-D-CSC-Segmente anhand ihres mittleren Grauwerts in die fünf angeführten Klassen. Aufgrund von Rauschen oder lokalen Artefakten werden in manchen Bildern fälschlicherweise kleine Einschlüsse einer Gewebeklasse in einem größeren Objekt einer anderen Gewebeklasse detektiert. Da diese kleinen Einschlüsse zu Problemen in der nachfolgenden Centerline-Bestimmung führen würden, werden sie über eine Nachbarschaftsanalyse detektiert und entfernt.

Nachdem nun für jeden Voxel bekannt ist zu welcher Gewebeklasse er gehört, kann ein Binärbild erzeugt werden, in dem kontrastmitteldurchströmtes Lumen Vordergrund und alle anderen Punkte Hintergrund sind. Auf diesem Binärbild wird eine euklidische 3-D-Distanztransformation durchgeführt. Hierbei muss darauf geachtet werden, dass bei der Berechnung der Distanztransformation die in der Regel anisotrope Auflösung der Daten miteinbezogen wird. Dies kann beispielsweise in dem schnellen Algorithmus von Meijster [7] durch geringe Modifikationen erreicht werden.

Das Ergebnis der Distanztransformation bildet die Grundlage für die Bestimmung der Centerline durch das Aortenlumen. Hierzu wird ein gerichteter gewichteter Graph aufgebaut, in dem die Voxel innerhalb des Lumens die Knoten bilden. Von jedem Knoten weisen 26 Kanten zu den Knoten der Nachbarvoxel im 3-D. Sei d_{max} das globale Maximum der Distanztransformation auf den Voxeln innerhalb des Lumens. Das Gewicht einer Kante ergibt sich aus der Differenz aus d_{max} und dem Wert der Distanztransformation am Voxel, das dem Zielknoten der Kante entspricht. Somit erhalten Kanten, die zu außen gelegenen Voxeln führen ein hohes Gewicht und Kanten zu in der Mitte des Lumens gelegenen Voxeln ein geringes Gewicht. Eine Shortest-Path-Suche mittels des Dijkstra-Algorithmus liefert die Centerline durch das Lumen deshalb als kürzesten Pfad zwischen den Knoten, die den durch den Benutzer vorgegebenen Start- und Endkoordinaten entsprechen.

Um kleine Ungenauigkeiten in der berechneten Centerline auszugleichen, wird diese durch wiederholtes Anwenden eines [1 2 1]-Filters geglättet. Die so erhaltene Mittelline erlaubt es, in regelmäßigen Abständen zur Aorta orthogonale 2-D-Schnittbilder mittels linearer Interpolation der Volumendaten zu generieren. Weiterhin wird ein Längsschnitt durch die entlang der Centerline gestreckte Aorta erzeugt. Während die orthogonalen Schnitte die lokale Ausdehnung von Lumen und Aneurysmasack zeigen, kann durch den Längsschnitt die globale Form des Aneurysmas erfasst werden.

3 Ergebnisse

Das vorgestellte Verfahren wurde auf 10 Datensätzen unterschiedlicher Patienten erfolgreich getestet. Dabei wurden auch präoperative Datensätze untersucht, auf denen das Verfahren ebenfalls anwendbar ist.

Abbilduns 1 zeigt ein Beispiel. Durch die nicht-orthogonale Ansicht erscheint die Aorta im Schnittbild stark ellipsenförmig verzerrt (Abb. 1a). Im orthogonal zur Centerline berechneten Schnitt an der selben Stelle ist der Aortenquerschnitt unverzerrt (Abb. 1c). Im Längsschnitt durch die gestreckte Aorta lässt sich die globale Form des Aneurysmas gut erfassen (Abb. 1c). Die Positionen im 3-D, an denen eine orthogonale Schicht erzeugt wird, sind durch eine weiße Linie visualisiert (Abb. 1d).

4 Diskussion

Das vorgestellte Verfahren ist robust in der Lage, CTA-Datensätze des menschlichen Abdomens zu analysieren und in eine leichter auswertbare Darstellung zu transformieren. Mit Hilfe der transformierten Darstellung ist die Messung des Aneurysmadurchmessers einfacher, schneller und genauer möglich. Weiterhin können globale Formveränderungen über Längsschnitte der Aorta einfach

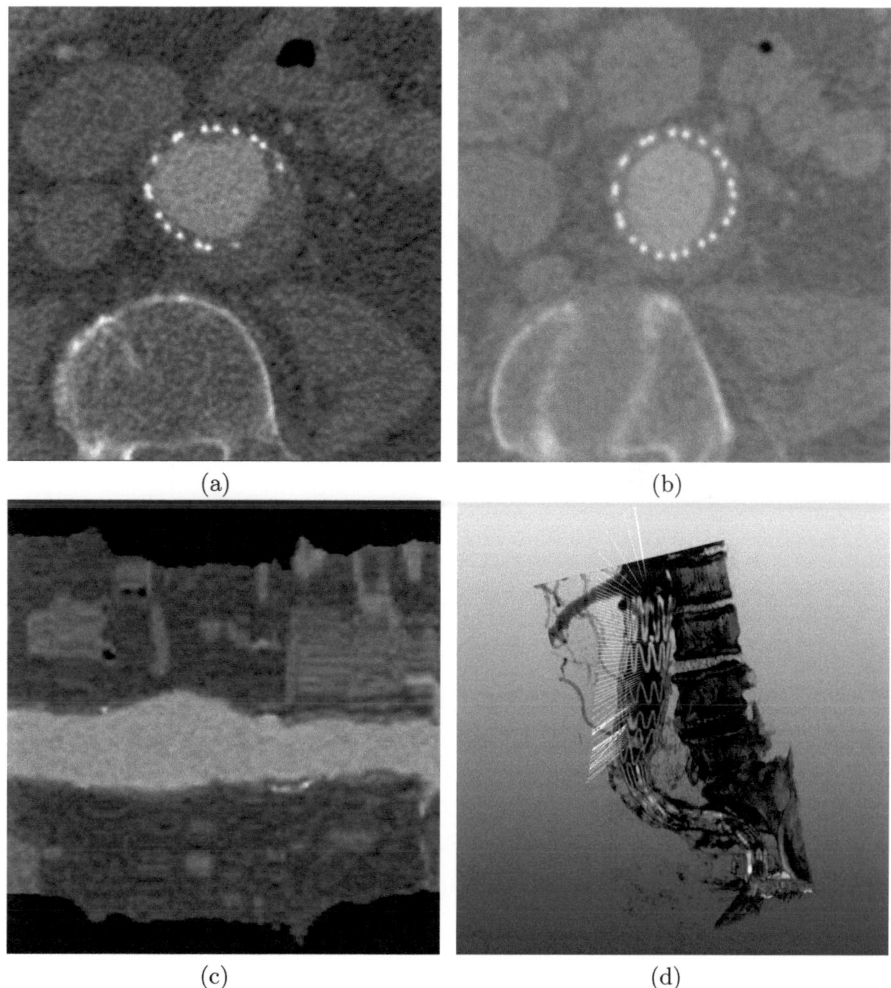

(a) (b) (c) (d)

Abb. 1. Aorta im axialen (a), orthogonalen (b) und Länsgsschnitt (c) sowie der dreidimensionale Aortenverlauf (d)

erkannt werden. Die Arbeit entsteht in enger Kooperation zwischen Radiologen des Bundeswehrzentralkrankenhaus Koblenz und Computervisualisten der Universität Koblenz-Landau, um ein Verfahren zu entwickeln, das auf die Bedürfnisse der potentiellen Anwender abgestimmt ist.

Während das Verfahren bisher nur die manuelle Analyse unterstützt, sollen in Zukunft Teilschritte der Nachkontrolle automatisiert werden, möglichst auch unter Ausnutzung programmierbarer Grafikhardware. Als erster Schritt bietet sich die automatische Bestimmung des Durchmessers des Aneurysmas an. Diese Messung kann dann nicht nur an der Stelle der maximalen Ausdehnung, sondern über die komplette Aneurysmalänge erfolgen. Ebenfalls wäre die Bestimmung des Aneurysmavolumens wünschenswert, das neben dem 2D-Durchmesser als weiterer Parameter für die Diagnostik dienen könnte.

Literaturverzeichnis

1. Olabarriaga SD, Rouet JM, Fradkin M, et al. Segmentation of thrombus in abdominal aortic aneurysms rrom CTA with nonparametric Statistical Grey Level Appearance Modeling. Med Image. 2005;24(4):477–85.
2. de Bruijne M, van Ginneken B, Viergever MA, et al. Interactive segmentation of abdominal aortic aneurysms in CTA images. Med Image Anal. 2004;8:127–38.
3. Kuwahara M, Hachimura K, Eiho S, et al. Processing of ri-angiocardiographic images. In: Preston K, Onoe M (ed): Digital Processing of Biomedical Images. 1976; p. 187–202.
4. Sturm P; IEEE Signal Processing Society. 3D-Color-Structure-Code: Segmentation by using a new non-plainness island hierarchy. Proc IEEE ICIP. 2004; p. 953–6.
5. Priese L, Sturm P, Wang H. Hierarchical cell structures for segmentation of voxel images. Lect Note Comp Sci. 2005;3540:6–16.
6. Zhang B, Hsu M, Dayal U. K-Harmonic means: A spatial clustering algorithm with boosting. Lect Note Comp Sci. 2001;2007:31–45.
7. Meijster A, Roerdink J, Hesselink W. A general algorithm for computing distance transforms in linear time. In: Mathematical Morphology and its Applications to Image and Signal Processing. Kluwer; 2000. p. 331–40.

Modellbasierte automatische Ermittlung des Gefäßdurchmessers in digitalen Fundusbildern

Georg Pisinger[1], Verena Lauren[2]

[1]Fakultät für Informatik und Mathematik, Universität Passau
[2]FORWISS, Universität Passau
Georg.Pisinger@uni-passau.de

Kurzfassung. Für die Diagnose krankhafter Veränderungen der Netzhaut ist die Bestimmung des Durchmessers der retinalen Blutgefäße sehr wichtig. Dieser Artikel befasst sich mit der automatischen Bestimmung des Gefäßdurchmessers im Subpixelbereich. Dieses Verfahren stützt sich dabei auf ein zweidimensionales Gefäßmodell. Der Vergleich mit existierenden Algorithmen zeigt, dass die neue Methode zu einer deutlichen Verbesserung der Ergebnisse führt.

1 Einleitung

Die Frühgeborenenretinopathie (RPM) ist eine Erkrankung, die überwiegend Kinder mit niedrigem Geburtsgewicht betrifft. Durch Fehlentwicklung der retinalen Blutgefäßen kann es zur strukturellen Veränderung der Netzhaut kommen, die Blindheit oder schwerwiegende Sehbehinderungen zur Folge haben, z.B. durch Netzhautablösung, Makulafalten, Refraktionsamblyopie usw. Die Ermittlung des Durchmessers retinaler Blutgefäße ist zur Diagnose von RPM unerlässlich. Mittels moderner bildgebender Untersuchungen (z.B. mit der RetCam 120, Massie Research Laboratories, Dublin, CA, USA) ist es möglich, digitale Fundusbilder guter Qualität aufzunehmen. Die Bildauswertung kann dann mit den heute zur Verfügung stehenden Methoden objektiv und weitestgehend automatisch geschehen. Obwohl es sich um Farbbilder handelt, wird meist nur der Grünkanal als Grauwertbild verwendet, da dort die Kontraste zwischen Gefäß und Hintergrund am größten sind.

Jedoch sind gerade im Bezug auf die Bestimmung des Durchmessers der Blutgefäße die bisherigen Verfahren zu ungenau. Eine Klasse von Methoden (z.B. [1]) versucht aus dem Grauwertprofil senkrecht zur Gefäßverlaufsrichtung den Durchmesser zu bestimmen. Die Verlaufsrichtung wird dabei aus den Pixeln der Gefäßzentrale geschätzt. Da diese aber nicht exakt bestimmt werden kann und das Grauwertprofil aufgrund von Digitalisierungs- und Quantisierungseffekten keine zuverlässigen Aussagen über den Gefäßdurchmesser liefert, sind diese Verfahren weniger gut geeignet.

Die Methode von Lowell et. al. [2] verwendet hingegen ein zweidimensionales geradliniges Gefäßmodell mit einem Gaußschen Querschnittsprofil. Grauwertschwankungen werden besser ausgeglichen und die Verlaufsrichtung wird in der

Approximation nachoptimiert. Jedoch zeigten Tests an realem Bildmaterial, dass dieses Verfahren den Durchmesser der Gefäße bis zu 20 % unterschätzt [3]. Zudem wird die Methode bei stärker gekrümmten Gefäßen immer ungenauer.

Daher wird in diesem Artikel ein zweidimensionales Gefäßmodell vorgestellt, welches sowohl geradlinige als auch gekrümmte Gefäßverläufe modellieren kann. Zudem werden schnelle Algorithmen zur Approximation dieser Modelle an gegebene Grauwertdaten vorgestellt.

2 2D-Gefäßmodelle

Die im Folgenden vorgestellten Gefäßmodelle basieren auf die in [4] eingeführte 2-Niveaupassung.

2.1 Definition der Gefäßmodelle

Seien $k, l \in \mathbb{N}$, $k, l > 0$. Weiter sei die Menge $M = [0, k] \times [0, l]$ ein Rechteck im $\mathbb{R}^2$ und $P = \{0, \dots, k-1\} \times \{0, \dots, l-1\}$ bezeichne die Menge aller Pixel eines Bildes. Für die Entstehung eines digitalen Bildes wird folgendes einfache Sensormodell verwendet:

Definition 1. *Sei* $A_{i,j} = [i, i+1] \times [j, j+1]$ *und* $\ell_{i,j}(f) = \int\limits_{A_{i,j}} f(x)\, d\lambda(x)$ *für* $(i, j) \in P$. *Dann ist* $\ell_{i,j}(f)$ *die Digitalisierung von* f *über dem Pixel* (i, j).

Die verwendeten Gefäßmodelle basieren auf Indikatorfunktionen auf Kreisringe und Streifen. Diese Mengen können als Differenz von konzentrischen Kreisscheiben und Halbebenen mit parallelen Randgeraden beschrieben werden. Ist also für $m \in \mathbb{R}^2$ und $r \in \mathbb{R}$ $K_{m,r} := \{x \in \mathbb{R}^2 | \|x - m\| \leq r\}$ die Kreisscheibe mit Mittelpunkt m und Radius r, so beschreibt $K_{m,r_2} \setminus K_{m,r_1}$ $(r_1 < r_2)$ einen Kreisring. Das Gefäßmodell für gekrümmte Gefäße wird dann beschrieben durch Funktionen aus dem Funktionenraum

$$\mathcal{K} = \{\alpha \cdot \mathbb{1}_{K_{m,r_2} \setminus K_{m,r_1}} + \beta \cdot \mathbb{1}_{M \setminus (K_{m,r_2} \setminus K_{m,r_1})} | \alpha, \beta \in \mathbb{R}, m \in \mathbb{R}^2, r_1 < r_2\}. \quad (1)$$

Diese Funktionen nehmen dabei innerhalb des Kreisrings konstant den Wert α an und außerhalb konstant den Wert β. Ebenso ist für $n \in S_1(0) := \{x \in \mathbb{R}^2 | \|x\| = 1\}$, $s \in \mathbb{R}$ $E_{n,s} := \{x \in \mathbb{R}^2 | \langle x | n \rangle \geq s\}$ eine Halbebene und $E_{n,s_1} \setminus E_{n,s_2}$ $(s_1 < s_2)$ beschreibt einen Streifen. Das Gefäßmodell für geradlinige Gefäße wird dann beschrieben durch Funktionen aus dem Funktionenraum

$$\mathcal{E} = \{\alpha \cdot \mathbb{1}_{E_{n,s_2} \setminus E_{n,s_1}} + \beta \cdot \mathbb{1}_{M \setminus (E_{n,s_2} \setminus E_{n,s_1})} | \alpha, \beta \in \mathbb{R}, n \in S_1(0), s_1 < s_2\}. \quad (2)$$

Ist nun $f \in \mathcal{K}$ bzw. $f \in \mathcal{E}$, so gibt es $A, B \subseteq \mathbb{R}^2$ mit $B \subseteq A$, $\alpha, \beta \in \mathbb{R}$ und $f = \alpha \cdot \mathbb{1}_{A \setminus B} + \beta \cdot \mathbb{1}_{M \setminus (A \setminus B)}$. Die Digitalisierung dieser Funktion f am Pixel

(i,j) ergibt sich dann zu

$$\begin{aligned}\ell_{i,j}(f) &= \alpha \cdot \int_{A_{i,j}} \mathbb{1}_{A\setminus B}(x)\, d\lambda(x) + \beta \cdot \int_{A_{i,j}} \mathbb{1}_{M\setminus(A\setminus B)}(x)\, d\lambda(x) = \\ &= \alpha \cdot F(A_{i,j} \cap (A \setminus B)) + \beta \cdot F(A_{i,j} \setminus (A \setminus B)) \overset{B\subseteq A}{=} \\ &= \alpha(F(A_{i,j} \cap A) - F(A_{i,j} \cap B)) + \beta(1 - F(A_{i,j} \cap A) + F(A_{i,j} \cap B)) = \\ &= \alpha(a_{i,j} - b_{i,j}) + \beta(1 - a_{i,j} + b_{i,j}). \end{aligned} \tag{3}$$

$F(X)$ bezeichne dabei die Fläche der Menge $X \subseteq \mathbb{R}^2$. Zudem werden die Abkürzungen $a_{i,j} := F(A_{i,j} \cap A)$ und $b_{i,j} := F(A_{i,j} \cap B)$ verwendet. Man beachte, dass die Mengen A, B und somit auch die Flächen $a_{i,j}$ und $b_{i,j}$ von den Parametern m, r_1, r_2 bzw. n, s_1, s_2 abhängen.

2.2 Approximation an Grauwertbilder

Seien nun für jedes Pixel $(i,j) \in P$ ein Grauwert $g_{i,j}$ gegeben. Nun soll das vorgestellte Gefäßmodell an ein Grauwertbild angepasst werden. Passung bedeutet, dass die Parameter derart gewählt werden müssen, dass die Differenz zwischen realen Grauwerten und den berechneten Grauwerten aus dem Sensormodell möglichst wenig abweichen. Aus Stabilitätsgründen wird dabei die Methode der kleinsten Quadrate verwendet, d.h. es wird

$$\phi(\alpha, \beta, m, r_1, r_2) := \sum_{(i,j)\in P} \Big(g_{i,j} - \big(\alpha(a_{i,j} - b_{i,j}) + \beta(1 - a_{i,j} + b_{i,j})\big)\Big)^2 \tag{4}$$

minimiert. Für $f \in \mathcal{E}$ minimiert man $\phi(\alpha, \beta, n, s_1, s_2)$. Solche Optimierungsprobleme können mit folgendem Satz gelöst werden. Aus Notationsgründen wird nur der Kreisringfall betrachtet. Der andere Fall verläuft völlig analog.

Theorem 1. *Sei* $N = |P|$ *und für* $(i,j) \in P$ *sei* $c_{i,j} = a_{i,j} - b_{i,j}$ *und* $W = N \sum_{(i,j)\in P} c_{i,j}^2 - (\sum_{(i,j)\in P} c_{i,j})^2$. *Ein Tupel* $(\alpha_0, \beta_0, m_0, r_{1,0}, r_{2,0})$ *ist genau dann ein lokales Minimum von* ϕ, *falls*

$$\alpha_0 = \frac{1}{W} \left(\sum_{(i,j)\in P} (1 - c_{i,j}) \sum_{(i,j)\in P} c_{i,j} g_{i,j} - \sum_{(i,j)\in P} c_{i,j}(1 - c_{i,j}) \sum_{(i,j)\in P} g_{i,j} \right) \tag{5}$$

und

$$\beta_0 = \frac{1}{W} \left(\sum_{(i,j)\in P} c_{i,j}^2 \sum_{(i,j)\in P} g_{i,j} - \sum_{(i,j)\in P} c_{i,j} \sum_{(i,j)\in P} c_{i,j} g_{i,j} \right) \tag{6}$$

sind und $(m_0, r_{1,0}, r_{2,0})$ *ein lokales Maximum der Funktion* $\psi : \mathbb{R}^2 \times \mathbb{R} \times \mathbb{R} \to \mathbb{R}$,

$$\psi(m, r_1, r_2) = \frac{1}{W} \sum_{(i,j)\in P} \left(c_{i,j} \sum_{(i',j')\in P} g_{i',j'} - \sum_{(i',j')\in P} c_{i',j'} g_{i',j'} \right)^2 \tag{7}$$

ist.

Beweis. Mit den Abkürzungen $c := (c_{0,0}, \ldots, c_{k-1,l-1})$, $e := (1, \ldots, 1)$ und $g := (g_{0,0}, \ldots, g_{k-1,l-1})$ folgt aus dem Theorem 1 in [4] als Bedingungen für ein lokales Minimum $(\alpha_0, \beta_0, m_0, r_{1,0}, r_{2,0})$ von ϕ

$$\alpha_0 = \frac{\|e-c\|^2 \langle c|\, g\rangle - \langle c|\, e-c\rangle \langle e-c|\, g\rangle}{\|c\|^2\|e-c\|^2 - \langle c|\, e-c\rangle^2}, \beta_0 = \frac{\|c\|^2 \langle e-c|\, g\rangle - \langle c|\, e-c\rangle \langle c|\, g\rangle}{\|c\|^2\|e-c\|^2 - \langle c|\, e-c\rangle^2} \tag{8}$$

Es ist

$$\|c\|^2\|e-c\|^2 - \langle c|\, e-c\rangle^2 = \langle c|\, c\rangle (\langle e|\, e\rangle - 2\langle e|\, c\rangle + \langle c|\, c\rangle) - \langle c|\, e\rangle^2 + 2\langle c|\, e\rangle \langle c|\, c\rangle - \langle c|\, c\rangle^2 = N\langle c|\, c\rangle - \langle c|\, e\rangle^2 \tag{9}$$

und ebenso leicht ergibt sich weiter

$$\alpha_0 = \frac{\langle e-c|\, e\rangle \langle c|\, g\rangle - \langle c|\, e-c\rangle \langle e|\, g\rangle}{N\langle c|\, c\rangle - \langle c|\, e\rangle^2}, \beta_0 = \frac{\langle c|\, c\rangle \langle e|\, g\rangle - \langle c|\, e\rangle \langle c|\, g\rangle}{N\langle c|\, c\rangle - \langle c|\, e\rangle^2}. \tag{10}$$

Nach Theorem 1 in [4] ist $(\alpha_0, \beta_0, m_0, r_{1,0}, r_{2,0})$ ein lokales Minimum von ϕ genau dann, wenn α_0, β_0 obige Gleichungen erfüllen und $(m_0, r_{1,0}, r_{2,0})$ ein lokales Maximum der Funktion $\psi : \mathbb{R}^2 \times \mathbb{R} \times \mathbb{R} \to \mathbb{R}$ ist mit $\psi(m, r_1, r_2) = \alpha_0 \langle c|\, g\rangle + \beta_0 \langle e-c|\, g\rangle$. Es folgt mit $\overline{g} = \sum_{(i,j)\in P} g_{i,j} = \langle e|\, g\rangle$

$$\begin{aligned}
&(\langle e-c|\, e\rangle \langle c|\, g\rangle - \langle c|\, e-c\rangle \langle e|\, g\rangle) \langle c|\, g\rangle + (\langle c|\, c\rangle \langle e|\, g\rangle - \langle c|\, e\rangle \langle c|\, g\rangle) \langle e-c|\, g\rangle = \\
&\langle e-c|\, e\rangle \langle c|\, g\rangle^2 + \langle c|\, c\rangle \langle e|\, g\rangle \langle c|\, g\rangle - \langle c|\, e\rangle \langle e|\, g\rangle \langle c|\, g\rangle + \\
&\langle c|\, c\rangle \langle e|\, g\rangle^2 - \langle c|\, e\rangle \langle c|\, g\rangle \langle e|\, g\rangle - \langle c|\, c\rangle \langle e|\, g\rangle \langle c|\, g\rangle + \langle c|\, e\rangle \langle c|\, g\rangle^2 = \\
&N\langle c|\, g\rangle^2 - 2\langle c|\, e\rangle \langle e|\, g\rangle \langle c|\, g\rangle + \langle c|\, c\rangle \langle e|\, g\rangle^2 = \\
&N\left(\sum_{(i,j)\in P} c_{i,j} g_{i,j}\right)^2 + \sum_{(i,j)\in P} c_{i,j}^2 \overline{g}^2 - 2\sum_{(i,j)\in P} c_{i,j} \sum_{(i,j)\in P} c_{i,j} g_{i,j} \overline{g} = \\
&\sum_{(i,j)\in P}\left(c_{i,j}^2 \overline{g}^2 - 2c_{i,j}\overline{g}\sum_{(i',j')\in P} c_{i',j'} g_{i',j'} + \left(\sum_{(i',j')\in P} c_{i',j'} g_{i',j'}\right)^2\right) = \\
&\sum_{(i,j)\in P}\left(c_{i,j}\overline{g} - \sum_{(i',j')\in P} c_{i',j'} g_{i',j'}\right)^2
\end{aligned} \tag{11}$$

Dies sind die Aussagen des Satzes. □

Die Werte $c_{i,j}$ können für gegebene Parameter m, r_1, r_2 bzw. n, s_1, s_2 sehr einfach unter Verwendung geometrischer Überlegungen berechnet werden. Nach Satz 1 können also die Parameter α und β aus dem Optimierungsproblem eliminiert werden. Bei der praktischen Implementierung wird auf die Menge der Zentralpixel der Gefäße aufgebaut, welche mit Hilfe eines Standardsegmentierungsverfahren bestimmt wurden. Da ein Gefäß nie ein gesamter Kreisring ist,

Abb. 1. Beispielquerschnitt zweier modellbasierter Verfahren

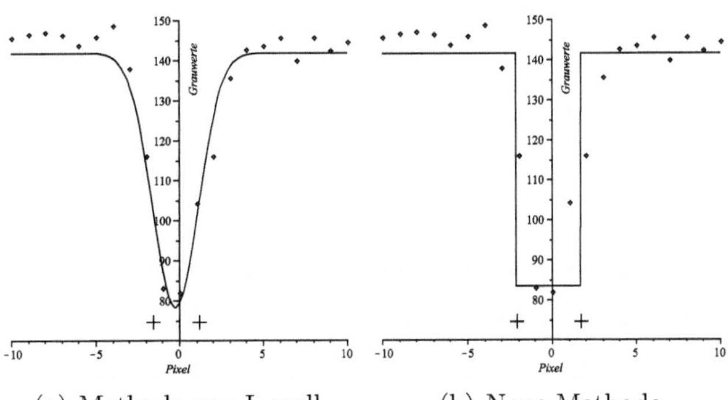

(a) Methode von Lowell (b) Neue Methode

wird die Passung nur in einer lokalen Umgebung des Zentralpixels angewendet. Ein lokales Optimum von ψ kann dann mit Hilfe des Levenberg-Marquardt Algorithmus berechnet werden. Eine vorherige Kreispassung an die Gefäßzentralpixel liefert gute Startwerte.

3 Ergebnisse und Ausblick

Zum Vergleich der Ergebnisse von der Methode von Lowell [2] und dem neuen Verfahren wurden alle Gefäße von 10 realen Bildern analysiert. Abb. 1 zeigt stellvertretend für eine Stelle die Grauwerte entlang eines Gefäßquerschnitts ($\diamond$) und die gepassten Gauss- und 2-Niveaufunktionen. (+) kennzeichnet jeweils den durch die Methode festgelegten Gefäßrand. Man sieht eindeutig, dass bei der Verwendung der Gaußfunktion der Gefäßdurchmesser unterschätzt wird. Ein Vergleich mit manuell gesetzten Gefäßrändern zeigt, dass die neue Methode ein solches Verhalten nicht mehr besitzt. Zur statistischen Analyse wurde ein gleichmäßig dickes Gefäß untersucht. Die ermittelten Gefäßdurchmesser aus lokalen Gefäßteilstücken ergaben bei der neuen Methode eine Streuung von 0.013, die wesentlich geringer als die Streuung von 0.027 des Verfahrens von Lowell.

In einem nächsten Schritt soll das Modell erweitert werden, damit Gefäße mit hellen Lichtreflexen entsprechend analysiert werden können.

Literaturverzeichnis

1. Chapman N, Witt N, Goa X, et al. Computer algorithms for the automated measurement of retinal arteriolar diameters. Br J Ophthalmol. 2001;85:75–9.
2. Lowell J, Hunter A, Steel D, et al. Measurement of retinal vessel widths from fundus images based on 2-D modeling. IEEE Trans Med Imaging. 2004;23(10):1196–1204.
3. Rassam SMB, Patel V, Brinchmann-Hansen O, et al. Accurate vessel width measurement from fundus photographs: A new concept. Br J Ophthalmol. 1994;78:24–9.
4. Pisinger G, Lauren V. Automated analysis of vessel diameters in MR images. In: Proc VIIP; 2004. p. 931–6.

Freehand 3-D Sonographic Measurement of the Superficial Femoral Artery

Dennis Sandkühler, Christian Sobotta, Matthias Samsel, Heinrich Martin Overhoff

Medical Engineering Laboratory, University of Applied Sciences Gelsenkirchen
Dennis.Sandkuehler@FH-Gelsenkirchen.de

Abstract. Visualization of vessels for diagnostics and intervention are usually done under fluoroscopic X-ray view using intravenous contrast agents, which has potential risks. To avoid this problem an ultrasound-based approach was investigated. The definition of reproducible geometric measures is important for image guided navigated implantations. Such measures can benefit from geometric body which approximate the vessels. We addressed the problem of fitting cylindric bodies to datasets by using a robust technique based on rejection strategies for irrelevant points and data sets.

1 Introduction

Generally catheterizations of vessels are made for findings of vascular diseases like vascular obliteration. Depending on whether vascular diseases are detected, balloon angioplasty or stent implantations are performed. Diagnostics and intervention are done under fluoroscopic X-ray view using intravenous contrast agents. Contraindications for the use of intravenous contrast agents are known allergic reaction, nephropathy or hyperthyreosis. However, 2-D sonography and especial Doppler sonography have already proven to visualize the vessel system sufficiently during an intervention [1, 2], avoid X-ray exposure as well as contrast agent application and this can be valuable alternative.

Three-dimensional ultrasound (3-D US) imaging techniques are already established for intra-operativ registration [3] and organ detection [4]. Since optical tracking system having line of sight problems the use of electromagnetic tracking devices for freehand 3-D US volume acquisition seems to be the best choice for this application even though position data have to be checked carefully [5, 6]. Especially, due to the absence of ultrasonic visible markers for identifying the length of balloon catheters and stent devices is problematic. In this pilot study, we investigated the problem of fitting geometric bodies to 3-D US image volumes of the femoral artery and the measurement of its geometry.

2 Materials and Methods

Three-dimensional ultrasound image volumes of the femoral artery of four patients with vascular diseases were acquired. For this purpose, a high-class conventional ultrasound imaging system (iU 22, Philips Medical Systems, Bothell, USA) with a linear 4-8 MHz probe was used together with an electro-magnetic localizer system (Aurora™, Northern Digital Inc., Waterloo, Ontario, Canada). Two six degrees-of-freedom sensors are attached to the transducer to locate the ultrasound probe position and to detect non-conformable position data. The sensor positions are recorded synchronously with 2-D ultrasound images during manually performed freehand sweeps (Fig. 1). The sweeps of the same anatomical structures are recorded several times to control the influence of small patient movements and possible investigator induced tissue deformations during data acquisition.

After recording of the image and position data, the 2-D images are segmented automatically. The segmentation process takes advantage of the colored Doppler data in the 2-D images and heuristics on anatomic plausibility of the vessel's continuity. Table 1 describes the segmentation algorithm in detail. The indices (a-d) correspond to the result-images in Fig. 2.

The segmentation results (Table 1) are scattered data from the structure's surface at voxel position $\mathbf{x}_{\text{volume}}$. Among the visual examination, for navigated intervention geometrically interpretation of segmented objects are necessary. To quantify the shape of the segmentation results and to remove erroneous data, cylindric bodies can be adapted, so that they fit to the data better than a small error ϵ. Since the points are in general considerably corrupted by segmentation and position measurement errors, the identification of the cylindric body's parameters is inherently instable. In this work we used an iterative approach to generate a robust, i.e. data insensitive identification. The robustification consists of the computation of cylindric reference bodies and the iterative discard of possible erroneous voxels. In this approach, we use a cylinder model for approximation of parts of the femoral artery system.

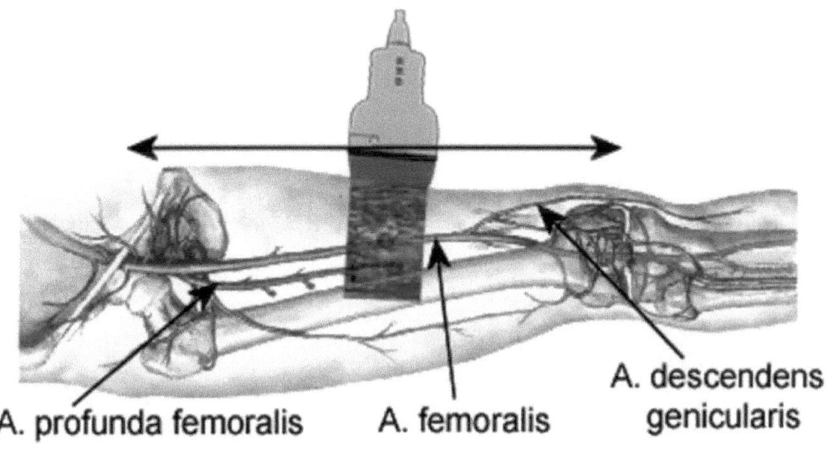

Fig. 1. Acquiring 3-D US image volumes of the femoral artery, modified from [7]

Table 1. Processing steps of automatic vessel detection

index	description
a	preprocessing: Enhance image contrast by using histogram stretching; noise reduction by using image despeckling
b	Detect circular Doppler data with radius between 20 and 60 pixels; outline the regions
c	After detecting the Doppler data border, a region growing algorithm is used to expand the segmentation to the artery wall
d	Transfer the segmentation results to images without Doppler data by using a heuristic estimation about artery geometry

N voxels $\mathbf{x}_{\text{volume}}(i)$, $i = 1, \ldots, N$ of the entire volume may approximate a cylinder jacket which is characterized by the cylinder-axis vector $\mathbf{x}_C$, the position vector $\mathbf{x}_0$ and the radius R of the cylinder. A least-squares-fit must be determined, such that the error of estimation is to be minimized. The optimum is found by discarding $\alpha\%$ of all N voxels and minimization of the functional $J(\Theta, \mathbf{x}_{\text{volume}})$ over the remaining voxels $j = 1, \cdots, N \cdot (1-\alpha)$ by an appropriate choice of the parameters $\Theta = (\mathbf{x}_C, \mathbf{x}_0, r)$.

$$J(\Theta, \mathbf{x}_{\text{volume}}) = \sum_{j=1}^{N\cdot(1-\alpha)} \left(\frac{|\mathbf{x}_C \times (\mathbf{x}_{\text{volume}}(j) - \mathbf{x}_0)|}{|\mathbf{x}_C|} - R \right)^2 = \sum_{j=1}^{N\cdot(1-\alpha)} e_j^2 \rightarrow \min$$

The algorithm is initialized by a principal component analysis (PCA) of all N voxels. Their center point $\mathbf{x}_{center}$ is a starting gues for $\mathbf{x}_0$. The eigenvector belonging to the largest eigenvalue gives the initial value for $\mathbf{x}_C$.

The following steps are processed:

- determine initial values $\mathbf{x}_0$ and $\mathbf{x}_C$ from PCA, $(\alpha = 0, j = 1 \cdots, N)$
- discard randomly $\alpha\%$ of all N voxels $(j = 1 \cdots, N \cdot (1-\alpha))$

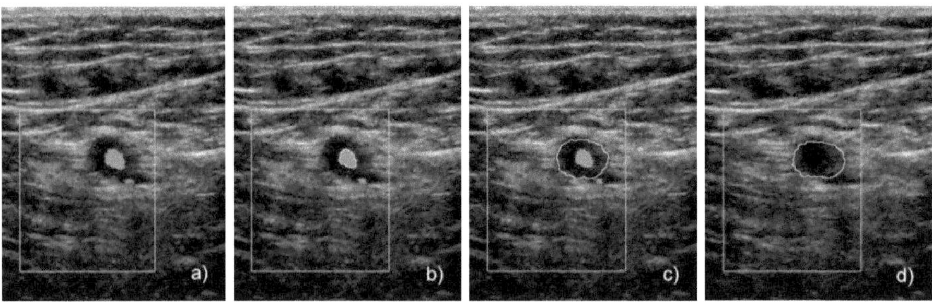

Fig. 2. Image segmentation (intermediary results): a) original ultrasound image, b) detect Doppler data, c) expand to artery wall, d) transfer to images without Doppler data

- find the best fit for all $N \cdot (1 - \alpha)$ remaining voxels by using Nelder-Mead-Simplex optimization [8]. If the minimization criterion of the numerical optimization algorithm is fulfilled [8], go to step 3, else generate new parameters $\mathbf{x}_0$ and $\mathbf{x}_C$, set $\alpha > 0$ and go to step (1)
- $\mathbf{x}_0, \mathbf{x}_C$ and R are the optimal cylinder parameters, J is a measure for the accuracy of the fit.

If the optimal cylinder parameters are found, the algorithm receives a new sample of N voxels from the volume.

To verify the approximation algorithm, corrupted datasets of β% of all segmented voxels where added to a manually corrected 3-D ultrasound volume. The corrupted datasets contain a set of normally distributed erroneous points $\mathbf{x}_{\text{noise}}$ over the entire volume.

3 Results

Image acquisition of all sweeps took less than 10 minutes for each patient. By positioning the patient in a stable supine position, the course of the A. iliaca externa, their bifurcation into A. femoralis and A. profunda femoralis as well as the bifurcation of the A. femoralis into the A. descendens genicularis can be recorded. The visualization of all US image sweeps of one patient showed slightly deformed and translated vessel shapes with a maximum deviation of 4 mm. The minimal diameter of automatically detected vessels by approximating with the cylinder model was 3 mm. The approximation algorithm is able to detect cylindrical vessels, adding up to $\beta = 5\%$ of noise (Fig. 3a) to the segmented ultrasound volume. The result are shown in Fig. 3c).

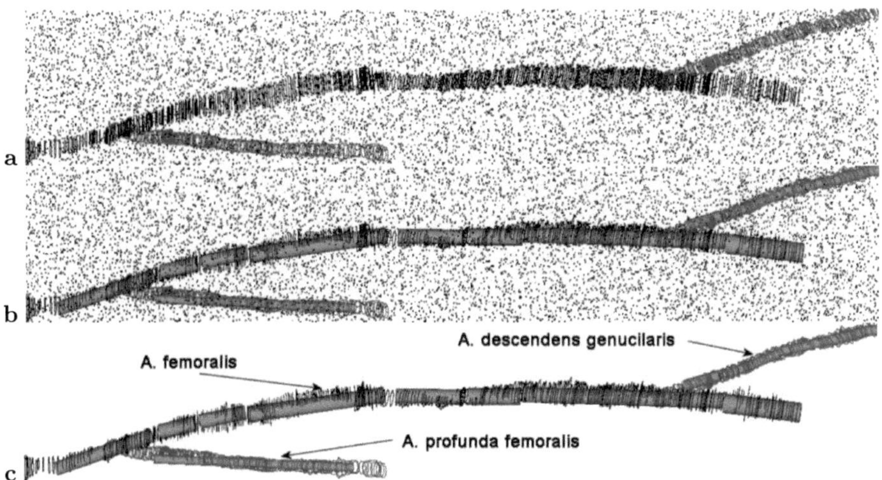

Fig. 3. Results of the approximation with the cylinder model by adding 5% noise to the data

4 Discussion

The presentability of the femoral artery in 3-D ultrasound volumes has proven to be quite successful. The vessel's geometries in two different US image volumes is reproducible up to 4 mm and can not be separated to image presentation under different acquisition orientations, segmentation errors or wanting patient fixation.The approach to define simple geometric bodies and to approximate them using data-robust algorithms seems to be applicable also for other anatomical structures and leads directly to a more robust image segmentation procedure.

References

1. Ritchie CJ, Edwards WS, Mack LA, et al. Three-dimensional ultrasonic angiography using power-mode Doppler. Ultrasound Med Biol. 1996;22(3):277–86.
2. Moriwaki Y, Matsuda G, Karube N, et al. Usefulness of color Doppler ultrasonography (CDUS) and three-dimensional spiral computed tomographic angiography (3D-CT) for diagnosis of unruptured abdominal visceral aneurysm. Hepatogastroenterology. 2002;49(48):1728–30.
3. Barratt DC, Penney GP, Chan CSK, et al. Self-calibrating 3D-ultrasound-based bone registration for minimally invasive orthopedic surgery. IEEE Trans Med Imaging. 2006;25(3):312–23.
4. Poon TC, Rohling RN. Three-dimensional extended field-of-view ultrasound. Ultrasound Med Biol. 2006;32(3):357–69.
5. Hummel J, Figl M, Kollmann C, et al. Evaluation of a miniature electromagnetic position tracker. Med Phys. 2002;29(10):2205–12.
6. Hastenteufel M, Vetter M, Meinzer HP, et al. Effect of 3D ultrasound probes on the accuracy of electromagnetic tracking systems. Ultrasound Med Biol. 2006;32(9):1359–68.
7. Netter FH. Interaktiver Atlas der Anatomie des Menschen. Novartis; 1999.
8. Nelder J, Mead R. A simplex method for function minimization. Comp J. 1965;7:308–13.

Automatic Detection of Air Holes Inside the Esophagus in CT Images

Andreas Fieselmann[1,2], Stefan Lautenschläger[2], Frank Deinzer[2], Björn Poppe[1]

[1]Medical Radiation Physics, University of Oldenburg, Oldenburg, Germany
[2]Siemens AG Medical Solutions, Forchheim, Germany
andreas.fieselmann.ext@siemens.com

Abstract. Air holes inside the esophagus can be used to localize the esophagus in computed tomographic (CT) images. In this work we present a technique to automatically detect esophageal air holes in this modality. Our technique is based on the extraction of a volume of interest, air segmentation by thresholding and classification of respiratory and esophageal air using a priori knowledge about the connectivity of air voxels. A post-processing step rejects wrong results from artifacts in the CT image. We successfully tested our algorithm with clinical data and compared the detection results of a human expert and our technique.

1 Introduction

The esophagus is a muscular tube with a diameter of approximately 10 mm. It passes from the pharynx through the mediastinum into the stomach and has direct contact with the left atrial posterior wall whereas the exact route varies individually [1]. It is important to know the position of the esophagus during atrial ablation therapy. This intervention treats atrial fibrillation by radiofrequency catheter ablation of the pulmonary veins inside the left atrium. If the power of the catheter at the contact area of the left atrium and the esophagus is too high, thermal injury of the esophagus may occur and a fistula that connects the esophagus and the left atrium can develop [2]. This situation is potentially fatal because air is able enter into the left atrium.

A segmentation of the esophagus is helpful to plan the ablation strategy and decrease the power at its contact area with the left atrium. Unfortunately, the contrast of the esophagus in medical images (cardiac CT, cardiac C-arm CT [3] or cardiac MRI) is low which makes edge-based segmentation difficult. A feature to identify the position of the esophagus are small air holes inside the esophagus (Fig. 1). They are a normal phenomenon and are visible in most CT images, although their number and sizes are highly variable.

Very few studies investigated the segmentation of the esophagus in tomographic images [4, 5, 6]. Rousson et *al.* [4] detect esophageal air holes to refine their segmentation result. *After* their segmentation algorithm has estimated a centerline of the esophagus low intensity voxels are detected in the neighborhood of the centerline. The complete air holes are obtained by means of a region growing algorithm. Two points on the centerline and a segmentation of the aorta and left atrium are needed as input to the algorithm. The two other studies [5, 6] use optic flow and deformable models respectively to segment the esophagus but do not detect esophageal air holes. Our technique detects esophageal air holes fully automatic without any user input and can be used to initialize an algorithm to segment the esophagus.

2 Materials and Methods

Our algorithm consists of three main steps which are described in the following sections and illustrated in Fig. 2.

2.1 Automated Extraction of a Volume of Interest

The algorithm confines all computations to a volume of interest (VOI) in order to decrease computational time and the number of wrong results in the subsequent analysis. It is extracted relative to a reference point $\boldsymbol{p} = (p_x, p_y, p_z)^T$ at the left atrium which is computed by projecting the center of mass of the left atrium onto its posterior wall. A segmentation of the left atrium is available because it is the primary organ of interest and always segmented before the esophagus in the clinical workflow.

We use a 2D rectangular region of interest centered at $(p_x + t_x, p_y + t_y)^T$ in all axial slices. The side lengths s_x, s_y and $\boldsymbol{t} = (t_x, t_y)^T$ are determined from a set of CT images such that the esophagus is always inside the VOI. Our parameters measured in mm and with orientation as shown in Fig. 1 are $\boldsymbol{t} = (-15, -20)^T$, $s_x = 100$ and $s_y = 100$.

2.2 Classification of Esophageal Air Holes

Most visible air in a cardiac CT scan exists inside the respiratory organs: the lungs, the bronchi and the trachea. This respiratory air constitutes one connected

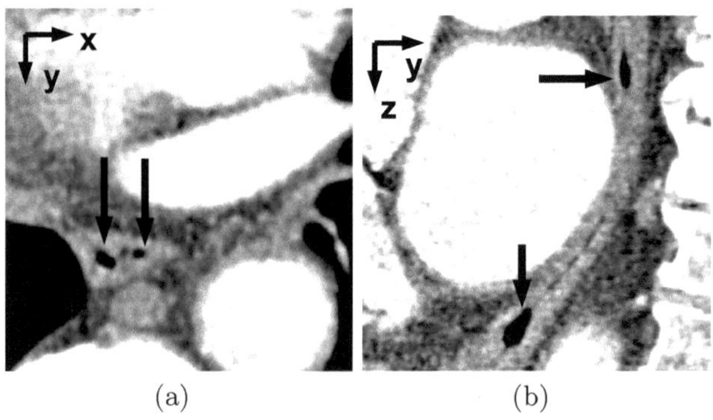

(a) (b)

Fig. 1. Cardiac CT images with esophageal air holes: (a) axial and (b) sagittal view

component. Another location in the mediastinum where air can exist is inside the esophagus.

Air has a very low Hounsfield unit (HU) value in CT images. In our algorithm the entire air is segmented by applying a threshold value I_{air} at -400 HU. This threshold value has been suggested by Kemerink et al. [7] to segment the lung parenchyma. All voxels with intensities below -400 HU are labeled as air.

In the next step the air is classified into respiratory or esophageal air. The respiratory air is classified using a 3D volume growing algorithm [8] whose seeds are placed at the left and right boundaries of the VOI at voxels that have been labeled as air. The output of the volume growing algorithm is subtracted from the initial air image. In the resulting image all air voxels not connected to the boundaries are still labeled. These voxels are classified as esophageal air. Finally, esophageal air holes are found by identifying connected components of esophageal air.

2.3 Post-processing

Artifacts in the CT image with low HU values can be misclassified as esophageal air. An important example are dark streaks due to beam hardening of the X-rays [9]. They occur very close to high intensity areas. These high intensity areas originate e.g. from the use of a contrast agent. Post-processing is needed to recognize and reject artifacts misclassified as esophageal air.

Our algorithm recognizes beam hardening artifacts by computing the image intensity histogram in a certain region around each esophageal air hole. If the histogram contains intensities greater than 600 HU then the air hole is rejected. The histogram region is determined by dilating the bounding box of the air hole isotropically by 5 mm.

3 Results

We validate our algorithm with 7 pre-interventional contrast-enhanced cardiac CT scans of patients treated with atrial ablation therapy. The scans were ac-

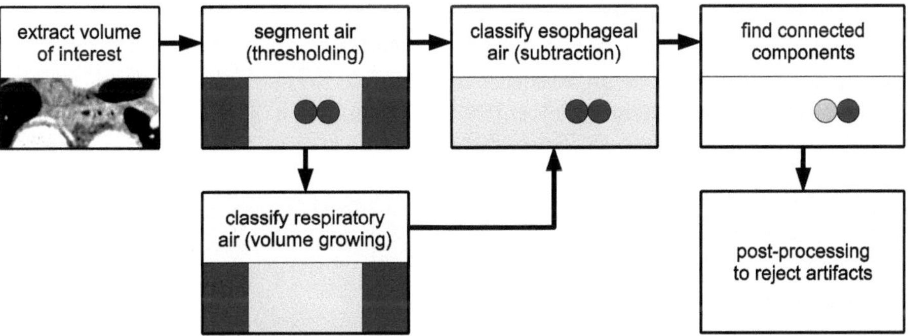

Fig. 2. Flow chart of the algorithm to detect esophageal air holes in a CT image

Table 1. Esophageal air holes detected by a human expert and the algorithm in 7 patient scans. Caudal and cranial are defined relative to the left atrial center

patient number	1	2	3	4	5	6	7
human expert							
number at caudal/cranial side	3/9	11/11	5/2	10/4	6/3	4/5	2/1
algorithm							
number at caudal/cranial side	3/2	4/4	5/1	7/0	4/0	0/1	2/0
misclassified esoph. air holes	0	0	1	0	0	0	0
number of rejected artifacts	19	16	0	25	8	41	4
minimum size in voxels	1	1	3	1	1	8	1
maximum size in voxels	6623	1859	9344	65	1694	8	3506

quired using a 16-slice MDCT scanner (SOMATOM® Sensation 16, Siemens AG Medical Solutions) with an in-plane resolution of approximately $0.35 \cdot 0.35$ mm^2 and a slice thickness of approximately 0.6 mm. A human expert labels all esophageal air holes manually and the left atrium is segmented using the software *syngo*® InSpace EP (Siemens AG Medical Solutions). We implement our algorithm in C++ using the open-source software library Insight Toolkit [10].

Our algorithm detects esophageal air holes in all 7 patient scans (Table 1) but misses air holes that have intensities greater than I_{air} which are found by the human expert. The number of misclassified air holes is very low and all beam hardening artifacts are successfully recognized and rejected. The sizes of detected air holes vary strongly. The minimum size is one pixel volume but this does not correspond to the true size of the air hole which contains some voxel intensities greater than I_{air}. The majority of air holes are found caudal to the left atrial center before the esophagus enters into the stomach. Fig. 3 shows air holes cranial (a-c) and caudal (d-f) to the left atrial center. The computational time is about 5 seconds for one patient scan.

4 Discussion

Our algorithm successfully detects esophageal air holes in cardiac CT scans and requires no input from the user. It makes use of the connectivity of respiratory air voxels which are not connected to esophageal air voxels. A possible extension of our algorithm is to use an adaptive threshold to segment the air. Because only a few air holes are sufficient to localize the esophagus it is not a high priority to detect all air holes.

The locations of air holes reveal the position of the esophageal lumen and the contour of the esophagus can be estimated using this knowledge. It is possible to visualize the air holes directly or use the air holes to initialize an algorithm to segment the esophagus.

Fig. 3. Regions of cardiac CT images with labeled esophageal air holes: (a-c) cranial of the atrial center, (d-f) caudal of the atrial center

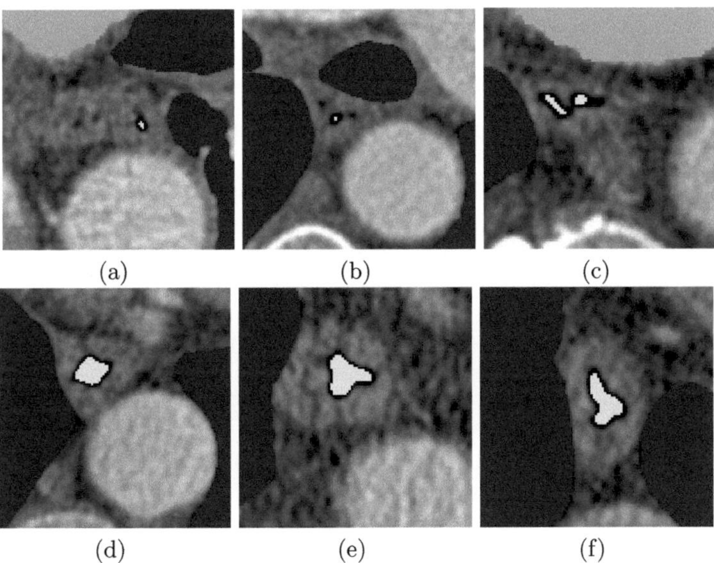

References

1. Tsao HM, Wu MH, Higa S, et al. Anatomic relationship of the esophagus and left atrium: Implication for catheter ablation of atrial fibrillation. Chest. 2005;128(4):2581–7.
2. Pappone C, Oral H, Santinelli V, et al. Atrio-esophageal fistula as a complication of percutaneous transcatheter ablation of atrial fibrillation. Circulation. 2004;109(22):2724–6.
3. Lauritsch G, Boese J, Wigström L, et al. Towards cardiac C-arm computed tomography. IEEE Trans Med Imaging. 2006;25(7):922–34.
4. Rousson M, Bai Y, Xu C, et al. Probabilistic minimal path for automated esophagus segmentation. Proc SPIE. 2006;6144:49–4H.
5. Huang TC, Zhang G, Guerrero T, et al. Semi-automated CT segmentation using optic flow and Fourier interpolation techniques. Comput Methods Programs Biomed. 2006;84(2-3):124–34.
6. Ragan D, Starkschall G, McNutt T, et al. Semiautomated four-dimensional computed tomography segmentation using deformable models. Med Phys. 2005;32(7):2254–61.
7. Kemerink GJ, Lamers RJS, Pellis BJ, et al. On segmentation of lung parenchyma in quantitative computed tomography of the lung. Med Phys. 1998;25(12):2432–9.
8. Handels H. Medizinische Bildverarbeitung. Stuttgart: Teubner; 2000.
9. Kalender WA. Computed Tomography. 2nd ed. Erlangen: Publicis Corporate Publishing; 2005.
10. Ibanez L, Schroeder W, Ng L, et al. The ITK Software Guide. 2nd ed. Kitware Inc.; 2005.

Digitale Subtraktion von kontrastiertem Stuhlmaterial für die virtuelle CT-Koloskopie

Zvonimir Mostarkic[1,2], Lutz Gündel[2], Bernd Freisleben[1]

[1]Fachbereich Mathematik und Informatik, Philipps-Universität Marburg
[2]Siemens Medical Solutions, Siemens AG, Forchheim
mostarkic@informatik.uni-marburg.de

Kurzfassung. In der virtuellen Koloskopie mittels CT-Daten werden Stuhlreste durch oral zugeführte Kontrastmittel hervorgehoben, um diese vom umliegenden Darmgewebe des Patienten abzugrenzen. Eine eindeutige 3D Befundung wird für den Radiologen ermöglicht, nachdem die Stuhlreste aus den Bilddaten entfernt und die Darmwände für den virtuellen Darmdurchflug nicht verdeckt werden. In diesem Beitrag wird ein Verfahren vorgestellt, welches ermöglicht, Stuhl- und Flüssigkeitsreste nachträglich aus Computertomographien zu subtrahieren, ohne dabei falscherweise Darmgewebe zu entfernen. Zum einen kommen dabei adaptive Schwellwerte zum Einsatz, die aus dem Histogramm des CT-Datensatzes gewonnen werden, und zum anderen werden mit einer Eigenwertanalyse der Hesse'schen Matrix Darmfaltenperforationen vermieden.

1 Einleitung

Die computertomographische (CT) Kolonographie ist als neue Befundungsmethode zur Darmpolypdiagnose entwickelt worden, da die klassische Koloskopie mit Endoskopeinsatz von vielen Patienten als unangenehm empfunden wird [1]. Bei der CT-Kolonographie wird der Kolon des zu untersuchenden Patienten vor der Computertomographie komplett entleert, da Stuhl- und Darmgewebe in CT-Daten auf ähnliche Werte abgebildet und somit nur sehr schwer unterschieden werden können. Als Folge würden Polypen, die von Stuhl umgeben sind, nicht erkannt werden. Das komplette Abführen des Stuhls wird jedoch wie bei der konventionellen Koloskopie als unangenehmer Bestandteil der Untersuchung empfunden [1]. Daher sind Protokolle für die Darmvorbereitung in der Entwicklung, nach welchen dem Patienten 48-24 Stunden vor der CT-Aufnahme bestimmte Kontrastmittel zusammen mit einem Nahrungsprogramm verabreicht werden, wodurch fäkales Material in den CT-Daten kontraststärker erscheint [2]. So ist es möglich, dass Stuhlreste im Darm verbleiben, die bei entsprechender Darmvorbereitung flüssig sind; dieses macht die Untersuchung für den Patienten angenehmer. Vor der Computertomographie wird dem Patienten Raumluft bzw. CO_2 insuffliert, damit die Darmwände nicht zusammenfallen.

Bisherige Ansätze zur digitalen Bereinigung des Kolons benutzen globale, manuell festzulegende Schwellwerte zur Stuhlsegmentierung [3, 4] oder schlagen vor, mit eindimensionalen Filtern, sog. Segmentierungsstrahlen, die Übergangsvoxel zwischen Luft und Stuhl zu erfassen [5, 6]. Diese Übergangsvoxel gehören zu den bei CT-Daten bekannten Teilvolumenartefakten (partial volume effect, PVE) [7]. Diese Ansätze reichen aufgrund von Bildrauschen und inhomogener Kontrastmittelverteilung jedoch häufig nicht aus, um das Stuhlmaterial fehlerlos zu entfernen. Zudem bewirken sie z.T. Darmfaltenperforationen oder deren Löschung.

In diesem Beitrag wird ein Verfahren vorgestellt, das die Stuhlreste aus CT-Bilddaten entfernt und eine anschließende virtuelle 3D-Befundung des Kolons (sog. virtueller Darmdurchflug) erlaubt, ohne die genannten Nachteile aufzuweisen. Das Verfahren besteht aus den Komponenten: (a) initiale Kolonsegmentierung, (b) Darmfaltenerhaltung und (c) Stuhloberflächendetektion. Experimente mit Datensätzen aus der klinischen Routine zeigen, dass das vorgeschlagene Verfahren qualitativ hochwertige Ergebnisse in akzeptabler Rechenzeit erzielen kann.

Der Beitrag ist folgendermaßen gegliedert. Abschnitt 2 stellt die entwickelten Methoden für die einzelnen Komponenten des Verfahrens vor. Experimentelle Resultate werden in Abschnitt 3 beschrieben. Abschnitt 4 fasst die Ergebnisse des Beitrags zusammen und gibt einen Ausblick auf zukünftige Arbeiten.

2 Material und Methoden

Der Abschnitt gliedert sich in die Beschreibung der initialen Kolonsegmentierung mit der Bestimmung des Schwellwertes zur Subtraktion des markierten Stuhls, der Methode zur Darmfaltenerhaltung, und abschließend der Stuhloberflächendetektion, d.h. der Erkennung der PVE-Voxel am Stuhl-Luft-Übergang.

2.1 Schwellwertbestimmung

Es wird davon ausgegangen, dass ein CT-Datensatz des Abdomens vorliegt, der den mit Gas insufflierten Kolon mitsamt kontrastverstärktem Stuhl enthält. Entsprechend der Hounsfield-Skala [7] werden Voxel v mit einem Wert $v \leq 900$ HU

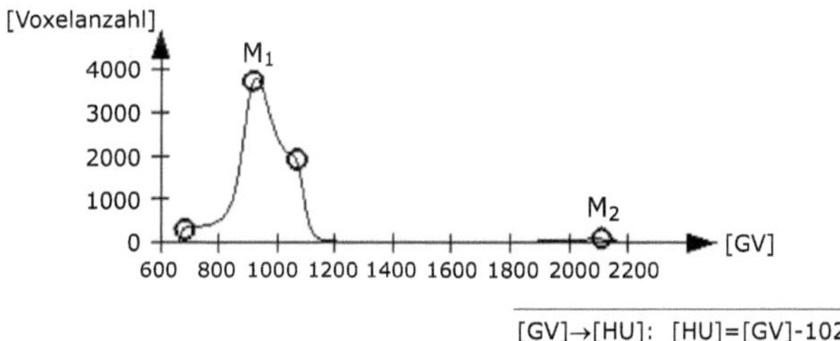

Abb. 1. Histogramm $h(d)$ des den gasgefüllten Kolon umgebenden Bereichs; der Schwellwert t_{tag} wird als Wert zwischen den Maxima M_1 und M_2 bestimmt mit $t_{\text{tag}} = (M_1 + M_2) \cdot 0,45$

(Hounsfield Units) (= HU-Wert von Gas) als potentielle gasgefüllte Kolonvoxel der Menge c_g zugewiesen. Die Menge c_g wird mit einer morphologischen Dilation erweitert zu $c_{gDil} = c_g \oplus dilstr$; das Strukturelement $dilstr$ ist eine mit Einsen gefüllte 13×13-Matrix. So ist durch die Anordnung von Luft und Stuhl im Kolon (Abb. 2.4 links) sichergestellt, dass genügend Bildbereiche zur gasgefüllten Kolon-Segmentierung hinzugenommen werden, die kontrastierten Stuhl enthalten. Aus dem Histogramm $h(d)$ der Voxelmenge $d = c_{gDil} - c_g$ kann der Schwellwert t_{tag} automatisch, adaptiv an den jeweiligen Bilddatensatz bestimmt werden, der weiter unten dazu herangezogen wird, um die Stuhlreste zu subtrahieren. Der Schwellwert wird auf einen Grauwert zwischen dem absoluten Maximum M_1 und dem lokalen Maximum M_2 im hinteren Bereich von $h(d)$ gesetzt (Abb. 2.1). M_1 umfasst die Darmwände und umliegendes Weichgewebe, welche zum großen Teil in d enthalten sind. Der empirische Wert $t_{\text{tag}} = (M_1 + M_2) \cdot 0,45$ hat sich als angebrachter Schwellwert für die Stuhlsubtraktion herausgestellt. Je nach Datensatz und Stuhlkontrastierung nimmt t_{tag} üblicherweise Werte im Bereich 200-400 HU an.

2.2 Darmfaltendetektion

Bevor die Subtraktion des Stuhls durchgeführt wird, werden zunächst die von Stuhl umgebenen Darmfalten detektiert. So wird gewährleistet, dass diese bei der anschließenden Stuhlsubtraktion durch eine Schwellwertoperation nicht perforiert bzw. entfernt werden. Darmfalten, die von markiertem Stuhl umgeben sind, können bedingt durch PVE in den Bilddaten höherwertiger und über dem Grauwertbereich von Gewebe erscheinen.

Der Darmfaltenerkennung liegt die Überlegung zu Grunde, dass die Grauwerte einer Darmfalte im Vergleich zu dem umliegenden, kontraststarken Stuhl ein lokales Minimum darstellen und über die Bestimmung der Extrema im Bild detektiert werden können. Erreicht wird dieses mit einem Filter, das mittels der Hesse'schen Matrix und den zweiten Ableitungen der Bildfunktion die Darmfalten vorsegmentiert [4].

Sei $g(x, y)$ die Bildfunktion einer Gauß-geglätteten axialen CT-Schicht. Ausgehend von der 2D Hesse'schen Matrix

$$H(g(x,y)) = \begin{bmatrix} \frac{\partial^2 g(x,y)}{\partial x^2} & \frac{\partial^2 g(x,y)}{\partial x \partial y} \\ \frac{\partial^2 g(x,y)}{\partial x \partial y} & \frac{\partial^2 g(x,y)}{\partial y^2} \end{bmatrix} \tag{1}$$

wird durch deren Hauptachsentransformation der Eigenwert λ_1 berechnet, der zum ersten Eigenvektor gehört. Alle Voxel v, für die gilt $\lambda_1 > t_{\text{svd}}$, sind mögliche von Stuhlmaterial bedeckte Darmfalten und werden der Menge c_{fold} zugeordnet. Dieses Vorgehen zur Lokalisierung von Darmfalten ist angeleht an Frangi's Blutgefäßhervorhebungs-Filter [8]. Eine mathematische Begründung kann dort gefunden werden. Im Gegensatz zu kontrastierten Blutgefäßen bei Frangi, die helle röhrenförmige Gebilde in dunklerer Umgebung darstellen, sind hier analog dazu die Darmfalten dunklere linienförmige Strukturen in hellerer Bildumgebung.

2.3 Detektion des Luft-Stuhl-Übergangs

Oberflächenvoxel des Stuhls am Übergang von Luft zu Stuhl, die wegen Teilvolumenartefakten von der Schwellwertoperation nicht erfasst werden, werden mittels des *Laplacian of Gaussian* (LoG) Kantenfilters entfernt. Dabei wird die Gradienteninformation des LoG genutzt, und nur diejenigen Voxel als PVE-Voxel klassifiziert, die in y-Richtung verlaufende Gradienten mit den größten Beträgen aufweisen. Es wird die Gegebenheit ausgenutzt, dass die flüssigen Stuhlreste durch die Gravitationskraft bedingt stets eine nahezu horizontale Oberfläche bilden und die Luft-Stuhl-Übergänge die „steilsten Kanten" in den Bilddaten darstellen.

2.4 Stuhlsubtraktion

Es folgt eine Schwellwertoperation, die alle Voxel v, mit $v > t_{\text{tag}}$ (Abschn. 2.1), als kontrastierten Stuhl aus den CT-Daten subtrahiert, indem sie die Bildwerte auf den von Gas setzt. Darmfaltensegmente c_{fold} (Abschn. 2.2) werden dabei nicht betrachtet. Ein 3D Regionen-Wachstums-Verfahren (RWV) vermeidet, dass nicht von der Subtraktion erfasste Teile des Stuhls als „im Kolon schwebende Inseln" übrig bleiben. Wegen Inhomogenitäten des Fäkalmaterials können solche Stuhlreste auftreten. Das RWV spürt sie als komplett von Gas umschlossene kleine Segmente auf und subtrahiert sie. Abschließend werden die durch die Subtraktion entstandenen, scharfen Kanten an den Darmwänden wie in [3] mit einem dreidimensionalen Gauß-Filter gefaltet, wodurch die Rekonstruktion der Mucosa und damit ein natürliches Erscheinungsbild der Darmwand erzielt wird.

3 Ergebnisse

Für die Evaluierung wurden 10 Datensätze aus der klinischen Routine mit je ca. 400-800 Schichten verwendet, sowie auch ein Phantomdatensatz. Die Stuhlreste wurden dabei in allen Datensätzen vollständig entfernt; verdeckte Polypen sichtbar und damit einwandfrei diagnostizierbar. Als Beispiel ist in Abbildung 2.4 eine multiplanare Rekonstruktion (MPR) einer Schicht gezeigt. Das linke Bild zeigt darin die typisch flüssigen Stuhlreste im Kolon des Patienten (hell dargestellt). Das rechte Teilbild zeigt dieselbe MPR nach der Stuhl-Subtraktion mit dem vorgestellten Verfahren; der Kolon ist in dem Fall nur mit Gas gefüllt. Die digitale

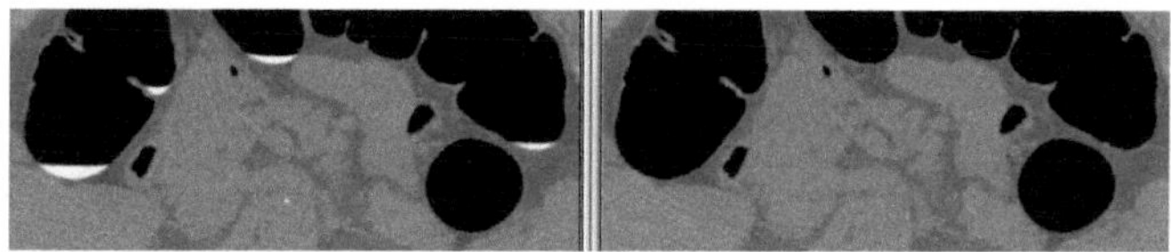

Abb. 2. Links: eine multiplanare Rekonstruktion (MPR) des mit kontrastreichen Stuhlresten gefüllten Kolon. Rechts: die gleiche MPR durch das vorgestellte Verfahren von den Stuhlresten gereinigt

Subtraktion benötigt mit der bisher nicht auf Laufzeit optimierten Methode für einen 512x512x500 (x-, y-, z-Achse) Voxel großen Datensatz knapp 3 Minuten - auf einem z.Zt. üblichen PC mit 2,4 GHz Prozessortakt, 2 GB Arbeitsspeicher, unter Windows XP(Reg TM).

4 Zusammenfassung und Ausblick

Das hier vorgestellte Verfahren ermöglicht es, Stuhl- und Flüssigkeitsreste in CT-Datensätzen zu detektieren und restefrei zu entfernen. Außerdem bleiben durch die Darmfaltenerkennung das Darmgewebe und auch kleine Polypen im Bild erhalten. Dies ist zwingend erforderlich, weil so die tatsächliche Morphologie des inspizierten Kolons erhalten bleibt.

Eine gradientenbasierte Glättung der Kolonoberfläche zur Mucosarekonstruktion wäre eine sinnvolle Erweiterung des Verfahrens, welches bisher einen normalverteilten Gauß-Filter einsetzt. Zu untersuchen ist, ob eine 3D-Erweiterung der Methode verbesserte Ergebnisse liefert. In [9] wird ein 3D-Ansatz für die Stuhlsubraktion vorgestellt, das bzgl. der Darmfaltendetektion Ähnlichkeiten mit dem hier vorgestellten Verfahren aufweist; allerdings wird dort keine Zeitangabe gemacht und die Detektion erfordert eine komplexere Berechnung.

Als nächster Schritt soll eine Differenzierung zwischen Knochenmaterial und kontrastiertem Stuhl eingeführt werden, so dass ossale Strukturen nicht entfernt werden. Das Entfernen beeinflusst die endoluminale 3D-Rekonstruktion des Kolon jedoch nicht, da Knochen und Kolonwände nicht direkt angrenzende Bereiche darstellen.

Literaturverzeichnis

1. Van Gelder RE, Birnie E, et al. CT colonography and colonoscopy: Assessment of patient preference in a 5-week follow-up study. Radiology. 2004;233(2):328–37.
2. Zalis ME, Hahn PF. Digital subtraction bowel cleansing in CT colonography. Am J Roentgenol. 2001;176:646–8.
3. Zalis ME, Perumpillichira J, Hahn PF. Digital subtraction bowel cleansing for CT colonography using morphological and linear filtration methods. IEEE Trans Med Imaging. 2004;23(11):1335–43.
4. Gündel L, Sühling M, Eckert H. Novel method for digital subtraction of tagged stool in virtual colonoscopy. Proc SPIE. 2008;6914. To appear.
5. Lakare S, Chen D, Li L, et al. Electronic colon cleansing using segmentation rays for virtual colonoscopy. Proc SPIE. 2002;4683:412–8.
6. Sato M, Lakare S, Wan M, et al. An automatic colon segmentation for 3D virtual colonoscopy. IEICE Trans Inform Sys. 2001;E84-D(1):201–8.
7. Buzug TM. Einführung in die Computertomographie. Springer, Berlin; 2004.
8. Frangi AF, Niessen WJ, Vincken KL, et al. Multiscale vessel enhancement filtering. Lect Notes Comp Sci. 1998;1496:130–7.
9. Cai W, Näppi J, et al. Digital bowel cleansing for computer-aided detection of polyps in fecal-tagging CT colonography. Proc SPIE. 2006;6144:690–8.

METK – The Medical Exploration Toolkit

Christian Tietjen[1], Konrad Mühler[1], Felix Ritter[2], Olaf Konrad[2], Milo Hindennach[2], Bernhard Preim[1]

[1]Institut für Simulation und Graphik, Otto-von-Guericke-Universität Magdeburg
[2]MeVis Research, Center for Medical Image Computing, Bremen
tietjen@isg.cs.uni-magdeburg.de

Abstract. In the following we will describe concept and realization of the Medical Exploration Toolkit – the METK. The METK is designed for loading, visualizing and exploring segmented medical data sets. It is a framework of several modules based on the free MeVisLab, a development environment for medical image processing and visualization. The framework is platform-independent and freely available. We will also present several different applications, developed with the METK.

1 Introduction

For many tasks in computer-aided medical visualization, it is not sufficient to display just one anatomical structure or to perform a simple volume rendering. Building applications for complex case analysis with advanced visualization techniques is still an extensive job. Low level libraries like VTK [1] are very flexible, but the application development for supporting a special task is very time consuming. Julius [2] and VolV [3] are based on VTK and Qt and provide a faster application development. However, the programming environment is still C++, thus, substantial programming knowledge is still required.

MeVisLab [4] provides an easy to learn, script based framework for medical image processing and visualization, based on modular visual programming. Among other libraries, VTK and Qt are also integrated. Thus, a full image processing and visualization pipeline can be used for application development without deep programming knowledge.

Currently, there is no general communication or data standard available in public with MeVisLab. Hence, newly designed visualization or exploration techniques need to be adapted for each application. Also simple tasks such as loading specific patient image data or the visualization of segmented structures require a deep knowledge of the used techniques. The Application Frame (AppFrame) facilitates the integration and testing of new algorithms and the development of application prototypes with MeVisLab that can be used in clinical environments [5]. While AppFrame indeed addresses generic issues such as DICOM image import and export, user-management, reporting, and documentation functionality, it does not provide advanced visualization and exploration techniques. In addition, the AppFrame is not available in public.

Hence, we developed the Medical Exploration Toolkit (METK) as a comprehensive collection of basic and advanced visualization and exploration techniques with a common communication protocol. These underlying structures are invisible for application developers. Thus, they can focus on application requirements and come up with complex applications using just a few METK modules. The METK is platform-independent and will be freely available at the end of 2007.

2 Materials and Methods

The METK is composed of five different layers: communication layer, database layer, visual processing layer, visualization layer and exploration layer (Fig. 2). For each layer, several METK modules are available that can be combined to networks, building up an application.

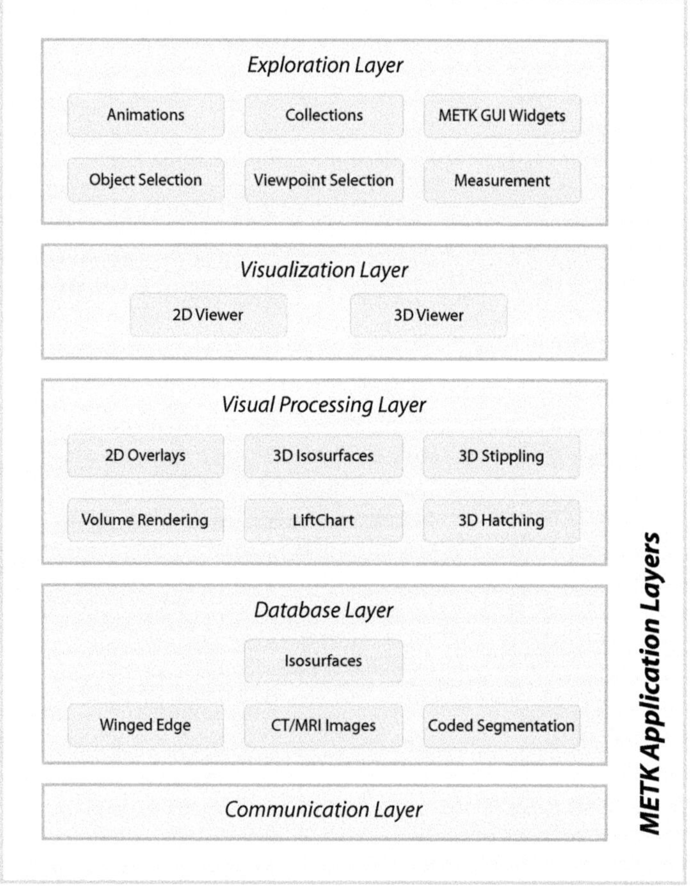

Fig. 1. Layer schema of the METK

The *communication layer* enables all modules to share events with other modules and to be notified about global events, like loading or closing a case. A case consists of original CT or MRI datasets with additional segmentation masks, descriptions about their anatomical affiliation and patient information. Also, visualization parameters may be stored. All METK modules can access and manipulate these data. So, if one module changes the color of a structure, all other METK modules may react on this event and may adjust their own settings. The main visualization properties are always shared to provide a synchronized visualization in all modes and viewers.

The *database layer* contains all necessary data: image data and segmentations masks, as well as isosurfaces and their winged edge data. The isosurfaces are generated by default, because they are needed at most. All other data may be made available optionally, if one visualization module needs it. Since the computation of an isosurface may be computationally expensive for some structures, it is possible to compute those surface only if necessary, e.g., if they are treated as visible. For setting up a new case or expanding an existing one, there are still several modules available in MeVisLab. The METK does not provide particular segmentation algorithms, like LiveWire or Watershed, that are already present in MeVisLab. It just provides functions for storing the retrieved segmentation information in a METK readable manner. The entire case must be provided in form of an XML file. The case data contains information about the segmented structures (e.g., type and color). The image data itself may be provided in one of many standard formats like DICOM, Analyze or RAW.

The *visual processing layer* interprets the data. Several visualization techniques are implemented, which are not part of the MeVisLab library. Isosurfaces may be displayed by shaded surfaces, silhouettes, stippling or hatching. Image data may be displayed as orthogonal 2D slices or as volume rendering. In both modes, the segmentation masks may be displayed by colored overlays or by tagged volume rendering. More advanced techniques like displaying LiftCharts [6] or distances to other structures are also available in 2D and 3D [7]. Every visualization technique may be turned on or off for every single structure. Thus, it is possible to render the whole scene with isosurfaces, but the pathologic structures with an additional silhouette.

The *visualization layer* displays and combines the visualization of each structure provided by the visual processing layer. It is possible to combine different visualization techniques in separated 2D and 3D viewers as well as in combined 2D/3D viewers. Simple screen shot facilities are also provided.

The *exploration layer* contains high level exploration techniques. The entire state of the METK database may be stored along with a short comment, a caption, a small thumbnail and a screen shot, referred to as a *collection*. A collection is later accessible for further explorations or presentations. Furthermore, the datasets may be explored by using automatically generated animations [8]. Those animations are described in a high-level manner and can be automatically reused for many similar cases. The development of application interfaces is supported with well designed METK widgets on the basis of Qt, e.g., for structure lists or panels to change visualization parameters. The navigation in 3D is supported by advanced techniques for automatic viewpoint selection [9], by intelligent object selection algorithms (if multiple semi-transparent structures are overlapping each other) and by facilities for structure measurement.

Only the communication and database layers are mandatory. All other modules are optional. However, it is possible to combine the functionalities of different modules. For example, it is possible to smoothly switch from one collection or the current viewing state to another collection by using animations.

We also developed a new technique for the efficient management of segmentation masks. Normally, segmentation masks of structures are saved in single files for each structure. This results in extensive memory consumption, because for complex operations like combined 2D overlay visualization of multiple structures, all segmentation masks needs to be hold in memory. To avoid that, a *coded segmentation* module was developed. The coded segmentation combines all segmentation masks derived from the same image in only one image. Each voxel value represents a combination of structures that the voxel belongs to. The information of relation between voxel values and belonging structures is stored in the case. The coded segmentation is especially useful for liver surgery, where all segmented structures are overlapping each other (e.g., tumor, Couinaud segment and vessels).

3 Results

As shown in Fig. 3(a), only four modules are necessary to load and display a spine case dataset with 34 different structures. The METKManager loads the case data and provides the obligatory isosurface data (Communication and Database Layer). METKIsosurface renders the isosurfaces with shaded surfaces (Visual Processing Layer) and the METKViewer3D finally displays the shaded isosurfaces (Visualization Layer). The METKStructureGroupBrowser enables the user to show or hide the different groups of structures or separate structures (Exploration Layer).

Currently, two applications based on METK are published, while more are in a pre-release development state. The NeckSurgeryPlanner [7] is a software assistant for pre-operative planning and visualization of neck dissections (Fig. 3(b)). The LiverSurgeryTrainer [10] is a training system to learn specific tasks for liver donor transplantations and tumor resections.

4 Discussion

The METK helps to develop basic applications very fast. It provides basic facilities like case management as well as advanced visualization and exploration techniques like stippling or viewpoint selection. No programming knowledge is necessary to set up high level applications. The resulting applications are as slim as possible, because the basic database and visualization layers are optional. The METK is platform-independent and will be freely available at www.metk.net.

Fig. 2. (a) Network of an application to explore segmented structures in 3D and to change their visibility. (b) A screen shot of the NeckSurgeryPlanner

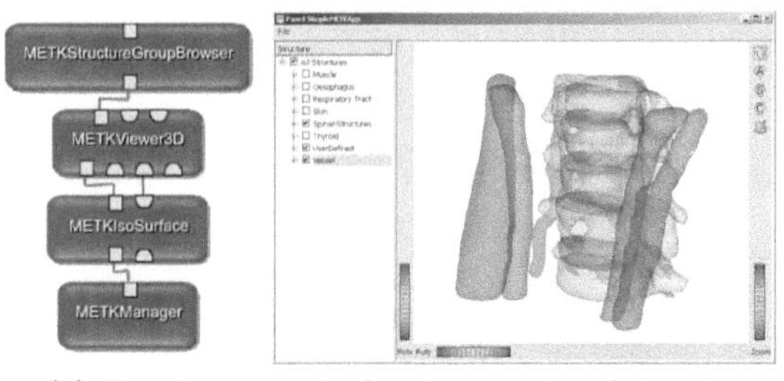

(a) Simple network showing a spine dataset.

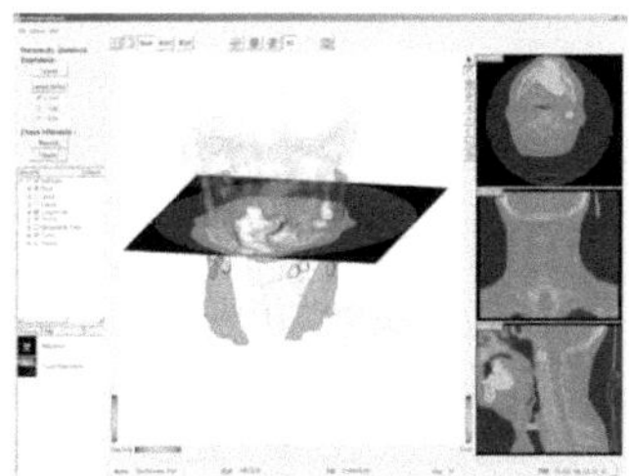

(b) NeckSurgeryPlanner

A great deal of work still needs to be done. A kind of METK self-management would be helpful. Some modules need the guaranteed existence of another, for example, the animation module needs a 3D viewer to render. When developing complex applications, the separation between case and application data is still a problem. For an application with multiple viewers, the viewer parameterization should be stored in the case, like image windowing information in DICOM, or separately, because it is undefined on loading the case in another application.

Acknowledgement. This work was supported by the BMBF in the framework of the SOMIT-FUSION project (FKZ 01|BE 03B) and by the Deutsche Forschungsgemeinschaft (DFG) (Priority Programme 1124, PR 660/3-1).

References

1. Kitware Inc . VTK Home Page; 2007. http://www.vtk.org.
2. Keeve E, Jansen T, Krol Z, et al. JULIUS: An extendable software framework for surgical planning and image-guided navigation. Proc MICCAI. 2001; p. 1336–7.
3. Pfeifle, M et al . VolV: Eine OpenSource-Plattform für die medizinische Visualisierung. In: Proc. CURAC; 2007. p. 193–6.
4. MeVis Research. MeVisLab Home Page; 2007. http://www.mevislab.de.
5. Rexilius J, Kuhnigk JM, Hahn HK, et al. An application framework for rapid prototyping of clinically applicable software assistants. In: GI Jahrestagung; 2006. p. 522–8.
6. Tietjen C, Meyer B, Schlechtweg S, et al. Enhancing Slice-based Visualizations of Medical Volume Data. In: EuroVis; 2006. p. 123–30.
7. Tietjen C, Preim B, Hertel I, et al. A Software-assistant for pre-operative planning and visualization of neck dissections. In: Proc CURAC; 2006. p. 176–7.
8. Mühler K, Bade R, Preim B. Adaptive script based animations for intervention planning. Proc MICCAI. 2006; p. 478–85.
9. Mühler K, Neugebauer M, Tietjen C, et al. Viewpoint selection for intervention planning. In: EuroVis; 2007. p. 267–74.
10. Cordes J, Mühler K, Preim B. Die Konzeption des LiverSurgery-Trainers. In: GI-Jahrestagung; 2006. p. 514–21.

GridIJ
Eine dynamische Grid Service Architektur für Bildverarbeitung

Alexander Frank, Rainer Stotzka, Thomas Jejkal, Volker Hartmann, Michael Sutter, Nicole Ruiter, Michael Zapf

Forschungszentrum Karlsruhe, Institut für Prozessdatenverarbeitung und Elektronik
alexander.frank@ipe.fzk.de

Kurzfassung. Die vorgestellte Architektur erleichtert wissenschaftlichen Benutzern den Zugriff auf Rechenkapazitäten innerhalb eines Grid ohne Vorkenntnisse der zugrundeliegenden Techniken. GridIJ ist eine Referenzimplementierung für die Bildverarbeitung. Dem Benutzer wird eine grafische Oberfläche bereitgestellt, die einen einfachen Zugriff auf Bildverarbeitungsalgorithmen in einem Grid erlaubt. Mit einem Java Interface kann die Funktionalität erweitert werden. Um die Architektur einzurichten sind zwei zusätzliche Web-Services in einem GT4 Container notwendig. Tests zeigen, dass die Architektur einen hohen Leistungsgewinn im Vergleich zur Ausführung auf einem Einzelplatzrechner ermöglicht.

1 Einleitung

Die Anforderungen an die Rechenkapazität in der medizinischen Bildverarbeitung steigen stetig an. Zum Beispiel sind in der klinischen Praxis, bei der Registrierung von Volumen, hunderte von zeitintensiven Einzelregistrierungen nötig.

Es gibt diverse Möglichkeiten diese Einzelregistrierungen auf mehrere Rechner zu verteilen um die Ausführungszeit zu verringern. Eine davon ist der Einsatz von Grid Technologie. Hierbei werden mehrere Rechner in einem Netzwerk über eine Middleware verbunden. Aus diesem Verbund werden freie Rechenkapazitäten für die Bearbeitung der Aufgabe genutzt. Der Benutzer benötigt dazu allerdings zusätzliches Wissen über die eingesetzte Technologie.

Es existieren bereits mehrere Ansätze welche die Arbeit mit einem Grid erleichtern sollen [1, 2, 3]. Die Erweiterung der Funktionalität benötigt aber immer noch viel Fachwissen und entsprechende administrative Rechte.

Die Grid-Middleware GT4 [4] bietet die Möglichkeit Web-Services bereitzustellen, in denen wissenschaftliche Funktionen realisiert werden können. Für die Integration neuer Web-Services in GT4 sind administrative Rechte auf dem Server notwendig. Dies ist selten für alle Mitarbeiter erwünscht. Die Installation eines neuen Web-Service macht es außerdem notwendig den GT4 Container neu zu starten und damit laufende Verarbeitungen anderer Benutzer zu unterbrechen.

Die Universität Marburg stellt zur Lösung dieses Problems den Hot Deployment Service (HDS) [5] bereit. Mit dessen Hilfe ist es möglich Web-Services dynamisch in einen laufenden GT4 Container einzubinden.

Das Ziel dieser Arbeit ist der Aufbau einer serviceorientierten Architektur, die Funktionen zur Bildverarbeitung bereitstellt und dynamisch erweitert werden kann. Benutzern, die neue Funktionalität erstellen wollen, soll dies ohne zusätzliches Wissen über die zugrundeliegende Technik ermöglicht werden.

2 Material und Methoden

GridIJ ist die Referenzimplementierung der o.g. Architektur. Als Grundlage für GridIJ dient die Bildverarbeitungssoftware ImageJ [6]. Mit ihr ist es möglich dem Benutzer eine interaktive Benutzeroberfläche auf der Clientseite und eine Sammlung von Bildverarbeitungsmethoden auf der Serverseite bereitzustellen. Dem Benutzer wird so ein einfacher Weg zur Beschleunigung der Bildverarbeitung bereit. Dafür benötigt er keine Kenntnisse über die zugrundeliegende Technik. Die Architektur besteht hauptsächlich aus drei Komponenten (Abb. 1):

Die GT4 Worker Nodes stellen die Rechenkapazität bereit. Jeder GT4 Worker Node beinhaltet mindestens einen GT4 Container, der durch den HDS und den GridNodeMonitor Service (GNMS) zusätzliche Funktionalität erhält. Der GNMS wird zur Ermittlung der Auslastung eingesetzt. Auf dem GT4 Worker Node wird per HDS ein Web-Service, genannt IJPlugin Service, installiert. Dieser Web-Service ist eine Laufzeitumgebung in der die Bildverarbeitung in Form von GridPlugins durchgeführt wird.

Ein GridPlugin ist ein Javaprogramm, das den Bildverarbeitungsalgorithmus eines Benutzers beinhaltet. Hierzu sind lediglich zwei Methoden zu implementieren.

Die *setupPlugin* Methode übergibt die Bilder an das GridPlugin. In der *run-Plugin* Methode wird die Bildverarbeitung durchgeführt. Als Argument erhält die Methode ein Properties Objekt mit den Parametern des GridPlugins.

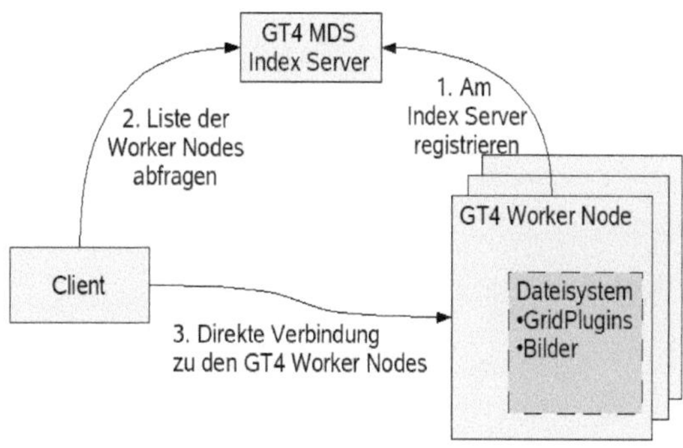

Abb. 1. Komponenten der Architektur mit initialem Verbindungsaufbau

Listing 83.1. Das GridPlugin Interface besteht aus zwei Methoden, in welche die Bildverarbeitungsfunktionen implementiert werden

```
public interface GridPlugin{
  public void setupPlugin(ImagePlus[] imgp);
  public String runPlugin(Properties arg);
}
```

Eine weitere Aufgabe des IJPlugin Service ist die Verwaltung der Daten auf dem GT4 Worker Node – einschließlich des Datentransfers.

Der GT4 MDS Index Server dient als Informationsspeicher. Er enthält die Adressen der verfügbaren GT4 Worker Nodes. Das bedeutet, dass sich sämtliche GT4 Worker Nodes zu Beginn am GT4 MDS Index Server registrieren müssen. Zur Erfüllung der Aufgabe wird das GT4 Monitoring and Discovery System (MDS) [7] eingesetzt.

Der Client stellt die Schnittstelle für den Benutzer bereit. Er verteilt die Daten selbstständig auf die verbundenen GT4 Worker Nodes. Des weiteren ist er für die Installation des IJPlugin Service zuständig. Die Verbindung zu den GT4 Worker Nodes stellt der Client nach folgendem Schema her:

1. Es wird eine Anfrage an den GT4 MDS Index Server gestellt, um eine Liste der verfügbaren GT4 Worker Nodes zu erhalten.
2. An den GNMS jedes GT4 Worker Nodes wird eine Anfrage zur Ermittlung der Auslastung gestellt.
3. Aus diesen Informationen wird eine Rangliste generiert, die es erlaubt die GT4 Worker Nodes mit der geringsten Auslastung zu priorisieren.
4. Ist die Verbindung hergestellt wird die Laufzeitumgebung in Form des IJPlugin Services installiert.

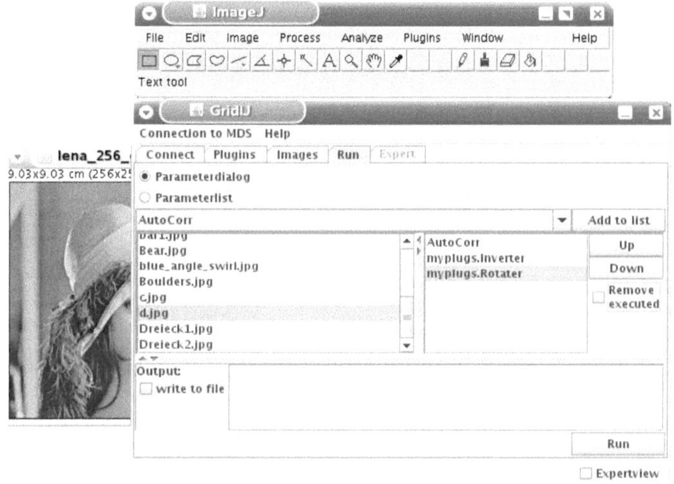

Abb. 2. Grafische Oberfläche von GridIJ mit geöffnetem run-Register

5. Der Benutzer gibt an welche Daten und GridPlugins er auf die GT Worker Nodes transferieren möchte.
6. Die GridPlugins werden auf der Clientseite zu einem linearen Workflow zusammengestellt und auf den GT4 Worker Nodes abgearbeitet.

Für den einfachen Zugang zur Architektur wird dem Benutzer von GridIJ eine grafische Oberfläche (Abbildung 2) zur interaktiven Bildverarbeitung bereitgestellt. Mit Hilfe dieser kann der Benutzer mit der Architektur interagieren indem er einen Workflow erstellt, diesen auf dem Grid ausführt und die Ergebnisse im Anschluss daran herunterlädt.

3 Ergebnisse

Zur Evaluierung der Architektur wurde ein Registrierungsalgorithmus in ein GridPlugin portiert. Die Portierung von dieser Standalone-Anwendung in ein GridPlugin dauerte weniger als zehn Minuten.

Der Algorithmus hat eine Verarbeitungszeit von ca. fünf Sekunden pro Bild. Dies wurde absichtlich so gewählt um den zusätzlichen Verwaltungsaufwand der Architektur zu untersuchen.

Die Evaluierung wurde auf einem Testbed von 16 GT4 Worker Nodes durchgeführt. Als Datensatz wurden 128 Bilder, mit einer Größe von jeweils 196 KByte, benutzt. Jeder Test wurde viermal ausgeführt und die Verarbeitungszeiten gemittelt. Die Zeiten wurden auf der Clientseite gemessen, daher werden sie vom langsamsten GT4 Worker Nodes bestimmt.

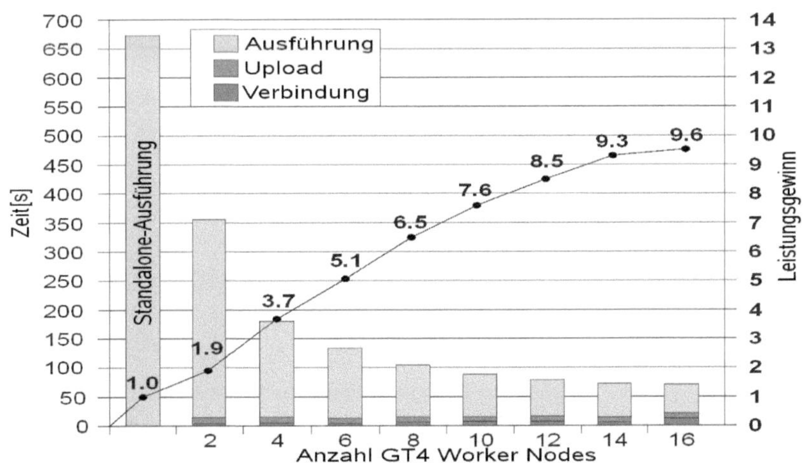

Abb. 3. Leistungsgewinn des Bildregistrierungsalgorithmus durch GridIJ

4 Diskussion und Schlussfolgerung

Der von der Architektur produzierte Verwaltungsaufwand beeinflusst die Verarbeitungszeit nur gering. Beim Umstieg vom Einzelplatzrechner auf ein Grid mit zwei GT4 Worker Nodes ist es bereits möglich die Verarbeitungszeit annähernd zu halbieren. Dieser Leistungsgewinn nimmt bei steigender Zahl der GT4 Worker Nodes durch den erhöhten Verwaltungsaufwand ab. In diesem Szenario kann man erkennen, dass der Leistungsgewinn ab 16 GT4 Worker Nodes, durch die geringe Laufzeit des Algorithmus, nur noch geringfügig zunimmt (Abbildung 3).

Es konnte somit gezeigt werden, dass die vorgestellte Architektur im Stande ist Bildverarbeitungsalgorithmen ohne zusätzlichen Aufwand für den Benutzer zu beschleunigen. Darüber hinaus kann sie auf weitere Problemstellungen, durch die Möglichkeit der einfachen Erweiterbarkeit der Funktionalität, angewandt werden. Für den Benutzer ist es dabei transparent auf welchen GT4 Worker Nodes seine Berechnungen durchgeführt werden. Er interagiert nur mit der grafischen Benutzeroberfläche von GridIJ.

Momentan wird der Zugriff auf die entstandene Implementierung verallgemeinert, so dass die Architektur ohne größere Schwierigkeiten auch in Programme wie MatLab, LabVIEW und Octave integriert werden kann. Dies ermöglicht ein breites Spektrum an Aufgaben abzudecken. Ein weiteres Projekt beschäftigt sich mit der Verwendung der Architektur zur Rekonstruktion von 3D-Volumen eines Ultraschall Computertomographen [8].

Literaturverzeichnis

1. Allen G, Davis K, Goodale T, et al. The grid application toolkit: Towards generic and easy application programming interfaces for the grid. Proc IEEE.
2. SAGA Research Group; 2007. http://forge.gridforum.org/projects/saga-rg/.
3. Arnold D, Agrawal S, Blackford S, et al. Users' Guide to NetSolve V1.4.1. Knoxville, TN: University of Tennessee; 2002. ICL-UT-02-05.
4. Foster I. Globus toolkit version 4: Software for service-oriented systems. Lect Note Comp Sci. 2005;3779:2–13.
5. Friese T, Smith M, Freisleben B. Hot Service Deployment in an Ad Hoc Grid Environment. Proc ICSOC. 2004; p. 75–83.
6. Rasband WS. ImageJ, US National Institutes of Health, Bethesda, MD, USA; 1997–2006. http://rsb.info.nih.gov/ij/.
7. Schopf JM, Pearlman L, Miller N, et al. Monitoring the grid with the Globus Toolkit MDS4. J Phys. 2006;46:521–5.
8. Stotzka R, Würfel J, Müller T. Medical imaging by ultrasound computer tomography. Proc SPIE. 2002; p. 110–9.

Qualitätszentrierte Softwareentwicklung in wissenschaftlichen Arbeitsgruppen
Auf dem Weg vom Prototypen zum Produkt

D. Maleike, J. Neuhaus, T. Heimann, M. Nolden, J. Poxleitner, M. Schöbinger, T. Schwarz, M. Seitel, I. Wegner, P. Wolber, H.-P. Meinzer, I. Wolf

Abteilung für Medizinische und Biologische Informatik, DKFZ Heidelberg
d.maleike@dkfz.de

Kurzfassung. Neue Bildverarbeitungsmethoden werden häufig hauptsächlich für Publikationszwecke entwickelt. Die Weiterentwicklung bis zur Verwendbarkeit für klinische Anwender erfordert zusätzlichen Aufwand und wird daher oft nicht weiter verfolgt. In dieser Arbeit wurden mehrere Bildanalyseverfahren unserer Abteilung konsequent zu einem stabilen und benutzbaren Softwareprodukt weiter entwickelt, so dass es für den Einsatz bei klinischen Partnern und als Demonstrationssoftware auf Messen verwendbar ist. Wir beschreiben das Vorgehen bei der Weiterentwicklung, welche Erfahrungen gemacht wurden und welcher zusätzliche Aufwand damit verbunden ist.

1 Einleitung

In wissenschaftlichen Abteilungen entstehende Bildverarbeitungsmethoden sind in der Regel Machbarkeitsstudien. Sie sind mehr auf Publikationen ausgerichtet als auf die Benutzung durch Nicht-Informatiker (z.B. Mediziner). Stabilität, eine angemessene Benutzeroberfläche und Integration in den klinischen Arbeitsablauf sind häufig untergeordnete Ziele. In diesem Beitrag haben wir mehrere fortgeschrittene Segmentierungs- und Analyseverfahren unserer Abteilung zu einem Softwareprodukt weiter entwickelt, das Ansprüchen an die Softwarequalität so weit genügt, dass es für umfangreiche Evaluationen durch klinische Partner und für Demonstrationen auf Messen geeignet ist. Die entwickelte Anwendung ist in die CHILI®-PACS-Workstation integriert. Die folgenden Abschnitte beschreiben die notwendigen Schritte auf dem Weg zu diesem Softwareprodukt und die gewonnenen Erfahrungen.

2 Material und Methoden

Die folgenden Abschnitte beschreiben die Werkzeuge und die Vorgehensweise, die in der Weiterentwicklung der Anwendungsmodule zu einem hochqualitativen Softwareprodukt verwendet wurden.

2.1 Medical Imaging Interaction Toolkit

Die Softwareentwicklung in unserer Abteilung ist auf das Medical Imaging Interaction Toolkit (MITK) aufgebaut. MITK ist ein Softwareframework für das Rapid Application Development im Bereich medizinischer Bildverarbeitung.

Versionsverwaltung Alle Entwickler arbeiten an einer gemeinsamen in zahlreiche Module aufgeteilten Quellcodebasis. Damit Änderungen bei der Vielzahl an Entwicklern nachvollziehbar bleiben, wird das Versionierungssystem Subversion eingesetzt. Es erlaubt das Kommentieren von Änderungen, Archivierung alter Versionen, sowie bei Bedarf das Auftrennen der Quellcodeversion in verschiedene parallele Entwicklungszweige (Branching).

Build Management Mit dem Ziel, Anwendungen „in die Klinik" zu bringen, ist es notwendig verschiedene Rechnerkonfigurationen zu unterstützen. Um dieses Ziel zu erreichen, wird das Continuous-Integration-Tool „Dart" aus ITK verwendet. Client-Rechner mit verschiedenen Betriebssystemen, Compilern und Bibliotheksversionen übersetzen jede Nacht die aktuelle Quellcodeversion und führen automatisierte Modul- und Anwendungstests aus. Fehler beim Kompilieren und Testen werden den Entwicklern, die für die entsprechende Codeänderung verantwortlich sind, automatisiert per Email mitgeteilt. Zusätzlich werden die Ergebnisse auf einer Webseite veröffentlicht. Fehler, die nur in bestimmten Konfigurationen auftreten, werden so zeitnah bemerkt. Außerdem steht immer eine aktuelle Binärversion für jede unterstützte Rechnerkonfiguration zur Verfügung.

Fehler-/Anforderungsverwaltung Zur Erfassung und Verwaltung von Fehlermeldungen (Bug-Reports) und Anforderungen (Feature-Requests) wird das Fehlerverwaltungssystem Bugzilla verwendet. Anwender und Tester können damit Fehlerberichte sowie neue Anforderungen an Entwickler senden. Die Entwickler können Fehlerberichte diskutieren, einem Verantwortlichen zuweisen, Anforderungen zu geplanten Meilensteinen zuordnen und die Bearbeitung der Fehler dokumentieren.

2.2 Vorgehensweise

Um das Ziel eines bedienbaren und stabilen Softwareprodukts zu erreichen, haben wir einen komplettenntwicklungsprozess von der Definition von Zielen, daraus abgeleiteten funktionalen und qualitativen Anforderungen bis zu deren Umsetzung und einer intensiven Qualitätssicherung durchlaufen. Die funktionalen Anforderungen ergaben sich aus einer Reihe von medizinisch relevanten Fragestellungen, die mithilfe der in der Abteilung bereits verfügbaren Software kurzfristig gelöst werden konnten. Als Zielsysteme wurden SUSE Linux 10.2 und Windows XP mit festgelegten Versionen der verwendeten Bibliotheken definiert.

Aus dem Ziel, dass die Software bei klinischen Partnern eingesetzt werden soll, wurden die beiden Qualitätsanforderungen „Benutzbarkeit" und „Zuverlässigkeit" abgeleitet. Um das Ziel „Benutzbarkeit" zu erreichen, wurde eine Menge einfacher Regeln für die Benutzeroberfläche definiert – nicht jedoch neue Bedienkonzepte eingeführt, weil dies in der Regel komplexe Änderungen bedeutet.

Durch Konzentration auf bereits existierende Softwaremodule war ein Großteil der funktionalen Anforderungen bereits erfüllt. Die noch fehlenden Teile wurden als erster Arbeitsschritt vervollständigt, so dass eine funktional vollständige Version der Software erstellt werden konnte. Parallel dazu wurde ein Demosystem auf einem Notebook eingerichtet, auf dem die Software dank eines lokalen PACS Servers mit anonymisierten Bilddaten auch ohne Netzwerkverbindung innerhalb der CHILI-PACS-Workstation laufen kann.

Nach Fertigstellung des ersten Prototypen wurde im Versionsverwaltungssystem ein neuer Entwicklungszweig eingerichtet, um die qualitative Weiterentwicklung von der parallel laufenden funktionalen Weiterentwicklung zu trennen. Der Prototyp wurde anschließend von einem Qualitätssicherungsteam auf die Qualitätsanforderungen hin getestet. Gefundene Fehler wurden mit dem Fehlerverwaltungssystem ausführlich dokumentiert und an die zuständigen Entwickler verteilt. Nach zwei Fehlerbehebungsrunden (je eine Woche) wurde eine Release-Kandidat-Version an ein auf 14 Personen erweitertes Testteam (davon zwei Mediziner) verteilt. Nach zwei weiteren Iterationen erfüllte die Software dann alle funktionalen und qualitativen Anforderungen und es konnte ein Release erstellt werden.

3 Ergebnisse

Diese Arbeit hat drei unterschiedliche, aber gleichermaßen wichtige Ergebnisse. Zum einen existiert nun ein stabiles Softwareprodukt, das an klinische Partner für Tests und Evaluationen herausgegeben werden kann. Zusätzlich wurde eine Vorgehensweise entwickelt, wie in einer wissenschaftlichen Abteilung der Übergang vom internen Prototyp zu einer extern verwendbaren Version machbar ist. Zusätzlich wurde durch die Arbeit auch der Aufwand quantifizierbar, der für die Weiterentwicklung eines Prototyps zu einem extern verwendbaren Softwareprodukt notwendig ist.

3.1 Die Softwaremodule

Das entwickelte Softwareprodukt besteht aus folgenden Anwendungsmodulen:

- *Bronchialbaumsegmentierung auf CT-Daten* mit einem Bereichswachstumsverfahrens, dessen Auslaufen in die Lunge automatisch detektiert wird [1].
- Interaktive *Lymphknotenvolumetrie auf CT-Daten* durch eine deformierbare Oberfläche mit Formwissen zum Monitoring über den Therapieverlauf [2].
- *Lungensegmentierung auf Cine-MR-Daten (3D+t)* über statistische Formmodelle. Beweglichkeit und Volumenverlauf der Lunge über die Zeit sind interessant für die Diagnose.

– *Herzventrikelvolumetrie auf MR-Daten* durch statistische Formmodelle, woraus klinische Maße wie die Ejektionsfraktion bestimmt werden können [3].
– *Modellierung der Herzklappenaufhängung (Annulus) auf zeitaufgelösten 3D-Ultraschall-Daten* durch interaktive Definition eines Splines. Dies kann die Grundlage für eine Prothesenauswahl bilden [4].
– *Leberresektionsplanung auf CT-Daten* aufgrund manueller Segmentierungen und Lebergefäß-Versorgungsgebietsberechnung [5].
– *Verkürzte Leber-OP-Planung auf CT-Daten* durch automatische Lebersegmentierung in ca. 2 Minuten [6] und manuelle Definition einer gekrümmten Schnittebene in volumenvisualisierten Lebergefäßen.
– *Gehirntumorvolumetrie auf MR-Daten* mittels interaktiver Graphcut-Segmentierung als Grundlage der Therapieplanung.

3.2 Erfahrungen aus dem Projekt

Die wesentlichen Erkenntnisse aus dem Projekt sind:

– Die Aufstellung medizinisch relevanter Fragestellungen zu Beginn hat sich als nützliche Grundlage für alle zu treffenden Entscheidungen im Projektverlauf erwiesen.
– Das Abspalten der qualitativen von der funktionalen Weiterentwicklung durch einen Branch im Versionsverwaltungssystem hat sich als nützlich erwiesen. Da Fehlerbehebungen in der Regel in beiden Entwicklungszweigen durchgeführt werden sollen, ergibt sich ein zusätzlicher Schulungsbedarf bzgl. des Versionierungstool.
– Bei der Kombination mehrerer Anwendungsmodule kann es zu Seiteneffekten kommen, z.B. dass ein Modul fälschlicherweise Daten eines anderen Moduls ändert oder löscht. Um diese Fehler zu finden, sollten die Module möglichst schnell zu einem Gesamtsystem integriert und als solches getestet werden. Hieraus lässt sich die Designregel ableiten, dass Module keine impliziten Annahmen über den Zustand ihrer Daten treffen dürfen, sondern diese bei jedem Zugriff auf Validität testen müssen.
– Mit Tests, bei denen mehrere Datensätze hintereinander bearbeitet werden, können Speicherlecks gefunden werden. Speicherlecks können unter anderen dadurch entstehen, dass ein Anwendungsmodul Daten eines anderen Moduls referenziert und so die Freigabe verhindert. Dies sollte ebenfalls durch eine Designregel verboten werden.
– Das manuelle Testen durch ein Testteam mit unterschiedlichen Hintergründen hat sich sehr bewährt. Damit sollte begonnen werden, sobald die Software eine Grundstabilität erlangt hat.

3.3 Aufwandsabschätzung

Tabelle 1 zeigt den geschätzten Aufwand für das Projekt. Hierbei ist hervorzuheben, dass der Aufwand für einen ersten Prototypen ebenso hoch ist wie die Weiterentwicklung zur Erfüllung der Qualitätsanforderungen.

Tabelle 1. Geschätzter Aufwand für die Erstellung des Softwareprodukts. Die Spalte „Entwicklungsstand" zeigt den geschätzten Zustand der Softwaremodule bezogen auf die funktionalen und qualitativen Anforderungen (vor Projektbeginn). Die Spalte „Entwicklungsaufwand" enthält die Arbeitszeit in Personentagen (8h-Tage) aufgeteilt in Aufwand zur Erfüllung der funktionalen und der Qualitätsanforderungen und in den Test- und Verwaltungsaufwand. Der Gesamtaufwand beträgt etwa ein Personenjahr

	Entwicklungsstand	Entwicklungsaufwand
Funktionale Anforderungen	65 %	126 Personentage
Qualitative Anforderungen	45 %	105 Personentage
Testen	—	10 Personentage
Verwaltung	—	13 Personentage
Gesamt		254 Personentage

4 Diskussion

Wir haben in dieser Arbeit ein stabiles Softwareprodukt entwickelt, das eine Auswahl der Forschungsarbeiten unserer Abteilung beinhaltet. Es wurde so weit entwickelt, dass es an klinische Partner herausgegeben sowie auf Messen als Demonstrationssystem gezeigt werden kann. Auf dem Weg zu einem einsetzbaren Produkt fehlt hier noch die Zertifizierung nach dem Medizinproduktegesetz. Hierfür ist beträchtlich mehr Aufwand notwendig, da bei einem solchen Vorhaben zusätzlich eine systematische Planung und Dokumentation nötig ist.

Das Projekt hat neben dem Softwareprodukt an sich vor allem Erfahrungen über das optimale Vorgehen und den benötigten Aufwand gebracht. Dies gilt es nun in Schulungsunterlagen den Entwicklern zugänglich zu machen und bei zukünftiger Projektplanung zu berücksichtigen.

Literaturverzeichnis

1. Wolber P, Wegner I, Heimann T, et al. Tracking und Segmentierung baumförmiger tubulärer Strukturen mit einem hybriden Verfahren. Proc BVM. 2008.
2. Maleike D, Fabel M, Tetzlaff R, et al. Lymph node segmentation on CT images by a shape model guided deformable surface method. Proc SPIE. 2008;Accepted.
3. Schwarz T, Heimann T, Wolf I, et al. 3D heart segmentation and volumetry using deformable shape models. Proc Comp Cardiol. 2007;In print.
4. Seitel M, Frank C, Simone RD, et al. Unterstützung der Planung von Mitralklappen-Annuloplastien mittels 4D-Echokardiographieaufnahmen. Proc CURAC. 2007; p. 283–6.
5. Meinzer HP, Thorn M, Cardenas CE. Computerized planning of liver surgery: An overview. Comput Graph. 2002;26(4):569–76.
6. Heimann T, Münzing S, Meinzer HP, et al. A shape-guided deformable model with evolutionary algorithm initialization for 3D soft tissue segmentation. Inf Process Med Imaging. 2007;20:1–12.

Konzept und Realisierung eines Zustandsmaschinen-Editors für Interaktionen medizinischer Bildverarbeitung mit Debug-Funktionalität

Daniel Stein, Marcus Vetter, Ivo Wolf, Hans-Peter Meinzer

Abteilung für Medizinische und Biologische Informatik,
Deutsches Krebsforschungszentrum, D-69120 Heidelberg
d.stein@dkfz.de

Kurzfassung. In diesem Beitrag wird ein Open-Source-Plug-In für die Entwicklungsumgebung Eclipse vorgestellt, mit dem ein Programmablauf in Form von Zustandsmaschinen grafisch modelliert werden kann. Außerdem bietet das Konzept mit der Debug-Funktion die Möglichkeit, während der Laufzeit einer Applikation alle verwendeten Zustandsmaschinen und deren Zustandsfolgen zu beobachten. Dadurch lassen sich erstellte Zustandsmaschinen auf ihre korrekte Arbeitsweise hin überprüfen. Durch die Debug-Funktion wird das Aufspüren von Fehlern im Programmdesign deutlich vereinfacht, was gerade für die Qualitätskontrolle von medizinischen Anwendungen wichtig ist. Die erstellten Zustandsmaschinen werden beim Speichern in eine XML-Beschreibung überführt. Diese kann von anderen Applikationen direkt weiter verwendet werden.

1 Einleitung

Die Vielfalt an Möglichkeiten, die während einer Interaktion medizinischer Applikationen entstehen, kann durch eine Mealy-Zustandsmaschine [1] abgebildet werden. In der Theorie sind alle Programme Zustandsmaschinen, unabhängig davon, ob sie speziell als Zustandsmaschine programmiert sind oder über Variablen, Bedingungen oder Schleifen direkt im Programm-Code implementiert sind [2]. Zum Beispiel kann ein Regionenwachstums-Algorithmus nur angewendet werden, wenn zuvor die Bedingung „Saatpunkt in einem Bild gesetzt“ erfüllt ist, was einem Zustand „Saatpunkt gesetzt“ entsprechen könnte. In diesen Zustand würde man über das Ereignis „neuer Saatpunkt“ kommen und aus diesem Zustand gäbe es dann einen Übergang mit dem Ereignis „Regionenwachstum starten“ in den Folgezustand. Deswegen geht der Trend dahin, den Programmablauf direkt in Form von Zustandsmaschinen zu entwerfen. So ist zum Beispiel IGSTK (Image-guided Surgical Toolkit) gerade dabei, ein Architecture Validation Toolset zu entwickeln, bei dem jeder Programm-Code zunächst als Zustandsmaschine dargestellt wird. Dies soll die Patientensicherheit bei der Verwendung medizinischer Software durch einen zuverlässigen und stabilen Programmablauf erhöhen [2, 3]. Jedoch ist das Erstellen von Zustandsmaschinen im Programm-Code sehr umständlich und bei einer wachsenden Anzahl an Zuständen auch sehr unübersichtlich [4].

Bei umfangreichen Zustandsmaschinen mit vielen Zuständen und Übergängen ist es mühsam und zeitaufwendig, Änderungen vorzunehmen. Zum Neuerstellen einer Zustandsmaschine muss der Ersteller den Ablauf dieser bereits im Kopf vorgeplant haben, um den Ablauf im Programm-Code implementieren zu können. In den meisten Fällen wird eine solche Zustandsmaschine noch auf dem Reißbrett entworfen, da auf Grund der Komplexität der Zustandsmaschine ein Diagramm zur Verdeutlichung des Ablaufs nötig ist. Mit Hilfe einer grafischen Oberfläche können komplexe Zustandsmaschinen schnell konstruiert, geändert und als Programm-Code gespeichert werden. Dies ermöglicht neuen Mitarbeitern ein schnelleres Einarbeiten in den Ablauf einer Zustandsmaschine.

Eventuell auftretende Entwurfsfehler, die erst bei Ablauf einer Anwendung unter Verwendung der Zustandsmaschine auftreten, sind im Programm-Code sehr schwer zu lokalisieren, da der Ablauf einer komplexen Zustandsmaschine anhand des Programm-Codes nur mühsam nachzuvollziehen ist. So entsteht für den Benutzer ein hoher Arbeitsaufwand, der mit Hilfe eines geeigneten Tools zum Debuggen von Zustandsmaschinen minimiert werden kann.

2 Methoden

Der entwickelte Zustandsmaschinen-Editor wurde in Java als Plug-In für die Entwicklungsumgebung Eclipse erstellt. Der Editor basiert auf dem bereits bestehenden Plug-In Graphical Editing Framework (GEF). Das GEF bietet eine Klassenbibliothek als Grundgerüst eines grafischen Editors.

Mit dem Zustandsmaschinen-Editor ist ein Programm entstanden, das sich in zwei Programmteile gliedert.

Der erste Teil ist ein Editor, mit dem Zustandsmaschinen grafisch modelliert werden können. Es können sowohl bestehende Zustandsmaschinen aus einer XML-Datei geöffnet, als auch eine neue XML-Datei angelegt werden. Der Programmablauf vom Öffnen einer XML-Datei bis zur Visualisierung einer Zustandsmaschine im Editor ist als Objektdiagramm in Abbildung 1 dargestellt. Zunächst wird mit Hilfe von JDOM die XML-Datei ausgelesen und die darin vorhandenen Zustandsmaschinen an die StateMachinesList übergeben. Aus dieser Liste können mehrere Editorfenster gleichzeitig geöffnet werden (Abb. 2). Dabei beinhaltet jeder Editor eine Zustandsmaschine, die aus mehreren verschiedenen Zuständen besteht. Jeder Zustand kann mehrere Übergänge mit jeweils einem Event besitzen, die jeweils mehrere Aktionen bewirken können. Im Editor stehen alle zur Bearbeitung von Zustandsmaschinen benötigten Funktionen zur Verfügung (Abb. 2). Zusätzlich können neue Zustandsmaschinen erstellt, nicht mehr benötigte gelöscht, sowie bereits bestehende kopiert und unter anderem Namen gespeichert werden. Nach dem Speichern werden alle vorgenommenen Änderungen automatisch in XML-Code konvertiert und in die XML-Datei geschrieben.

Der zweite Teil des Programms wurde entwickelt, um eventuelle Modellierungsfehler festzustellen. Hierbei handelt es sich um einen Debugger, der parallel zum Betrieb einer Applikation ausgeführt wird. Dabei wird eine Client-Server-Verbindung zwischen dem Zustandsmaschinen-Editor und der Applikation aufgebaut. Der Zustandsmaschinen-Editor dient als Server, die Applikation als Client. Die Applikation sendet alle von ihr benutzten Zustandsmaschinen und alle bei ihr eingehenden Ereignisse an den Zustandsmaschinen-Editor. In diesem kann die gewünschte Zustandsmaschine geöffnet werden. Es werden der aktuelle Zustand und der aktuelle Übergang durch eine rote Hinterlegung markiert. Zusätzlich erhält der Benutzer die Möglichkeit, den Zustand der Zustandsmaschine zu einem früheren Ereignis zu beobachten. Dies ermöglicht dem Benutzer den gesamten Ablauf einer Zustandsmaschine zu einer aufgetretenen Ereignisfolge noch einmal nachzuvollziehen.

3 Ergebnisse

Mit dem Zustandsmaschinen-Editor wurde ein Open-Source-Programm erstellt, das sich auf einfache Art und Weise in die ebenso frei verfügbare Entwicklungsumgebung Eclipse einbinden lässt. Mit Hilfe der grafischen Oberfläche wird das Erstellen, Bearbeiten, Refactoring und Reengineering von Zustandsmaschinen nicht nur beschleunigt, sondern auch deutlich übersichtlicher und einfacher (Abb. 2).

Durch die integrierte Debug-Funktion, die alle benutzten Zustandsmaschinen und Ereignisse einer Applikation registriert, steht ein nützliches Tool zur Aufspürung von Designfehlern innerhalb einer Zustandsmaschine zur Verfügung.

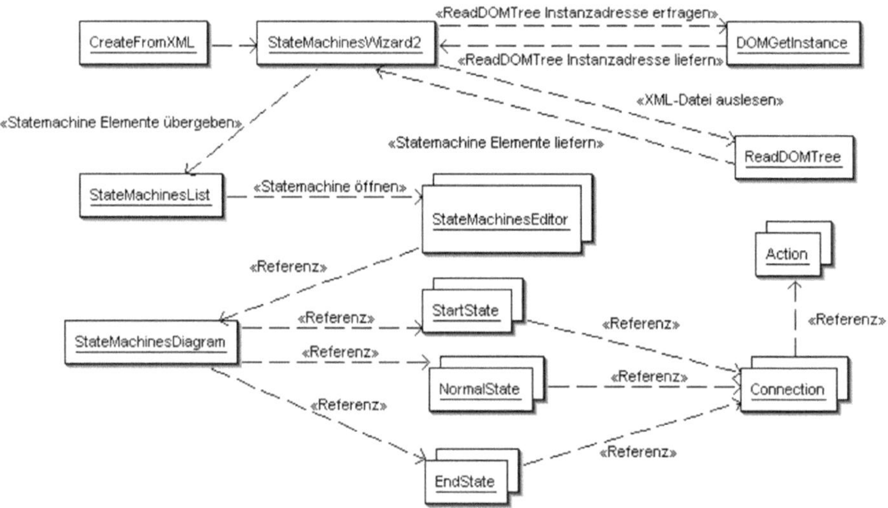

Abb. 1. Objektdiagramm: Ablauf des Zustandsmaschinen-Editor-Plug-Ins vom Öffnen einer XML-Datei bis zur Visualisierung einer Zustandsmaschine im Editor

Im Medical Imaging and Interaction Toolkit (MITK) [5] ist der Editor, sowie die Debug-Funktion bereits erfolgreich im Einsatz um neue Zustandsmaschinen zu definieren und komplexe Abläufe zu überprüfen und nachzuvollziehen. Es zeigen sich bereits die erwarteten Vorteile beim Refactoring, sowie beim Reengineering von bestehenden Zustandsmaschinen.

4 Diskussion

Durch das hier vorgestellte Tool wird es möglich sein, Zustandsmaschinen einfach, schnell und übersichtlich zu entwerfen. Des Weiteren steht mit der Debug-Funktion ein Tool zur Verfügung, mit dem man den Ablauf einer Zustandsmaschine während der Laufzeit der entwickelten Applikation auf die korrekte Arbeitsweise hin überprüfen kann.

Der Zustandsmaschinen-Editor wurde in Java mit der Programmieroberfläche Eclipse programmiert, da mit Hilfe dieser Open-Source-Entwicklungsumgebung ein neues Plug-In mit wenig Aufwand installiert und sofort genutzt werden kann. Als Programmiersprache wurde Java gewählt, weil Eclipse selbst in Java programmiert ist und sich die definierten Ziele in Java am besten verwirklichen ließen. Hinzu kommt, dass für Eclipse mit dem Graphical Editing Frame-

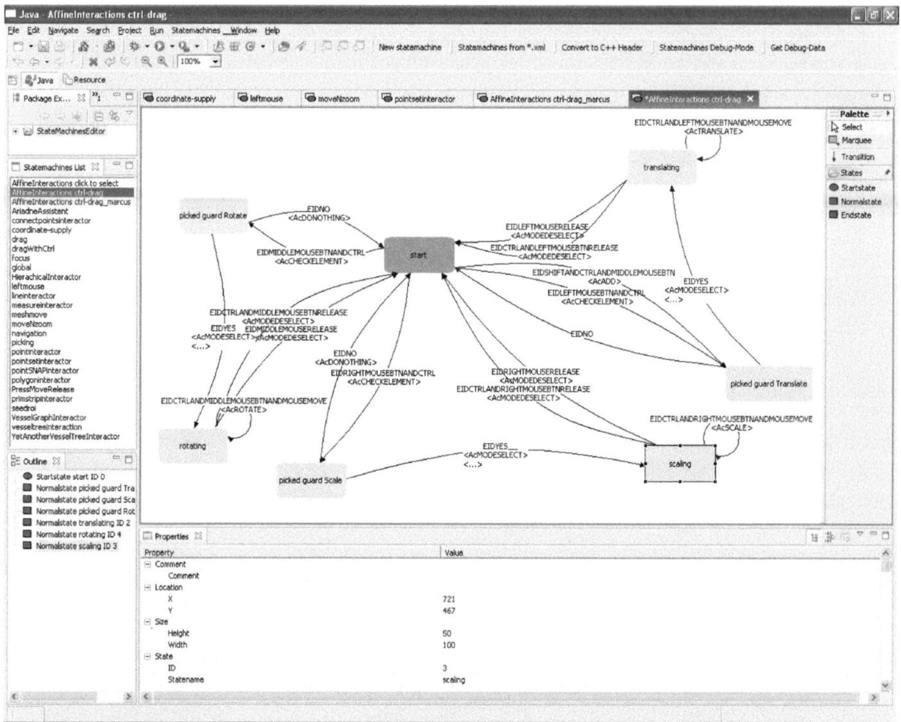

Abb. 2. Möglicher Aufbau der Benutzeroberfläche des Zustandsmaschinen-Editors

work (GEF) bereits ein in Java geschriebenes Plug-In zur Verfügung steht, das die Rahmenfunktionen zur Erstellung eines grafischen Editors bietet.

Das Konzept, die Zustandsmaschinen im XML-Format zu speichern, macht den Editor unabhängig von der Programmiersprache der Applikation, die diese Zustandsmaschinen nutzt. Die entstehende XML-Datei kann in jede Applikation, die Zustandsmaschinen im XML-Format verwendet, eingebunden werden.

Durch die Client-Server-Architektur zwischen dem Editor und der Applikation, die die Zustandsmaschinen verwendet, wird auch bei der Debug-Funktion die Unabhängigkeit zwischen Applikation und Editor gewahrt. In der Applikation muss nur ein passender Client implementiert werden, der sich mit dem als Server agierenden Editor verbindet. Dadurch, dass der Editor und die Applikation in verschiedenen Threads ablaufen und die Applikation nur die verwendeten Zustandsmaschinen und auftretenden Ereignisse an den Editor schickt, ändert sich die Performanz nicht wesentlich.

Der entstandene Zustandsmaschinen-Editor ist open-source und mit dem MITK zusammen frei verfügbar. Eine Installationsanleitung ist im Internet: http://www.mitk.org/documentation/doxygen/StatemachineEditor.html.

Literaturverzeichnis

1. Mealy GH. A method for synthesizing sequential circuits. Bell System Techn J. 1955;34(5):1045–79.
2. Gary K, Kokoori S, David B, et al. An architecture validation toolset for ensuring patient safety in an open source software toolkit for image-guided surgery applications. In: IJ - MICCAI Open Science Workshop. The Insight Journal; 2006.
3. Cheng P, Zhang H, Kim HS, et al. IGSTK: Framework and example application using an open source toolkit for image-guided surgery applications. Proc SPIE. 2006;6141:590–8.
4. Wegner I, Vetter M, Wolf I, et al. Ein generisches Interaktionskonzept mit Undo für die medizinische Bildverarbeitung. Proc BVM. 2004.
5. Wolf I, Vetter M, Wegner I, et al. The medical imaging interaction toolkit (MITK). Proc SPIE. 2004;5367:16–27.

Evaluating the Performance of Processing Medical Volume Data on Graphics Hardware

Matthias Raspe, Guido Lorenz, Stefan Müller

Institute for Computational Visualistics,
University of Koblenz-Landau (Campus Koblenz)
mraspe@uni-koblenz.de

Abstract. With the broad availability and increasing performance of commodity graphics processors (GPU), non-graphical applications have become an active field of research. However, leveraging the performance for advanced applications combining hardware and software implementations is more than just efficient shader programming: the data transfer is often the main limiting factor. Therefore, we will investigate in the applicability of commodity graphics hardware for medical data processing, and propose a GPU-based framework for representing computations on volume data. Also, we will show the clear performance gain of different operations compared to CPU algorithms and discuss their context. Not only the much higher performance of hardware implementations is attractive, but also the fact that the computation results can be visualized directly, i.e., without introducing an overhead and thus allowing for literally interactive applications.

1 Introduction

With the advances in computer graphics hardware during the last few years, the computational performance of such commodity hardware is able to clearly outperform modern multi-core processors. As shown recently in [1], many areas are able to benefit from the computing performance of programmable graphics processors (GPU). In medical application, however, visualization tasks are still the primary use for graphics hardware.

While many general purpose applications have been successfully addressed, image processing remains a particularly interesting field due to the architecture of graphics hardware. Being optimized especially for two-dimensional textures, processing such image data is obvious and achieves optimal performance. However, lots of image data, especially the medical field is acquired and processed volumetrically, i.e., as three-dimensional data.

This imposes several issues for applications targeting at graphics hardware. First, the available on-board memory becomes critical for large volume data produced by modern imaging systems. Also, 3D textures are not very flexible as they usually do not allow for direct write access, thus preventing their use as render targets. However, the main problem is still the data transfer to and especially from the graphics memory, with volume data intensifying the issue due to the additional dimension. For certain applications, however, this is not as problematic as it might seem. As Langs et al. [2] have shown by using the graphics hardware for filtering large volumes representing video frames and thereby achieving a performance several orders of magnitudes faster than commercial CPU implementations. Köhn et al. [3] have implemented image registration algorithms on the GPU and also report a clear performance gain being only flawed by some graphics driver limitation.

In order to evaluate the discussion for processing (medical) volume data, we will compare different types of operations with respect to their runtime performance as CPU and GPU implementations, respectively. Therefore, our GPU-based framework "Cascada"that is already used in the context of medical segmentation (see [4]) regards computation processes at a more abstract level and handles processing and visualization tasks uniformly. The cross-platform system also provides basic functionality for handling (medical) volume data and integrates different visualization techniques and input devices.

2 Material and Methods

2.1 Overview of the GPU-based Framework

The system for (general purpose) GPU programming focuses on processing volume data, mainly from tomographic imaging systems such as CT or MRI. The algorithms are represented in a hierarchical structure, consisting of:

- *Sequences* encapsulate procedures ranging from simple thresholding operations to iterative algorithms or visualization components
- Sequences consist of multiple *passes* that resemble shader programs being executed by rendering geometry
- *Shader programs* combine the different types of shaders (currently: vertex and fragment programs) with an additional infrastructure for handling parameters, concatenation, etc.

For efficient data handling, we use basically two complementing approaches. First, the data is represented as volumes packed into RGBA-tuples, thus allowing for direct rendering into the volume and exploiting the SIMD (Single instruction, multiple data: processing four data items simultaneously) architecture of GPUs. Therefore, four successive slices of the scalar volume (or four DICOM slices) are combined into one RGBA slice. For both backward compatibility and better performance, the system additionally uses a two-dimensional representation of the volumetric data as introduced by Harris et al. [5]. As shown in [2], the time for accessing the flat-3D texture by converting the 3D texture coordinates into the 2D address is even less than direct 3D access for basic interpolation modes. All representations of the volume data are converted and loaded to/from the GPU only on demand, i.e., expensive operations are kept at a minimum.

At the level of render passes in our hierarchical representation, the system does not distinguish between processing and visualization steps. The only difference is the target of the pass/sequence (i.e., offscreen/onscreen buffer) which can be changed during runtime, if needed. Therefore, the system implicitly allows for displaying the results of algorithms while they are computed, with a negligible performance overhead on modern graphics hardware, as shown in [4]. Currently, our system provides several volume visualization modes, with standard MPR (multi-planar reformation) and direct volume rendering by means of GPU raycasting.

2.2 Performance Comparison

In order to provide some measure for the efficiency of our framework, we have compared its processing performance with MeVisLab [6], a widely used software system for efficient medical data processing and visualization. Although "Cascada"also provides software implementations of the algorithms, it is not optimized in this regard. Let alone the fact that comparing a system with itself is not meaningful and transferable at all. Most of MeVisLab's core algorithms are based on an image processing library that, in combination with the powerful frontend, allows for flexible and rapid development of applications. However, the system does not utilize programmable graphics hardware, except for visualization purposes and simple modifications of primarily visual results via shader programs.

As mentioned before, an important factor for leveraging the performance of GPUs is the amount of data transfer relative to the processing. Basically, a much better performance can be achieved by loading the data once to the graphics card's memory and compute as much as possible there. This is also preferable for the simultaneous visualization of the results during computation.

We have set up two different scenarios for comparing the systems. The first one is intended to show the performance at operations with different levels of computational complexity, ranging from simple thresholding to gradient computation in a 3D neighborhood. The second performance test (figure 1) aims at mimicking a reasonable procedure for volume processing, so the focus is on combining different operations while limiting data transfer to the extent needed.

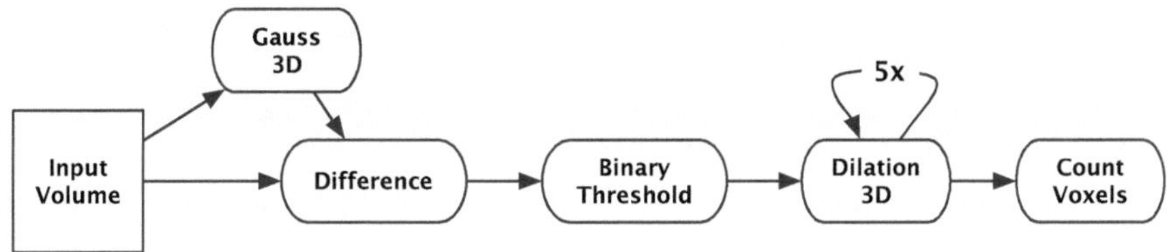

Fig. 1. Test setup for evaluating the performance of some pipeline consisting of different types of operations

Table 1. Computation times in seconds for the two data sets (CT scan/MRI scan). The GPU version excludes data transfer from/to the video memory and is averaged over multiple runs

Operation	MeVisLab	Cascada (all)	Cascada (GPU)
Binary	0.73 / 0.21	1.9 / 0.55	0.038 / 0.011
Gradient 2D	10.1 / 2.9	2.6 / 0.7	0.06 / 0.017
Gradient 3D	14.9 / 3.9	2.6 / 0.72	0.059 / 0.018
Gauss 2D	1.36 / 0.37	2.48 / 0.73	0.061 / 0.017
Gauss 3D	3.65 / 1.01	2.59 / 0.78	0.09 / 0.026

Table 2. Single computation times in seconds for the two data sets (CT scan/MRI scan). The GPU version includes the shader and all setup steps between the stages; the initial upload is omitted as it is addressed in table 1. Total time does not include loading the data for both platforms

Operation	MeVisLab	Cascada (GPU)	∅ speedup
Gauss+Difference	3.6 / 1.48	0.74 / 0.23	5.5
Binary Threshold	0.7 / 0.23	0.125 / 0.049	5.2
Dilation 3D (5x)	27.12 / 7.6	1.14 / 0.343	23
Count Voxels	1.1 / 0.7	0.33 / 0.078	6
Total	32.9 / 10.8	2.41 / 0.76	14

All the experiments have been performed on an Intel Core2Duo (2.4 GHz) with 2 GB RAM and an Nvidia Geforce 8800 GTS with 640 MB of VRAM. For MeVisLab we have used the latest SDK version (1.5.1) available from their website with default settings. We have applied the algorithms in both applications on the same datasets: a $512 \times 512 \times 223$ CT scan (DICOM files), and an MRI scan $256 \times 256 \times 256$ (raw volume), both with 16 bit values.

3 Results

In the following tables, we have gathered all the timings from the aforementioned experiments. The first table shows some details on the single operations with increasing complexity (no neighborhood, 4/6-neighborhood, and 8/26-neighborhood, respectively). In addition to their behaviour in the different dimensions, the transfer overhead is measured in detail.

The second table gives an overview of some reasonable concatenation of varying operations. No additional time for data transfer and/or conversion is measured here, as both systems work in their appropriate format for subsequent execution. We have also integrated special caching modules in MeVisLab to decouple the different steps and allow for comparable measuring.

4 Discussion

As can be seen in the preceding tables, the GPU is able to clearly outperform CPU implementations for all operations with speedups of up to 250, even for non-trivial algorithms. In contrast, including the additional time for the data transfer to and from the GPU reveals the severe impact on the performance: depending on the type and dimensionality of the operation, and the size of the volume the software implementation can surpass the GPU's performance in this case. Aside from several optimizations that are left as future work for the GPU system to tackle this issue, reloading the whole volume in every stage is not very likely to be needed. Therefore, the second scenario has been set up to provide a more "real life"workflow, with the GPU being more than one order of magnitude ahead of CPU implementations and thus being well suited for the computationally demanding field of medical image processing.

Of course, there is still room for improvement and investigation, aside from just technical optimization. Software performance is not only measured in raw computing performance, but also in programming effort where a research system as Cascada cannot cope with established platforms. Also, graphics hardware vendors have already started to simplify the use of their hardware by regarding GPUs more as devices than purely graphics oriented hardware. However, the key advantage of using graphics hardware also for computation, namely the visualization "for free"will be harder to use then. Regarding the fast development cycles of graphics hardware, the performance advantage will most likely be increasing as can be easily seen from speedups with past hardware generations.

References

1. Owens JD, Luebke D, Govindaraju N, et al. A survey of general-purpose computation on graphics hardware. Comput Graph Forum. 2007;26(1):80–113.
2. Langs A, Biedermann M. Filtering video volumes using the graphics hardware. Lect Note Comp Sci. 2007;4522:878–87.
3. Köhn A, Drexl J, Ritter F, et al. GPU accelerated image registration in two and three dimensions. Proc BVM. 2006; p. 261–5.
4. Raspe M, Wickenhöfer R, Schmitt F. Visualisierungsgestützte 3D-Segmentierung und Quantifizierung von Bauchaortenaneurysmen. Proc CURAC. 2007; p. 197–200.
5. Harris MJ, Baxter WV, Scheuermann T, et al. Simulation of cloud dynamics on graphics hardware. Proc ACM SIGGRAPH/EUROGRAPHICS Conf Graph Hardware. 2003; p. 92–101.
6. MeVis. MeVisLab: A Development Environment for Medical Image Processing and Visualization; 2007. http://www.mevislab.de.

Detection of Focal Cortical Dysplasia Lesions in MRI Using Textural Features

Christian Loyek[1], Friedrich G. Woermann[2], Tim W. Nattkemper[1]

[1]Applied Neuroinformatics, Faculty of Technology, Bielefeld University, Bielefeld
[2]Bethel Epilepsy Center, Mara Hospital, Department MRI, Bielefeld
cloyek@techfak.uni-bielefeld.de

Abstract. Focal cortical dysplasia (FCD) is a frequent cause of medically refractory partial epilepsy. The visual identification of FCD lesions on magnetic resonance images (MRI) is a challenging task in standard radiological analysis. Quantitative image analysis which tries to assist in the diagnosis of FCD lesions is an active field of research. In this work we investigate the potential of different texture features, in order to explore to what extent they are suitable for detecting lesional tissue. As a result we can show first promising results based on segmentation and texture classification.

1 Introduction

Focal cortical dysplasia (FCD) [1], a disorganisation of cortical development, is an important cause of medically intractable partial epilepsy. In medically resistant epilepsy patients, only surgical removal of the dysplastic lesions leads to significant reduction or cessation of seizures. High-resolution magnetic resonance imaging (MRI) has improved detection of FCD in the past years and has allowed more patients to undergo resective surgery. However, visual analysis and identification of FCD is a challenging task and strongly depends on the experience and expertise of the observer.

In a large number of cases, FCD lesions can not clearly be distinguished from healthy cortex and often remain unrecognised in standard radiological analysis [2]. Even for experienced radiologists it is difficult to descry the subtle characteristics with which FCD lesions are displayed in MR images. This motivates the question whether a computerized quantitative analysis will be capable to reliably detect these lesions.

In a few previously published approaches it was shown that an observer independent, quantitative analysis of MRI data has potential to assist in the diagnostics of FCD [3, 4]. Even though the proposed methods increase the sensitivity for FCD, the results are often associated with an increased number of false positive (FP) results [5]. This is due to the fact that the proposed methods are based on visual MRI characteristics [6] which can not clearly be linked to FCD lesions.

In this work, we investigate the potential of machine learning based classification of texture features for the purpose of detecting local structures in MR

Table 1. Features considered in this study can be separated into three groups

Statistical	Grey level co-occurrence	Grey level run-length
x_1^{S} = mean	x_1^{CO} = contrast	x_1^{RL} = short run emphasis
x_2^{S} = median	x_2^{CO} = homogeneity	x_2^{RL} = long run emphasis
x_3^{S} = variance	x_3^{CO} = inverse difference	x_3^{RL} = grey level distribution
x_4^{S} = skewness	x_4^{CO} = energy	x_4^{RL} = run-length distribution
x_5^{S} = kurtosis	x_5^{CO} = entropy	x_5^{RL} = run percentage
x_6^{S} = energy		
x_7^{S} = entropy		

images. We demonstrate that our features are able to recover lesional tissue within single cases with a low number of false positives, even for cases which are not easy to identify for the expert eye.

2 Materials and Methods

MRI scanning was performed on a 1.5 Tesla scanner (Siemens Magnetom Symphony, Erlangen, Germany) equipped with a standard head coil. The analysis comprises T1-weighted 3D-sequences (MPRAGE, TR = 11.1 msec, TE = 4.3 msec, slice thickness 1.5 mm, FOV 201 mm $\times$ 230 mm, matrix 256 $\times$ 256, voxel size 0.9mm $\times$ 1.5mm $\times$ 0.9mm) which were provided by the Bethel Epilepsy Center in Bielefeld, NRW. All images include a histologically confirmed FCD lesion. Each lesion was manually labeled by an experienced neuroradiologist.

2.1 Features

One possibility to describe texture is to calculate statistical moments based on the grey level histogram of a region or a window. In literature, statistical features are often called *first-order texture features*. Seven statistical measures have been extracted according to [7] (table 1, first column).

To account for second order texture properties we additionally apply one of the most well-known methods of texture analysis: grey-level co-occurrence matrices (COM) proposed by Haralick et al. [8]. A COM counts the relative occurrences of voxel pairs in an image window that have certain intensity values and that are seperated by a voxel distance d^{COM} in a relative direction α^{COM}. Based on the cost statistics different features can be computed as described in [8]. Five of the most common COM features are selected (table 1, second column).

We further extend the set of features by using a run-length-based technique as proposed by Galloway [9]. It calculates characteristic textural measures from grey-level run lengths in different image directions α^{RLM}. The third column in table 1 shows the five scalar features derived from the grey-level run length matrices (RLM).

2.2 Experimental Setup

For each analysed image an *inner-case-classification-setup* is performed. Inner-case classification aims to determine to what extend the applied texture features are suitable to detect FCD lesions within a single image. The setup has three steps:

- *Image Preprocessing:* In order to exclusively consider voxels of the cortex, the images are previously segmented into grey matter (cortex), white matter and cerebrospinal fluid using a standard algorithm described in [10] implemented in the statistical parametric mapping software (SPM2). For the calculation of the co-occurrence and the run-length features, the number of image grey values were reduced to 32 values.
- *Feature Extraction:* Each cortex voxel $v \in \Omega$ with position (l, m, n) is associated with a feature vector $\mathbf{x}_{lmn}$ which combines all scalar texture measures above-mentioned and can be formulated as

$$\mathbf{x}_{lmn} = (x_1^{\mathrm{S}}, ..., x_7^{\mathrm{S}}, \bar{x}_1^{\mathrm{CO}}, ..., \bar{x}_5^{\mathrm{CO}}, \bar{x}_1^{\mathrm{RL}}, ..., \bar{x}_5^{\mathrm{RL}})^{\mathrm{T}} \tag{1}$$

  All values of $\mathbf{x}_{lmn}$ are calculated within a $7 \times 5 \times 7$-window with $v(l, m, n)$ as the center voxel. In the case of the COM, we selected the distance $d^{\mathrm{COM}} = 1$ and directions $\alpha^{\mathrm{COM}} = 0°, 45°, 90°, 135°$ within coronal slices. This results in four COMs, each representing one special direction. Thus, for each COM a set of five derived features is obtained (table 1, second column). In order to make the features invariant to the angle α, each feature value $x_1^{\mathrm{CO}}, ..., x_5^{\mathrm{CO}}$ of the four COMs is averaged and finally described by $\bar{x}_1^{\mathrm{CO}}, ..., \bar{x}_5^{\mathrm{CO}}$. The values $\bar{x}_1^{\mathrm{RL}}, ..., \bar{x}_5^{\mathrm{RL}}$ of $\mathbf{x}_{lmn}$ are obtained in the same way using $\alpha^{\mathrm{RLM}} = 0°, 45°, 90°, 135°$ for the run-length directions.
- *Training & Classification:* Voxels have to be classified depending on whether they represent the class of normal cortex (label $y = -1$) or the class of lesional cortex (label $y = 1$). For this purpose, we randomly extracted a training dataset $\Gamma = \Gamma_{\mathrm{N}} \cup \Gamma_{\mathrm{L}} = \{\mathbf{x}_i, y_i)\}, i = 1, ..., k$ with Γ_{L} being a subset of lesional tissue signals and Γ_{N} being a subset of normal tissue signals. A support vector machine (SVM) with a gaussian kernel was trained using Γ. Finally, all cortex voxels $v \in \Omega \setminus \Gamma$ are classified based on the trained SVM.

3 Results

Our method is applied to five different cases, i.e. subjects. In each case the FCD lesion was marked by an expert (author F.G.W.). The accuracy is assessed by computing sensitivity (SE) and specificity (SP) as shown in table 2. Results for one particular case are illustrated in figure 1. Figure 1(a) shows a coronal slice of an original T1-weighted image including the expert label. Our method generates three-dimensional classification maps which visualise the class of the voxels assigned by the SVM (figure 1(b)), white regions indicate lesional characteristics whereas grey voxels represent tissue classified as normal. Figure 1(c) shows an overlay of the original image and regions classified as lesional tissue.

Table 2. The sensitivity (SE) and specificity (SP) values of the classification of five different cases

	subject 1	subject 2	subject 3	subject 4	subject 5
SE	0,946	0,904	0,846	0,960	0,982
SP	0,865	0,892	0,734	0,880	0,922

4 Discussion

We propose a quantitative approach using local texture features for the inner-case detection of focal cortical dysplasia lesions in MRI. The used features are powerful enough to allow automatic discrimination of normal cortex and lesional cortex tissue. In this work the proposed classification setup is only applied on an inner-case study to verify whether the features are suitable to find a lesion, however within the same image.

Using texture features we successfully detect lesional tissue in each of the applied cases which is confirmed by the increased SE values. Figure 1(b) and 1(c) exemplarily point out that the main part of the lesion is correctly classified. Furthermore, figure 1(b) demonstrates that only a small fraction of voxels is classified as false positives (see table 2 for sensitivity and specificity values for the remaining cases).

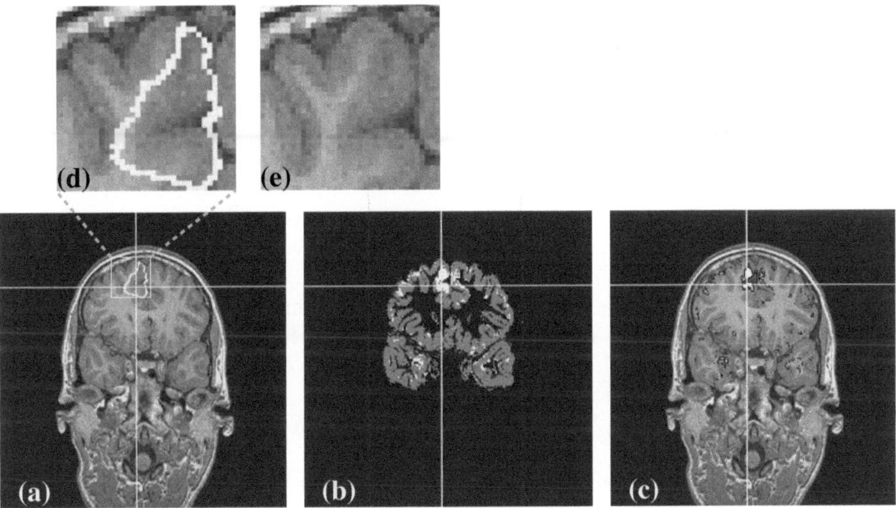

Fig. 1. Images describing results of subject 2. (a) Slice of the original T1-weighted MRI including a marking hand-labeled by an expert. (b) Classification map. (c) Overlay of the original image and the regions classified as lesional tissue. (d) and (e) show a magnification of the lesion

The classification setup is applied on previously segmented cortex tissue which is of particular importance for the classification accuracy. In the beginning of the study, the whole image was used for training the SVM, but this led to significantly inferior classification results. A major fraction of image information which was learned by the SVM is not important for this classification problem.

Different neighborhood sizes for the feature extraction are tested. A window size of $7 \times 5 \times 7$ leads to the best results. In order to overcome the problem of voxel anisotropy, only five slices in y-direction are considered.

The quantisation of the images in order to compute the COM and RLM features leads to a major performance increasement than using the original number of grey values. The conclusion that follows is that two much details, i.e. number of grey values, suppress the general differences between the types of tissue.

We perform the classification based on single feature approaches, i.e. statistical features, COM features and RLM features (see columns in table 1). The results point out that using single feature methods leads to an inferior classification accuracy than merging the feature sets. As a conclusion, FCD lesions contain both first- and second-order properties which enable their discrimination from normal cortex tissue. The results of this work can be considered as a necessary basic condition for realising a real CAD (computer aided diagnosis) setup which has to be analysed regarding generalisation in future studies.

Acknowledgement. The work is funded by the Bielefeld University.

References

1. Taylor D, Falconer M, Bruton C, et al. Focal dysplasias of the cerebral cortex in epilepsy. J Neurol Neurosurg Psychiatry. 1971;34:369–87.
2. Tassi L, Colombo N, Garbelli R, et al. Focal cortical dysplasia: Neuropathological subtypes, EEG, neuroimaging and surgical outcome. Brain. 2002;125:1719–32.
3. Huppertz H, Grimm C, Fauser S, et al. Enhanced visualization of blurred gray-white matter junctions in focal cortical dysplasia by voxel-based 3D MRI analysis. Epilepsy Res. 2005;67:35–50.
4. Colliot O, Antel S, Naessens V, et al. In vivo profiling of focal cortical dysplasia on high-resolution MRI with computational models. Epilepsia. 2006;47(1):134–42.
5. Woermann F, Brandt C, Schaumann-von Stosch R. Neuroradiologische Diagnostik in der Epileptologie. Akt Neurol. 2004;31:60–72.
6. Barkovich A. Pediatric Neuroimaging. Williams + Wilkins, Philadelphia: Lippincott; 2000.
7. Pratt W. Digital Image Processing. New York: John Wiley & Sons; 1991.
8. Haralick R, Shanmugam K, Dinstein I, et al. Textural features for image classification. IEEE Trans System Man Cybern. 1973;3(6):610–21.
9. Galloway M. Texture analysis using gray level run lengths. Comp Graph Image Process. 1975;4:172–9.
10. Ashburner J, Friston K. Multimodal image coregistration and partitioning: A unified framework. Neuroimage. 1997;6:209–17.

Automatic Segmentation of the Cortical Grey and White Matter in MRI Using a Region-Growing Approach Based on Anatomical Knowledge

Christian Wasserthal[1], Karin Engel[1], Karsten Rink[1], André Brechmann[2]

[1]Otto–von–Guericke University, Magdeburg, Germany
[2]Leibniz Institute for Neurobiology, Magdeburg, Germany
karsten@isg.cs.uni-magdeburg.de

Abstract. We propose an automatic procedure for the correct segmentation of grey and white matter in MR data sets of the human brain. Our method exploits general anatomical knowledge for the initial segmentation and for the subsequent refinement of the estimation of the cortical grey matter. Our results are comparable to manual segmentations.

1 Introduction

The analysis of the functional organisation of the cortical areas, as assessed by anatomical and functional MRI, requires a precise segmentation of the grey and white matter in the anatomical data. The automatic segmentation of the cortex is a complex task for two main reasons. First, the inter–subject variability of the human brain anatomy restricts the use of general anatomical knowledge. Second, image artifacts, such as partial volume effects and inhomogeneities of the scans, complicate the separation between grey and white matter regions. Several methods have been applied in recent years to estimate gray and white matter volumes (semi)automatically on MRI [1]. The most popular methods separate intensity histograms which are assumed to be composed of a grey matter distribution and a white matter distribution [2]. The data is then classified directly, or the parameters of the two distributions determine the intensity range for region growing approaches [3]. Other methods include active contours and surfaces [4, 6, 5].

Our algorithm consists of a number of basic methods which resolve the complex task utilising general anatomical knowledge. The algorithm allows for a fully automatic and fast segmentation of the grey and white matter regions.

2 Method

We use an algorithm that allows for a segmentation of the grey and white matter in Talairach transformed MR data sets of the human brain.

The 3d–anatomical T1–weighted MRI were scanned on a 1.5 Tesla head scanner (GE Medical Systems). Using the commercial software BrainVoyager [7] the

16 bit data sets have been converted to 8 bit and transformed to match the standard brain of the Talairach atlas [8] (Fig. 1(a) and 1(e)).

The result of our algorithm is a segmentation in 3D where each voxel x of the data set is assigned one of four labels. These labels are l_W for white matter, l_G for grey matter, l_B for background and l_V for ventricles.

A histogram analysis gives an estimate for the mean value of the white matter intensity E_W, a lower intensity limit for the white matter t_W and an upper threshold for the cerebrospinal fluid (CSF) t_{CSF}.

In order to get a histogram that is suitable for computing the parameters for the regions of interest, we only use voxels within an ellipsoid Ω_1 (Fig. 1(b)), whose parameters are derived from the Talairach proportional grid (Fig. 1(a)) to give an approximation of the cerebrum.

Then, all voxels x with $x < t_{CSF}$ are set to l_B. The CSF in the ventricles gets another label l_V, because the meaning of the background label does not apply here. Given the Talairach proportional grid, the ventricles can easily be located and labeled using a region–growing (Fig. 1(f)). We use two ellipsoids Ω_2 to approximate the eye regions (Fig. 1(e)). The brightest 15% of these areas are set l_B, i.e. background, to avoid problems in the following step of our algorithm.

From our approximation of the cerebrum, Ω_1, in combination with the calculated mean E_W, a small area within the white matter is automatically assigned as seed voxels for a second region growing process. White matter voxels are now segmented based on intensity and minimum distance to background (Fig. 1(c)). More specifically, $x = l_W$ if $x > t_W \wedge min\{d(x, y = l_B)\} \geq 3mm$. The second criterion is based on anatomical knowledge about the brain, that grey matter has a thickness of $3 - 5mm$, even if the data suggest otherwise. This criterion

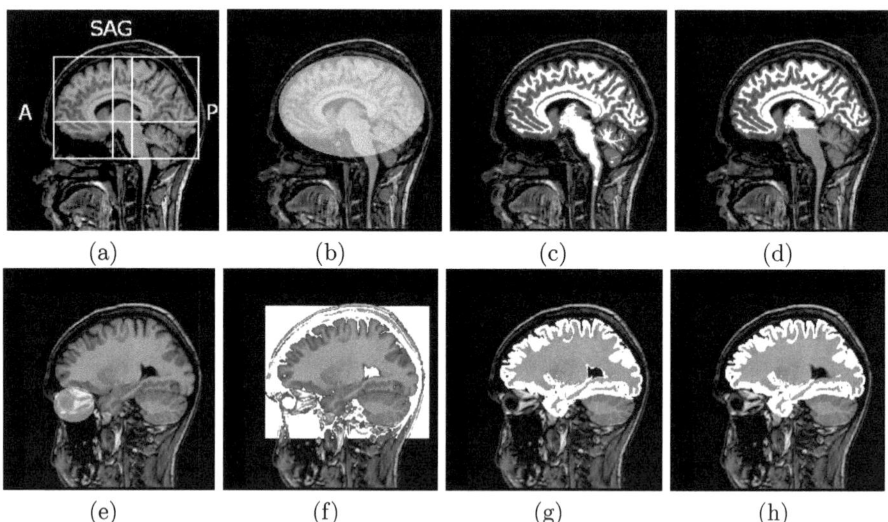

(a) (b) (c) (d)
(e) (f) (g) (h)

Fig. 1. Figures 1(a) and 1(e) present two sagittal slices from one of the data sets. For a detailed description of the intermediate segmentation results (Section 2)

does not apply to the region around the ventricles, where white matter directly borders CSF. Since voxels of this region are assigned the label l_V instead of l_B, this poses no problem to our algorithm. The masking of the eyes was necessary because these high intensity regions touch the brain.

Now we apply a flooding algorithm initialised on the bottom-most voxel $x = l_W$ of the data set, which is in our case always situated in the spinal cord. The algorithm counts in every axial slice i voxels $x_i = l_W$ connected to the spinal cord and sets every voxel $x_i = l_B$ if $\frac{\#x_{i+1}}{\#x_i} < \theta$. Once the flooding reaches the cerebrum, the number of connected white matter voxels in a slice increases significantly and the algorithm stops. Because of this increase, any threshold $100 < \theta < 10000$ gives the same result. Note, that this still allows for white matter voxels below the final flood level in other parts of the brain. Using this simple rule we remove all voxels within the spinal cord and the cerebellum and retain a clean segmentation of the white matter (compare Figs. 1(c) and 1(d)).

In the next step, any unlabelled voxels x with $min\{d(x, y = l_W)\} < 6mm$ are set l_G, i.e. grey matter (Fig. 1(g)). This is a reasonable choice as these voxels have not been labelled as background and are still within the expected range for grey matter. All other still unlabelled voxels are set to l_B. In a number of postprocessing steps we now reduce the number of misclassified voxels. Via a connected component analysis voxels that represent fat, ventricles or meninges are identified and set to l_B. By now, we can easily calculate a mean value E_G from a more reliable set of voxels $x = l_G$ and can change the label of any $x = l_W$ with $|x - E_G| < |x - E_W|$ to l_G (Fig. 1(h)). Finally, all $x = l_V$ can be set l_B, so that all voxels that are not grey or white matter are now labelled as background.

3 Results

Five data sets were available for the evaluation. The quality of the data varied with respect to signal–to–noise ratio and grey level inhomogeneities. A gold standard was given in terms of manual segmentations of four transversal example slices per data set. Additional reference segmentations were computed by using the software BrainVoyager [7], which relies on a comparable segmentation approach and is of widespread use in the neuroimaging community. These segmentations were generated independently by one neurobiologist and one trained expert.

3.1 Performance and Robustness in Parametrisation

The segmentation using BrainVoyager includes the isolation of the brain by applying standard Talairach masks, as well as a histogram–based grey and white matter classification. The masking is followed by nonlinear smoothing and region growing within the segmented volume. The cortex boundary is then improved using morphological operations [3]. For reasons of comparability to our algorithm, we didn't include the inhomogeneity correction usually performed in BrainVoyager by an expert.

For the segmentation with BrainVoyager user interactions were required in one of the five cases. If parameter values, e.g. the threshold for separating grey and white matter, were poorly specified the segmentation failed. Small variations in the parameter values led to significant alterations in the segmentations. The whole segmentation process (without any topological corrections) took the trained user about 300 seconds on a standard PC (3.2 GHz Pentium 4).

Our algorithm is fully automatic and requires no user interaction. In our approach, parametrisation of the different region growing steps is more robust, because it is less data driven but utilises anatomical information, e.g. distance–to–surface priority. In contrast to BrainVoyager, no smoothing for reducing the variation in the grey and white matter signal intensity is needed. Computational time of the whole algorithm on a data set with 256^3 voxels is about 65 seconds. Note, that the postprocessing steps take about 50 seconds, while the large part of the segmentation can be computed very fast due to the simple algorithms.

3.2 Assessment of the Segmentation Results

A visual inspection of the segmentation results by another two experts indicate that our segmentations are of high quality even in regions of low contrast, e.g. the occipital lobe (Fig. 2).

To evaluate the accuracy of our segmentation, we assembled a quantitative analysis based on the slices of the five data sets for which a gold standard was available. Our analysis showed, that the accuracy of our segmentation is comparable with the accuracy of the manual segmentations (Table 1). In contrast, the

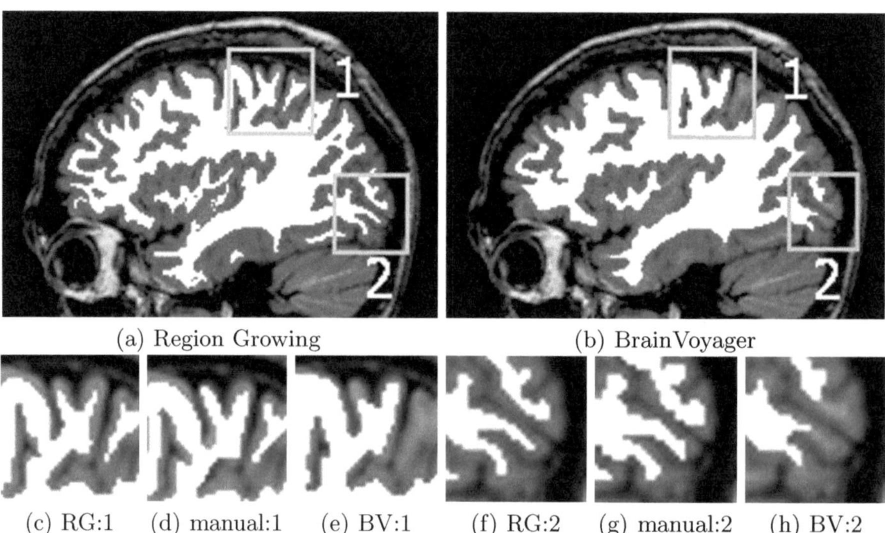

(a) Region Growing (b) BrainVoyager

(c) RG:1 (d) manual:1 (e) BV:1 (f) RG:2 (g) manual:2 (h) BV:2

Fig. 2. Comparison of our algorithm with a BrainVoyager segmentation: representative slice (a,b); particulary difficult regions from the slice (c-h); further examples at http://isgwww.cs.uni-magdeburg.de/bv/rgapplett/

Table 1. Quantitative assessment of the segmentations using BrainVoyager and our Region–Growing approach based on anatomical knowledge. We computed the (mean ± standard deviation of the) Hausdorff–distance d_H and the Mean Squared Distance d_M of the grey–white matter boundaries to compare the segmentation results with the expert's segmentations of example slices of five data sets (in mm)

	Data set	1	2	3	4	5
d_H	BrainVoyager	17.9 ± 7.9	17.3 ± 6.2	14.0 ± 5.7	16.7 ± 4.5	17.3 ± 4.8
	Region–Growing	7.4 ± 2.7	7.5 ± 2.6	9.0 ± 5.4	9.3 ± 2.0	10.2 ± 3.3
d_M	BrainVoyager	16.8 ± 12.2	14.5 ± 10.7	10.9 ± 6.8	21.0 ± 6.8	15.6 ± 10.2
	Region–Growing	1.7 ± 0.8	1.2 ± 0.4	1.5 ± 0.5	3.3 ± 1.7	3.8 ± 0.9

BrainVoyager segmentations clearly underestimate the white matter and miss white matter of gyri which can be easily identified (compare for example Figs. 2(c) and 2(d)).

4 Discussion

We presented a technique for the segmentation of grey and white matter in MRI data using a modified region growing process. By incorporating general anatomical knowledge in a sequence of simple segmentation steps we obtained robust and fully automatic segmentation results. These results are comparable to the manual segmentations of trained experts.

References

1. Pham D.L., Xu C. and Prince J.L.: Current methods in medical image segmentation. Ann Rev of Biomed Engineering 2(1) 2000:315–337.
2. Mangin JF, Coulon O, Frouin V. robust brain segmentation using histogram scale-space analysis and mathematical morphology. Lect Note Comp Sci. 1998;3175:1230–41.
3. Kriegeskorte N, Goebel R. An efficient algorithm for topologically correct segmentation of the cortical sheet in anatomical MR volumes. NeuroImage. 2001;14:329–46.
4. Davatzikos C, Bryan N. Using a deformable surface model to obtain a shape representation of the cortex. IEEE Trans Med Imag. 1996;15(6):785–95.
5. Goldenberg R, Kimmel R, Rivlin E, et al. Cortex segmentation: A fast variational geometric approach. IEEE Trans Med Imag 2002;21(12):1544–51.
6. Dale A, Fischl B, Sereno M. Cortical surface–based analysis: 1. Segmentation and surface reconstruction. NeuroImage 1999;9:179–94.
7. Goebel R. Brain Voyager 2.0: From 2D to 3D fMRI analysis and visualization. NeuroImage 1997;5:635, http://brainvoyager.com
8. Talairach J, Tournoux P. Co-Planar Stereotaxic Atlas of the Human Brain. Stuttgart: Thieme 1988

Model-Based Segmentation of Cortical Regions of Interest for Multi-subject Analysis of fMRI Data

Karin Engel[1], André Brechmann[2], Klaus Toennies[1]

[1]Otto-von-Guericke University, Magdeburg, Germany
[2]Leibniz Institute for Neurobiology, Magdeburg, Germany
engel@isg.cs.uni-magdeburg.de

Abstract. The high inter–subject variability of human neuroanatomy complicates the analysis of functional imaging data across subjects. We propose a method for the correct segmentation of cortical regions of interest based on the cortical surface. First results on the segmentation of Heschl's gyrus indicate the capability of our approach for correct comparison of functional activations in relation to individual cortical patterns.

1 Introduction

The current approach in functional brain imaging is to average the data across subjects and map the resulting brain activation on a standard brain (i.e. Talairach or Montreal Neurological Institute (MNI)). A prerequisite for the precise localisation of functional areas, however, is to correctly register any given brain volume to the brain template used as standard space. Different registration methods are used to compensate either only the brain size by linear transformation or the relative location and shape of gross anatomical structures, i.e. prominent sulci and gyri, by non–linear transformations both implemented in fMRI analysis software like SPM (http://www.fil.ion.ucl.ac.uk/spm/) or BrainVoyager (http://brainvoyager.com). Current registration methods, however, do not adequately consider inter–individual differences in configuration of specific brain regions, e.g. the auditory cortex (AC) [3]. The alternative approach is to define subject–specific regions of interest (ROI) by using a combination of anatomical landmarks and clusters of brain activation obtained in functional imaging studies [1, 6]. So far, the observer–dependent and time–consuming nature of the manual delineation of ROI represents a tradeoff for the advantages (better spatial specificity and improved statistical power) of this approach.

Therefore, we developed a hierarchical Finite Element Model of the auditory cortical folding pattern and applied it to the automatic surface–based labeling of Heschl's gyrus [4]. Here, we use our model for segmentation of the landmark–oriented auditory ROI described in [1, 6]. This provides a reliable surface–based comparison of auditory functional activations across subjects.

2 Method

We use an algorithm that allows for the sequential segmentation of landmark–related cortical ROI based on the cortical surface. Functional activations are analysed and classified at a regional level.

2.1 Definition and Segmentation of the ROI

Our algorithm utilises the properties of the cortical surface, represented as flat maps (Fig. 1(a)). This firstly requires the inner cortical surface (white – grey matter boundary) to be extracted based on the exact segmentation of the grey and white matter according to [8]. The triangulated cortical surface of each hemisphere is then processed to create flat maps using BrainVoyager.

The empirical system of landmark–related ROI serves to parcellate the AC into four areas with known differential activation [1, 6]. The ROI form adjacent territories in the individual hemispheres in relation to the anatomical landmarks depicted in Fig. 1(b). ROI T1 follows the course of Heschl's gyrus (HG) on its anteromedial rim and extends on the lateral aspect of gyrus temporalis superior (lGTS). TA covers planum polare anterior to HG, T2 is centered to Heschl's sulcus (HS), and T3 covers the posterior planum temporale (PT).

A collection of finite element models (FEM) [7, 4] represents the structural decomposition of the auditory cortical folding pattern into different gyri and

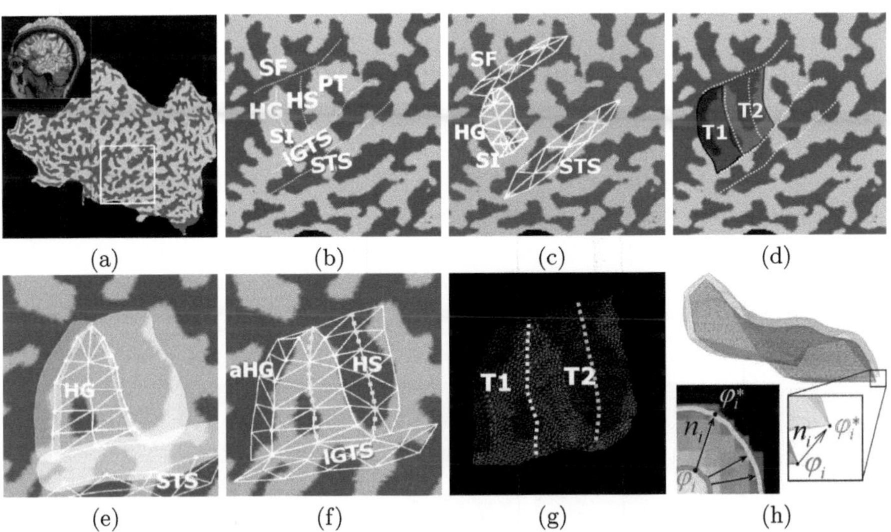

Fig. 1. Identification of anatomical landmarks and surface–based segmentation of auditory ROI. Our algorithm utilises the properties of 2D flat maps of the cortical surface (a) and detailled (b)–(g). Color indicates gyri (light), sulci (dark) and background (black). Each flat map vertex φ_i is associated with its position on the 3D folded cortical surface (h)

sulci, namely HG - which may or may not show a sulcus intermedius (SI) -, Sylvian Fissure (SF) and sulcus temporalis superior (STS). It represents HG as the central part of the hierarchical FEM of the AC (Fig. 1(c)). Automatic segmentation of the landmarks in the individual flat maps can be accomplished by a combination of the dynamic FEM with an evolutionary strategy, as described in [4], or with user interaction (Sec. 3).

The temporal lobe is then further subdivided. In this work, we are only interested in T1 and T2 (Fig. 1(d)), i.e. labeling of HS, the anteromedial rim of HG (aHG) and lGTS completes our parcellation. The shape models of HG and STS – which are segmented in the previous step of our algorithm – define expectation maps for the adjacent HS, aHG and lGTS (Fig. 1(e)). These are likewise represented as dynamic FEM. The algorithm initialises the FEM based on the parametrisation of the HG and STS model, i.e. it uses the final displacements of the matched shape models' boundary nodes (Fig. 1(f)).

Based on the segmented anatomical landmarks, the temporal lobe of each individual subject can be easily parcellated into the two auditory ROI. Therefore, flat map vertices segmented by the FEM of aHG, HG and HS are combined. Finally, ROI T1 and T2 are separated by the medial axis nodes of the HG model. Each flat map vertex φ_i is now assigned label l_b for background, or contributes to the inner cortical surface of ROI $r \in \{T1, T2\}$, i.e. $\varphi_i = l_r$ (Fig. 1(g)). The corresponding outer cortical surface of ROI r is represented by vertices $\{\varphi_i^* = l_r\}$, which are estimated by sampling the pre–segmented grey matter along the surface normals n_i (Fig. 1(h)). The voxels enclosed by $\{\varphi_i = l_r\}$ and $\{\varphi_i^* = l_r\}$ constitute the 3D–ROI masks used for analysis of fMRI data.

2.2 Surface-Based ROI Analysis of the fMRI Data

The activation profiles for all voxels v_j within a ROI mask are extracted and modeled using the general linear model [5]. Contrasting with the standard voxel–level analyses, the statistical tests are performed on the regional activations. Activation clusters exceeding a spatial extent of 8 contiguous voxels at the given significance level, e.g. $p < .001$, are considered for further analyses.

In our case, we are interested in comparing the activation patterns within ROI across subjects. The clustered functional volumes are therefore projected

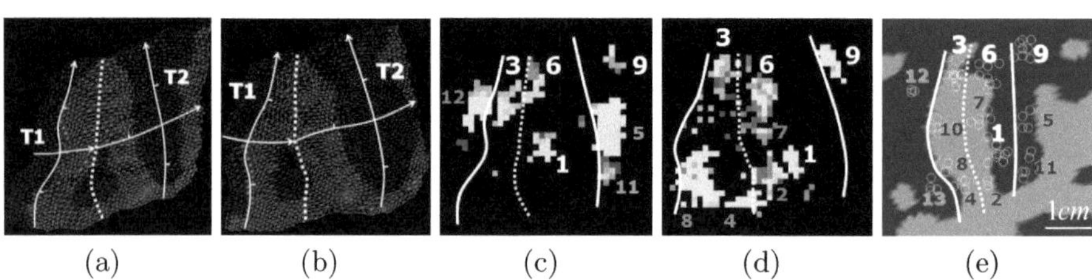

Fig. 2. Classification of functional activations: auditory ROI T1 and T2 in left hemisphere (LH) for two different subjects (a)–(d); activations are displayed in resolution of voxels v_j (c), (d); activation peaks for nine subjects mapped onto a template (e)

Table 1. The (mean ± standard deviation of the) Hausdorff–distance δ_H of the 2D ROI boundaries and the region overlap ω of the 3D ROI masks were computed for comparison with the expert's segmentations of nine data sets

ROI	T1, LH	T2, LH	T1, RH	T2, RH
δ_H in *mm*	0.12 ± 0.1	0.19 ± 0.12	0.1 ± 0.09	0.16 ± 0.11
ω in %	95.0 ± 2.9	94.1 ± 3.6	94.5 ± 4.0	94.0 ± 4.1

onto the individual cortical surfaces. We employ two different volume–to–surface projection methods which define a mapping $M : \varphi_i \mapsto v_j$. The first method is to consider each vertex $\varphi_i = l_r$ of the 3D inner cortical surface of ROI r and assign to it the activation of the voxel with which it intersects (M_I). Second, the activation along the entire grey matter thickness of the ROI is considered. It is defined by pairs of vertices ($\varphi_i = l_r, \varphi_i^*$) (Fig. 1(h)). The maximum activation along this segment is mapped to φ_i (M_{TS}).

A local, object–centered coordinate system is established in each individual data set by the model–based segmentation of the ROI. This allows for the detailed classification of the activations based on the spatial position w.r.t. the coordinates. In our case, activations within T2 can be differentiated by their relation to the medial axis nodes of the HS model, which constitute the y–coordinate (lateral–medial). Linear interpolation of the nodal displacements along the boundaries of the HG and HS models establishes the x–coordinate (anterior–posterior) within T2. Equivalent clusters within T1 can be identified based on the x–coordinate which is defined similarly based on the boundaries of aHG and HG. The nodes which are shared by the aHG and HG models represent the y–coordinate (lateral–medial) within T1 (Figs. 2(a) and 2(b)).

3 Results

The two auditory ROI in the left and right hemispheres (LH and RH) were parcellated for nine subjects. A gold standard was given in terms of manual segmentations of the ROI in 2D (on the flat maps) and in the 3D MRI data sets.

3.1 Quality and Performance of the ROI Mask Segmentation

In this work, we interactively initialised the prototypical finite element meshes which represent the shape and structural configuration of HG, (SI), SF and STS (Fig. 1(c)). More specifically, instances of the hierarchical FEM of the auditory folds were placed close to the position of the landmark SF in each individual flat map and adequately scaled, i.e. two mouse clicks were required for initialisation. This allows examining the adequacy of our segmentation method based on correctly identified landmarks HG, SF and STS (note, that FEM of HS, aHG and lGTS are initialised automatically). For all data sets segmentation of ROI T1 and T2 in 2D stopped after $7-20$ seconds. While manual delineation of the ROI in a 3D MRI data set took a trained expert $45-70$ minutes, the 3D–ROI masks were computed in about 30 seconds on a standard PC (3.2GHz P4, Matlab/C). As given in Table 1, our segmentations are comparable with the gold standard in 2D (which proves correct extrapolation of the individual ROI boundaries) and 3D (which shows accuracy in sampling the ROI's grey matter volume).

3.2 Surface-Based fMRI ROI Analysis

To proof our concept of surface–based labeling of functional activations, we applied our method to the auditory fMRI study of Deike et al. [2]. We used the M_{TS} mapping before labeling of the activation clusters, because we found that at average 67% more activation in the cortical grey matter was captured compared with the mapping M_I.

While usually a ROI analysis computes the coordinate of the activation peak in standard space, our method considers any ROI activations and computes several candidates for fields of specific functionality. Moreover, the contribution of individual activations can be analysed w.r.t. the group average ROI activations. In our case, the inter–subject comparison of activation patterns relies on labels which represent relations to anatomical landmarks. Figures 2(c) and 2(d) show multiple labeled clusters of auditory activation for two subjects. Dotted and solid lines represent HG and the y–coordinates of T1 and T2, respectively. Figure 2(e) shows activation peaks of identical clusters in all nine subjects mapped to a template based on the displacements of the parametric ROI model in the individual and template cortical surfaces. Clusters with equivalent labels varied of up to $8mm$ in standard space. However, the spatial configuration was consistent among subjects (for example, clusters 1,3,6 and 9 were present in all nine subjects, cluster 12 in three subjects), which suggests functional correspondence.

4 Discussion

Using our hierarchical deformable shape model, individual landmark–related ROI can be segmented almost automatically and very precisely. The parametric ROI model supports a detailed functional parcellation of the human neocortex.

References

1. Brechmann A, Baumgart F, Scheich H. Sound–level–dependent representation of frequency modulations in human auditory cortex: A low noise fMRI study. J Neurophys 2003; 87: 423–33
2. Deike S, et al. Auditory stream segregation relying on timbre involves left auditory cortex. Neuroreport 2004; 15(9): 1511–4
3. Desai R, et al. Volumetric vs. surface–based alignment for localization of auditory cortex activation. Neuroimage 2005; 26: 1019–29
4. Engel K, Brechmann A, Toennies K. A two–level dynamic model for the representation and recognition of cortical folding patterns. Proc IEEE ICIP 2005; 297–300

5. Friston K, et al. Statistical parametric maps in functional imaging: A general linear approach. Human Brain Mapping 1995; 2: 189–210
6. Gaschler-Markefski B, et al. Definition of human auditory cortex territories based on anatomical landmarks and fMRI activation. In: Dynamics of Speech Production and Perception, IOS-Press 2006; 5–16
7. Sclaroff S, Pentland A. Modal matching for correspondence and recognition. IEEE Trans Pattern Anal Mach Intell 1995; 17(6): 545–61
8. Wasserthal C, et al. Automatic segmentation of the cortical grey and white matter in MRI using a region growing approach based on anatomical knowledge. Proc BVM 2008;

Probabilistic Tracking of Virus Particles in Fluorescence Microscopy Image Sequences

W.J. Godinez[1,2], M. Lampe[3], S. Wörz[1,2], B. Müller[3], R. Eils[1,2], K. Rohr[1,2]

[1]BIOQUANT, IPMB, University of Heidelberg, Germany
[2]Dept. of Bioinformatics and Functional Genomics, DKFZ Heidelberg, Germany
[3]Department of Virology, University of Heidelberg, Germany
wgodinez@ieee.org

Abstract. Fluorescence time-lapse microscopy is a powerful technique for observing the spatial-temporal behavior of viruses. To quantitatively analyze the exhibited dynamical relationships, tracking of viruses over time is required. We developed probabilistic approaches based on particle filters for tracking multiple virus particles in time-lapse fluorescence microscopy images. We employed a mixture of particle filters as well as independent particle filters. For the latter, we have developed a penalization strategy to maintain the identity of the tracked objects in cases where objects are in close proximity. We have applied the approaches to synthetic images and quantified their performance. We have also successfully applied the approaches to real microscopy images of HIV-1 particles and have compared the tracking results with ground truth from manual tracking.

1 Introduction

The aim of our work is to study the dynamic behavior of the human immunodeficiency virus (HIV) based on live cell microscopy using fluorescently labelled virus particles. Tracking single virus particles yields quantitative information that contributes to the understanding of viral processes (e.g., cell entry). To obtain statistically sound conclusions, many individual particles must be automatically tracked. However, tracking virus particles is challenging. Problems are due to the small size of viruses as well as their complex motion behavior. Also, one has to cope with the large number of virus particles, the relatively high level of cell autofluorescence, as well as a relatively low signal-to-noise ratio.

In previous work on *virus tracking*, a *deterministic* two-step paradigm encompassing virus localization and motion correspondence has been typically employed. For localization, most approaches employ a maximum intensity search strategy, where intensity maxima are associated with virus particles (e.g., [1]). For motion correspondence, approaches that consider the motion of all viruses via graph-theoretical algorithms have been used (e.g., [2]). In contrast to the deterministic schemes, *probabilistic* approaches additionally include a spatial-temporal filter. An approach using a pool of Kalman filters has been presented in [3]. However, the steps of object localization and spatial-temporal filtering are uncoupled. This entails that temporal information is not used for localization, and analogously image information is not directly used by the filter to estimate the position of an object. In contrast to the Kalman filter, the particle filter, which has been introduced to the field of computer vision in [4], exploits more efficiently the image and temporal information encoded in an image sequence. An approach using a mixture of particle filters for virus tracking has been presented in [5]. There, however, only a fixed number of objects could be tracked. Generally, the number of objects changes over time (e.g., objects enter the field of view).

In this contribution, we introduce probabilistic approaches for tracking multiple viruses in fluorescence microscopy time-lapse images. We have developed two approaches based on particle filters, namely an approach using a *mixture of particle filters* and an approach using *independent particle filters*. In contrast to the former scheme, the latter approach can track a variable number of objects. We address the problem of filter merging that arises when using independent particle filters via a penalization mechanism based on a deterministic motion correspondence algorithm. The developed approaches are fully automatic and have been successfully applied to synthetic image sequences as well as to real microscopy image sequences displaying HIV-1 particles.

2 Materials and Methods

In our approaches, tracking is formulated as a Bayesian sequential estimation problem. At time step t, the aim is to estimate the state $\mathbf{x}_t$ of a virus given a sequence of measurements $\mathbf{y}_{1:t}$. By modeling the temporal behavior using a *dynamical model* $p(\mathbf{x}_t|\mathbf{x}_{t-1})$ and incorporating image information via a *measurement model* $p(\mathbf{y}_t|\mathbf{x}_t)$, a Bayesian filter estimates the *posterior* distribution $p(\mathbf{x}_t|\mathbf{y}_{1:t})$ via stochastic propagation and Bayes' theorem:

$$p(\mathbf{x}_t|\mathbf{y}_{1:t}) \propto p(\mathbf{y}_t|\mathbf{x}_t) \int p(\mathbf{x}_t|\mathbf{x}_{t-1})p(\mathbf{x}_{t-1}|\mathbf{y}_{1:t-1})d\mathbf{x}_{t-1}$$

An estimate of $\mathbf{x}_t$ can be obtained from the posterior $p(\mathbf{x}_t|\mathbf{y}_{1:t})$, which, in our case, is estimated using a particle filter. This algorithm approximates the posterior with a set $\{\mathbf{x}_t^i; w_t^i\}_{i=1}^{N_s}$ of N_s random samples $\mathbf{x}_t^i$ (the 'particles') that are associated with importance weights w_t^i. In the case of tracking multiple objects that have a similar appearance, multiple modes arise in the posterior distribution. Although a particle filter can in principle handle such a distribution, in practice the filter cannot maintain the multimodality over several time steps [4, 6]. To address this problem, one may model the posterior $p(\mathbf{x}_t|\mathbf{y}_{1:t})$ as a non-parametric M-component *mixture model*:

$$p(\mathbf{x}_t|\mathbf{y}_{1:t}) = \sum_{m=1}^{M} \pi_{m,t} p_m(\mathbf{x}_t|\mathbf{y}_{1:t})$$

where $\pi_{m,t}$ denotes the weight of the *m-th* component [6]. Each $p_m(\mathbf{x}_t|\mathbf{y}_{1:t})$ is approximated using a set of particles $\{\mathbf{x}_t^i; w_t^i\}_{i\in\tau_m}$, where τ_m is the set of indices indicating which particles belong to component m, and particles are allocated using a clustering mechanism. Note that $\sum_{m=1}^{M} |\tau_m| = N_s$, where $|\cdot|$ denotes the set size operator. The estimation performance deteriorates as the number of objects increases, since N_s remains constant, i.e., fewer particles are allocated to each component.

Alternatively, one may track multiple objects by instantiating one *independent particle filter* per object. In this case, for each filter, an independent set of particles of size N_s is used. Failures arise when objects are in close proximity, since the filters converge towards the object with the best likelihood $p(\mathbf{y}_t|\mathbf{x}_t)$. To address this problem, we propose a novel penalization strategy comprising three steps: first, the approach determines objects that are in close proximity. This reduces to finding cliques in an undirected graph, where the vertices are given by the filtered position estimates of the objects, and an edge is said to join two vertices if the distance between the positions of two objects is below a certain value. The second step determines the most plausible position $\hat{\mathbf{x}}_t$ for each object in each clique by seeking modes in the probability density function that is induced by merging all particles of all filters of a clique. The plausible positions are assigned to each object via a global nearest neighbor approach [1]. In some cases (e.g., when objects merge), a plausible position might not be found for an object. In this case, this object is not further considered in the penalization scheme; the filter may merge temporarily with another filter. In the third step, the weights of particles that are relatively distant to the most plausible position $\hat{\mathbf{x}}_t$ of an object are assigned lower values via a Gaussian function; given the lower weights, the resampling step of the particle filter might discard the penalized particles.

3 Results

We have applied our approaches to synthetic as well as real microscopy image sequences. To automatically detect virus particles, we employ either the spot-enhancing filter (SEF) [7] or 2D Gaussian fitting (GaussFit) and combine them with the particle filter approaches. The approaches using a mixture of particle filters (MPF) can only track objects that enter the field of view at time step $t = 0$, while those using independent particle filters (IPF) can track objects that enter the field of view at any time step. To measure the performance, we used the tracking accuracy defined as $P_{\text{track}} = \frac{n_{\text{track,correct}}}{n_{\text{track,total}}}$, which reflects the ratio between the number of correctly computed trajectories $n_{\text{track,correct}}$ and the number of true trajectories $n_{\text{track,total}}$. The value for $n_{\text{track,correct}}$ is computed as the weighted sum of the percentage of tracked time steps $r_{\text{tracked},i}$ for each *i-th* true trajectory: $n_{\text{track,correct}} = \sum_{i=1}^{n_{\text{track,total}}} w_i r_{\text{tracked},i}$, where the weight w_i is given by a Gaussian function, which takes as its argument the number of correctly computed trajectories $n_{\text{track},i}$. The weighting scheme is introduced to penalize computed trajectories that are broken. Note that $P_{\text{track}} \in [0, 1]$.

We validated the approaches based on several synthetic image sequences. Here, we describe the experimental results obtained for one image sequence. This

Table 1. Description of real microscopy image sequences

	Dimensions	No. of time steps	No. of objects
Seq. 1	256 × 256	250	23
Seq. 2	512 × 512	200	15
Seq. 3	512 × 512	400	43

Table 2. Tracking performance P_{track} for real microscopy image sequences

	SEF&MPF	GaussFit&MPF	SEF&IPF	GaussFit&IPF
Seq. 1	84.82%	81.95%	86.73%	82.61%
Seq. 2	84.64%	85.64%	93.54%	93.54%
Seq. 3	50.62%	49.04%	74.64%	67.76%

sequence consists of 100 images (256×256 pixels, 16-bit) displaying 20 synthetic particles. The SNR level is 4.55 and the noise model was assumed to be Poisson distributed. The quantitative experimental results are as follows: SEF&MPF achieves 79.28%, GaussFit&MPF attains 80.00%, SEF&IPF yields 85.65%, and GaussFit&IPF achieves 90.13%.

We also validated the algorithms using real microscopy image sequences. In these sequences, fluorescently labeled HIV-1 particles were imaged using a fluorescence wide-field microscope. Fluorophores were excited with their respective excitation wavelengths and movies were recorded with a frequency of 10Hz [8]. Ground truth for the virus positions was obtained by manual tracking using the commercial software MetaMorph. The quantitative experimental results for three sequences are presented in Table 2. Each sequence consists of 200 up to 400 frames (Table 1). Sample images of tracking results for the real sequence "Seq. 3" are shown in Fig. 1. Analogously to the experiments using synthetic data, it turns out that the approaches using IPF yield a higher tracking accuracy than those using MPF.

4 Discussion

Our experimental results suggest that the approaches based on independent particle filters (IPF) outperform those using a mixture of particle filters (MPF). The reason for this is twofold. First, since the MPF allocates a different number of particles to each object via a clustering mechanism, poor estimation results are obtained for those objects with few allocated particles. The clustering mechanism may generate non-compact clusters, which lead to inaccurate position estimates, in particular, for objects that lie in close proximity. In contrast, the IPF not only uses a constant number of particles for each object, but also copes with problems induced by the proximity of objects via our penalization scheme. Second, since the MPF cannot track a variable number of objects, its performance is reduced. In contrast, the IPF is able to handle a variable number of objects.

In summary, we have developed probabilistic approaches based on particle filters for tracking multiple viruses in microscopy image sequences. Our quantita-

Fig. 1. Tracking results for two approaches for the real microscopy image sequence "Seq. 3" (time step $t = 140$). For both approaches, an enlarged section delineated with a black rectangle is shown next to the original image

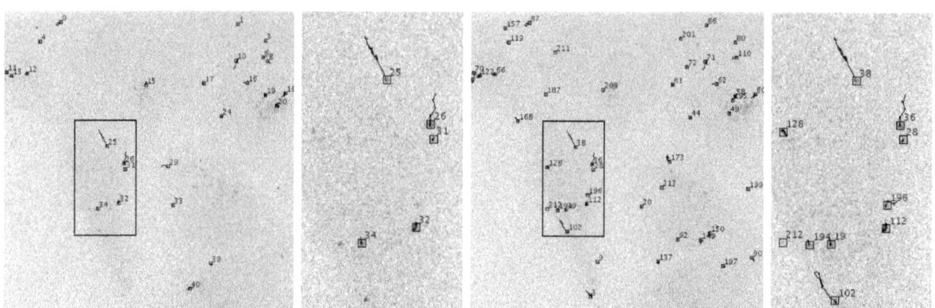

SEF&MPF: Original image and section SEF&IPF: Original image and section

tive experimental results based on synthetic and real microscopy image sequences show that the approaches yield a good tracking performance. The superior performance of our approach using IPF in combination with the novel penalization scheme suggests that this approach is well-suited for solving the problem of multiple object tracking.

Acknowledgement. Support of the BMBF (FORSYS) project VIROQUANT gratefully acknowledged.

References

1. Sbalzarini IF, Koumoutsakos P. Feature point tracking and trajectory analysis for video imaging in cell biology. J Struct Biol. 2005;151(2):182–95.
2. Schutz GJ, Schindler H, Schmidt T. Single-molecule microscopy on model membranes reveals anomalous diffusion. Biophys J. 1997;73(2):1073–80.
3. Arhel N, Genovesio A, Kim K, et al. Quantitative four-dimensional tracking of cytoplasmic and nuclear HIV-1 complexes. Nat Methods. 2006;3(10):817–24.
4. Isard M, Blake A. CONDENSATION: Conditional density propagation for visual tracking. Int J Computer Vis. 1998;29(1):5–28.
5. Godinez WJ, Lampe M, Wörz S, et al. Tracking of virus particles in time-lapse fluorescence microscopy image sequences. Proc BVM. 2007; p. 6–10.
6. Vermaak J, Doucet A, Pérez P; IEEE. Maintaining multi-modality through mixture tracking. Proc ICCV. 2003; p. 1110–6.
7. Sage D, Neumann FR, Hediger F, et al. Automatic tracking of individual fluorescence particles: Application to the study of chromosome dynamics. IEEE Trans Image Process. 2005;14(9):1372–82.
8. Lampe M, Briggs JAG, Endress T, et al. Double-labelled HIV-1 particles for study of virus-cell interaction. Virology. 2007;360(1):92–104.

Automated Analysis of siRNA Screens of Virus Infected Cells Based on Immunofluorescence Microscopy

Petr Matula[1,2], Anil Kumar[3], Ilka Wörz[3], Nathalie Harder[1,2], Holger Erfle[4], Ralf Bartenschlager[3], Roland Eils[1,2], Karl Rohr[1,2]

[1]BIOQUANT, IPMB, University of Heidelberg, [2] Dept. Bioinformatics and Functional Genomics, Biomedical Computer Vision Group, DKFZ Heidelberg
[3] Department of Molecular Virology, University of Heidelberg
[4] BIOQUANT, University of Heidelberg
p.matula@dkfz.de

Abstract. We present an image analysis approach as part of a high-throughput microscopy screening system based on cell arrays for the identification of genes involved in Hepatitis C and Dengue virus replication. Our approach comprises: cell nucleus segmentation, quantification of virus replication level in cells, localization of regions with transfected cells, cell classification by infection status, and quality assessment of an experiment. The approach is fully automatic and has been successfully applied to a large number of cell array images from screening experiments. The experimental results show a good agreement with the expected behavior of positive as well as negative controls and encourage the application to screens from further high-throughput experiments.

1 Introduction

Viruses need to enter cells and exploit their cellular machinery to produce own copies. Classical virology has focused on the virus itself, thereby neglecting critically important processes of the host cells [1]. Our ultimate goal is to develop a high-throughput microscopy screening system for genome-wide identification of cellular genes potentially involved in virus entry and replication, which is expected to lead to improvements in antiviral treatments. The general aim of our study is to develop approaches for automated analysis of images from genome-wide screens (with more than 20,000 genes generating more than 100,000 fluorescence images). Key tasks in this application are cell nucleus segmentation, detection of regions with transfected cells, and quantification of the virus infection level. The approaches should be efficient, robust, and fully automatic.

In recent years, a number of approaches for cell nuclei or whole cell segmentation based on fluorescence microscopy or other microscopy techniques have been reported (e.g., [2, 3, 4]). In *high-throughput* applications, approaches based on adaptive thresholding [5, 6] proved to give good results for cell nuclei segmentation, especially if the nuclei are not clustered. To separate clusters of nuclei, watershed-based approaches are often employed (e.g., [6]).

In this contribution, we describe an image analysis approach as part of a high-throughput system for genome-wide identification of cellular genes that are important for Hepatitis C and Dengue virus replication. Currently, to our best knowledge, there exists no image analysis system for quantifying viral signals given a large number of images on per cell basis, i.e. which measures the status of virus replication in transfected cells only, and combines the results from many different and repeated experiments to produce reliable statistics. In particular, we propose novel approaches (1) for the segmentation of cell nuclei based on gradient thresholding, (2) for the localization of regions with transfected cells within cell array images, and (3) for cell classification based on the infection level with application to quality assessment of an experiment.

2 Materials and Methods

The input data in our application consists of two-channel microscopy images of small interference RNA (siRNA) cell arrays [7] on which transfection reagents and different siRNAs are spotted in a grid pattern (Fig. 1a). We have developed an approach that comprises the following five main steps: (1) cell nuclei segmentation in channel 1 (Fig. 1b), (2) measurement of the level of viral protein expression in channel 2 stained by immunofluorescence (Fig. 1c), (3) detection of siRNA spot areas with transfected cells (Fig. 1d), (4) classification of cells based on their infection status, and (5) quality assessment of an experiment.

- *Segmentation:* To segment cell nuclei we use a gradient thresholding approach. We determine cell nucleus boundary regions by combining information from a gradient magnitude image and an image obtained by applying the Laplacian of Gaussian. This approach was previously applied for the segmentation of characters for text recognition [8]. In comparison to [8] we introduce the following post-processing steps. First, we apply connected component labeling and remove small and large objects. Then, the remaining objects are

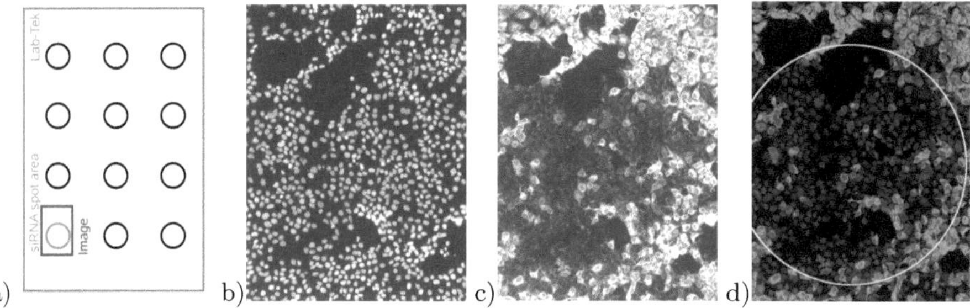

Fig. 1. Image data. (a) Cell array with $M \times N$ siRNA spot areas, (b) Image of cell nuclei for one spot area (channel 1), (c) Corresponding viral protein expression (channel 2), (d) Overlay of both channels and marked spot area

conditionally dilated while preventing merging with other components. Afterwards, holes in objects are filled (Fig. 2a). Finally, cell nuclei are identified in segmented objects by applying size and circularity criteria.

- *Quantification:* The virus replication level is quantified for each nucleus in its neighborhood by computing the mean of the intensities in the virus channel (channel 2). We have implemented and compared three different approaches for defining the neighborhood of nuclei: simple dilation (Fig. 2b), restricted dilation by influence zones (IZ) (Fig. 2d), and region growing in IZ (Fig. 2e). The latter two approaches rely on a partition of an image into IZ of each nucleus (Fig. 2c), which was computed using a seeded watershed transform of the inverted virus channel with the nuclei as initial seeds.
- *Localization:* Only those cells that come in contact with siRNA molecules should be quantified and therefore a circular region with transfected cells of known diameter must be localized in each image. Our approach consists of three steps: (1) finding the position of a circle of known diameter that has maximal difference between the mean virus expression level of cells inside and outside the circle, (2) selecting those positions that have expression level differences within a valid range, and (3) fitting of a grid with known parameters. Spot diameter and grid parameters are known from the siRNA spotting process. The valid range in step 2 was determined by simulations.
- *Classification:* To detect differences in virus infection level we use a measure denoted as infection rate ratio: $IRR = IR_i/IR_N$, where IR_i is the percentage of virus infected cells in siRNA spot area i and IR_N is the normal virus infection rate, i.e. the percentage of infected cells without knocked-down genes. To compute infection rates, the cells must first be classified as infected or non-infected. For classification we use the mean intensity in the virus channel in the neighborhood of a cell nucleus. The classification threshold was determined by maximizing the difference of infection rates in positive and negative controls. In positive controls the protein production level is blocked and therefore the signal is reduced. In negative controls the level of virus replication is not altered.
- *Quality Assessment:* A large number of images need to be analyzed to derive sound statistics. Since some of the images may be of poor quality (e.g., out-

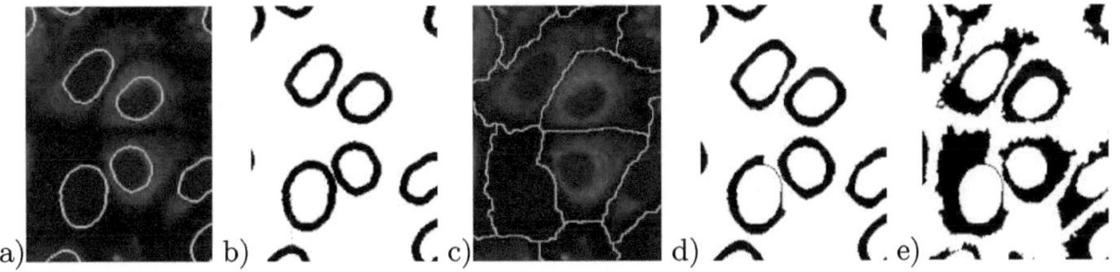

Fig. 2. Segmentation results for an image section. (a) Cell nuclei (blue), viral protein expression (red) with overlaid segmented nuclei, (b) Neighborhoods obtained by dilation, (c) Influence zones (IZ), (d) Constrained dilation by IZ, (e) Region-growing inside IZ

of-focus, no cells in certain areas, image artifacts) we need to exclude them. We perform quality checks on two levels: (1) on the whole experiment level and (2) on the single image level. On the whole experiment level, the main criterion is the difference between infection rates in positive and negative controls. If the difference is too small, the whole experiment is excluded. On the single image level, images with too small or a too large number of cells as compared to the average number of the whole experiment are excluded.

3 Results

Prior to applying the overall approach, we performed an evaluation of our approach for cell nuclei segmentation. To obtain ground truth, two experts marked cell nuclei in 8 randomly selected real images from 4 different experiments (2243 nuclei in total). We compared the results of our approach with that of adaptive thresholding by Otsu's method [5]. With our approach we were able to segment more than 94% of all nuclei whereas Otsu's method yielded only about 80%. We also studied the performance of the three approaches for defining the cell nucleus neighborhood. For each approach, we computed infection rate ratios (IRRs) for two experiments with 384 images each. The results of all three approaches were similar. Therefore we use the simplest approach based on dilation.

We have applied the overall approach to more than 20,000 images of Hepatitis C (HCV) and Dengue Virus (DV) infected screens. The overall results of 10 repeated experiments of an HCV screen (grid 6×6) and of 4 repeated experiments of a DV screen (grid 12×32) are presented in Fig. 3. Positive and negative controls are marked in Fig. 3a with light and dark gray bars and in Fig. 3b,c

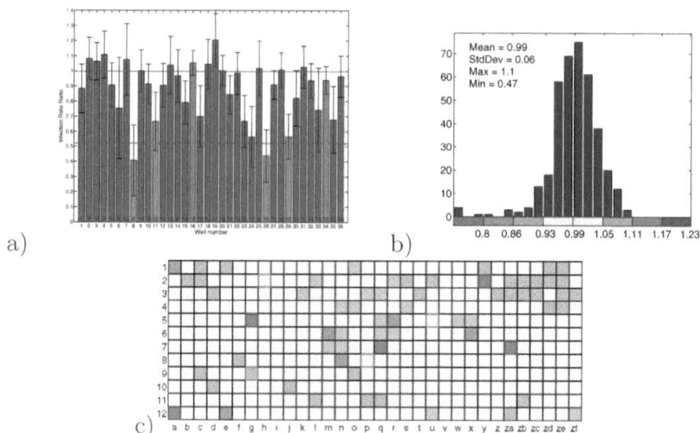

Fig. 3. Infection rate ratios computed from screening experiments. Results averaged (a) from 10 repeated experiments of an HCV screen, and (b, c) from 4 repeated experiments of a DV screen. The infection rate ratio is represented by gray tones (see the gray tone scale below the histogram)

they are marked at positions (a12, g5, q7, za7) and (g9, h2, p8, u5), respectively. It turned out that we obtain a good agreement with a reduced IRRs in positive controls as compared to IRRs in negative controls. Besides positive controls, reduced IRRs were also observed in other siRNA spot areas. This indicates the applicability of the whole approach.

4 Discussion

We have described an approach for the identification of genes involved in Hepatitis C and Dengue virus replication based on high-throughput screening experiments. The whole approach relies on (1) a novel gradient-based approach for segmentation of cell nuclei in fluorescence microscopy images, which increases the number of correctly segmented objects compared to adaptive thresholding, (2) combination of model-based circular region fitting and grid fitting for the localization of siRNA spot regions, which allows to exclude non-transfected cells, and (3) cell classification based on the infection level. The overall approach allows to fully automatically quantify a large number of images on single cell basis. The obtained results are in good agreement with the expected behavior and encourage the application to images from other high-throughput experiments, in particular, from genome-wide screens.

Acknowledgement. This work has been funded by the BMBF (FORSYS) project VIROQUANT.

References

1. Dam EM, Pelkmans L. Systems biology of virus entry in mammalian cells. Cell Microbiol. 2006;8(8):1219–27.
2. Wählby C, Lindblad J, Vondrus M, et al. Algorithms for cytoplasm segmentation of fluorescence labelled cells. Anal Cell Pathol. 2002;24:101–11.
3. Würflinger T, Stockhausen J, Meyer-Ebrecht D, et al. Robust automatic coregistration, segmentation, and classification of cell nuclei in multimodal cytopathological microscopic images. Comput Med Imaging Graph. 2004;28(1–2):87–98.
4. Elter M, Daum V, Wittenberg T. Maximum-intensity-linking for segmentation of fluorescence-stained cells. Proc MIAAB. 2006; p. 46–50.
5. Harder N, Mora-Bermúdez F, Godinez WJ, et al. Automated analysis of the mitotic phases of human cells in 3D fluorescence microscopy image sequences. Lect Note Comp Sci. 2006;4190:840–8.
6. Li F, Zhou X, Ma J, et al. An automated feedback system with the hybrid model of scoring and classification for solving over-segmentation problems in RNAi high-content screening. J Microsc. 2007;226(2):121–32.
7. Erfle H, Simpson JC, Bastiaens PIH, et al. siRNA cell arrays for high-content screening microscopy. Biotechnol. 2004;37(3):454–62.
8. Gonzalez RC, Woods RE. Digital Image Processing. Prentice Hall; 2002.

Determination of Contrast Sensitivity for Mammographic Softcopy Reading

Dörte Apelt, Heinz-Otto Peitgen

MeVis Research GmbH, Bremen
doerte.apelt@mevis.de

Abstract. Research of visual perception of luminance differences is an important basis for understanding the perception of complex patterns. We introduce a new approach for determining the contrast sensitivity function (CSF) in front of the complex anatomical structures of mammograms. For this purpose a sinusoidal pattern and digits are used as target items. The approximation to contrast thresholds is done by a psychophysical staircase procedure and is performed for a selection of spatial frequencies.

1 Introduction

The processing of contrast is a fundamental element in the visual pattern recognition. The quality of perceived structural properties of a mammogram depends on the presentation of the images, both from the technical parameters (size, maximum contrast of the monitor, gray value depth etc.) and ambient conditions (e.g. illuminance), and on the visualization method.

In psychological perception research contrast sensitivity is mainly investigated by use of sinusoidal patterns in front of a homogeneous image background [1]. It is not clear how results of those investigations attend to contrast sensitivity in front of a complex background.

In mammography the mapping of luminance differences is studied by test patterns like CDMAM phantoms [2] or by simulated or extracted mammographic lesions [3], and appropriate contrast detail diagrams. The CDMAM phantom permits a standardized assessment of the imaging properties of a system, although it disregards the complex anatomical structure of mammograms. On the other hand the use of lesions in different contrast levels together with a mammogram takes into account anatomical noise, but has the disadvantage that the results of an investigation strongly depend on the radiological expertise of the observers.

In this paper an approach is presented, that combines the advantages of using a standardized test pattern with that of a realistic complex mammographic image background.

2 Material and Methods

2.1 Target Items: Gabor Patterns and Digits

For the discrimination task a Gabor pattern is presented in a mammogram on an area of about 2.5 cycles per degree (visual angle) and for a time of 720 ms (Fig. 1). Contrast, orientation and spatial frequency of the pattern are varied. For the identification task the observer is confronted with digits as target items. The location of the items is marked by a fixation circle. The task of the observer is to focus on the given areal and to pay attention to given properties of the target item. After every presentation of the item the observer has to state the perceived orientation respectively digit. Each measurement starts with a significantly above threshold contrast. Dependent on the observers' answer the contrast is increased or decreased by a defined step width. The observer has to decide between 4 possible orientations respectively 10 possible digits, but furthermore he has the option to answer nothing seen (Unforced Choice Task, UWUD procedure [4]).

During the experiment the contrast is modified by a factor $f > 0$, which results in a change of the amplitude. For every pixel the factor marks the difference between the target item and the background.

2.2 Hypotheses

Three hypotheses are examined in the experiment:

- A CSF that is determined with a homogeneous background does not allow implications for a CSF with a complex image background, because the complex background involves higher cognitive processing of the visual input (tested for the discrimination task).
- The shape of the CSF is similar for mammograms with different tissue characteristics (tested for the discrimination task).
- The CSF for Gabor patterns (discrimination task) has a higher level than the CSF for digits (identification task).

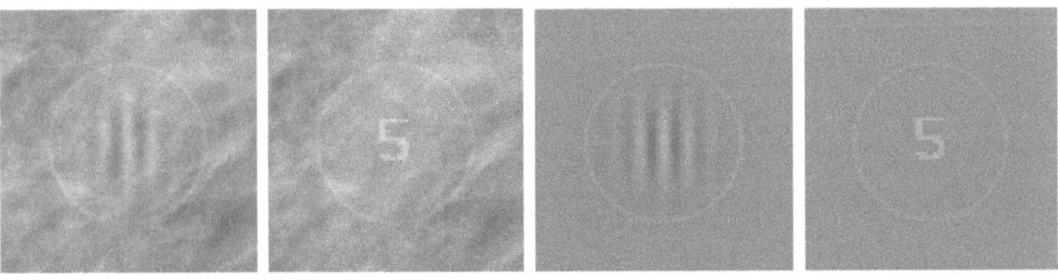

Fig. 1. Parts of the presented images with examples of the used target items (Gabor pattern, digit) with a mammographic respectively homogeneous background

2.3 Observers and Experimental Setup

Eight observers without radiological qualification participated in the experiment. The age range was between 25 and 65 years. The experiment was arranged in a room at an illumination of 10 lx (measured from viewers position with Gossen MavoLux 5032C). The observer was sitting in circa 57 cm distance of two 5K grayscale displays. On the left screen the target item was presented. The mammogram and the position of the item were not modified during the course of the measurement. Moreover the window level settings were fixed.

In the first 15 minutes measurements of contrast thresholds were conducted ongoing, to follow the adaptation to the luminance. For the last measurement in this period a uniform adaptation level of the observers can be expected (though individual differences in the reached adaptation levels can not be excluded). This measurement was used to check the hypotheses.

The determination of contrast thresholds was done with different images. Fig. 2 shows the corresponding parts of the images, where the items were presented.

3 Results

The main results of the experiment are shown graphically in Fig. 3, 4 and 5. Fig. 3 shows the contrast sensitivity functions of two observers P1 and P2 for a homogeneous and a mammographic image background. In both cases the CSF on homogeneous background is higher than on tissue. The contrast sensitivity functions of the same two observers but for different tissues are given in Fig. 4. The difference in contrast sensitivity for Gabor pattern and digits is shown in Fig. 5.

4 Discussion

For all observers the contrast sensitivity is significantly higher on a homogeneous background than on a tissue background with its anatomical noise. An explicit statement regarding the level and the shape of the CSF on tissue can not be derived from the CSF on homogeneous background. On tissue the CSF is less uniform (Fig. 3).

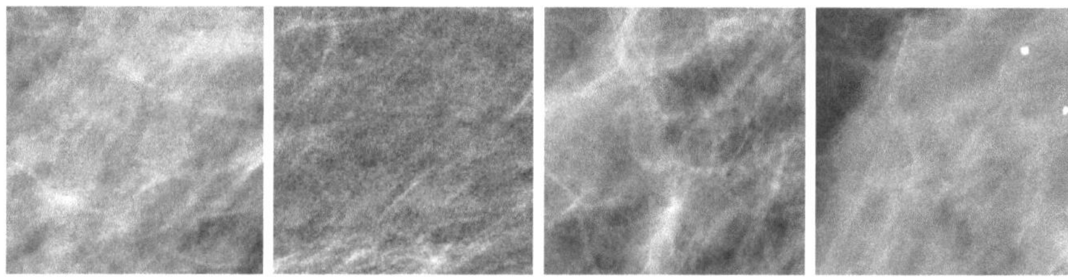

Fig. 2. Parts of the four presented mammograms with different properties in the structure of tissue

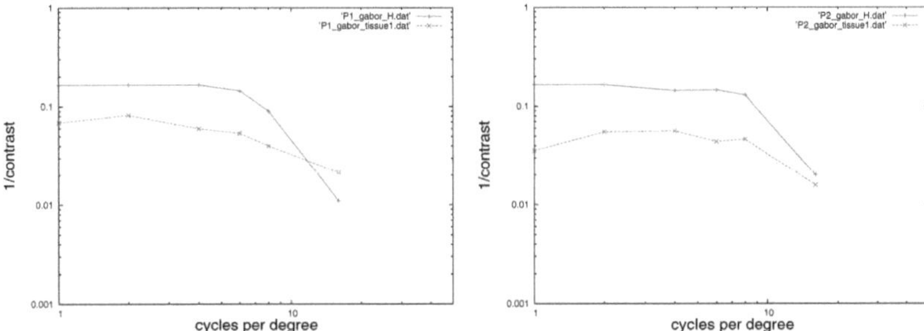

Fig. 3. Relation of the CSF for homogeneous background to CSF for tissue background; left: results of observer P1; right: results of observer P2

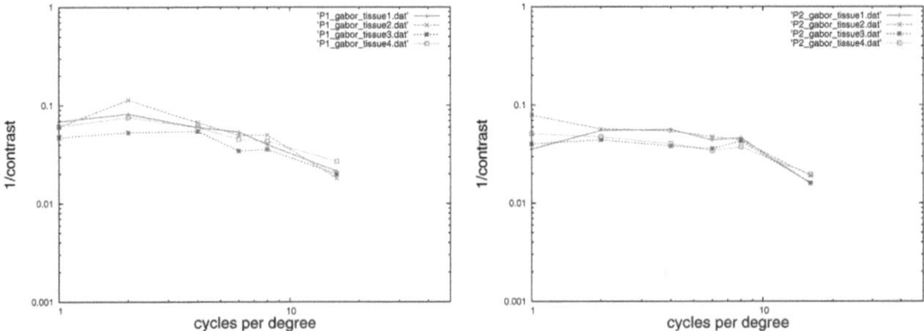

Fig. 4. CSF for 4 different mammographic images (cp. Fig. 2); left: results of observer P1; right: results of observer P2

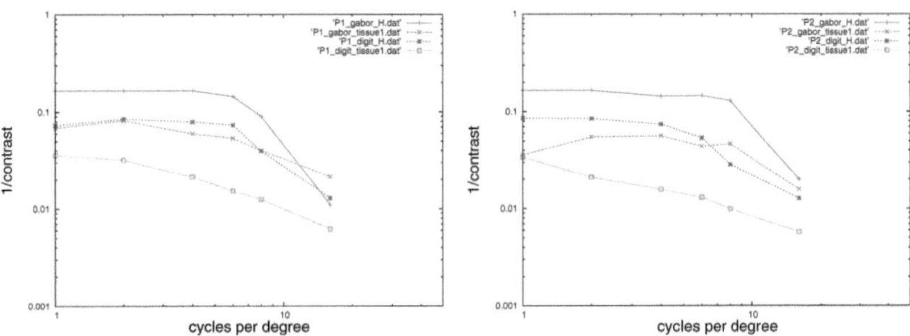

Fig. 5. Relation between CSF for digits to CSF for Gabor pattern on homogeneous and tissue background; left: results of observer P1; right: results of observer P2

The run of the CSF curve is similar for mammograms with different tissue characteristics (Fig. 4). An analysis of the image parts with a quadrature filter showed a similar frequency distribution. It is striking that the CSF is slightly higher on radiolucent tissue, which appears more homogeneous than the other tested tissues (bright curve in Fig. 4). The results of the eight observers confirm the second hypothesis, and let assume that an analysis of the CSF for a tissue background is slightly depending on the selected mammographic image.

As expected, the CSF is higher for the discrimination task than for the identification task (Fig. 5). For the identification of the digits higher cognitive processes are required. This is evident for both a homogeneous background as well as for a tissue background.

Studying the CSF in a mammographic context opens new possibilities for a psychophysical analysis of the contrast sensitivity depending on individual preferences, ambient conditions in the reading room, visualization methods and the design of application, e.g. with regard to luminance distributions in the field of view. This may support the diagnostic certainty in reporting breast cancer.

References

1. Barten PGJ. Contrast Sensitivity of the Human Eye and Its Effects on Image Quality. SPIE Press Monograph Vol. PM72; 1999.
2. Fletcher-Heath L, Metter RV. Quantifying the performance of human and software CDMAM phantom image observers for the qualification of digital mammography systems. Proc SPIE. 2005; p. 486–98.
3. Burgess AE, Jacobson FL, Judy PF. Mass discrimination in mammography: Experiments using hybrid images. Acad Radiol. 2003;10:1247–56.
4. Kaernbach C. Adaptive threshold estimation with unforced-choice tasks. Percept Psychophys. 2001;63(8):1377–88.

Kategorisierung der Beiträge

Primärfunktion des Verfahrens

Art des Projektes

Autorenverzeichnis

Stichwortverzeichnis

Anzeige

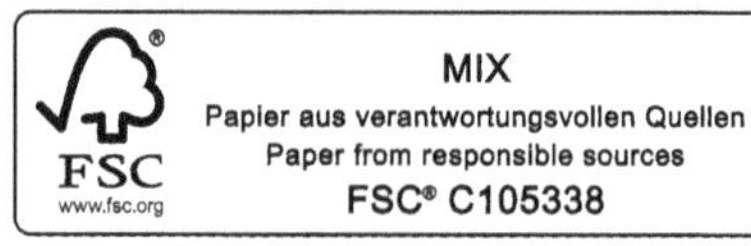

If you have any concerns about our products, you can contact us on
ProductSafety@springernature.com

In case Publisher is established outside the EU, the EU authorized representative is:
Springer Nature Customer Service Center GmbH
Europaplatz 3, 69115 Heidelberg, Germany

Printed by Libri Plureos GmbH
in Hamburg, Germany